W0106250

The Use of Human Cells for the Evaluation of Risk from Physical and Chemical Agents

NATO Advanced Science Institutes Series

A series of edited volumes comprising multifaceted studies of contemporary scientific issues by some of the best scientific minds in the world, assembled in cooperation with NATO Scientific Affairs Division.

This series is published by an international board of publishers in conjunction with NATO Scientific Affairs Division

A	**Life Sciences**	Plenum Publishing Corporation
B	**Physics**	New York and London
C	**Mathematical and Physical Sciences**	D. Reidel Publishing Company Dordrecht, Boston, and London
D	**Behavioral and Social Sciences**	Martinus Nijhoff Publishers
E	**Applied Sciences**	The Hague, Boston, and London
F	**Computer and Systems Sciences**	Springer Verlag
G	**Ecological Sciences**	Heidelberg, Berlin, and New York

Recent Volumes in Series A: Life Sciences

Volume 54—Leukotrienes and Prostacyclin
edited by F. Berti, G. Folco, and G. Velo

Volume 55—Durable Resistance in Crops
edited by F. Lamberti, J. M. Waller, and N. A. Van der Graaff

Volume 56—Advances in Vertebrate Neuroethology
edited by Jörg-Peter Ewert, Robert R. Capranica, and David J. Ingle

Volume 57—Biochemical and Biological Markers of Neoplastic Transformation
edited by Prakash P. Chandra

Volume 58—Arterial Pollution: An Integrated View on Atherosclerosis
edited by H. Peeters, G. A. Gresham, and R. Paoletti

Volume 59—The Applications of Laser Light Scattering to the Study of Biological Motion
edited by J. C. Earnshaw and M. W. Steer

Volume 60—The Use of Human Cells for the Evaluation of Risk from Physical and Chemical Agents
edited by Amleto Castellani

Volume 61—Genetic Engineering in Eukaryotes
edited by Paul F. Lurquin and Andris Kleinhofs

Volume 62—Heart Perfusion, Energetics, and Ischemia
edited by Leopold Dintenfass, Desmond G. Julian, and Geoffrey V. F. Seaman

The Use of Human Cells for the Evaluation of Risk from Physical and Chemical Agents

Edited by

Amleto Castellani

Casaccia Center for Nuclear Studies
Rome, Italy

Springer Science+Business Media, LLC

Proceedings of a NATO Advanced Study Institute on
the Use of Human Cells for the Assessment of
Risk from Physical and Chemical Agents,
held August 24–September 5, 1981,
in Pisa, Italy

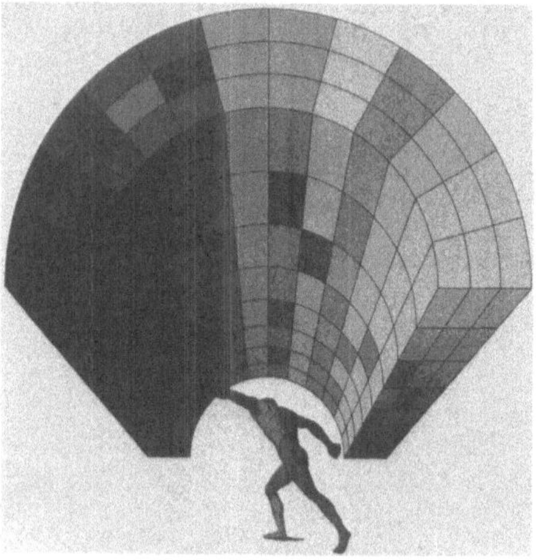

Library of Congress Cataloging in Publication Data

Main entry under title:

The Use of human cells for the evaluation of risk from physical and chemical agents.

(NATO advanced science institutes series. Series A, Life sciences; v. 60)
"Published in cooperation with NATO Scientific Affairs Division."
"Proceedings of a NATO Advanced Study Institute on the Use of Human Cells for the Assessment of Risk from Physical and Chemical Agents, held August 24–September 5, 1981, in Pisa, Italy."
Bibliography: p.
1. Carcinogenicity testing—Congresses. 2. Mutagenicity testing—Congresses. I. Castellani, Amleto. II. NATO Advanced Study Institute on the Use of Human Cells for the Assessment of Risk from Physical and Chemical Agents (1981: Pisa, Italy) III. North Atlantic Treaty Organization. Scientific Affairs Division. IV. Series. [DNLM: 1. Mutagenicity tests—Methods—Congresses. 2. Carcinogens—Analysis—Congresses. 3. Radiation effects—Congresses. 4. Cytological technics—Congresses. QY 95 N279u 1981]
RC268.65.U83 1983 616.99′4071′0287 83-2429
ISBN 978-1-4757-1119-6 ISBN 978-1-4757-1117-2 (eBook)
DOI 10.1007/978-1-4757-1117-2

© 1983 Springer Science+Business Media New York
Originally published by Plenum Press New York in 1983
Softcover reprint of the hardcover 1st edition 1983

All rights reserved. No part of this book may be reproduced, stored in a retrieval system, or transmitted in any form or by any means, electronic, mechanical, photocopying, microfilming, recording, or otherwise, without written permission from the Publisher

PREFACE

In this volume are collected 30 papers, 9 round table discussions and 11 communications presented at the ASI Course on "The use of human cells for the evaluation of risk from physical and chemical agents", sponsored by NATO and organized by ENEA.

The aim of the Course was to present different scientific approaches and technical advices in order to get dose-effect relationships which are the basis for risk evaluation. The scientific background which is behind this approach was extensively discussed.

Emphasis has been given to the use of human cells or human data in order to attempt to have a correct and realistic evaluation of the damage in humans.

There are many criticisms on the use of animal data for human risk evaluation because of differences between species and between strains within the same species: differences in metabolism, activation processes and DNA repair ability makes uncertain the extrapolation of animal data to humans.

Also data obtained using specific strains or highly inbred strains in order to reduce the variance are not applicable due to the heterogeneity of the human population connected with individual responses. In this respect only the use of human cells enable us to detect the individual variability and to identify sensitive subpopulations that would be at greater risk.

My appreciation to Pieranita and Alberto Castellani for the assistance during the meeting and to Giuseppe Biondi for his help in some of the editorial work.

Ameleto Castellani

Department of Health and
Environment Protection
ENEA, CRE, Casaccia
Rome, Italy

CONTENTS

LECTURES

ROUND TABLES

COMMUNICATIONS

WHAT DO WE MEAN BY THE EXPRESSION: RISK-ASSESSMENT?

J. D. Jansen

SIRM B.V.
Group Toxicology
P. O. Box 162, 2501 AN
The Hague, Netherlands

English is a wonderful scientific language because it is easy to coin a word or expression which describes clearly for all fellow researchers the goal of a new field of research, in other words that what the researchers would clearly like to know. As soon as we do know, the picturesque word or expression is changed into a scientifically accurate pseudo-greco-roman expression which is precisely defined, explained in the textbooks and from then onwards of no further interest to the creative researcher who is interested in discovering the unknown. However, for exactly the same reason English is also a hazardous language when different branches of science have to cooperate. This is because the specialist in one branch is apt to assume, consciously or subconsciously, that the expressions used in another branch describe achievements instead of goals for understanding.

An illustrative example of risk-assessment has been given by David Okrent in an excellent publication on Social Risk [1] - 3 people crossing the Atlantic in a rowing boat face a hazard of drowning, 300 people crossing the Atlantic in an oceanliner face the same hazard of drowning. It may be added that the oceanliners also face well-documented hazards of fire, fatal collision with other ships or icebergs and the passengers risk accidents from falling. The maximum societal hazard of the oceanliner is 100× higher than the maximum societal hazard of the rowing boat. As far as I know, there are no documented hazards from crossing the Atlantic in a rowing boat (which feat has been performed only once or perhaps twice). From this very concrete example, Okrent nor anybody else will "conclude" that crossing the Atlantic by rowing boat is safer than or preferable to crossing by oceanliner.

Nevertheless, in less concrete examples (e.g., comparing hazards of energy from coal with those of nuclear energy or risk-assessment of saccharin) people do come to such conclusions using lines of reasoning which are less obviously wrong because the "assumptions" are more abstract and hence less transparently wrong.

An example of the potential hazards of colorful expressions in genetics is given by the term "mutational load." The significance of this term seems immediately obvious to the outsider, primarily by its emotional and descriptive impact. However, a geneticist is hard pressed to give a satisfactory definition of what is meant, partly as a consequence of the absence of any known environmental effect on genetic disease [2, 3, 4] not even in the children born to the Hiroshima and Nagasaki survivors [5]. Because of this situation, Charlotte Auerbach, in 1975, gave a timely warning to the ranking of substances in order of (genetic) risk "because it will create the impression that our conclusions are meaningful, whereas in reality they are so full of uncertainties as to be practically meaningless" [16]. Her warning is still as valid in 1981 and was indeed repeated yesterday by Dr. Arlett.

In carcinogenesis research the expression risk-analysis is of course widely used. To the outsider and sometimes the legislator, the expression seems to mean that one determines the risk that somebody will develop a cancer of a specified site when he is exposed for a specified duration to a specified dosage of a defined chemical.

This can be done and has been done for smoking cigarettes. It has been done by Williams for a new aromatic amine, i.e., 4-aminobiphenyl which was considered for manufacture in the UK. This aromatic amine was already in production in the USA since 1938 without - at that time - any known carcinogenic hazard. As a result of Williams's analysis, epidemiologic research was initiated in the USA and Williams's quantitative prediction proved extraordinarily precise. Let us analyze why these 2 examples of correct quantitative analysis were possible - (they are the only two examples I know of):

(a) the risk-analysis of cigarette-smoking is based on a large-scale human experiment on more than 50,000 Americans [7] and a similar experiment on British doctors and not at all on animal experiments [8]. In fact, animal experiments at the time, would lead to the conclusion that cigarette-smoking does not constitute a carcinogenic hazard which is why many experimental cancer researchers doubted the validity of the epidemiologic data at a time that their results were already obvious, at least in retrospect. Of course, retrospective analysis is always a particularly satisfactory way of analyzing scientific problems because we can feel so clever in decrying those who could not yet discern the - now - obvious at the time.

(b) Williams's risk analysis of the hazard of 4-aminobiphenyl was based on:

(i) his own intimate knowledge of manufacturing conditions in the USA and UK at that time;

(ii) his own extremely tragic knowledge of the hazard of β-naphthylamine manufacture under UK conditions of manufacture;

(iii) a comparison in suitable experimental animals of the carcinogenicity of β-naphthylamine and 4-aminobiphenyl. (β-naphthylamine is not carcinogenic in rats, therefore both were tested in dogs.)

We can conclude that quantitative risk-analysis of a human carcinogen is possible, provided the evidence, additional to an independent of the animal data alone is available.

A frequently cited example of the possibilities of risk-analysis is vinylchloride monomer. As you may recall, Maltoni reported in 1974 on the occurrence of angiosarcomas in rats, mice, and hamsters, inhaling different concentrations of vinylchloride monomer (VCM). The effect was dose-related and appeared down to very low concentrations of VCM. Independently and at approximately the same time, a hospital physician and a local company doctor were alerted by the third case of angiosarcoma over a number of years, all in workers at a local PVC plant [10]. Angiosarcoma is a very rare disease - about 20-25 cases per year being recorded in the entire USA [11]. It was known at that time to be caused by Arsenic and Thorotrast. In this case the animal experiments accurately predicted that there was a hazard to humans. However, it is questionable whether the animal experiments also predicted the size of the hazard [12, 13, 14]. Up till now, that is seven years after discovery and enormous publicity, about 90 cases of angiosarcoma have been discovered in the entire VCM Industry outside the Communist World, covering more than 20,000 workers (although many or most of these were only exposed for a comparatively short period). All or almost all cases occurred in the very small plants built before the sixties, when because of the very great technical difficulties involved exposures were also immense and led to a number of cases of lethal asphyxiation (which occurs after exposure to about 50% (not ppm) or more of VCM). In summary, in animal experiments VCM looks like one of the most potent carcinogens but in man it looks as if colossal concentrations are necessary before a carcinogenic hazard occurs and it is possible that the Chemical Industry had eliminated the carcinogenic hazard of VCM by normal Technological development even before they were aware of the existence of such a hazard. This optimistic evaluation is by no means established: it is still well possible that angiosarcomas will develop at plants built after 1960 with a longer latency period. More importantly, it is not excluded that VCM may also cause other tumors than angiosarcoma in man. In this case there is a distinct difference between the concepts in the USA and Europe. European epidemiology has not shown the brain and lung tumors of the American investigation. This is not simply a question of whose epidemiology is "better": with the exception of the UK and Denmark, European epidemiology is certainly worse than the USA because of the absence of reasonable cancer registers. However, the brain and lung tumors would probably have been found if indeed present. Due to the absence of good cancer registries in most Industrial Europe, it may be impossible to definitely answer this question other than in the UK. However, if a credible positive answer would be obtained, then the entire risk-assessment of VCM might change. Whatever quantitative data are obtained in the future, the qualitative correctness of the animal data is beyond doubt.

It is unlikely that anybody would have doubted the qualitative prediction of dose-related carcinogenic effects in 3 animal species as demonstrated for VCM by Maltoni.

The same applies to nitrosamines: at a not so recent count, diethylnitrosamine was found highly carcinogenic in every experiment in a total of 14 species and strains, including monkeys and apes [15]: it would be very surprising if such a compound was not carcinogenic in men sufficiently exposed. However, accepting the high probability that the qualitative prediction is correct, does not automatically imply acceptance of a quantitative prediction. In public health considerations the latter prediction is frequently the most important one.

For PVC manufacture, the question of quantitative correlation between experimental data and human experience is not of overriding importance since Industry and Society can live with the measures taken up till now. However, for nitrosamines, the same question is of the greatest practical importance: nitrosamines are virtually ubiquitous and also produced within the human body. The nitrosamines and nitrosamides together can produce virtually the entire spectrum of human cancer and together they are the only class of known experimental carcinogens which could conceivably cause an important part of the now occurring cancers. The absence of human data is not too surprising in view of the difficulty of defining groups of people who differ in their exposure to these compounds. There are several theories which try to explain the origin of some human cancer in terms of nitrosamines. The fundamental difficulty of all these theories is that even if they are qualitatively all completely true for man (which has not been proven), there is as yet no possibility to conclude whether they explain an insignificant part of the current incidence or whether they explain the larger part or perhaps even the greatest part of the cancer concerned. (I am speaking about specific cancers such as stomach cancer and colon cancer.) Under these circumstances, it would be of greatest importance if quantitative or semi-quantitative data could be developed for the human carcinogenicity of specific nitrosamines.

Another example of the importance of quantitative assessment of carcinogens are the aflatoxins. Aflatoxin B_1 is one of the most potent liver carcinogens in the rat. In South Asia and Africa the (high) incidence of liver cancer is well correlated with aflatoxin exposure and a dose-response curve in humans can be constructed in these continents [17].

The considerations quite rightly sufficed to convince authorities in the developed world that aflatoxin exposures should be reduced and indeed this has been possible without great social or technical problems being encountered. However, a few, not yet well established data make scientific certainty less than absolute.

(i) aflatoxin B_1 is not carcinogenic for mice under normal experimental conditions [18] (it is when newborn mice are exposed [19];

(ii) aflatoxin seems to be metabolized by human liver even slower or less efficiently than by mouse liver [20];

(iii) high incidences of liver cancer occur only in those countries with a high incidence of hepatitis B.

(iv) liver cancer does not seem to be a great problem in the countries of South and Middle America [21] even though aflatoxin was originally discovered in peanuts from Brazil.

None of the four arguments are particularly convincing and several can be wrong or differently explained (especially the last argument). However, together they constitute a real possibility that perhaps aflatoxin is only carcinogenic in people affected by hepatitis B. This hypothesis has not received wide attention in the developed world where indeed the practical implications are small. However, in view of the present feasibility of vaccination against hepatitis B [22, 23], the question is of very great importance for several undeveloped countries which might find eradication for viral hepatitis a possible goal to achieve but severe restriction of aflatoxin-intake almost impossible before a relatively very great increase in wealth is achieved in these countries.

Until now, we have only discussed compounds which certainly produce cancer in man or at least are extremely likely to produce cancer in men sufficiently exposed. This situation dramatically changes in the face of conflicting experimental data. One such conflict was discussed with aflatoxin. The more common possibility is exemplified by the currently rapidly increasing range of compounds which produce liver or lung tumors in mice but not in other species. Many countries treat or have treated such compounds as if they are carcinogenic to man. This may be or may not be good Public Policy. However, such decisions have nothing to do with Science or with Risk Assessment because in these cases we must prefer the prediction from one animal species above the contrary prediction from another animal species and, as Cairns has rightly pointed out in his recent publication in Nature [24], usually we have no scientific basis for preferring the prediction from one species above a contrary prediction from another species. However, developments mainly of the last decade or last 5 years enable us to develop some arguments which may help in deciding whether such compounds may be a carcinogenic hazard to man under the conditions of human exposure:

(1) None of these compounds is known to be carcinogenic to man [25]. The evidence for this statement varies between non-existent and weak but is strong and convincing for two such compounds, i.e., Isoniazid [26, 27] and Phenobarbitone [28, 29]. The phenobarbitone data are especially convincing because they have been obtained on 8100 epileptics who were treated for life at dosages which produce measurable microsomal stimulation of the liver in man; moreover their epidemiological status was regularly updated until the latest publication covered 35 years of follow-up and each update reinforced the conclusions of the previous ones.

(2) Clayson has cogently argued that standard carcinogenicity tests cannot distinguish between promotors and complete carcinogens if the same tumors which seem to be caused by the test compounds also occur in the controls [30]. This particularly applies to many mice-strains used in testing which show a high incidence of liver and/or lung tumors in the controls. Because the incidence of human cancer seems largely affected by the presence or absence of promotors or inhibitors in the diet [31], the distinction between a promotor and complete carcinogen is not at all identical with the distinction between safety and hazard. However, some promotors seem to act only at concentrations well above those encountered by humans (phenobarbitone and saccharin might be examples) whereas others might be effective under human conditions (estrogens for alleviating menopausal symptoms might be an example).

(3) Most, but not all of these compounds are negative in mutagenic tests. The evidence for this statement ranges from weak (few tests have been conducted on phenobarbitone and there is evidence that phenobarbitone is not metabolized under the conditions of these tests) to strong (dieldrin). Consequently, according to a recent advice to the Dutch Health Authorities [32]

and according to a recent Working Group convened by the International Agency for Research on Cancer in Lyon, the results of such tests in mice only are not considered to establish carcinogenic activity unless independent information indicates such an activity [33]. Yet another example has been given yesterday by Dr. Legator in this course when discussing benzene: if benzene would be introduced as a new compound, i.e., without the benefit of the extensive human experience I doubt whether it would have great difficulties in passing the regulators: negative in the Ames Test and all other mutagenic tests (which have been done - not very many), only positive in chromosome aberrations in mice but not in Chinese Hamsters and, as recently found, also negative in another strain of mice which reacts positive on most known mutagens.

An entirely different aspect of Risk-Assessment is provided by the continuing series of assessment of the risks of taking the contraceptive pill [34, 35]. This series of assessments is clearly needed, of the highest importance and a tribute to the power of modern epidemiology [34], coupled with astute observation by observant physicians [35]. In a Dutch publication it was noted that the crude incidence of Down's syndrome was almost halved in the Netherlands and this was related to the drop in pregnancies in women above 35 years of age [36], presumably because of the use of the "pill." The same situation in the USA (a drop of 30-40% in the crude rate) was noted in a footnote in an American publication [37]. When I asked genetic epidemiologists from other countries they all confirmed the general phenomenon and added: but that is not a risk, therefore irrelevant for a risk-evaluation. Yet, the largely unrecorded partial disappearance of the burden of Down's syndrome may well represent a larger, more important, social effect than all the real risks together which have hitherto been associated with the pill. I am hesitant to use that other well-meaning and popular expression of risk-benefit equation in this context, mainly because the real benefits of using the pill are far wider, greater and also more personal. However, I do want to stress the grossly incomplete and therefore possibly grossly misleading picture which may result from only making a risk-assessment. Even if the risk-assessment is quantitatively precise (which it almost never is and mostly not at all), the assessment may force attention to such a small part of the entire change brought about by the compound or action being assessed that the resulting focus may be socially and humanly entirely wrong.

Risk-assessment is an extremely important but hardly developed scientific endeavor. Very often it is nothing more than extremely precise but meaningless calculations based on assumptions which are so wide that they must be wrong sometimes, many times, or even nearly always. However, definite and clear progress can be made, provided that we apply the same scientific rigor in our endeavor as we would apply to any other science and provided that we separate definitions, knowledge and assumptions as rigorously as Peto and Doll have done in their recent publication on the avoidable risks of cancer in the USA [38]. This may well be considered to be the definitive publication on the risk of cancer, not in the sense that it will not be changed by subsequent findings - on the contrary, I sincerely hope that it will become such a seminal publication that it will be quickly outdated by a spate of research generated by it. However, it can be considered definitive in the sense that for the first time, clear definitions of each issue are given, the limits of our knowledge have been reasoned and explained and, for the first time reasonable maximum and minimum limits have been given for each estimate. From now on, anybody will have to challenge their estimates with arguments or new data - both excellent ingredients for creative scientific progress.

Finally, I would like to give a few parameters within which each risk-assessment has to operate:

-	risk of dying	$\sim$1.0
-	risk of dying from cancer	$\sim$0.25 (in developed countries, strongly dependent on age distribution and average age of death)
-	risk of contracting bladder cancer for a small group of distillers	1.0
-	risk of dying from radiation induced cancer in survivors of Hiroshima and Nagasaki	$\sim$0.01-0.02 (as percentage of natural deaths until 1974).

I fully agree with Doll and Peto's admonition that "the detection of occupational hazards should [38] have a higher priority in any program of cancer prevention than their proportional importance might suggest" (because the risk to the small group involved may be very high). Yet I do want to emphasize that the overall cancer risk in a developed society is large and that the study of measures to lower that risk with 10-50% or more is at the very least as important as the further attempts to "calculate" risks of 100,000 or even less. Such studies of how to lower the cancer risks are now feasible for a number of sites [31, 38] but are pursued by a pitifully small number of researchers and are held up by legislative complications (which prohibit combining personal data with mortality data) in nearly the entire European continent (the UK and Denmark being shining exceptions which have therefore been able to contribute to an extraordinary degree to the epidemiological insights so ably analyzed by Doll and Peto).

REFERENCES

1. D. Okrent, Comment on Societal Risk, Science, 208:372-375 (1980).
2. H. B. Newcombe, Quantitative assessment of induced genetic ill-health in humans as a model for assessing genetic risks from chemicals, in: Bora, ed., Proc. Int. Symposium on Chemical Mutagenesis, Human Population Monitoring and Genetic Risk Assessment, Elsevier/North Holland Biochemical Press (in press).
3. H. B. Newcombe, Problems of assessing risk versus mutations, Genetics 92 (May suppl.) S199-S201 (1979).
4. J. V. Neel, H. Mohrenweiser, C. Satoh, and H. B. Hamilton, A consideration of two biochemical approaches to monitoring human populations for a change in germ cell mutation rates, in: Berg, ed., Genetic damage in man caused by environmental agents, Academic Press, New York (1979).
5. J. V. Neel, C. Satoh, H. B. Hamilton, M. Otake, K. Goriki, T. Kageoka, M. Fujita, S. Neriishi, and T. Asakawa, Search for mutations affecting protein structure in children of atomic bomb survivors: preliminary report. Proc. Natl. Acad. Sci. USA, 77:4221-4225 (1980).
6. C. Auerbach, The effects of six years of mutagen testing on our attitude to the problems posed by it, Mutation Res., 33:3-10 (1975).
7. E. Cuyler-Hammond and L. Garfinkel, Tobacco Epidemiology - A simulated animal experiment, in: Coulston, Shubik, eds., Human Epidemiology and animal laboratory correlations in chemical carcinogenesis, Ablex Publ. Comp., Norwood, New Jersey, USA (1980).
8. C. J. Kensler, S. P. Battista, and P. S. Thayer, Animal models for the study of tobacco carcinogenesis, in: Coulston, Shubik, eds., Human Epidemiology and animal laboratory correlations in chemical carcinogenesis, Ablex Publ. Comp., Norwood, New Jersey, USA (1980).
9. C. Maltoni and G. Lefemine, Carcinogenicity bio-assays of vinylchloride, I. Research plans and early results, Environm. Res., 7:187-405 (1974).
10. J. L. Creech, Jr., and M. N. Johnson, Angiosarcoma of liver in the manufactureof polyvinylchloride, J. Occup. Med., 16:150-151 (1974).
11. L. Makk, F. Delmore, J. L. Creech, L. L. Ogden, E. H. Fadell, C. L. Sangster, J. Clanton, M. N. Johnson, and W. H. Christopherson, Clinical and morphological effects of hepatic angiosarcoma in vinylchloride workers, Cancer, 37:149-163 (1976).
12. P. J. Gehring, P. C. Watanabe, and C. N. Park, Resolution of Dose-Response Toxicity Data for Chemicals Requiring Metabolic Activation, e.g., vinylchloride, Toxicol. Appl. Pharmacol., 44:581-591 (1978).
13. P. J. Gehring, P. G. Watanabe, and C. H. Park, Risk of angiosarcoma in workers exposed to vinylchloride as predicted from studies in rats, Toxicol. Appl. Pharmacol., 49:15-21 (1979).

14. A. Butcher, J. G. Filser, H. Peter, and H. M. Bolt, Pharmacokinetics of vinylchloride in the Rhesus monkey, Toxicol. Letters, 6:33-36 (1980).
15. P. N. Magee, R. Montesano, and R. Preusmann, N-Nitroso compounds and related carcinogens, in: Searle, ed., Chemical Carcinogens, Am. Chem. Soc., Washington, D.C. (1976).
16. G. N. Wogan, S. Paglialunga, and P. M. Newberne, Carcinogenic effects of low dietary levels of aflatoxin B_1 in rats, Food Cosmet. Toxicol., 12:681-685 (1974).
17. C. A. Linsell and F. G. Peers, Field studies on liver cell cancer, in: Hiatt, Watson, and Winsten, eds., Origins of Human Cancer, Cold Spring Harbor Lab. (1977).
18. G. N. Wogan, Aflatoxin carcinogenesis, in: Busch, ed., Methods in cancer research, Academic Press, New York (1973).
19. P. M. Newberne, Carcinogenicity of aflatoxin contaminated peanut meals, in: Wogan, ed., Mycotoxins in foodstuffs, M.I.T. Press, Cambridge, Massachussetts (1965).
20. D. P. H. Hsieh, J. T. Wong, Z. A. Wong, C. Michas, and B. H. Reubner, Hepatic Transformation of aflatoxin and its carcinogenicity, in: Hiatt, Watson, and Winsten, eds., Origins of Human Cancer, Cold Spring Harbor Lab. (1977).
21. R. L. Gross and P. M. Newberne, Naturally occurring toxic substances in food, Clin. Pharm. Ther., 22:680-697 (1977).
22. L. I. Lutwick, Relation between aflatoxin, hepatitis-B virus and hepatocellular carcinoma, The Lancet, 755-757 (1979).
23. Anon., Hepatitis-B vaccine passes first major test, Science, 210:760-762 (1980).
24. J. Cairns, The origin of human cancers, Nature, 289:353-357 (1981).
25. J. D. Jansen, The predictive value of tests for carcinogenic and mutagenic activity, in: Deichmann, ed., Toxicology and Occupational Medicine, Elsevier/North Holland, New York (1979).
26. J. D. Jansen, J. Clemmesen, and K. Sundaram, Isoniazid - an attempt at retrospective prediction, ICPEMC publication No. 4, Mutation Res., 76:85-112 (1980).
27. G. R. Howe, J. Lindsay, E. Coppock, and A. B. Miller, Isoniazid exposure in relation to cancer incidence and mortality in a cohort of tuberculosis patients, Int. J. Epidemiol., 8:305-312 (1979).
28. J. Clemmesen and S. Hjalgrim-Jensen, Epidemiological studies of medically used drugs, Arch. Toxicol. Suppl., 3:19-25 (1980).
29. J. Clemmesen and S. Hjalgrim-Jansen, Does Phenobarbital cause intracranial tumors? A follow-up through 35 years, Ecotoxicol. and Environm. Safety, 5:255-260 (1981).
30. D. B. Clayson, Carcinogens and carcinogenesis enhancers, Mutation Res., in press (1981).
31. J. H. Weisburger, On the etiology of gastro-intestinal tract cancers with emphasis on dietary factors, in: Emmelot, Kriek, eds., Environm. Carcinogenesis, Elsevier/North Holland Biochemical Press, Amsterdam (1979).

32. R. Kroes, Animal Data, interpretation and consequences, in: Emmelot, Kriek, eds., Environm. Carcinogenesis, Elsevier/North Holland Biochemical Press, Amsterdam (1979).
33. Int. Agency for Research on Cancer, Long-term and Short-term screening assays for carcinogenes: a critical appraisal, IARC Monographs, Lyon, Suppl., 2:72-73 (1980).
34. M. P. Vessey, Contraceptive Methods: risks and benefits, Brit. Med. J., Sept., 721-722 (1978).
35. E. T. Mays, Sex Steroids and Hepatic Growth, in: Coulston, Shubik, eds., Human Epidemiology and Animal Laboratory Correlations in Chemical Carcinogenesis, Ablex Publishing Comp., Norwood, New Jersey, USA (1980).
36. D. Hoogendoorn, Aanzienlijk dalend aantal kinderen met mongolisme, Ned. T. Geneesk. (summary in English), 112:1119-1120 (1978).
37. F. B. Hook, Human teratogenic and mutagenic markers in monitoring about point sources of pollution, Envirnonm. Res., 25: 178-203 (1981).
38. R. Doll and R. Peto, Avoidable risks of cancer in the US, J. Natl. Cancer Inst., 66:1195-1308 (1981).

THE SEARCH FOR CRITERIA TO ASSESS THE RISKS RESULTING FROM EXPOSURE TO CARCINOGENIC AGENTS

Umberto Saffiotti

Laboratory of Experimental Pathology
Division of Cancer Cause and Prevention
National Cancer Institute
Frederick, Maryland

INTRODUCTION

The increasingly rapid developments of toxicological research in the last few decades confronted us with the problem of correlating new scientific knowledge with its public health implications. Progressively more attention has been given to the nature of "self-replicating toxic effects," such as mutagenicity and carcinogenicity, in comparison with the "terminal toxic effects" studied by traditional toxicology [1]. Self-replicating toxic effects usually have the following characteristics: a) their appearance is delayed, often by a period of time as long as one-half or more of the lifetime of the host; b) the frequency of the expression of injury (e.g., tumor incidence) in the exposed population is directly correlated with the intensity of the exposure, but the intensity of the induced pathology (e.g., tumor growth and spread) is independent of the intensity of the exposure to the toxic agent; and c) the manifestations of toxicity are due to the proliferative response of a new altered cell population. Terminal toxic effects, on the other hand, usually have these different characteristics: a) they appear early after exposure to the toxic agents, b) the intensity of the induced pathology is directly correlated with the intensity of the toxic exposure, and c) the manifestations of toxicity are due either to altered functional products of the target tissues or to degenerative changes or death of the target cells themselves. For terminal toxic effects, it has often been possible to determine the human risk quantitatively by direct observation of individuals exposed to different dose levels of a toxic agent, within a relatively short time from their exposure. In many cases, when toxic symptoms started to occur at a given level of exposure, the exposure could be lowered and the symptoms would regress or disappear. When dealing with delayed self-replicating effects such as carcinogenesis, however, human observation of the effect is often possible only after a long time from the beginning of exposure and by that time preventive intervention may no longer be possible for that population (although the experience can be used to prevent exposures in subsequent cohorts).

Methods have therefore been sought to predict such delayed risks well in advance of irreparable human exposure, qualitatively at first and then possibly on a reliable quantitative basis. The difficulties of the latter estimate are the main subject of the present discussion, which is primarily concerned with carcinogenic risks from chemical agents. The following three aspects will be addressed: a) Identification of carcinogens and estimates of their number; b) Risk evaluation criteria; and c) Attribution of human cancer risks to different etiological factors and their concurrent roles.

IDENTIFICATION OF CARCINOGENS AND ESTIMATES OF THEIR NUMBER

Research on chemical carcinogens, from the early studies with coal tar and then with isolated polycyclic aromatic hydrocarbons, always revealed a strong implicit interest in the human risk aspect. This interest became more and more relevant with the discoveries of many other chemical classes of carcinogens which also involve significant human exposure, such as aromatic amines and azo-dyes, hormones, alkylating agents, N-nitroso compounds, hydrazines, metal compounds, mycotoxins, halogenated hydrocarbons, and several others. Since the early days, research on the biological and biochemical effects of carcinogens was coupled with the development of animal models for their experimental study. Much of the initial work on carcinogen identification was based on the use of relatively few biological models for carcinogenesis, mainly mouse skin tumor induction by repeated skin applications, rat liver tumor induction by feeding and induction of subcutaneous sarcomas in either species by topical injection. The test conditions were often poorly defined and the number of animals in each test group was often small (e.g., 15 to 20), so that the sensitivity of the test systems was very limited. Yet, even by such relative crude tests, major classes of carcinogens were identified and several fundamental biological characteristics of the carcinogenic process were discovered. By the mid 1950s, the systematic use of animal bioassays was recommended as the method of choice for the detection of suspected environmental carcinogens [2-5]. It was recognized that no a-priori assumption of safety could be made for environmental chemicals without a minimum of testing [2] and this "principle" became the basis for a revision of the laws and regulations intended to protect the population from carcinogenic risks; initially the emphasis was on the identification and control of intentional food additives (e.g., the 1958 Delaney clause on food additives in USA legislation) but later it extended to food contaminants, drinking water contaminants, environmental pollutants, occupational hazards, toxic consumer products and toxic substances in general.

As the public health implications of carcinogenesis research and bioassays on new chemicals became more widely recognized, the 1960s and early 1970s saw the emergence of the problem of setting sufficient standards for the design and conduct of carcinogenesis bioassays. Following broad consensus on basic bioassay criteria at the international level [6], and the experience of a large bioassay program organized in the USA by the National Cancer Institute, detailed guidelines for carcinogenesis bioassay in rodents were developed [7] and widely adopted in different countries [8, 9]. The validity and reliability of long-term animal carcinogenesis bioassays rests on many detailed criteria of experimental design, pathology evaluation and statistical analysis, which were recently extensively reviewed [10-12]. While these methods for long-term *in vivo* testing became established and generated many new detailed bioassay reports [13], it was clearly recognized that they had many limitations, including their 3-4 year practical time commitment [14], their high cost, and the need for extensive animal facilities with adequate chemical hazard controls.

Research advances in cell biology and genetics however opened up a major alternative approach, with the development of short-term *in vitro* biological systems capable of detecting the chemical induction of neoplastic transformation of cells in culture and of mutagenicity in bacterial or mammalian cells [9, 15-17]. The use of these systems is still the object of validation and evaluation research, but their role is widely recognized as a valuable complement to *in vivo* systems, especially for mechanism studies. The results of extensive tests in the last decade revealed the carcinogenic activity of a number of widely used chemicals, and caused considerable and often excessive public concern (a typical expression of this concern is the remark, heard among the uninformed public, that "everything causes cancer").

Estimations were made of the number of chemicals involved in this problem on the basis of available data [18, 19]. Order of magnitude differences characterize the total number of known chemicals (5×10^6), the number of chemicals involving significant human exposure ($6\text{-}7 \times 10^4$), the estimated number of all existing carcinogens (5×10^3 to 5×10^4, with great uncertainty), the estimated number of these that involve significant human exposure ($1\text{-}5 \times 10^3$, also with considerable uncertainty), the number of chemicals so far tested in animals for carcinogenicity ($4\text{-}7 \times 10^3$, depending on test criteria), the number of animal-tested chemicals considered as suspect carcinogens (1400 to 2800 depending on criteria), the number of animal-tested positive carcinogens (800 to 900 depending on criteria), the estimated number of these positive carcinogens that involve significant human exposure from any source (300 to 500) or from occupational sources (200 to 300), down to the number of carcinogens for which there is positive human evidence from epidemiologic studies (20 to 40). Such order of magnitude perspective on these estimates [18] suggests that research priorities can be focused on a relatively small number of chemicals for which experimental evidence is clearly positive but human evidence is not available. It is especially for these agents that future research utilizing human tissues and cells can bring particularly valuable contributions.

RISK EVALUATION CRITERIA

The association of potential human cancer risks with exposure to agents that are demonstrably carcinogenic in animal test systems was suggested quite early in the course of carcinogenesis research. Epidemiologic evidence preceded experimental confirmation for such classic carcinogens as tars and other combustion products, aromatic amines, metal compounds as well as ionizing radiation. Thus, epidemiologic evidence of risk was often a stimulus for experimental research. Recently, however, with the rapid expansion of experimental carcinogenesis studies in a variety of biological models, the reverse sequence is occurring more often: substances that are demonstrated to be carcinogenic in animal systems are later shown to be carcinogenic for human populations by epidemiologic methods (e.g., aflatoxin and vinyl chloride). It is to be hoped that many experimentally identified carcinogens will never obtain epidemiologic confirmation because protective measures, taken on the basis of experimental evidence, will prevent epidemiologically detectable human cancer increases.

The problem of carcinogenic risk evaluation from experimental data has been underlying public health concerns in this area for many years, especially since low level exposures to environmental carcinogens were recognized to occur in very large populations [19]. The correlation of experimental animal carcinogenesis bioassay results with esimated human risk has received the particular attention of mathematical statisticians who have analyzed the shape of the dose-response relationships in carcinogenesis from both human and experimental animal observations. Several mathematical models were proposed to fit the available response data (usually representing fairly high dose levels) in the hope that they could accurately predict the hypothetical response at low dose levels. A strong incentive towards such attempts came from a special public health orientation that sought to adjust technical controls to a calculated "safe level" of exposure, rather than to the much more difficult concept of "minimum technologically feasible level." The other alternative, eliminating the exposure altogether, was only possible in certain cases or for certain routes of administration, but often remained a theoretical goal.

The critical difficulty in the selection of statistical models of extrapolation from high to low dose is represented by the fact that different models can give widely divergent low-dose extrapolations based on the same high dose data. An important distinction was made in recent analyses of the problem of risk evaluation, namely that the use of these mathematical models should be limited to quantitative projections of dose-effect relationships within a given biological system, but could not be used to replace a qualitative evaluation of functional, metabolic, anatomic or any other biological differences between the system in which the data are obtained and the one for which the extrapolation is intended. This point was particularly stressed in recent reports [10-12] and must always be considered to avoid dangerous oversimplifications. In general, a linear model of dose response is currently favored as both prudent and realistic, although there are cases where it can generate underestimations of risk. Several recent reviews deal with these complex problems, and provide additional references [9, 10, 12, 20-25].

The attempt to express risk estimates with a single numerical index is related to the proposal by Meselson and Russell in 1977 [26] that a single numerical value for the mutagenicity of an agent in the Ames assay on Salmonella would be representative as an index of carcinogenic "potency" in animal bioassay. The assumption that the "potency" in the "most sensitive" tested animal species would correspond to that in the human species was previously proposed by a committee chaired by Meselson in 1975 [27]. I have already reviewed the inadequacies of this approach [12]. The fallacy of the concept of carcinogenic "potency" of a chemical, given as a numerical expression, is evident when one considers that carcinogenesis is the result of a chemical-biological interaction and therefore dependent of highly variable host factors. I like to avoid the term "potency" with its implied rigidity and rather refer to "observed levels of effects" which obviously apply only to the biological systems in which they were observed.

A strong and valid criticism of the single numerical approach to risk estimates based on extrapolation from animal data was recently published by a committee of the National Research Council [24]. This committee also attempted to avoid some of the pitfalls of the use of "potency" estimates by proposing the use of a "Carcinogenic Activity Indicator" limited to animal data only and never to be extrapolated to humans: its main purpose is to compare values derived for different compounds in animals under proper conditions. Confidence intervals provide ranges of values for such comparisons within a biological system.

The problem remains a difficult one. No scientifically valid direct methods have yet been found to offer a reliable quantitative numerical estimate of carcinogenic risk for a given human population on the basis of data derived from other biological systems.

A major problem derives from variations in metabolic rates in different systems; mathematical model research has started to address such problems [22].

ATTRIBUTION OF HUMAN CANCER RISKS TO DIFFERENT ETIOLOGIC FACTORS AND TO THEIR CONCURRENT ROLES

The identification of the role of different causative factors in the induction of cancer in a population is an important aspect of risk assessment. In the absence of a wide basis of substantial factual evidence, a great deal of speculative discussion has recently developed on this issue. I recently reviewed this problem and proposed a new way of considering it [18, 19], as summarized below.

Two different approaches have been taken in the past to analyze this problem. One approach consists of apportioning the total number of cancers among a number of causative factors by attributing each cancer to only one cause: in this way the sum of the fractions attributed to individual factors adds up to 100%. This approach has been based mostly on currently available epidemiologic data with their inherent limitations [28, 29]. This approach therefore tends to exclude from consideration the role of those hundreds of test-positive carcinogens mentioned above, for which there is human exposure but no available epidemiologic information on human effects.

The other alternative approach recognizes the role of many concurrent causative factors and therefore allows for a wide overlap of the fractions of total cases attributed to each factor. A critique of the "one-effect, one-cause" approach and arguments in support of a multifactorial approach to cancer risk attribution were contributed in 1978 by investigators from the U.S. Department of Health, Education, and Welfare in their testimony to the Occupational Safety and Health Administration [30]. This document stimulated much additional debate and further recognition of the interplay of different etiologic factors, although the tendency of several authors, even in the recent literature, remains that of apportioning their "best estimate" of the risk to "prevalent" factors separately, so as to add them up again to 100% [31] or near 100% [32].

The conceptual framework I have suggested [18, 19] allows for the interplay of multiple factors in the causation of all cancers and does not force reduction of the role of one factor by making allowance for another. The model provides estimates of the relative role of each of several categories of factors concurring to the causation of the total cancer incidence or mortality in a given population. It was developed to illustrate causative factors involving total cancer incidence (including non-melanoma skin cancer) for a distribution of cancer types such as is currently observed in the total USA population. The percent contribution of each category of factors is estimated mostly on the basis of epidemiologic evidence of past effects. The sum of all the contributions of individual categories of causative factors is several times higher than 100% (e.g., 600-700%).

For each category of factors, segments of the total population will be affected with different intensities: a segment may be affected predominantly while another may receive only a "background" contribution. A range of intensities thus characterizes the role of each factor in the total cancer incidence distribution. The intensity spectra of each concurrent factor are overlaid to determine the total effect. If some categories of factors (e.g., inhaled factors) are subdivided into smaller concurrent exposure classes (e.g., polycyclic hydrocarbons, N-nitroso compounds and inorganic compounds, all nearly ubiquitous factors) the number of overlays proportionally increases; if one were to consider each percentage of the population affected by each individual compound, the total would add up to many times 100%.

It remains difficult to distinguish exposure to potential carcinogens from actual causative effects, especially when considering low-level effects combining to increase the background risk. This problem is particularly suitable for a research effort utilizing the new methods for studies on human tissues and cells exposed to carcinogens [33-35].

The proposed model considers some categories of factors as being involved in the causation of all cancers: they are genetic factors (including species, sex, age, and other genetically determined characteristics), nutritional factors and "unknown" factors. Other types of factors involve exposure in nearly all cases but their causative role is likely to be less frequent; the following categories of factors are listed here, excluding their occupational component: physical agents, inhaled agents and dietary and other environmental chemicals. Other categories of agents are estimated to be present only in a fraction of the total cancers, such as occupational factors, non-genetic sexual and hormonal factors and infectious factors.

The combination of factors proportionally responsible for the induction of various cancers in a population derives from the intensity with which each factor interplays with the others. When all other factors concur to provide a highly "susceptible" condition just minimally below the level that determines a detectable cancer response, even a minimal increase in a single factor can constitute the sufficient condition that causally determines the onset of cancer. Conversely, when concurrence of all factors is effective in determining cancer induction, reduction of the intensity of one factor alone may lower the total intensity of the sum of the factors to a point where the cancer induction effect is no longer detectable.

Our ability to influence the various factors towards an ineffective combination (resulting in cancer prevention) depends on two aspects. One is our knowledge and ability to predict the relative contribution of different components of the total effect (risk assessment) and consequently to predict which change of individual factors is most likely to contribute to cancer prevention. The other aspect is our ability to intervene to implement the preventive change. Research approaches now offer unprecedented opportunities to move closer to these goals.

REFERENCES

1. U. Saffiotti, Scientific bases of environmental carcinogenesis and cancer prevention: developing an interdisciplinary science and facing its ethical implications, J. Toxicol. Environ. Health, 2:1435 (1977).
2. International Union Against Cancer, Report of Symposium on potential cancer hazards from chemical additives and contaminants to foodstuffs, Acta Unio Intl. Contra Cancrum, 13:170 (1957).
3. P. Shubik and J. Sice, Chemical carcinogenesis as a chronic toxicity test. A review, Cancer Res., 16:728 (1956).
4. Food Protection Committee, Food and Nutrition Board, Problems in the evaluation of carcinogenic hazards from the use of food additives, Cancer Res., 21:429 (1961).
5. Fifth Report of the Joint FAO/WHO Expert Committee on Food Additives, Evaluation of carcinogenic hazards of food additives, WHO Tech. Rept. Series, 220 (1961).
6. I. Berenblum, ed., Carcinogenicity Testing, UICC Tech. Rept. Series (1969).
7. J. M. Sontag, N. P. Page, and U. Saffiotti, Guidelines for carcinogen bioassay in small rodents, NCI Tech. Rept. Series, No. 1, DHEW Publ. No. (NIH)76-801 (1976).
8. Health and Welfare, Canada, The testing of chemicals for carcinogenicity, mutagenicity, and teratogenicity, Health and Welfare, Ottawa, Canada (1973).
9. International Agency for Research on Cancer, Long-term and short-term screening assays for carcinogens: A critical appraisal, IARC Monographs on the Evaluation of the Carcinogenic Risk of Chemicals to Humans, Supp. 2, IARC, Lyon (1980).
10. Interagency Regulatory Liaison Group, Work Group on Assessment, Scientific bases for identification of potential carcinogens and estimation of risks, J. Natl. Cancer Inst., 63:241 (1979).
11. U. Saffiotti, Identification and definition of chemical carcinogens: Review of criteria and research needs. J. Toxicol. Environ. Health, 6:1029 (1980).
12. U. Saffiotti, The problem of extrapolating from observed carcinogenetic effects to estimates of risk for exposed populations. J. Toxicol. Environ. Health, 6:1309 (1980).

13. R. A. Griesemer and C. Cueto, Jr., Toward a classification scheme for degrees of experimental evidence for the carcinogenicity of chemicals for animals, in: "Molecular and Cellular Aspects of Carcinogen Screening Tests," R. Montesano, H. Bartsch, and L. Tomatis, eds., IARC, Lyon (1980).
14. U. Saffiotti and N. P. Page, Releasing carcinogenesis test results: Timing and extent of reporting, Med. Pediatr. Oncol., 3:159 (1977).
15. R. Montesano, H. Bartsch, and L. Tomatis, Screening tests in chemical carcinogenesis, IARC Scientific Publ. No. 12, International Agency for Research on Cancer, Lyon (1976).
16. U. Saffiotti and H. Autrup, eds., In vitro carcinogenesis. Guide to the literature, recent advances and laboratory procedures. NCI Carcinogenesis Tech. Rept. Series No. 44, DHEW Publ. (NIH)78-844 (1978).
17. "Methods for carcinogenesis tests at the cellular level and their evaluation for the assessment of occupational cancer hazards." Proceedings of the Meeting of the Scientific Committee, Fondazione Carlo Erba, Milan (1977).
18. U. Saffiotti, The multifactorial origin of cancer: A proposed model for studies on the interaction of multiple concurring factors (submitted for publication).
19. U. Saffiotti, Occupational carcinogens in relation to the multifactorial origin of cancer: Experimental pathology approaches, Proc. Internat. Symposium on Prevention of Occupational Cancer, Helsinki, ILO, Geneva (1981) (in press).
20. D. G. Hoel, D. W. Gaylor, R. L.Kirschstein, U. Saffiotti, and M. A. Schneiderman, Estimation of risks of irreversible, delayed toxicity, J. Toxicol. Environ. Health, 1:133 (1975).
21. U. Saffiotti, Experimental identification of chemical carcinogens, risk evaluation and animal-to-human correlations, Environ. Health Perspect., 22:107 (1978).
22. M. W. Anderson, D. G. Hoel, and N. L. Kaplan, A general scheme for the incorporation of pharmacokinetics in low-dose risk estimation for chemical carcinogenesis: Example - vinyl chloride, Toxicol. Appl. Pharmacol., 55:154 (1980).
23. T. C. Campbell, Chemical carcinogens and human risk assessment, Fed. Proc., 39:2467 (1980).
24. Committee on Prototype Explicit Analyses for Pesticides, National Research Council, "Regulating pesticides," National Academy of Sciences, Washington, D.C. (1980).
25. W. J. Nicholson, ed., "Management of Assessed Risk for Carcinogens," Ann. New York Acad. Sci., Vol. 363, New York (1981).
26. M. Meselson and K. Russell, Comparison of carcinogenic and mutagenic potency, in: "Origins of Human Cancer," H. H. Hiatt, J. D. Watson, and J. A. Winsten, eds., Cold Spring Harbor Laboratory, Cold Spring Harbor, New York (1977).

27. Environmental Studies Board, National Research Council, Carcinogenesis in man and laboratory animals, in: Pest Control: An Assessment of Present and Alternative Technologies. Vol. 1. Contemporary Pest Control Practices and Prospects, National Academy of Sciences, Washington, D.C. (1975).
28. E. L. Wynder and G. B. Gori, Contribution of the environment to cancer incidence: An epidemiologic exercise, J. Natl. Cancer Inst., 58:825 (1977).
29. J. Higginson and C. S. Muir, Environmental carcinogenesis: Misconceptions and limitations to cancer control, J. Natl. Cancer Inst., 63:1291 (1979).
30. K. Bridbord, P. Decoufle, J. F. Fraumeni, D. G. Hoel, R. N. Hoover, D. P. Rall, U. Saffiotti, M. A. Schneiderman, and A. C. Upton (contributors), National Cancer Institute, National Institute of Environmental Health Sciences and National Institute for Occupational Safety and Health, Estimates of the fraction of cancer in the United States related to occupational factors, Testimony submitted on September 15, 1978, to the U.S. Occupational Safety and Health Administration on proposed regulations for the identification, classification and regulation of toxic substances posing a potential occupational carcinogenic risk to humans, OSHA, Washington, D.C. (1978).
31. J. Higginson, Multiplicity of factors involved in cancer patterns and trends, J. Environ. Pathol. Toxicol., 3:113 (1980).
32. R. Doll and R. Peto, The causes of cancer: Quantitative estimates of avoidable risks of cancer in the United States today, J. Natl. Cancer Inst., 66:1191 (1981).
33. U. Saffiotti and C. C. Harris, Carcinogenesis studies on organ cultures of animal and human respiratory tissues, in: Carcinogens: Identification and Mechanisms of Action, A. C. Griffin and C. R. Shaw, eds., Raven, New York (1979).
34. L. M. Franks and C. B. Wigley, eds., "Neoplastic Transformation in Differentiated Epithelial Cell Systems in vitro," Academic Press, London (1979).
35. C. C. Harris, B. F. Trump, and G. D. Stoner, eds., "Methods in Cell Biology," Vol. 21, Normal Human Tissue and Cell Culture, Academic Press, New York (1980).

SOME COMMENTS ON THE USE OF HUMAN CELLS FOR ESTIMATES OF RISK

Colin F. Arlett

MRC Cell Mutation Unit
University of Sussex
Falmer, Brighton
Sussex N1 9QG, England

INTRODUCTION

The credibility of estimates of risk can be placed in context by the essentially pessimistic but nevertheless realistic comments of others. Auerbach [1] in reviewing the difficulties of determining genetic hazards concluded that:

"The estimation of risk is a dangerous procedure because it will create the impression that our conclusions are meaningful, whereas in reality they are so full of uncertainties as to be practically meaningless."

Cumming [2] has recently debated the question "is risk assessment a science?" He concludes that while it is not a science *per se* it must produce answers because decisions will be made with or without its input. What those who practice risk assessment must do, however, is to utilize the scientific method. I propose providing some examples where human cells have been used and where they show that estimates using data from non-human cellular systems might prove completely misleading.

RISKS ASSOCIATED WITH GENETIC DISEASES

Examples where human cells have been used to estimate risks as a consequence of environmental hazards are limited so that it seems appropriate to consider first examples where there is no semantic debate relating to the definition of risk and where some unequivocal answers can be provided using tests which operate at the level of the cell.

The Lesch-Nyhan syndrome

Simple pedigree genetics indicate that the Lesh-Nyhan (L-N) syndome is an X-linked recessive condition with a low frequency of occurrence [3, 4]. The affected males have an excessive excretion of uric acid and are seen to be almost completely or partially lacking in hypoxanthine guanine phosphoribosyl transferase (HGPRT) activity [5, 6]. Such individuals are easy to recognize at the level of the single cell since the absence of HGPRT activity can be measured by a failure to take up ^{3}H hypoxanthine. This, in turn, means that an affected foetus can be easily recognized and, if so desired, aborted. Clearly this would make no difference to the frequency of such individuals in the population because of their ability to reproduce. What is important is the ability to recognize carriers, sisters and the mother. These can be recognized because the female skin is a mosaic as a consequence of the Lyonization process [7], the X chromosome is switched off in a particular cell apparently at random. Thus sisters who have a 50% probability of carrying the gene can be monitored by a simple autoradiographic procedure at the cellular level. A noncarrier sister (or brother) has no at risk progeny but offspring of a carrier sister will have, proportionally, one normal and one carrier daughter and one normal and one L-N son. If carrier daughters can be persuaded either not to reproduce or not to bear further carriers and given that there is no detectable mutation frequency then the gene may easily be eliminated.

Xeroderma Pigmentosum (XP)

The phenotype of this autosomal recessive [8] condition is concerned with sun-sensitivity and an enhanced frequency of skin cancer [9]. The frequency of the homozygotes in the Western World is 1 in 250,000 and in Japan it is more common, 1 in 40,000 [10]. The majority of the afflicted individuals have defects in the excision of UV-induced DNA lesions [11], a minority class are defective in daughter-strand repair processes [12]. Since it is an autosomal recessive condition the probability of a single individual within a sib-ship being affected is 0.25. The excision repair defect can be detected at the level of the single cell and has made it possible to detect XP individuals following amniocentesis and thus make possible an abortion [13]. The daughter-strand repair defect can potentially be measured in a sample of a relatively low number of cells and again might be used in cell populations derived from amniocentesis.

Ataxia-telangiectasia (A-T)

A second autosomal recessive condition which has a frequency of homozygotes in the USA of 1 in 40,000 [14] is A-T. This condition shows an increased tendency towards cancer and an enhanced induced and spontaneous chromosome fragility [15]. Giannelli [16] has felt able to use chromosome fragility as the basis of a test for A-T in amniotic cell cultures. The risk for each pregnancy is 1 in 4 from a mating of heterozygotes so this represents a condition where it is very worthwhile assaying for the A-T phenotype. Although all fibroblast cultures from A-T which have been tested show a marked hypersensitivity to the lethal effects of ionizing radiation [17] the test itself is too time consuming to be appropriate for amniotic cells.

Hungtington's Disease (HD)

The potential for success with XP and A-T where homozygotes can be detected *in utero* and thus aborted is of some significance but as was the case with LN such a course of action cannot reduce the frequency of the gene since afflicted individuals are unlikely to reproduce. The aim with these three conditions is to reduce the sum of human suffering. An extension of this same philosophy to dominant conditions has some more important implications with respect to eliminating the gene. Huntington's disease is such an autosomal dominant disease present at a frequency of 1 in 10,000 [18] in Northern Europe. It is a particularly distressing dementia where, as a consequence of its late onset afflicted individuals have usually had their children before the onset of recognizable clinical symptoms [19]. Half the offspring would be similarly afflicted the whole sib-ship being at risk.

There are reports indicating that cells from HD patients are hypersensitive to the lethal action of ionizing radiation [20, 21] or N-methyl-N'-nitro-N-nitrosoguanidine (MNNG) [22]. Our first series of experiments showed that HD fibroblasts from the Camden culture collection could be distinguished from normals [20] with respect to their sensitivity to γ-irradiation. A further investigation revealed that some HD fibroblast cultures were sensitive to ionizing radiation but others were not. The present status of our data indicate that the radiation response test is not sufficiently sensitive to permit the discrimination of HD cell strains from normals. The results with MNNG also need repeating in other laboratories since we are unable to confirm the sensitivity of either HD or A-T cell strains to this agent [23]. In principle the primary aim of detecting HD pre-symptomatically and thus preventing the reproduction of the gene is still attainable. Other dominant, late onset, cancer prone diseases such as familial polyposis coli [24] are also potentially amenable to similar approaches.

USE OF RODENT CELLS TO ESTIMATE HUMAN GENETIC RISK

The more usual problem we are faced with is the question "does compound X present a risk?" It can be relatively easy to answer the question but that is insufficient for the questioner really wants to know whether the risk is sufficiently great to be defined as a hazard. An example where an attempt has been made to answer the question in full for man follows from the study of the possible genetic consequences of PUVA therapy [25]. 8-Methoxypsoralen (8-MOP) is clearly mutagenic for bacteria when combined with UVA indicating a somatic risk [26]. The possibility of a genetic risk follows from the demonstration that 8-MOP is mutagenic in E. coli and Salmonella tester strains in the dark [27]. 8-MOP is capable of reaching the gonads and Steiner et al. [28] have shown that human beings have a considerable variation of psoralen in serum. Our own data [29] show that 8-MOP in the dark is weakly mutagenic for both Chinese hamster V79 and mouse lymphoma L5178Y cells. Using a combination of pharmokinetics and the mutation data Bridges [25] has estimated that the genetic risk for PUVA treatment is likely to give rise to one new human mutant every 60 years. This seems to be an entirely acceptable risk attendant on the benefits of this therapy.

In emphasizing the fragility of this estimate Bridges [25] pointed out the possibility that human cells and, therefore, beings, might not behave like rodent or mouse cells. There are a number of reasons for supposing that this might be the case. Metabolism is different between mouse and man and there are large differences in repair capacity, for example, mouse cells are very low in the ability to excise UV or "UV like" damage [30] when compared with human cells.

An appropriate example where human cells do not respond like mouse cells follows from our investigation of the mutagenic activity of 1-8 dinitropyrene (DNP). This agent has been shown to be an extremely potent frame shift mutagen in Ames tests [31] and it is of possible environmental significance since nitropyrenes may be present in diesel exhausts. Since in both Salmonella and E. coli it acts either by some novel reductase or as a direct acting mutagen we attempted to measure its mutagenic activity in mammalian cells. DNP was seen to be non-toxic [32] at the highest possible concentrations with both L5178Y mouse lymphoma cells and both normal and XP human fibroblasts. The XP cells were used as an excision defective human analogue of L5178Y.

In the L5178Y cells DNP produced clear dose response curves for the induction of mutants resistant to 6-thioguanine, ouabain, methotrexate, excess thymidine and 1-β-D arabinofuranosylcytosine [32]. It is undoubtedly mutagenic. The presence of the ouabain resistant mutants suggests that NDP is not acting as a frame-shift mutagen in these mouse cells as it does in bacteria. For the human cells we are only able to measure the induction of 6-thioguanine resistance. No such resistant mutants have been detected after treatment with DNP indicating that it is not mutagenic for human cells. A potentially trivial explanation for the difference is that DNP is not metabolized by human cells. Metabolism, however, may still occur in vivo in other human cell types. Whatever the final outcome of the genetic toxicity evaluation of 1-8 dinitropyrene, it illustrates a clear difference at the cellular level between man, mouse, and bacteria.

CONCLUSION

Human cells can be used to detect individuals at risk in some families segregating disadvantageous genes. A consideration of the example with DNP would suggest that estimating genotoxic risk is a difficult business and that human cells may not always behave like rodent cells in culture. We emphasize that much caution should be exercised when extrapolating from data obtained with non-human cells to man.

ACKNOWLEDGEMENTS

I am indebted to Professor B. A. Bridges for many helpful comments.

REFERENCES

1. C. Auerbach, The effects of six years of mutagen testing on our attitude to the problems posed by it, Mutation Res., 33:3 (1975).
2. R. B. Cumming, Is risk assessment a Science?, Risk Analysis, 1:1 (1981).
3. M. Lesch and W. L. Nyhan, A familial disorder to uric acid metabolism and central nervous system function, Am. J. Med., 36:561 (1964).
4. W. L. Nyhan, J. Pesek, L. Sweetman, D. G. Carpenter, and C. H. Carter, Genetics of an X-linked disorder of uric acid metabolism and cerebral function, Pediat. Res., 1:5 (1967).
5. J. E. Seegmiller, F. M. Rosenbloom, and W. N. Kelley, Enzyme defect associated with a sex-linked human neurological disorder and excessive purine synthesis, Science, 155:1682 (1967).
6. W. N. Kelley, Hypoxanthine-guanine phosphoribosyl transferase deficiency in the Lesch-Nyhan syndrome and gout, Fed. Proc., 27:1047 (1968).
7. M. F. Lyon, Sex chromatin and gene action in the mammalian X-chromosome, Am. J. Hum. Genet., 14:135 (1962).
8. V. A. McKusick, Mendelian Inheritance in Man, Catalogs of Autosomal Dominant, Autosomal Recessive, and X-linked Phenotypes, John Hopkins Univ. Press, Baltimore-London (1975).
9. K. H. Kraemer, Xeroderma pigmentosum, in: "Clinical Dermatology," D. J. Dennis, R. L. Dobson, and J. McGuire, eds., (Unit 19.7: Vol. 4), Harper and Row, Hagerstown (1980).
10. H. Takebe, Y. Miki, T. Kozuka, J.-I. Furuyama, K. Tanaka, M. S. Sasaki, Y. Fujiwara, and H. Akiba, DNA repair characteristics and skin cancers of xeroderma pigmentosum patients in Japan, Cancer Res., 37:490 (1977).

11. J. E. Cleaver, Defective repair replication of DNA in xeroderma pigmentosum, Nature, 218:652 (1968).
12. A. R. Lehmann, S. Kirk-Bell, C. F. Arlett, M. C. Paterson, P. H. M. Lohman, E. A. de Weerd-Kastelein, and D. Bootsma, Xeroderma pigmentosum cells with normal levels of excision repair have a defect in DNA synthesis after UV-irradiation, Proc. Natl. Acad. Sci., USA, 72:219 (1975).
13. C. A. Ramsy, T. M. Coltart, S. Blunt, S. A. Pawsey, and F. Giannelli, Prenatal diagnosis of xeroderma pigmentosum, Lancet, 2:1109 (1974).
14. M. Swift, Malignant disease in heterozygous carriers, Birth Defects, Orig. Artic. Ser., X11:133 (1976).
15. D. G. Harnden and B. A. Bridges, Ataxia-telangiectasia (A-T) - a model of cancer susceptibility, in: "Ataxia-telangiectasia - a cellular and molecular link between cancer, neuropathology and immune deficiency," B. A. Bridges and D. G. Harnden, eds., John Wiley and Sons, London (1981).
16. F. Giannelli, J. A. Avery, M. E. Pembrey, and S. Blunt, Prenatal exclusion of ataxia-telangiectasia, in: Ataxia-telangiectasia - a cellular and molecular link between cancer, neuropathology and immune deficiency," B. A. Bridges and D. G. Harnden, eds., John Wiley and Sons, London (1981).
17. C. F. Arlett and S. A. Harcourt, Survey of radiosensitivity in a variety of human cell strains, Cancer Res., 40:926 (1980).
18. P. R. Vessie, On the transmission of Huntington's chorea for 300 years: The Bures family group, J. of Nerv. and Ment. Dis., 76:553 (1932).
19. E. D. Bird, A. J. Caro, and J. B. Billing, A sex related factor in the inheritance of Huntington's chorea, Ann. of Human Genet., 37:255 (1974).
20. C. F. Arlett and W. J. Muriel, Radiosensitivity in Huntington's chorea cell strains: a possible pre-clinical diagnosis, Heredity, 42:276 (1979).
21. C. F. Arlett, Presymptomatic diagnosis of Huntington's disease, Lancet, i:540 (1980).
22. D. A. Scudiero, S. A. Meyer, B. E. Clatterbuck, R. E. Tarone, and J. H. Robbins, Hypersensitivity to N-methyl-N'-nitro-N-nitrosoguanidine in fibroblasts from patients with Huntington's disease, familial dysautonia, and other primary neuronal degenerations, Proc. Natl. Acad. Sci. USA, 78:6451 (1981).
23. I. A. Teo and C. F. Arlett, The response of a variety of human fibroblast cell strains to the lethal effects of alkylating agents, Carcinogenesis (in press).
24. T. Muto, H. J. R. Bussey, and B. C. Morson, The evolution of cancer of the colon and rectum, Cancer, 36:2251 (1975).
25. B. A. Bridges, An estimate of genetic risk from 8-methoxypsoralen photochemotheraphy, Human Genet., 49:91 (1979).
26. S. Igali, B. A. Bridges, M. J. Ashwood-Smith, and B. R. Scott, Mutagenesis in E. coli IV. Photosensitization to near ultraviolet light by 8-methoxypsoralen, Mutation Res., 9:21 (1970).

27. B. A. Bridges and R. P. Mottershead, Frameshift mutagenesis in bacteria by 8-methoxypsoralen (methoxsalen) in the dark, Mutation Res., 44:305 (1977).
28. I. Steiner, T. Prey, F. Gschnait, J. Washiittl, and F. Greiter, Serum level profiles of 8-methoxypsoralen after oral administration, Arch. Dermatol. Res., 259:299 (1977).
29. C. F. Arlett, J. A. Heddle, B. C. Broughton, and A. M. Rogers, Cell killing and mutagenesis by 8-methoxypsoralen in mammalian (rodent) cells, Clin. and Expt. Dermatol., 5:147 (1980).
30. I. G. Walker and D. F. Ewart, Repair synthesis of DNA in HeLa cells and L-cells following treatment with methylnitrosourea or ultraviolet light, Can. J. Biochem., 51:148 (1973).
31. H. S. Rosenkranz, E. C. McCoy, D. R. Sanders, M. Butler, K. K. Kiriazides, and R. Mermelstein, Nitropyrenes: isolation, identification and reduction of mutagenic impurities in a carbon black and toners, Science, 209:1039 (1980).
32. C. F. Arlett, J. Cole, B. C. Broughton, J. Lowe, and B. A. Bridges, Mutagenic effects in human and mouse cells by a nitropyrene, AUI/BNL Symposium of the Genetic Effects of Air-Borne Agents (in press).

THE STRAUSS-ALBERTINI TEST FOR DIRECT ENUMERATION OF DRUG-RESISTANT PERIPHERAL BLOOD LYMPHOCYTES

G.H.S. Strauss

Centre for Medical Research and MRC Cell Mutation Unit
University of Sussex
Brighton, England

Our objective in developing the Strauss-Albertini test was to provide a direct technique for assessing the in vivo incidence of mutant cells arising amongst circulating lymphocytes in animals and man. The test is an early attempt at direct estimation of genotoxic risk from environmental agents. My present intention is to review the development and primary applications of the test, update the method, and nurture interest in this seminal system. Except where indicated otherwise, I performed the experiments described here while a graduate student at the College of Medicine, University of Vermont (USA).

The test, in essence, is an offshoot of human cell in vitro test systems that rely upon the ability to select, quantify, and isolate mutants occurring in cultures spontaneously or following exposure to test mutagens (Albertini and De Mars, 1973; Thilly et al., 1976). The marker phenotype commonly used in these systems is purine-analogue resistance conferred as a result of DNA damage to the X-chromosomal gene (Hpt locus) responsible for the purine salvage enzyme, hypoxanthine-guanine phosphoribosyltransferase (HGPRT) (E.C.2.4.2.8). Normal cells die following phosphorylation of purine base analogues, whereas mutants deficient in HGPRT activity survive because they can utilize the de novo pathway for purine base processing in DNA synthesis. The X-linked recessive Lesch-Nyhan (L-N) syndrome is largely the consequence of germinally inherited mutations at Hpt and has provided the prototype HGPRT-deficient cell. Fibroblasts from L-N individuals grow in the presence of purine analogues at concentrations grossly cytotoxic to normal cells (De Mars, 1971).

To obviate questions concerning the metabolic realism and target relevancy of in vitro systems, we sampled directly from humans and tested for L-N-like cells. Peripheral blood lymphocytes (PBLs) are an obvious choice of specimen material, because they are easily accessible, they receive exposure to conditions extant throughout the body, and their behaviour under conditions of short-term culture has been well characterized.

Our initial experiments were designed to study the behaviour of L-N PBLs with regard to phenotypic expression under selective culture conditions. We extended earlier studies (Albertini and De Mars, 1974) which showed that although mosaicism exists in PBLs from L-N heterozygotes, it is limited (presumably by negative selective pressure in vivo). Dancis et al. (1978) reported that mosaicism does not exist in PBLs from L-N heterozygotes; however, these investigators did not recognize the sensitivity limits of their detection method. We performed liquid scintillation spectrophotometry on PBL cultures stimulated to tritiated thymidine (^{3}H-Tdr) incorporation by phytohaemagglutinin (PHA) in the presence of the purine analogue 8-azaguanine (AG). To be distinguished from the normal phenotype by this method, an L-N heterozygote must carry at least 1% mutant blood cells (Albertini and De Mars, 1974).

To test PHA-stimulated PBLs in the absence of the purine analogue 6-thioguanine (TG) and in the presence of two concentrations of TG, we used standard lymphocyte culture conditions, labelling with ^{3}H-Tdr at 72 h and terminating at 96 h (see Strauss and Albertini, 1979a, for a complete description of the original method). The results for PBLs from a normal individual, an L-N heterozygote, and an L-N male are expressed in Figure 1 as counts per minute as a function of molar concentration of TG.

The PBLs from each of the individuals were stimulated vigorously, in accord with our expectations for members of the population at large. At 2 x 10^{-4} M TG, cells from the L-N male showed virtually complete resistance to the drug, whereas there was partial inhibition at 2 x 10^{-3} M. In contrast, PBLs from the normal individual were inhibited completely at both doses of TG. The responses of the PBLs from the L-N female indicated that at the lower dose of TG, an identifiable minority population of L-N variants existed among a great majority of cells that behaved normally; at the higher concentration of TG, the L-N variants were indistinguishable from normal cells. It was clear that at very high concentrations of TG, the resistance of L-N cells was not absolute, and that a selective concentration of 2 x 10^{-4} M TG allowed L-N variants and normal cells to be distinguished. We concluded that the scintillation spectrophotometric assay could

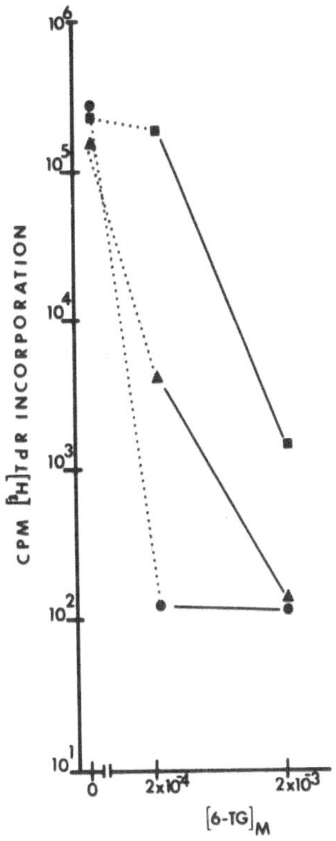

Figure 1. Incorporation of ^{3}H-Tdr in the presence of TG by PHA-stimulated PBLs from a normal male (●), an L-N heterozygote (▲), and an L-N male (■).

not estimate the proportion of L-N cells with sufficient sensitivity to be useful as a test for variants occurring at a frequency of much less that 0.01. With this in mind, we decided to develop an enumerative assay method.

We envisaged an approach that would employ a short culture period during which PBLs would be exposed to PHA and TG separately and together, to determine how many of the cells that can be activated by PHA are able to do so in the presence of TG. To design an accurate quantitative assay, we had first to study the kinetics of cell division and loss in PHA-stimulated, TG-inhibited cultures. A major barrier to enumerating PHA-treated lymphocytes is agglutination of the cells, which makes straightforward microscopic scanning for incidence of blast transformation impossible. To overcome this difficulty, we used a technique for producing free nuclei from the clumped lymphocytes.

Cultures of PBLs from a normal person were established at a density of 10^6 mononuclear cells per cubic centimeter of medium, and comparative counts of free nuclei were performed over time with an electronic particle counter (Coulter, ZBI model) and an haemocytometer. Results of this exercise were published elsewhere (Strauss and Albertini, 1979a). In summary, when cells were incubated with PHA alone, DNA synthesis was perceptable by 24 h, but numbers of nuclei remained unchanged for at least 42 h. During the period 42 to 48 h, numbers of nuclei began gradually to increase, reaching an additional 50% by 72 to 96 h. In contrast, nuclei from cultures treated with TG alone, those treated with TG and PHA, and those left untreated persisted up to 96 h with no overall gains or losses. On the basis of this information, we designed a culture protocol which, for the purpose of evaluating the products of in vivo genetic events, would provide sufficient time for vigorous DNA synthesis while denying any opportunity for cell division in vitro. The method we used in our earliest applications of the test can be found elsewhere (Strauss and Albertini, 1977, 1979a; Strauss et al., 1979, 1980). I now present a revised version that takes into account the recent finding that PBLs cycling at the time of biopsy can appear as TG-resistant (TG^r) variants. These cells, known as "phenocopies", may have resulted in overestimation of variant frequencies determined for normal individuals and those at risk. Preliminary results indicate that the phenocopies can be eliminated by freezing the PBL specimens before they are tested (R.J. Albertini, personal communication).

Venous blood is withdrawn into a syringe containing 0.1 ml heparin (1000 units/ml for injection without preservative) per 10 ml blood and mixed 1:1 with Hanks' balanced salt solution to which 2% heparin and 1% penicillin/streptomycin (100 units/ 100 µg/ml) have been added (HBSS). Density gradient separation of PBLs is achieved using lymphoprep with centrifugation for 10 min at 800 x g. The white-blood-cell layer is removed, washed with HBSS, and resuspended in medium for cryopreservation consisting of 70 volumes RPMI 1640 medium with 24 mM HEPES buffer, 0.2% heparin, and 1% penicillin/streptomycin; 20 volumes of pooled human AB plasma (heat-inactivated at 56°C for 20 min); and 10 volumes dimethyl sulphoxide. The cells are concentrated at a density of about 10^6/ml of the freezing medium, placed in plastic 1.5-ml Nunc tubes, and cooled in gas-phase nitrogen at -1°C/min. Cells can be stored for long periods in liquid nitrogen prior to testing. The frozen cells are thawed rapidly by rolling in the hands, and they are twice washed by addition of HBSS (at first dropwise), followed by centrifugation and resuspension. After washing, the cells are resuspended in complete medium (80% RPMI 1640 medium with 24 mM HEPES buffer + 20% AB plasma) containing reconstituted Bacto-Phytohemagglutinin-M at 0.025 cc/ml, to a density of 1.1 x 10^6 viable mononuclear cells/ml. Due to differential survivability of lymphocyte subtypes, viability and recovery must be at least 90%, for reliable results. Either TG from a Swinnex-filtered stock solution of 2 x 10^{-3} M in 0.5% Na_2CO_3, or 0.5% Na_2CO_3, is added at 0.1 ml to each 0.9-ml cell suspension containing PHA, in point-bottom screw-capped centrifuge tubes. Cultures are prepared in triplicate and incubated in a humidified 5% CO_2 atmosphere at 37°C for 30 to 36 h. For the final 6 h of incubation, 1 µCi ^{3}H-TdR (sp.act. 2.1, New England Nuclear) is added to each culture.

Before 42 h of incubation have elapsed, cultures are terminated by the addition of 4 ml 0.1 M citric acid to each culture tube. Citric acid treatment followed by vortexing produces free nuclei by rupturing the cellular membranes without damaging the nuclei, when followed by proper fixation. The tubes are vortexed and centrifuged at 600 x g for 10 min. The supernatants are removed, 5 ml of methanol-acetic acid (5:1) fixative are added, followed by vortexing, and the tubes are centrifuged as before. The supernatants are removed completely, and the pellets are then resuspended in 0.2 ml of fixative, in which they are left to stand, tops tightened, at 4°C for at least 3 h. Much care should be taken to avoid a change in the acidity of the fixative by evaporation of methanol until the moment the nuclear suspensions are added to slides. Within 24 h of fixation, cellular membranes are ruptured by triturating the pellet fraction with a 1-ml syringe bearing a 25-gauge spinal tap needle. At this point, an 0.025-ml sample of the nuclei in fixative is counted using an electronic particle counter (Coulter, ZBI model), and the remaining nuclei are carefully added to one of three 15- x 15-mm coverslips that previously have been affixed with Permount to a glass microscope slide. It is essential to rinse the syringe carefully between samples to avoid cross contamination.

Slides are allowed to air dry, then stained with 1% aceto-orcein for about 2 min and rinsed well, first with distilled water and then with running tap water. For autoradiography (in total darkness), the slides are dipped en masse into NTB-2 (Kodak) undiluted emulsion pre-warmed to 43°C, allowed to air dry, and exposed in dark boxes at a temperature no higher than -20°C for no less than 24 h, but usually for a week. After the exposure period, the slide boxes are warmed to room temperature and then developed with D19 (Kodak) 4 min, stopped in 1% acetic acid 1 min, and fixed in hypo (Kodak) 5 min. The processed slides are rinsed in distilled water and allowed to dry before each coverslip is dabbed with immersion oil to "clear" the emulsion.

Figure 2 is a photomicrograph (100 X) of an autoradiograph of nuclei from a PHA-stimulated culture prepared as described above. The dissociated nuclei are evenly distributed, and labelled nuclei are easily distinguishable from those unlabelled. From cultures containing PHA only, 2500 nuclei are counted differentially by medium-power microscopy, and a labelling index (LI) is calculated as the percent positive cells. Nuclei from cultures treated with TG in addition to PHA are scanned completely at low power, and all positive nuclei (confirmed by viewing at medium power) are counted. The LI is calculated using the Coulter-counter estimate as the number of negative cells present. The TG^r PBL variant frequency (Vf) is then determined as the ratio of the LIs, such that

$$\frac{\text{LI (PHA + TG)}}{\text{LI (PHA)}} = \text{Vf}.$$

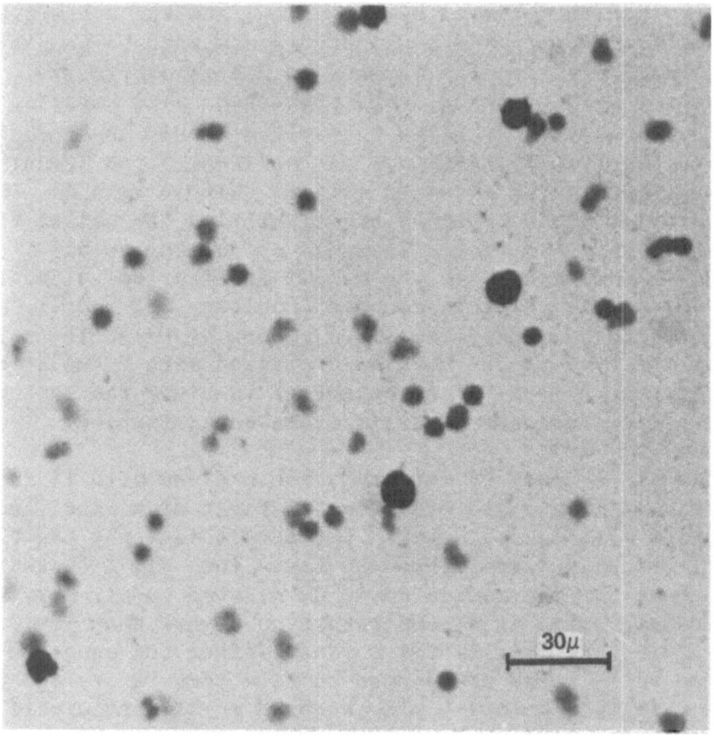

Figure 2. Autoradiograph of nuclei from a PHA-stimulated PBL culture.

When we performed the mass scintillation assay for PHA-stimulable, TG^r PBLs (Figure 1), we also tested the same normal individual, L-N heterozygote, and L-N male using the enumerative system to determine their variant TG^r PBL frequencies. The results of this experiment are shown in Figure 3. Frequencies of 9.0×10^{-5} and 4.5×10^{-5} were calculated for the normal individual at 2×10^{-4} M and 2×10^{-3} M TG, respectively (these points represent a low plateau following a precipitous fall from frequencies observed at 2×10^{-5} M TG and lower concentrations) (Strauss and Albertini, 1979a; Strauss et al., 1980). In contrast, PBLs from the L-N male again showed nearly complete resistance to TG, with a variant frequency of 7.5×10^{-1} in the presence of 2×10^{-4} M TG, whereas at 2×10^{-3} M TG, their frequency fell to 3.5×10^{-3}. PBL resistance to TG again was found to be intermediate in cells from the L-N female, for whom variant frequencies of 1.8×10^{-3} at 2×10^{-4} M TG and 2.7×10^{-4} at 2×10^{-3} M TG were determined.

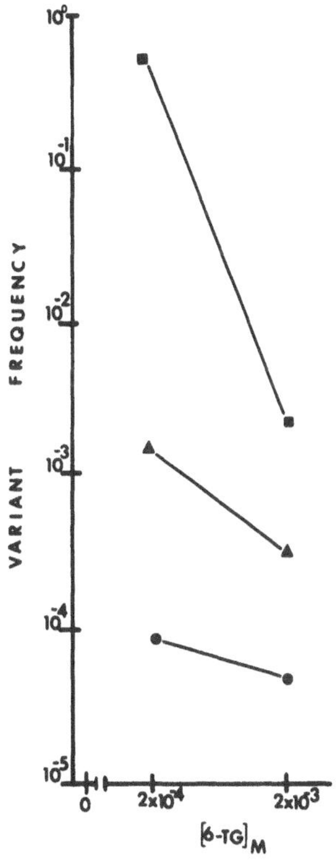

Figure 3. Frequencies of TG^r PBLs in a normal male (●), an L-N heterozygote (▲), and an L-N male (■).

The enumerative assay clearly detects and quantitates mosaicism for the L-N mutation in PBLs from L-N heterozygotes (Strauss et al., 1980). Compared with the enumerative approach, scintillation spectrophotometry of mass cultures falls short markedly, because it cannot distinguish between minimal ^{3}H-Tdr incorporation by many cells and maximal activity on the part of a small number of cells. Although the nuclei of active PBLs are labelled unambiguously and can be identified easily among extremely large numbers of TG-sensitive (TG^s) PBLs, we were concerned that if in vitro metabolic co-operation occurs (Subak-Sharpe et al., 1979), it might prevent detection of TG^r PBLs. To test the effectiveness of our system in detecting rare TG^r PBLs within a majority population of TG^s PBLs, we prepared cultures containing artificial mixtures of nil, 10^{-5}, 10^{-4}, 10^{-3}, 10^{-2}, 10^{-1}, and 5 PBLs from an L-N male in majority populations of PBLs from a normal individual. The cultures were treated with a selective concentration of 2×10^{-4} M TG and assayed autoradiographically as described above. Results of this reconstruction experiment appear in Figure 4.

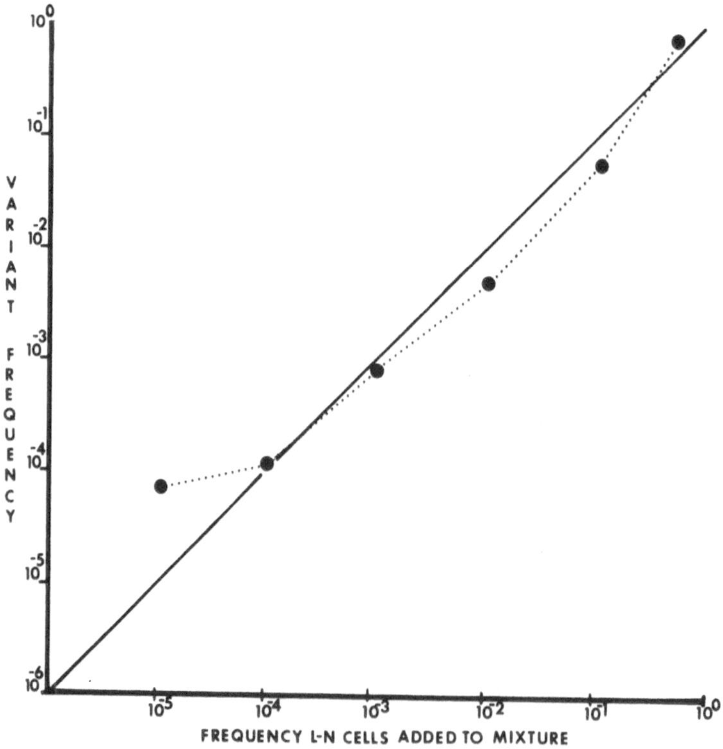

Figure 4. Detected frequency of TG^r PBLs as a function of frequency of L-N cells added to culture (●). Solid line represents the expected recovery frequencies.

The experimental variant frequencies were near to theoretical expectations except in the case of the culture containing 10^{-5} L-N cells. Our expectation at this low frequency point was distorted by our failure to take into account the spontaneous frequency of variants among 10^6 PBLs from the normal individual (which was determined to be 5.5×10^{-5}). The sum of spontaneous and added TG^r PBL frequencies accounted for the apparent discrepancy. The results of this experiment suggested that selection against the mutant phenotype did not occur in vitro and did not decrease efficiency of recovery in the present system.

Next we determined the frequencies of TG^r PBLs in healthy, non-L-N individuals who were not considered to be at risk from environmental mutagens. In 71 experiments, 31 individuals were tested at 2×10^{-3} M TG, and in 98 experiments, 63 individuals were tested at 2×10^{-4} M TG. About 20% of these individuals were tested at both concentrations of TG. The people tested ranged in age from 11 to 75 years. The median frequency of TG^r PBLs at 2×10^{-3} M TG was 1.0×10^{-4} (the mean was 1.3×10^{-4}, and the 10th and 90th percentiles were 5×10^{-5} and 1.5×10^{-4}, respectively). At 2×10^{-4} M TG, the median frequency was 1.1×10^{-4} (the mean was 1.3×10^{-4}, and the 10th and 90th percentiles were 6.1×10^{-5} and 2.1×10^{-4}, respectively). No correlation between age of donor and variant frequency was found. We hypothesized that because many of the pertinent PBLs are long-lived, failure of TG^r PBLs to accumulate with time may be accounted for, in part, by in vivo selection against the well-differentiated cell. In the case of the L-N heterozygotes, we assume that the absence of true Lyonization is the result of negative selective pressure both at the stem-cell level (McKeran et al., 1974) and against PBLs at advanced stages of maturity.

While continuing to develop a cumulative variant-frequency registry for normal individuals (controls), we commenced a study of a heterogeneous group of cancer patients receiving various chemotherapeutic agents, usually in combination over variable time courses. Also, some of the patients were being given X-ray treatments. In the initial study, most solid tumours were represented, but haematological malignancies were excluded. Twenty normal controls and 11 treated cancer patients were tested at 2×10^{-4} M TG, while cells from 24 controls and 42 treated cancer patients were studied at 2×10^{-3} M TG. Data from this study are presented as a scattergram in Figure 5. The average variant frequency at 2×10^{-3} M TG for normal controls was 8.7×10^{-5}, and at 2×10^{-4} M it increased slightly to 1.3×10^{-4}.

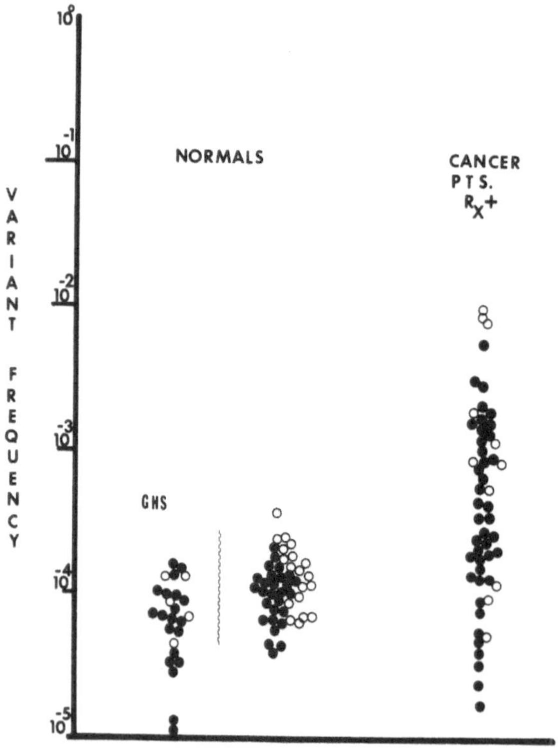

Figure 5. Frequency of TG^r PBLs in a heterogeneous group of cancer patients (right column), a group of normal controls (center column), and a single healthy individual (left column), determined at 2 x 10^{-4} M TG (●) and 2 x 10^{-3} M TG (o). Each point represents the results from one or more studies on an individual.

The values from the single control tested five times at 2 x 10^{-4} M TG and 20 times at 2 x 10^{-3} M, except for the outlying low frequencies from two tests, showed variability and a range similar to what was seen within the control group. For the treated cancer patients, however, the distributions of variant frequencies at both TG concentrations were clearly different from those of the controls. Of 11 patients tested at the lower concentration, 8 showed variant frequencies higher than that of the highest normal control tested at the same concentration. In agreement with this, of 42 patients tested at 2 x 10^{-3} M TG, 26 showed frequencies higher than the highest seen in a normal person tested at that TG concentration.

Figure 6 illustrates the relationship between the labelling indices of non-inhibited PHA-stimulated cultures and variant frequencies. From this information, we concluded that elevated variant frequencies in cancer patients were not necessarily correlated with labelling indices lower than in controls, and that in this regard the groups did not differ. Clearly, PBLs from cancer patients responded normally to PHA.

Considering that most antineoplastic therapies in use today are known to damage DNA (Bender and Young, 1978), it is not surprising to find elevated variant frequencies in the treated group. The extreme variability of variant frequencies within this

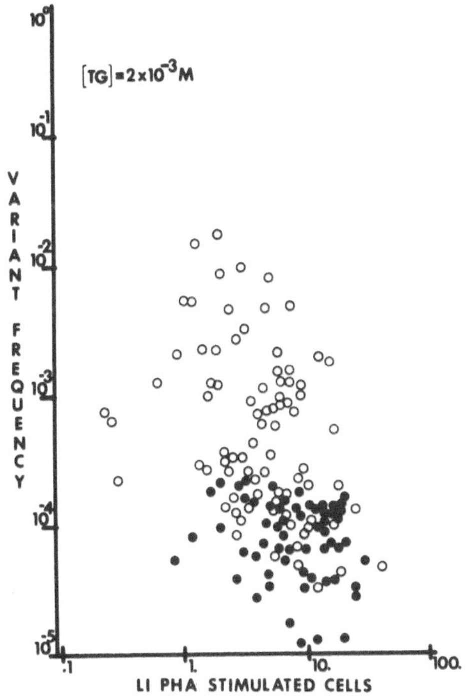

Figure 6. Variant frequency from individual tests as a function of labelling index (LI) in treated cancer patients (o) and normal controls (●) tested at 2 x 10^{-3} M TG.

group is also expected, considering the heterogeneous nature of the contributing factors.

Preliminary studies (Strauss and Albertini, unpublished results) indicated that untreated breast-cancer patients, about to undergo surgery, showed elevated TG^r PBL frequencies. This may have been an effect of causal agents such as carcinogens on PBLs directly, and/or it may have been produced through an interaction of PBLs with tumour-associated factors. Further studies are required to increase our understanding of these phenomena. Interestingly, when the first of these breast-cancer patients had received her initial course of adjuvant chemotherapy following surgical treatment, her variant frequency, initially determined to be above normal, at 6.7×10^{-4}, had increased to 1.6×10^{-3}.

For several studies recently completed or now in progress, we have used a longitudinal approach, whereby each individual is monitored and assessed in terms of personal baseline values. I discuss our long-term studies of PUVA-treated individuals in another contribution to this volume.

John Louras, working in Dr. Richard Albertini's laboratory, conducted a longitudinal test series to determine TG^r frequencies in a group of cancer patients before and during radiotherapy. Representative results for two patients who were given pelvic irradiation (3000 rads cumulative over three weeks and 4250 rads cumulative over four weeks) indicated that although each showed elevated variant frequencies prior to treatment (3.5×10^{-4} and 1.7×10^{-3}), both showed gradual increases during treatment, reaching maximum frequencies (7.0×10^{-3} and 1.1×10^{-2}, respectively) within several days of discontinuation of treatment. During this period the patients continued to respond normally to PHA, so the increases in variant frequencies were directly related only to the observed absolute increases in TG PBLs (Louras and Albertini, personal communication).

Tony Quinn, also working in Albertini's laboratory, found that to determine variant frequencies in Fisher rat PBLs, one must use a total incubation period of 68 h and proceed essentially in the same fashion as for humans (personal communication). He treated groups of rats with cyclophosphamide doses of nil, 3.0, 6.0 or 10.0 mg/kg/day over a period of 6 weeks; although the side effects of this potent drug resulted in severe lymphocytopoenia and decreased labelling indices, definite dose-related elevations in variant frequency were seen in all groups. The untreated rats showed a constant set of variant frequencies in approximately the same range as determined for humans (Strauss and Albertini, 1979b; Albertini, 1979).

We also performed experiments to determine frequencies of TG^r PBLs in dogs that had received or donated renal allografts and were given purine-analogue immunosuppressants. Although we discontinued these studies for technical reasons related to the surgical procedures, we did measure variant frequencies two times before the transplant and five times after the transplant in one recipient and one donor. We found that although both animals received azathioprine and showed variant frequencies in the normal range (as determined in humans) before the procedure, only the recipient showed elevated variant frequencies after the transplant, and these were sustained during the remaining test period. A second animal receiving a transplant showed normal variant frequencies in the two tests prior to transplant and an elevation in variant frequency approaching one order of magnitude on the third test occasion, but died from surgical trauma soon thereafter (Strauss and Albertini, unpublished results).

Except in L-N individuals, the presence of TG^r cells in humans is, for the most part, unimportant to health except where purine analogues are used therapeutically. Prospective evaluations we conducted using human renal transplant recipients provided further insights as to the nature of the TG^r PBLs. Figure 7 is a schematic of the clinical course of an individual who was grafted with a cadaveric kidney, which failed due to chronic rejection. These data are representative of results from 20 individuals we have tested who suffered similar fates. We also have studied individuals who were fortunate to have received well-matched grafts from living related donors. Although variant frequency always increased shortly after grafting, it gradually returned to only moderate elevations. The present system may therefore be developed for use in monitoring the efficacy of azathioprine as an immunosuppressant for transplantation. Vastly elevated variant frequencies in renal graft recipients are evidence for <u>in vivo</u> amplification, through cell division, of the mutant phenotype. We believe that our ability to establish long-term PBL cultures in medium containing 2×10^{-4} TG provides evidence for the analogous <u>in vitro</u> process.

We used two approaches in developing long-term lines from PBLs. In the first instance, we took PBLs from normal donors and from a transplant patient having a very high variant frequency, and infected the cultures with Epstein-Barr virus B95-8 in the presence and absence of TG. Though PBLs from each donor transformed and grew well in the absence of TG, only the PBLs from the transplant patient developed into an established B-cell line in the presence of TG (Strauss and Albertini, 1979a; Albertini, 1979). Ron Lane, in our laboratory, obtained similar results using T-cell growth factor to propagate a T-cell line from the

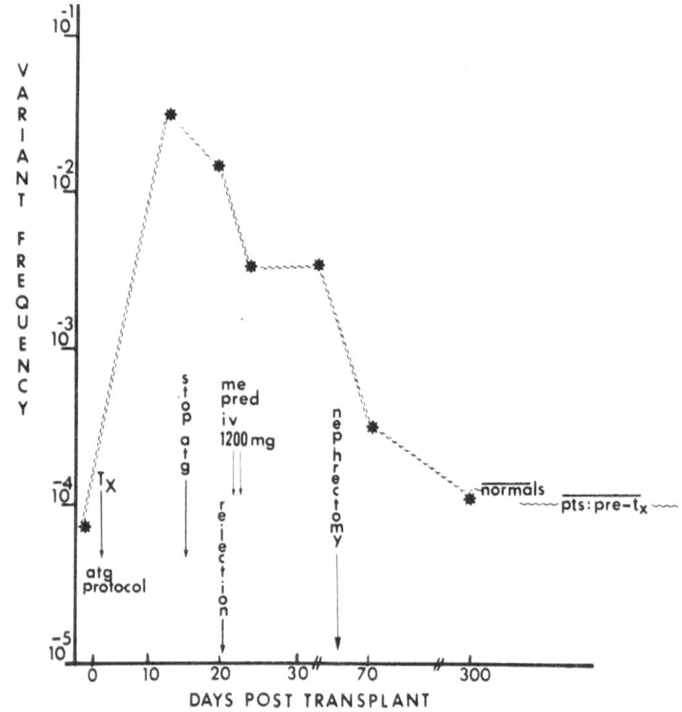

Figure 7. Frequency of variant PBLs in an individual receiving a kidney and treatment with antithymocyte globulin (atg) and the purine analogue azathioprine. The individual was treated for rejection with methyl prednisone (me pred) 20 days post transplant. The mean values for 63 normal individuals (normals) and 20 pre-treatment patients (pts:pre-t_x) are indicated.

PBLs of a renal graft recipient. Both of these culture methods can be used to isolate and characterize further the TG^r PBLs after cloning.

To define the variants further, we tested TG^r PBLs for senstivity to HAT medium (HAT^s phenotype). HAT medium contains hypoxanthine and aminopterin (a folic acid antagonist) to poison endogenous purine synthesis, so that normal cells retaining HG-PRT activity survive, and thymidine is added because the inhibitor also blocks endogenous thymidine synthesis. L-N and type-I-induced TG^r mutant fibroblasts are HAT^s, whereas type-II-induced mutants are not (De Mars and Held, 1972). Briefly, all TG^r PBLs from normal individuals were found to be HAT^s (degree of HAT^s estimated as the difference between TG^r PBL variant frequency and TG^r PBL HAT^r variant frequency). We found 98% of TG^r PBLs from an L-N heterozygote, 66% of TG^r PBLs from a renal transplant recipient, and 86% of TG^r PBLs from a PUVA-treated psoriatic patient to be HAT^s. These results strengthen our belief that TG^r PBLs are, for the most part, very much like L-N type-I mutants.

We believe that most important among various factors contributing to the dramatic rises in the TG^r PBL frequencies of renal transplant recipients (all of whom received azathioprine) is the phenomenon of proliferation of drug-resistant cells in response to antigenic stimulation. This appears to be especially significant where disparity between graft and recipient is great and probably represents *in vivo* selection in favour of the mutant cell. We presume that mutant lymphocytes arising in this fashion will be able to respond with high specificity against histoincompatible cells of the graft. It may be possible to administer the folic acid antagonist methotrexate (MTX) sequentially, in combination with a purine analogue, to counter dangerous elevations of TG^r PBL populations, which may indicate imminent rejection of a graft. In the case of HAT^s L-N type-I cells, such a strategy might result in drug-induced immunological tolerance, through cycle-specific killing driven by antigenic stimulation. A precedent for this approach may be chemotherapy for childhood acute lymphocytic leukemia (ALL), wherein TG and MTX are often used together. When we tested PBLs from children suffering from ALL during the part of the sequence when only TG was given, we found greatly elevated variant frequencies which fell near to or below normal immediately following administration of MTX. We saw similar patterns in other diseases for which MTX was used in combination with various drugs, although the results were not as dramatic as with ALL (Strauss and Albertini, 1979a).

Two important features of the Strauss-Albertini test, especially with regard to longitudinal evaluations, are its brief latency and patency periods. The phenototypic expression of TG^r PBLs according to this test is complete within only several days following mutagenic exposures. The length of this period (and the magnitude of genotoxic damage observed) must depend, to some degree, upon the extent of specific and non-specific killing of PBLs, as well as upon related states of lymphopoiesis. The persistence of the changes also must depend upon these factors plus the operation of negative selection mechanisms. The changes appear to last only days or weeks following discontinuation of exposure to selective and/or inductive agents, according to the results of our longitudinal studies. However, more information is needed further to characterize the TG^r PBLs.

Because the Strauss-Albertini test uses human material, it is not necessary to extrapolate results from another species to the human case. The question of whether the somatic-cell changes observed are genetic or epigenetic remains to be settled definitively. If TG^r PBLs are indicators of somatic-cell genetic damage, the Strauss-Albertini test may have a role to play in retrospective monitoring for environmental contaminants, in testing of agents that have passed through in vitro screening tests, and in making cost-benefit analyses for therapeutic agents. The problem of individual susceptibility to mutagenic hazards also may be addressed, ultimately, when changes in TG^r PBLs can be linked to genic health. We hope to be able to extrapolate results from humans to animals, and then to use the rat system to predict the effects of putative mutagens on humans.

Various modifications of the Strauss-Albertini test are possible. While in the Medical Research Council's Cell Mutation Unit, I have developed a promising variation on our theme that may be applicable to in vivo monitoring. The method relies on the use of T-cell growth factor (TCGF) to detect, quantify, and clone TG^r-T PBLs that can grow continuously, while maintaining their normal T-cell functions. Using a series of monoclonal antibodies, we have characterized lines developed so far as containing exclusively mature thymus-derived lymphocytes. We have successfully completed a series of recovery experiments using PBLs from L-N individuals, and we have detected, with high sensitivity, rare L-N PBLs in majority populations of TG^s PBLs in medium containing TG and TCGF. Also, we have used the lymphocyte clonal assay to enumerate TG^r mutant lymphocytes occurring in normal individuals. These early results compare favourably with those from the Strauss-Albertini test performed in parallel. The TG^r continuous T-lymphocyte (CTL) clones, produced using limiting dilutions of lymphocytes with TCGF as a mitogen, have provided material for further characterizations of mutant cells and for immunological determinations of their functional abilities. Further, CTLs should be useful in assays for genotoxic effects after in vitro exposures to putative mutagens. We hope to be able to compare results after in vivo and in vitro exposures in both animals and man. Our efforts to develop the lymphocyte clonal assay as a direct mutagenicity test system are described elsewhere (Strauss, in press).

I acknowledge with deep gratitude the unfaltering dedication and persistence with which my friends Jayne Deane, Carol Czina, and Debbie Czina served as technical assistants during my time in Dr. Albertini's laboratory. I should like to thank Drs. Albertini and Louras for sharing their recent, unpublished data.

The author is currently supported by the British Cancer Research Campaign.

REFERENCES

Albertini, R.J., 1979, Direct Mutagenicity testing with peripheral blood lymphocytes, in: "Banbury Report 2, Mammalian Cell Mutagenesis: The Maturation of Test Systems", A.W. Hsie, J.P. O'Neill, and V.K. McElheny, eds., Cold Spring Harbor Laboratory Press, Cold Spring Harbor.

Albertini, R.J., and De Mars, R., 1973, Detection and quantification of X-ray induced mutation in cultured diploid human fibroblasts, Mutation Res., 18:199.

Albertini, R.J., and De Mars, R., 1974, Mosaicism of peripheral blood lymphocyte populations in females heterozygous for the Lesch-Nyhan mutation, Biochem. Genet., 11:397.

Bender, R.A., and Young, R.C., 1978, Effects of cancer treatment on individual and generational genetics, Seminars in Oncology, 5:46.

Dancis, J. Berman, P.H., Jansen, V., and Balis, M.E., 1978, Absence of mosaicism in the lymphocyte in X-linked congenital hyperuricemia, Life Sci., 7:587.

De Mars, R., 1971, Genetic studies of HGPRT deficiency and the Lesch-Nyhan syndrome with cultured human cells, Fed. Proc. 30:944.

De Mars, R., and Held, K., 1972, The spontaneous azaguanine-resistant mutants of diploid human fibroblasts, Humangenetic, 16:87.

McKeran, R.O., Howell, A., Andrews, R.M., Watts, R.W.E., and Arlett, C.F., 1974, Observations on the growth in vitro of myeloid progenitor cells and fibroblasts from hemizygotes and heterozygotes for "complete" and "partial" hypoxanthine-guanine phosphoribosyltransferase deficiency, and their relevance to the pathogenesis of brain damage in the Lesch-Nyhan syndrome, J. Neurol. Sci., 72:183.

Strauss, G.H.S., in press, Direct mutagenicity testing: The development of a clonal assay to detect and quantitate mutant lymphocytes arising in vivo, in: "Banbury Report 13, Indicators of Genotoxic Exposures in Man and Animals," V.K. McElheny, ed., Cold Spring Harbor Laboratory Press, Cold Spring Harbor.

Strauss, G.H., and Albertini, R.J., 1977, 6-Thioguanine resistant lymphocytes in human peripheral blood, in: "Progress in Genetic Toxicology," D. Scott, B.A. Bridges, and F.H. Sobels, eds., Elsevier/North-Holland, Amsterdam.

Strauss, G.H., and Albertini, R.J., 1979a, Enumeration of 6-thioguanine resistant peripheral blood lymphocyte frequencies in man as a potential test for somatic cell mutation arising in vivo, Mutation Res., 41:353.

Strauss, G.H., and Albertini, R.J., 1979b, Longitudinal determination of 6-thioguanine resistant blood lymphocyte frequencies in individuals receiving 8-methoxypsoralen and long-wave ultraviolet light treatment (PUVA), Environ. Mutagen, 1:152.

Strauss, G.H., Albertini, R.J., and Allen, B.J., 1980, An enumerative assay of purine analogue resistant lymphocytes in women heterozygous for the Lesch-Nyhan mutation, Biochem. Genet. 18:529.

Strauss, G.H., Albertini, R.J., Krusinski, P.A., and Baughman, R.D., 1979, 6-Thioguanine resistant peripheral blood lymphocytes in humans following psoralen, longwave ultraviolet light (PUVA) therapy, J. Invest. Dermatol., 73:211.

Subak-Sharpe, J.H., Burk, R.A., and Pitts, J.D., 1979, Metabolic co-operation between biochemically marked mammalian cells in tissue culture, J. Cell. Sci., 4:353.

Thilly, W.G., De Luca, J.G. Hoppe, I.V.H., and Penman, B.W., 1976, Mutation of human lymphoblasts by methylnitrosourea, Chem. Biol. Interact., 15:33.

INDUCTION OF SISTER CHROMATID EXCHANGE BY CHEMICAL MUTAGENS

Paul E. Perry

MRC Clinical and Population Cytogenetics Unit
Western General Hospital
Edinburgh EH4 2XU
Scotland

INTRODUCTION

Cytogenetics underwent something of a revolution in the mid 1970s with the development of new techniques for the visualization of sister chromatid exchange (SCE). One of the reasons for the excitement was the observation that many chemical mutagens elicted dose dependent increases in the frequency of SCEs, and since these events proved to be simple to score and the analysis of only twenty or so cells per dose point was usually sufficient for statistical purposes, this method showed considerable advantages over the conventional cytogenetic method of assessing chromosome damage, aberration scoring. There are, however, important differences between SCE and aberrations, and this is reflected in the uses we can make of these phenomena in mutagen and carcinogen identification, and in the assessment of risk.

Before going on to discuss the possible use of SCE in risk assessment I should like firstly to discuss briefly the history of SCEs and the methods available for their analysis in *in vitro* and *in vivo* situations.

SCEs were first described by Taylor (1958) who found that if cells were allowed to replicate their DNA once in the presence of ^{3}H-thymidine, and then again in the absence of the isotope, autoradiographs made at the ensuing mitosis showed the metaphase chromosomes to be composed of one labelled and one unlabelled chromatid as a result of semiconservative replication of DNA. Symmetrical switches in the silver grain labelling between the chromatids were sometimes observed and these Taylor called sister chromatid ex-

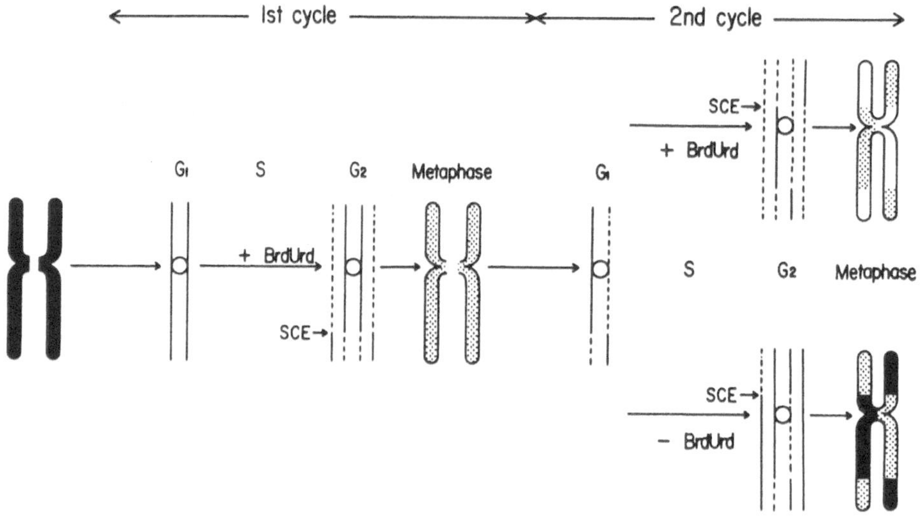

Fig. 1. Diagrammatic representation of differential BrdUrd incorporation into sister chromatids, and SCE. SCEs occurring during both the first and second cycles are detectable in second division cells. BrdUrd may be incorporated during both cell cycles, or during only the first followed by a second cycle in its absence.

changes. Unlike structural chromosome aberrations, no overall change in morphology of the chromosomes was involved and in conventionally stained chromosome preparations SCEs are therefore not distinguishable. The identification of SCEs by autoradiographic methods did not lend itself readily to questions concerning the frequency of SCEs, particularly where high frequencies were concerned, because the technique lacked resolution and was tedious. Advances in SCE methodology came with the development of simple techniques that replaced ^{3}H-thymidine with bromodeoxyuridine (BrdUrd) as the label and autoradiography with fluorescent and/or Giemsa staining techniques (Latt, 1973; Perry and Wolff, 1974) as the detection method. These new methods surpassed the resolution of the former techniques and for this reason most of our present knowledge about the influence of chemical and physical agents upon SCE has been gained in the last 6 or 7 years.

To achieve the necessary differential staining of the sister chromatids, the cells must undergo either two cell cycles in the presence of BrdUrd, or else one cycle in BrdUrd followed by a further cycle in its absence (see Fig. 1). The difference in the level of substitution between the chromatids is detected as dim versus intense fluorescence with fluorescent dyes, or light versus dark magenta staining with Giemsa. We should note at this point that the

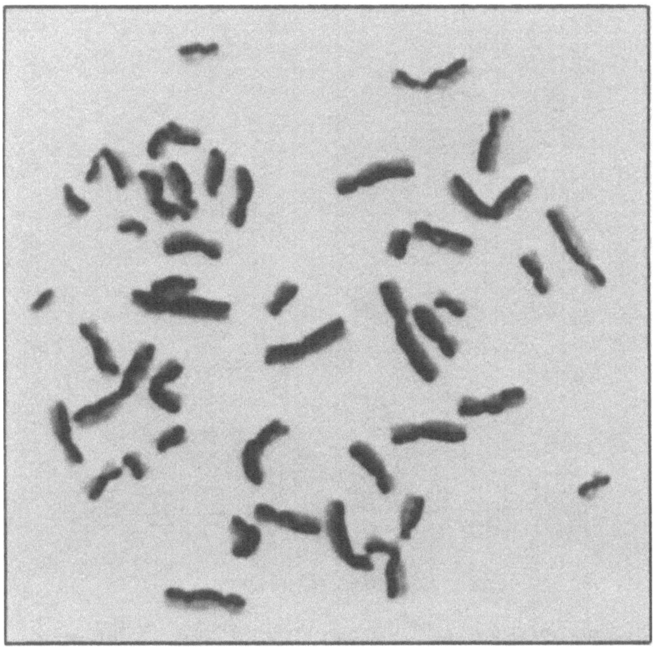

Fig. 2. SCEs in a human peripheral blood lymphocyte stained by the fluorescence plus Giemsa technique (Perry and Wolff, 1974).

number of SCes observed in cells treated according to this scheme is the sum over the 2 cell cycles and the value must be halved to give an approximation of the SCE occurring during each cell cycle.

Soon after the advent of the new staining techniques it was reported that a variety of chemical mutagens gave dose dependent increases in the incidence of SCE in CHO cells (e.g., Perry and Evans, 1975) and in cultured human lymphocytes (Solomon and Bobrow, 1975). The SCE methodology was soon extended to encompass chemicals that require in vivo metabolic activation either by the addition of 'S9-mix' to cultured cells (Stetka and Wolff, 1976a; Natarajan et al., 1976) or by the development of in vivo SCE assays in which BUdR was administered to the test animal and the SCE incidence analyzed in some replicating tissue such as bone marrow (Vogel and Bauknecht, 1976) spermatogonial cells (Allen and Latt, 1976) regenerating liver (Allen et al., 1978) or cheek pouch cells (Shuler and Latt, 1978).

RELATION SCE TO MUTATION AND TRANSFORMATION

Overall, a reasonable correlation exists between the SCE data and mutagenicity or carcinogenicity data, although certain exceptions are known. For example, x-irradiation and the cytostatic

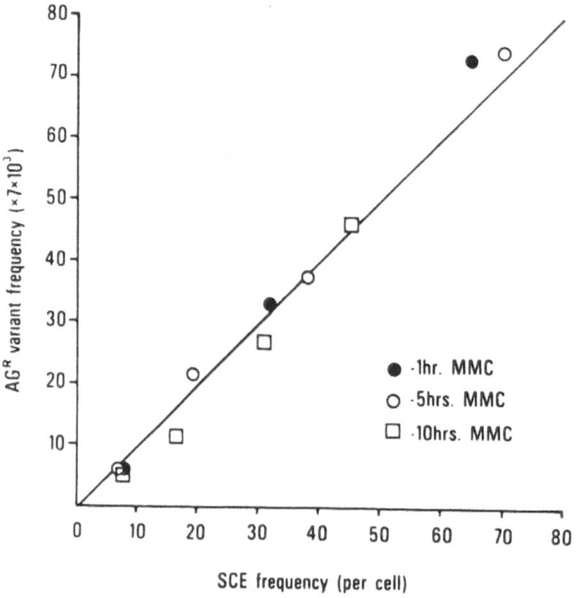

Fig. 3. Relation between AG^R variants and SCE frequency in human lymphocytes exposed to Mitomycin C for 1, 5, and 10 h at various concentrations over the range 10^{-9} M to 10^{-6} M (from Evans and Vijayalaxmi, 1981).

drug bleomycin are potent mutagens and cause chromosome structural damage, yet they have only a weak SCE-inducing ability even at comparatively high dose levels (Perry and Evans, 1975). For this reason SCEs in conjunction with structural chromosome damage would seem to offer a more comprehensive cytogenetic assay. Clearly, for some agents SCE data alone will give us neither a quantitative nor qualitative estimate of DNA damage.

There is no direct evidence relating SCE with mutation although superficially both phenomena are more compatible with cell survival, which is in contrast to structural chromosome damage which is frequently cell lethal. Carrano et al. (1978, 1979) compared the induction of 8-azaguanine resistant variants in CHO cells with the induction of SCE and observed linear correlations for several chemicals, although the slope was different for each. Further linear correlations between variant frequency and SCEs have recently been reported in chinese hamster cells (Siriani and Huang, 1980) and cultured human lymphocytes (Evans and Vijayalaxmi, 1981), and in some cases a numerical comparison has been attempted (Carrano et al., 1978; Evans and Vijayalaxmi, 1981; see Fig. 3). If the SCE:mutation ratio obtained _in vitro_ may be extrapolated to cells _in vivo_ the possibility arises that mutation rate in Man could be predicted from _in vitro_ or _in vivo_ SCE results (Carrano et al., 1978).

Relevant to this discussion is the recent report linking the alkylation of specific DNA bases with the induction of SCE in Chinese hamster V79 cells (Swenson et al., 1980). It was found that the production of 06-alkylguanine by various alkylating agents correlated with the induction of SCE and with mutagenesis in V79 cells, thus supporting the suggestion that SCE and mutagenesis can result from a common DNA lesion.

Significantly, a positive linear relationship has recently been reported between carcinogen induced SCE and neoplastic cell transformation in cultured Syrian hamster embryonic cells (Popescu et al., 1981), and it remains to be seen whether further work will support the validity of this important finding.

THE NATURE OF THE LESION THAT GIVES RISE TO SCE

There is good evidence that SCE occur during the DNA synthesis phase of the cell cycle, but the DNA damage that eventually results in SCE can be caused by treatment at any stage of the cell cycle. This suggests that the lesions responsible for SCE production persist in the cell at least until the DNA synthesis phase. Wolff et al. (1974) showed that after UV irradiation of Chinese hamster ovary (CHO) cells at various stages of the cell cycle, an intervening period of DNA synthesis was necessary before an increase in SCE occurred. Irradiation in G_2 did not produce an increase in SCE at the immediately ensuing metaphase, but an increase was observed in the second metaphase after exposure. Thus for UV-irradiation some of the lesions that give rise to SCE are long-lived and persist until the S phase when SCE formation occurs.

There is also evidence that the SCE inducing lesions produced by many chemicals can persist for some length of time. For example, Wolff (1978) found that ethylmethanesulfonate, methylmethanesulfonate, 4-nitroquinoline-1-oxide and N-acetoxyacetylaminofluorene all induced SCEs in both the first and second cycle following pulse chemical treatment. Latt and Loveday (1978) reported that alkylations induced by 8-methoxypsoralen plus UV-irradiation persist, and cause SCE, for several cycles in CHO cells, and Ishii and Bender (1978) found that SCEs were still induced 3 cell cycles after mitomycin-C treatment of human lymphocytes in vitro.

These findings have important implications when we come to consider the use of SCE in dosimetry and risk estimation, because the human material of choice, the circulating peripheral blood lymphocyte, is in an arrested Go stage of the cell cycle and can, to some extent, store damage that has occurred some weeks, months, or even years previous to cytogenetic examination. In the case of ionizing radiation this catalogue of past exposure can be read with some precision by scoring structural chromosome aberrations at the first mitosis following mitogenic stimulation. Can we do the same with SCEs?

TRANSIENT EXPOSURE TO CHEMICAL MUTAGENS

Most data indicate that SCEs are not a good measure of transient exposure. Firstly, there is now abundant evidence from patients undergoing cyclophosphamide and adriamycin cytostatic chemotherapy that a significant elevation in the SCE frequency occurs in lymphocytes assayed immediately after drug treatment but this is usually followed by a return to the pretreatment SCE control level a few days later (Perry and Evans, 1974; Lambert et al., 1978, 1979; Natarajan et al., 1978; Nevstad, 1978). Moreover, this transient increase in SCE frequency with drug treatment is repeated with each readministration of the drug. On the other hand, it is apparent that while the majority of anti-cancer drugs follow the above pattern it is not universal. For example, 1-(2-chloroethyl)-3-cyclohexyl-1-nitrosourea (CCNU) causes an elevation of SCE that may persist in some individuals for eight to sixteen weeks (Lambert et al., 1979). The reason for the transient increase with some drugs and prolonged increase with others is unknown, although several factors could be responsible. The gradual decline could be due to slow depletion of the chemical in vivo by metabolism and excretion but this cannot account for the transient increase seen in rabbits injected with EMS (Stetka and Wolff, 1976b), as this chemical has a half life in serum-containing medium of only 2.2 h (Jensen et al., 1977). The decline could also be due to the repair of the long-lived lesions in vivo or to removal of the damaged cells from the bloodstream and replacement with undamaged cells. Lambert et al. (1979) suggest that the relatively slow and incomplete repair of DNA damaged by CCNU and its ability to induce DNA interstrand cross-links and DNA-protein cross-links may be responsible for the prolonged SCE increase observed with this agent.

CHRONIC EXPOSURE TO CHEMICAL MUTAGENS

The dose levels to the lymphocytes of the chemicals used in cancer chemotherapy is high compared with the concentration of environmental mutagens to which individuals are unknowingly exposed and we might query, with some justification, whether SCE are capable of detecting chronic low dose exposure. In fact several lines of evidence suggest that measurement of SCE incidence may be of some value in investigations of this nature.

Stetka et al. (1978) reported that repeated weekly intraperitoneal administration of the direct acting mutagen mitomycin-C to rabbits initially gave small increases in SCE within one day of injection, followed by a return to control levels within one week. After the fourth injection the elevated SCE level failed to return to the control level and persisted for several weeks thereafter. Exposure of the animals to the same total dose given as a single injection resulted in a transient increase only. Overall, repeated exposure was at least as effective as acute exposure in eliciting

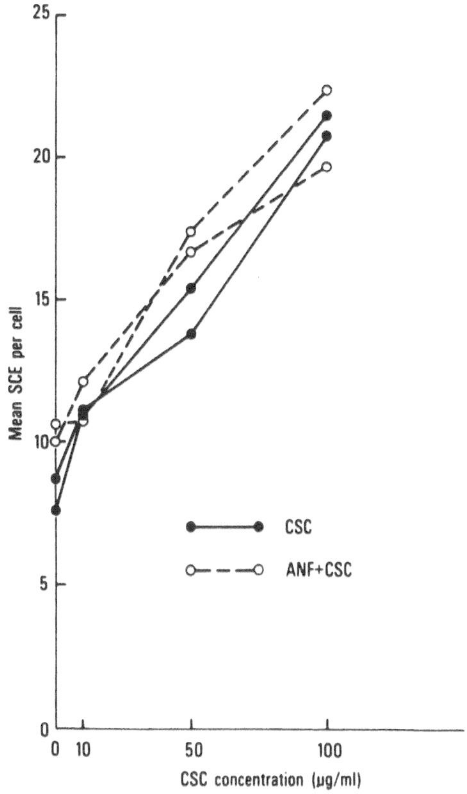

Fig. 4. Induction of SCE by cigarette smoke condensate (CSC). The metabolic inhibitor α-naphthoflavone (ANF) does not affect the SCE response and hence the compounds responsible for SCE induction must be direct acting (from Hopkin and Perry, 1980).

long-lived SCEs in vivo and it was proposed that SCE might therefore provide a valuable assay for detection of low level chronic chemical mutagen exposure even when the individual is not available for testing until some time after the exposure has taken place.

There are now several published reports concerning the SCE levels in individuals exposed to chronic low doses of mutagenic agents. For example, it has been found that technicians engaged in laboratories performing hormone analysis exhibited an average lymphocyte SCE frequency of 19.7 SCE per cell compared with the control group mean of 13.5 SCE per cell (Funes-Cravioto et al., 1977). Furthermore, four children of two female technicians working during pregnancy also showed a significantly increased average level of 15.8 SCE per cell. In this laboratory considerable amounts of or-

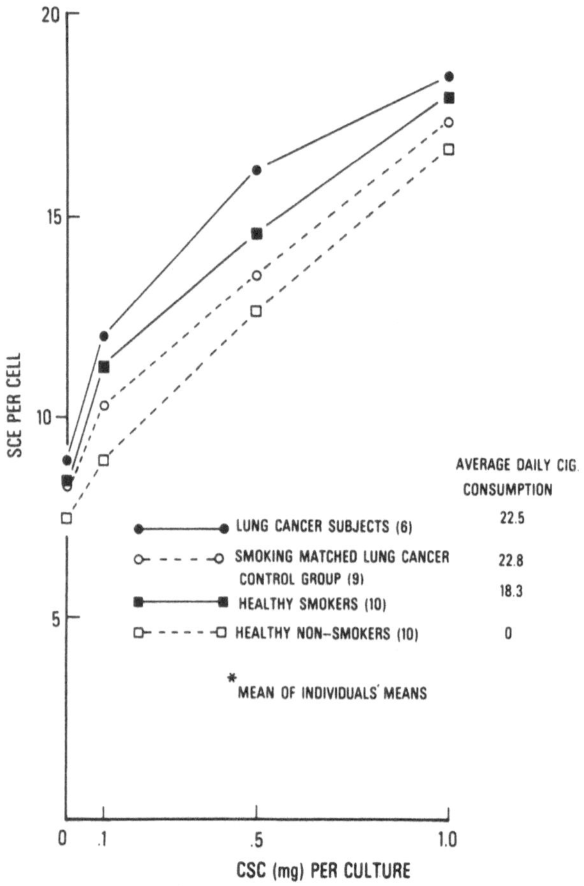

Fig. 5. Within group pooled mean SCEs (mean of individual means) at different concentrations of cigarette smoke condensate (CSC) (from Hopkin and Evans, 1980).

ganic solvents were used and benzene was considered the most likely cause of the observed effects. Other reports have also recently appeared concerning the cytogenic effects of exposure to vinyl chloride monomer (VCM). Kucerova et al. (1979) analyzed blood samples from nine workers who had been exposed to relatively high (20-150 ppm) exposure levels of VCM and found an increased mean SCE level of 13.8 SCE/cell in the exposed population compared with a control level of 9.41 SCE per cell. Anderson et al. (1981) have studied a larger number of workers exposed to lower VCM levels and observed only a small increase in SCE compared with the control group. This increase was not statistically significant whereas the level of chromosomal aberrations showed a considerable increase over the control level. Thus in situations of very low chronic exposure, or where considerable time has elapsed since the exposure occurred, SCE analysis may be of only limited value.

Table 1. SCE Induction by Benzo(a)pyrene in Cultured Mouse Embryos at 7.5 Days of Gestation (from Galloway et al., 1980)

BP	Nonresponsive		Responsive	
μM	AKR/J	DBA/2J	Balb/C	C3H
0	4.5 ± 0.3	12 ± 0.7	6.6 ± 0.3	8.6 ± 0.6
0.1	11 ± 0.4	13 ± 0.7	22 ± 0.5	23 ± 0.6
1.0	9.7 ± 0.5	19 ± 0.7	39 ± 0.9	47 ± 3.0
3.0	6.9 ± 0.7		51 ± 1.7	68 ± 2.1
10	12 ± 0.6		64 ± 1.1	

An example of individuals exposed to chronic high concentrations of a proven mutagen is afforded by cigarette smokers who inhale the tobacco smoke. Although mutagenic products can be detected in the urine of inhaling cigarette smokers, there is little direct information regarding the reaction of cigarette smoke with the DNA of cells in vivo. Cigarette smoke condensate is a potent inducer of SCEs in Chinese hamster and human cells in vitro (see Fig. 4) and so we should expect equivalent DNA damage in the exposed cells of the lung. Several recent reports have compared the incidence of SCE in lymphocytes of smokers and nonsmokers and while some investigations claim no difference in the SCE values (Hollander et al., 1978; Ardito et al., 1980; Crossen and Morgan, 1980) others indicate a small but consistent and significant increase in the cells of cigarette smokers (Lambert et al., 1978; Krishna-Murthy, 1979; Hopkin and Evans, 1980). Overall, when factors such as age, drug intake, and smoking habits are taken into account, an average SCE elevation of approximately one per cell occurs with every twenty cigarettes smoked each day.

Hopkin and Evans investigated the in vitro response of lymphocytes from healthy smokers and nonsmokers and smoking lung cancer patients to cigarette smoke condensate (Fig. 5) and found that healthy smokers exhibited slightly higher yields of SCE than nonsmoking controls, but slightly lower yields than the smoking lung cancer patients.

SCE IN EMBRYOS

Finally I would like to mention some experiments in the mouse that have used SCE analysis to detect chromosome damage in embryos exposed to carcinogen. Inducible metabolism of benzo(a)pyrene in the mouse is controlled by the Ah locus, and this inducibility is inherited as a Mendelian autosomal dominant trait that is expressed in most adult tissue. However, since too little material is available for biochemical analysis in the mouse embryo, there has been considerable debate over the expression of the inducible enzyme system in utero.

Galloway et al. (1980) found that inducible $7^1/_2$ day gestation mouse embryos of Ah^b/Ah^d genotype cultured in the presence of benzo-(a)pyrene responded with a large increase in the incidence of SCE compared with non inducible Ah^d/Ah^d embryos (see Table 1). Thus embryos at a critical stage of organogenesis may be at risk from exposure to polycyclic hydrocarbons and other chemicals metabolized by this inducible enzyme system. There is no clear evidence that a parallel situation exists in man as no correlation has yet been found between benzo(a)pyrene induced SCE and the human Ah locus (Schonwald et al., 1977; Rudiger et al., 1976).

In conclusion, SCE would seem to have several virtues in the assessment of exposure and risk but one cannot deny that there are also some drawbacks. They are attractive to the cytogeneticist and seem to bear a close relationship with mutation and cell transformation in vitro. They also provide a useful guide in situations of transient exposure yet are of only limited use in the identification of chronic low dose exposure to chemical mutagens. A greater understanding of the lesions responsible for SCE and the multitude of factors that may effect the reponse in vitro and in vivo may allow us to interpret SCE data more fully.

REFERENCES

Allen, J. W., and Latt, S. A., Analysis of sister chromatid exchange formation in vivo in mouse spermatogonia as a new test system for environmental mutagens, Nature, 260:449 (1976).

Allen, J. W., Shuler, C. F., and Latt, S. A., BrdU tablet methodology for in vivo studies of DNA synthesis, Somat. Cell Genet., 4:393 (1978).

Anderson, D., Richardson, C. R., Purchase, I. E. H., Evans, H. J., and O'Riordan, M. L., Chromosomal analysis in vinyl chloride exposed workers: comparison of the standard technique with the sister chromatid exchange technique, Mutat. Res., 83:137 (1981).

Ardito, G., Lamberti, L., Ansaldi, E., and Ponsetto, P., Sister-chromatid exchanges in cigarette-smoking human females and their newborns, Mutat. Res., 78:209 (1980).

Carrano, A. V., Thompson, L. H., Lindl, P. A., and Minkler, J. L., Sister chromatid exchange as an indicator of mutagenesis, Nature, 271:551 (1978).

Carrano, A. V., Thompson, L. H., Stetka, D. G., Minkler, J. L., Mazrimas, J. A., and Fong, S., DNA crosslinking, sister chromatid exchange and specific locus mutations, Mutat. Res., 63: 175 (1979).

Crossen, P. E., and Morgan, W. F., Sister chromatid exchange in cigarette smokers, Hum. Genet., 53:425 (1980).

Evans, H. J., and Vijayalaxmi, Induction of 8-azaguanine resistance and sister chromatid exchange in human lymphocytes exposed to mitomycin-C and x-rays in vitro, Nature, 292:601 (1981).

Funes-Craviot, F., Kolmodin-Hedman, B., Lindsten, J., Nordenskjold, M., Apaţa Gayon, G., Lambert, B., Norberg, G., Olin, R., and Swenson, A., Chromosome aberrations and sister chromatid exchanges in workers in chemical laboratories and a rotoprinting factory and in children of women laboratory workers, Lancet, ii:322 (1977).

Galloway, S. M., Perry, P. E. Meneses, J., Nebert, D. W., and Pedersen, R. A., Cultured mouse embryos metabolize benzo(a)pyrene during early gestation: genetic differences detectable by sister chromatid exchanges, Proc. Natl. Acad. Sci. USA, 77: 3524 (1980).

Hollander, D. H., Tockman, M. S., Liang, Y. W., Borgaonkar, D. S., and Frost, J. K., Sister chromatid exchanges in the peripheral blood of cigarette smokers and in lung cancer patients and the effect of chemotherapy, Hum. Genet., 44:167 (1978).

Hopkin, J. M., and Evans, H. J., Cigarette smoke-induced DNA damage and lung cancer risks, Nature, 283:338 (1980).

Hopkin, J. M., and Perry, P. E., Benzo(a)pyrene does not contribute to the SCEs induced by cigarette smoke condensate, Mutat. Res., 77:377 (1980).

Ishii, Y., and Bender, M., Factors influencing the frequency of mitomycin C-induced sister chromatid exchanges in 5-bromodeoxyuridine substituted human lymphocytes in culture, Mutat. Res., 51:411 (1978).

Jensen, E. M., LaPolla, R. J., Kirby, P. E., and Harworth, S. R., In vitro studies of chemical mutagens and carcinogens, I. Stability studies in cell culture medium, J. Natl. Cancer Inst., 59:941 (1977).

Krishna Murthy, P. B., and Prema, K., Sister-chromatid exchanges in oral contraceptive users, Mutat. Res., 68:149 (1979).

Kucerova, M., Polivkova, Z., and Batora, J., Comparative evaluation of the frequency of chromosomal aberrations and the sister chromatid exchange numbers in peripheral lymphocytes of workers occupationally exposed to vinyl chloride monomer, Mutat. Res., 67:97 (1979).

Lambert, B., Linblad, A., Nordenskjold, M., and Werelius, B., Increased frequency of sister chromatid exchanges in cigarette smokers, Hereditas, 88:147 (1978).

Lambert, B., Ringborg, U., and Lindbad, A., Prolonged increase of sister-chromatid exchanges in lymphocytes of melanoma patients after CCNU treatment, Mut. Res., 59:295 (1979).

Latt, S. A., Microfluorometric detection of deoxyribonucleic acid replication in human metaphase chromosomes, Proc. Natl. Acad. Sci. USA, 70:3395 (1973).

Latt, S. A., and Loveday, K. S., Characterization of sister chromatid exchange in induction by 8-methoxypsoralen plus near UV light, Cytogenet. Cell Genet., 21:184 (1978).

Natarajan, A. T., Van Buul, P. P. W., and Raposa, T., An evaluation of the use of peripheral blood lymphocyte systems for assessing cytological effects induced in vivo by chemical mutagens, in: "Mutagen-induced chromosome damage in man," H. J. Evans and D. C. Lloyd, eds., University Press, Edinburgh, England (1978).

Natarajan, A. T., Tates, A. D., Van Buul, P. P. W., Meijers, M., and De Vogel, N., Cytogenetic effects of mutagens/carcinogens after activation in a microsomal system in vitro. I. Induction of chromosome aberrations and sister chromatid exchanged by diethylnitrosamine (DEN) and dimethylnitrosamine (DMN) in CHO cells in the presence of rat liver microsomes, Mutat. Res., 37:83 (1976).

Nevstad, N. P., Sister chromatid exchanges and chromosome aberrations induced in human lymphocytes by the cytostatic drug adriamycin in vivo and in vitro, Mutat. Res., 57:253 (1978).

Perry, P., and Evans, H. J., Cytological detection of mutagen-carcinogen exposure by sister chromatid exchange, Nature, 258:121 (1975).

Perry, P. E., and Searle, C. E., Induction of sister chromatid exchange in Chinese hamster cells by the hair dye constituents 2-nitro-*p*-phenylenediamine and 4-nitro-*o*-phenylenediamine, Mutat. Res., 56:207 (1977).

Perry, P. E., and Wolff, S., New Giemsa method for differential staining of sister chromatids, Nature, 261:156 (1974).

Popescu, N. C., Amsburgh, S. C., and DiPaolo, J. A., Relationship of carcinogen induced sister chromatid exchange and neoplastic cell transformation, Int. J. Cancer, 28:71 (1981).

Rudiger, H. W., Kohl, F., Mangeles, W., Von Wichert, P., Bartram, C. R., Wohler, W., and Passarge, E., Benzpyrene induced sister chromatid exchanges in cultured human lymphocytes, Nature, 262: 290 (1976).

Schonwald, A. D., Bartram, C. R., and Rudiger, H. W., Benzpyrene induced sister chromatid exchanges in lymphocytes of patients with lung cancer, Hum. Genet., 36:261 (1977).

Schuler, C. F., and Latt, S. A., Sister chromatid exchange test in Chinese hamster cheek pouch mucosa, J. Dental Res., 578:211 (1978).

Siriani, S. R., and Huang, C. C., Comparison of induction of sister chromatid exchange, 8-azaguanine and ouabain-resistant mutants by cyclophosphamide, ifosfamide and 1-(pyridyl-3)-3,3-dimethylthriazene in Chinese hamster cells cultured in diffusion chambers in mice, Carcinogenesis, 1:353 (1980).

Solomon, E., and Bobrow, M., Sister chromatid exchanges: A sensitive assay of agents damaging human chromosomes, Mutat. Res., 30:273 (1975).

Stetka, D. G., Minkler, J., and Carrano, A. V., Induction of long-lived chromosome damage as manifested by sister chromatid exchange in lymphocytes of animals exposed to mitomycin-C, Mutat. Res., 51:383 (1978).

Stetka, D. G., and Wolff, S., Sister chromatid exchanges as an assay for genetic damage induced by mutagenic carcinogens, I. In vivo test for compounds requiring metabolic activation, Mutat. Res., 41:333 (1976a).

Stetka, D. G., and Wolff, S., Sister chromatid exchanges as an assay for genetic damage induced by mutagenic carcinogens, II. In vitro test for compounds requiring metabolic activation, Mutat. Res., 41:343 (1976b).

Swenson, D. H., Harbach, P. R., and Trzos, R. J., The relationship between alkylation of specific DNA bases and induction of sister chromatid exchange, Carcinogenesis, 1:931 (1980).

Taylor, J. H., Sister chromatid exchanges in tritium labelled chromosomes, Genetics, 43:515 (1958).

Vogel, W., and Bauknecht, T., Differential chromatid staining by in vivo treatment as a mutagenicity test system, Nature, 260: 448 (1976).

Wolff, S., Chromosomal effects of mutagenic carcinogens and the nature of the lesions leading to sister chromatid exchange, in: "Mutagen-induced chromosome damge in man," H. J. Evans and D. C. Lloyd, eds., University Press, Edinburgh, England (1978).

Wolff, S., Bodycote, J., and Painter, R. B., Sister chromatid exchanges induced in Chinese hamster cells by UV irradiation of different stages of the cell cycle: The necessity for cells to pass through S, Mutat. Res., 25:73 (1974).

DOSE-RESPONSE RELATION OF CHROMOSOME ABERRATIONS

J. D. Jansen

SIRM B.V.
Group Toxicology
The Hague
Netherlands

First of all I want to make clear that I am not a geneticist and even less a cytogeneticist. There are many people here who know far more than I do about the subject. I can only give the view and experience of a very interested scientific outsider. However, much of my time has been spent in trying to determine the human relevance of chromosome aberrations and in trying to ensure the protection of human health in manufacturing plants.

Therefore, I hope that the discussion will give some tentative answers to the following questions:

(a) are chromosome aberrations an important source of human disease?

(b) is there evidence that chromosome aberrations in somatic cells are related to human disease?

(c) why do we measure the incidence of chromosome aberrations in lymphocytes?

(d) what are the pitfalls in measuring the incidence of chromosome aberrations?

(e) is there a dose-response relationship for chromosome aberrations?

(f) what is the future potential for measuring the rate of chromosome aberrations?

1. ARE CHROMOSOME ABERRATIONS AN IMPORTANT SOURCE OF HUMAN DISEASE?

Genetic disease is commonly considered to be responsible for a large part of the total human disease burden. A precise percentage cannot be given:

(a) because genetics frequently determines only a (small) part of observed disease which occurs also in the absence of specific genetic susceptibility. As an example, sporadic cases of monolateral retinoblastoma, a malignant tumor of the eye in infants, are 90% nonhereditary whereas bilateral retinoblastoma is a dominant hereditary disease [1, 2].

(b) because a great number of genetically based "aberrations" can be recognized but do not affect health or sometimes only under exceptional circumstances (e.g., congenital absence of plasmacholinesterase, apparent only after treatment with muscle relaxants [3]). The means of diagnosing such genetic "aberrations" are increasing rapidly and it is reasonable to assume that in the end everybody will be found to be aberrant somewhere in the sense of falling outside the "norm" of the country. Of course the line between serious disease and no-disease is fluid and subjective: e.g., to what extent do you include cosmetic handicaps which do not affect physical health?

(c) because the total "burden" of genetic disease is unknown.

Nevertheless, a "reasonable" estimate is that 10% of a cohort of newborns will at some time during its life-span exhibit a disease in which there is a significant genetic component [4]. A large part of these diseases will be very serious (Down's syndrome, achondroplasia, etc.), requiring institutional treatment for life which sometimes hardly differs in life expectancy from normal populations. On this basis the social impact of genetic disease may well be larger than the social impact of cancer. In this context it may be significant that the decision-makers in society who decide on the distribution of funds for research are afraid of dying from cancer themselves whereas in the nature of things these same decision-makers have already been spared a serious burden of genetic disease. Within this overall impact of serious genetic disease, chromosome aberrations play a large part. The precise part in terms of fertilized germ cells is difficult to define, as is apparent from the drawing by Emil Witschi (Fig. 1) [5]. Witchi estimates that under favorable circumstances only 30% of the fertilized eggs will develop into a normal living baby.

Among live births, Hook and Hamerton [6, 7, 8] reported about 6 per 1000 chromosome abnormalities, about half of which are "of

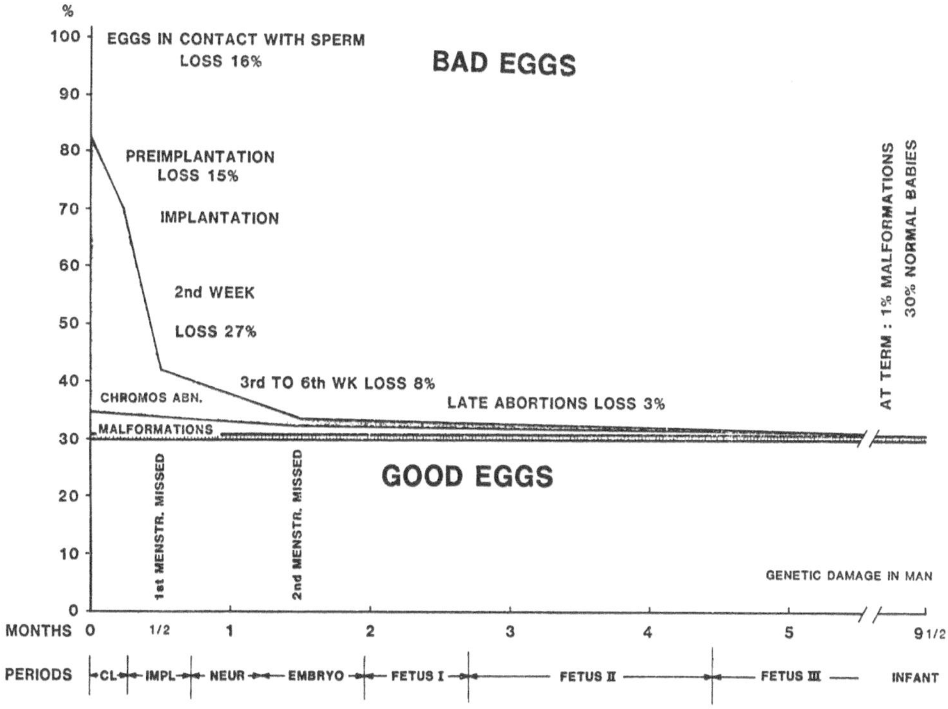

Fig. 1 (from Ref. 7).

clinical significance." Down's syndrome is the most frequent chromosome aberration which is phenotypically detectable and has a rate of about 1 in 1000 live births in the USA [8]. The crude rate of Down's syndrome varies strongly with the maternal age composition of the newborns in the population and has dropped in the USA [8] and Holland [9] by about 30-50%, largely or entirely due to the introduction of the "pill" which has greatly reduced the number of unwanted or unexp-cted pregnancies in women at higher age groups.

The rather lengthy discussion has been given to illustrate that:

(a) chromosomal aberrations in germ-cells are an important source of serious genetic disease [7];

(b) rather important changes in the crude incidence of genetic diseases take place with time although these changes are not recorded in most countries [2, 8, 9], and

Table 1. Malignancy and Specific Somatic Cytogenetic Abnormality in Affected Tissues (Ref. 5)

Malignancy	Chromosome abnormality
Chronic myelogenous leukemia	22q-, translocation (Ph'+)
Meningioma	22 monosomy
Burkitt's lymphoma	$14q^+$
Dysgerminoma and gonadoblastoma	(8q translocation in non-Africans)
Retinoblastoma	xo/xy
Wilm's tumor-aniridia	13q14 deletion
	11p13 deletion

(c) there is no known relation between any "mutagenic" chemical and chromosomal aberrations in germ-cells. Even in an intensively investigated cohort of 17,000 children born to "proximally exposed" parents in Hiroshima and Nagasaki (proximally exposed defined as a conjoint exposure of the parents to about 115 rem) in comparison with an equal cohort of children born from parents whose mean conjoint exposure was estimated at <1 rem has failed to give any evidence of an increase in genetic disease or survival. The incidence of Down's syndrome was even lower in the children of the exposed parents [10]. (For a discussion see Hook and Porter [11] and Newcombe [12].)

This last point certainly cannot be made in the sense that there is no connection. In this context it is relevant to repeat the remarks by Neel et al. [13] who reported on their search for point mutations affecting protein structure in children of atomic bomb survivors. Their preliminary report did not establish that the mutation rate in the survivors was increased (although the data were compatible with such an increase). They went on to say that "they did not consider (their) study as a test of the hypothesis that mutations were produced but rather as an effort to provide a responsible estimate of the magnitude of the genetic effects that must be assumed to have occurred (my underlines)."

2. IS THERE EVIDENCE THAT CHROMOSOME ABERRATIONS IN SOMATIC CELLS ARE RELATED TO HUMAN DISEASE?

It is known that survivors of Hiroshima and Nagasaki, even 30 years after the event, still show an increased rate of chromosome aberrations [14]. Even workers who were exposed to permissible rates of radiation were shown to slowly accumulate chromosome aberrations [15]. However, there is no known relation between aberrations and disease even though the Japanese specifically looked for it in atomic bomb survivors [16] (it must be stated that scientifically the Japanese study was unsatisfactory for unavoidable organizational reasons as explained by the authors).

There are specific, rare, tumors which are closely associated with and probably causally related to highly specific chromosome lesions [7] (Table 1). Moreover, many known carcinogens are known to cause chromosome aberrations (e.g., vinylchloride [17, 18, 19], benzene [20, 21, 22], several cytostatics). Styrene is not thought to be a carcinogen but seems also to cause chromosome aberrations in heavily exposed workers [23, 24] (who also were exposed to different chemicals).

Summarizing, there is no good evidence that chromosome aberrations in somatic cells cause disease although some highly specific lesions are closely related to equally highly specific diseases.

3. WHY USE BLOOD LYMPHOCYTES FOR MEASUREMENT OF CHROMOSOME ABERRATIONS?

The technique for culturing blood lymphocytes is well developed although important details such as duration of cultivation and others are still not universally standardized, leading to important quantitative differences in outcome between some laboratories [26]. The technique is deceptively simple in terms of equipment and can be readily applied by many laboratories. However, the application and subsequent interpretation requires scientific expertise and lack of bias of the highest order. Obtaining a blood sample is a relatively easy procedure so that repeat analyses are possible in the same subject. For animal investigations this is one of the very few methods permitting repeat analyses. The method was used and developed as the most sensitive to record exposure to radiation in man. It still is the most sensitive method to determine exposure to carcinogens in man although new biochemical and molecular biologic methods may well supersede it for measuring exposure to specific chemicals. You will hear about such methods from Dr. Osterman-Golkar. These new methods usually have to be developed for each chemical separately whereas the measurement of chromosome aberrations is more generally applicable. The price paid for general applicability is, more difficulties in interpretation. Chromosome aberrations in essentially non-dividing cells such as lymphocytes are in themselves without any clinical significance. The interest comes from the possibility of quantitative evaluation and from the quite reasonable assumption that aberrations in lymphocytes are likely to be accompanied by aberrations in other cells in which tumors could possibly develop. The assumption that such aberrations would also develop in the germ-cells is less obvious in view of the existence of the blood-testes barrier in man [25]. We may make such measurements for different purposes:

(a) to follow the course of treatment with cytostatics of cancer patients,

(b) to obtain background data on chromosome aberrations of a geographically defined population,

(c) to check the health of an industrially exposed population as one part of the Occupational Health Program.

The following discussion will mainly concentrate on this latter aspect.

4. PITFALLS IN MEASURING CHROMOSOME ABERRATIONS

Many pitfalls are known and can therefore frequently be corrected by proper design of the investigation. The most obvious pitfall is subjective observer error [8, 29]. Therefore, it is essential that blood samples are coded and contain both exposed and control samples. It is equally essential that the investigator checks and discusses his findings with collaborators who are not directly involved in the investigation. If these essential precautions are not taken, the results may be largely or entirely worthless unless an enormous effect is registered as in cancer patients being treated with cytostatics. Even with the greatest caution, interlaboratory variations in the scoring of chromatid or chromosome gaps are so large that they are frequently not even recorded [26]. The variations arise out of the difficulty of avoiding personal bias, as well as out of slight differences in sample preparations. Therefore, Natarajan and Obe place most importance on the recording of exchanges, and intensive cooperation between some of the best laboratories in Europe has now resulted in essentially interchangeable data on the basis of which intercountry comparisons are now becoming possible [26]; more will be said on this subject under the heading of future potential.

In addition, the following factors are known to increase the frequencies of chromosome aberrations:

(a) alcoholism: long-term extreme alcoholism is necessary for an obvious effect [27]. This may not greatly affect industrial populations although population investigations have to consider this aspect.

(b) smoking [27, 28] has an important effect on chromosomal aberrations: therefore smoking habits have to be taken into account in comparing exposed and controls.

(c) virus infections: these can cause a serious and usually reversible increase in chromosome aberrations [26]. Usually, virally induced changes are easy to recognize and the situation can be corrected by analysis of a later sample. Such infections and especially the non-reported use of therapeutic drugs are the major possible sources of confusion in longitudinal studies, i.e., when people serve as their own control before and after exposure to an industrial chemical. These pitfalls are not easy to take into account because information from patients on the use of therapeutic drugs is notoriously unreliable, both in terms of the kind of drug prescribed and in terms of quantity taken.

(d) The effect of age on the incidence of chromosome aberrations is well known and can therefore be fully taken into account. A prime example of use of this knowledge is Evan's classical publication on the effect of very low doses of radiation [15].

(e) Reversibility: It is known that even 30 years after the Hiroshima and Nagasaki bombing [14] or after radiation of Ankylosing Spondylitis patients, increased chromosome aberrations are still apparent [29]. There are also convincing data on individuals (not on groups) that previous exposure to benzene may result in chromosome aberrations which persist for many years. However, most of the other chemicals (as known up till now) cause mainly aberrations which disappear after some weeks or at most some months.

Dr. Perry has referred to the fact that SCEs do not persist. In this comparison, chromosome aberrations tend to persist for a longer period. However, it is important to realize that only relatively few chemicals have been properly investigated. Therefore it is yet impossible to generalize and it may be that one chemical acts quite differently from another. Hence, several authors have found no effect from the use of cytostatics in cancer patients on the frequency of chromosome aberrations [30]. These negative findings can be reconciled with the positive data from other investigators who followed cancer patients before, during and after treatment: depending upon the chemical used, the clearcut effects of cytostatics disappear from a few weeks to a few months after treatment [26]. It is common parlance to say that "repair" has occurred and it is known that an active repair process does occur in lymphocytes. However, in a specific investigation it is usually impossible to distinguish between active repair and the possibility that the affected lymphocytes disappear from the blood circulation.

One further difficulty may appear in interpreting results from chromosome analyses in industrial populations: such results are frequently compared with results of air analyses with the intent to establish a quantitative correlation between exposure and chromosome aberrations. In itself, this attempt is important and should be encouraged. However, in our experience it is seldom or never possible to do so with any precision with industrial chemicals for the following reasons:

(a) We do not know whether chromosome aberrations are caused by rare peak-exposures or by the time-weighted average exposure to an industrial chemical [31].

(b) It is very difficult to measure the actual exposure of a worker. A good industrial hygiene effort may indicate the time-weighted average exposure for the average worker with some degree of precision; however, peak exposures, especially "accidental" peak exposures, are very difficult to estimate, precisely because they do not occur during "normal" operations. This difficulty applies especially to Petrochemical plants which largely operate in the open air: under those conditions "normal" exposures will frequently approach zero although "accidental" exposures may reach virtually any concentration. (I do not refer to large accidents but to relatively large deviations from normal operations.) These extremes are considerably reduced in chemical plants which are enclosed within a building.

(c) Sometimes it is possible to use personal samplers. In theory such samplers should give an accurate record of the time-weighted average exposure of the individual workers. However, we regularly found that exposures calculated from personal samplers were lower than calculated from industrial hygiene measurements of ambient working air. We ascribe all or most of the difference between these two measurements to something akin to a placebo effect of medicine: the worker who knows that his personal exposure is measured will probably unconsciously tend to be more careful.

The possibily most intractable difficulty has been reserved for the last and that is the definition of a "control" population. About 4 years of hard work in one particular complex of manufacturing plants, combined with increasing information from other population groups in the same country has given us some preliminary insight into the kind and number of aberrations to be expected in an ideal control group. The first study was related to vinylchloride workers. Not unexpectedly, in view of the extremely low exposure at that time, no indication of an increase in chromosome aberrations [18] was found. We even found a much lower incidence of aberrations than in the control group. Inspection of the "control" group revealed that some workers were exposed to ECH, a known clastogen. However, later investigations showed that also ECH-exposures under our industrial conditions did not cause chromosome aberrations. We then noticed some very high incidences in controls who were working in the Medical Department. Further investigations showed that these incidences were due to therapeutic drugs. Currently, the vinylchloride group still shows the lowest incidence of chromosome aberrations of any group of workers within the manufacturing complex. However, regular weeding out of "improper" controls has given us a better idea of the incidence in an entirely "nonexposed" control group. "Nonexposed" in this sense of course also applies to life-style. Recently, we investigated a group of office workers, who were not occupationally exposed at all but belonged to a different social group. This group has now taken over in our experience as the group with the lowest incidence of chromosome aberrations.

I am telling this prolonged story in order to illustrate that the ideal control group does not exist but can only be defined with increasing precision when many more directly comparable population data are available.

5. IS THERE A DOSE-RESPONSE RELATIONSHIP FOR CHROMOSOMAL ABERRATIONS?

This questions cannot be answered in a formal manner because, apart from radiation, I am not aware of any investigation in vivo of a chemical which could answer this question precisely. In radiation, the dose-response curve is so well known that chromosome aberrations are used to determine the extent of short-term high exposures. However, with chemicals it is clear that "high" exposures produce a "great" increase in chromosome aberrations and it is equally clear that reduction in exposure results in a number of chromosome aberrations which is similar to unexposed controls. Failure to realize this dose-reponse relation results in comments in the literature about "conflicting" data on the capacity of compounds to induce chromosome aberrations [8].

Indeed, there are really conflicting data which are in fact based on one set of unsatisfactory data. For instance, many chemicals have been implicated to cause chromosome aberrations on the basis of tests which did not include controls or where observer bias was not excluded, to name only two of the most common mistakes. In other words: several publications are only "conflicting" because one of them was in reality worthless.

However, cases remain of so-called "conflicting" results by excellent researchers: in nearly all cases the one investigation was performed on heavily exposed workers and the other on workers with very low exposures. Given the known occurrence of repair in lymphocytes [26] and their long duration of the nondividing period, the existence of a no-effect level for chromosome aberrations from chemicals would not be unexpected.

In my view, it seems reasonably established by experiences, that there is a definite no-effect level for the induction of chro-

Table 2. Incidence of Exchange Aberrations (Ref. 28)

	Berlin	Edinburgh
Control	11.3×10^{-4}	32.5×10^{-4}
Smokers	68×10^{-4}	63.6×10^{-4}

Table 3. Exchange Aberrations $\times 10^{-4}$ (Ref. 26, 28)

Obe	:	11.6	(in Berlin)
Natarajan	:	7.33	(in Netherlands)
Ivanov	:	8.7	(in Bulgaria)
alcoholics	:	48.4	(viz., 9.6 in controls)
smokers	:	68.0	(in Berlin, viz., 11.3 in controls)
		63.6	(in Edinburgh, viz., 32.5 in controls)
VCM 20-30 ppm	:	97	
1 ppm	:	3	(viz., 4 in controls)

Data from A. T. Natarajan and G. Obe, Ecotoxic. and Environm. Safety 4:468-481 (1980); data on smokers from H. J. Evans, Environm. Carcinogenesis 329-344 (1979)

mosome aberrations. It might be that this no-effect level is due to the low sensitivity of the test and consequently is a purely statistical artifact. This point cannot be proven one way or the other but does not seem likely: there are many occasions where the aberrations in a well-monitored "exposed" group were actually lower than in the control group and very low in comparison with other population data. Also, cancer patients after treatment clearly return to their pretreatment incidence of aberrations and they do so rapidly; this seems difficult to reconcile with a view of a linear increase of chromosome aberrations with any exposure no matter how small, the smaller increases merely remaining undetectable because of statistical considerations.

6. THE FUTURE POTENTIAL FOR THE MEASUREMENT OF CHROMOSOME ABERRATIONS

Currently there are a number of first-class laboratories in Europe which use commensurate techniques and obtain directly comparable results. To my, doubtless incomplete, knowledge, such laboratories exist in West Germany, UK, and Holland. This means that obtaining comparable population data in these countries becomes a a real possibility. Already now, interesting comparisons can be made which as yet defy explanations as the comparison by Evans [28] between smokers and nonsmokers given in Table 2.

In this table the point of interest is not the similarity between the smokers but the fact that Edinburgh "controls" have almost 3× the aberrations of controls in West Berlin. Does that mean that the population in Berlin is "healthier?" or do they drink less alcohol? Or does this only mean "normal" differences to be expected from "normal" sample variations? Smokers were matched to controls in each city and apparently unintentionally "matched" between cities.

For a more general impression, Table 3 gives a composite view of findings from comparable studies. Within industries, the measurement of chromosome aberrations will remain for some time to become a most welcome and sensitive tool for monitoring the health of exposed workers despite the enormous labor involved (very roughly about 100 samples/trained operator/year) and despite the nonspecific nature of the results.

Interpretation of the results in terms of risk assessment is impossible. However, an increase in chromosome aberrations does mean at the least that the hereditary apparatus of some somatic cells has been affected and that steps should be taken to avoid such a situation.

In addition, we may hope that population studies may suggest genetic or environmental origins of the apparent differences between populations or population groups in the incidence of chromosome aberrations and aberrations due to occupational exposure can be quantitatively compared with increases which result from lifestyle influences.

Hook, the epidemiologist of the New York State - North Eastern Chromosome Registry is sceptical about "the sensitivity of chromosomal disease to environmental hazards" [7]. However, as apparent from his own publications, the contribution of the registery of New York State to the understanding of the possible origins of chromosomal disease is already substantial. It is very likely that comparable registries in other countries, using comparable techniques would uncover as yet completely unsuspected causes of chromosomal disease, be they environmental or not.

To sum up:

(1) the measurement of chromosome aberrations cannot or not yet be used for risk estimation,

(2) the method is extremely laborious and therefore not usable as a convenient routine,

(3) the problem of defining a suitable control group is a major one,

(4) the method must be used by highly qualified and experienced researchers; if not, it will cause more confusion than insight [7, 8].

However, despite this enumeration of difficulties, it still seems the most sensitive and effective method to ensure the safety of workers who are exposed to low concentrations of a carcinogen or to detect workers who are inadvertently exposed to an unknown carcinogenic hazard.

Its use in monitoring populations has hardly begun but will most probably yield most important insights.

REFERENCES

1. J. J. Mulvihill, Congenital and genetic diseases, in: Fraumeni, ed., Persons at High Risk of Cancer, Academic Press, New York (1975).
2. E. Matsunaga, Collection and evaluation of existing data on the incidence and prevalence of genetically determined disease (excluding chromosomal aberrations) in man, ICPEMC working paper, Mutation Res., in press.
3. K. Berg, Inherited variation in susceptibility and resistance to environmental agents, in: Berg, ed., Genetic Damage in Man Caused by Environmental Agents, Academic Press, New York (1979).
4. J. R. Miller, personal communication.
5. J. German, Clinical implications of chromosome damage, in: Berg, ed., Genetic Damage in Man Caused by Environmental Agents, Academic Press, New York (1979).
6. E. B. Hook and J. L. Hamerton, The frequency of chromosome abnormalities detected in consecutive newborn studies, in: Hook and Porter, eds., Population Cytogenetics: Studies in Humans, Academic Press, New York (1977).
7. E. B. Hook, The contribution of chromosome abnormalities to human morbidity and mortality and some comments upon surveillance of chromosome mutation rates, in: Bora, ed., Chemical Mutagenesis, Human Population Monitoring, and Genetic Risk Assessment, to be published by Elsevier/North Holland, Amsterdam.
8. E. B. Hook, Human teratogenic and mutagenic markers in monitoring about point sources of pollution, Environm. Res., 25:178-203 (1981).
9. D. Hoogendoorn, Aanzienlijk dalend aantal kinderen met mongolisme, Ned. T. Geneesk., 122:1119-1120 (1978).
10. W. J.Schull and J. V. Neel, Maternal radiation and mongolism, Lancet 1:537-538 (1962).

11. E. D. Hook and I. H. Porter, Human population genetics - comments on racial differences in frequency of chromosome abnormalities, putative clustering of Down's Syndrome and radiation studies, in: Hook and Porter, eds., Population Cytogenetics: Studies in Humans, Academic Press, New York (1977).
12. H. B. Newcombe, Problems of assessing risks versus mutations, Genetics, 92:5199-5201 (1979).
13. J. V. Neel, C. Saton, H. B. Hamilton, M. Otake, K. Goriki, T. Kageoka, M. Fujita, S. Neriishi, and J. Asakawa, Search for mutations affecting protein structure in children of atomic bomb survivors: Preliminary report, Proc. Natl. Acad. Sci. USA, 77:4221-4225 (1980).
14. T. Sofuni, H. Shimba, K. Ohtaki, and A. A. Awa, A cytogenetic study of Hiroshima atomic bomb survivors, in: Evans and Lloyd, eds., Mutagen-Induced Chromosome Damage in Man, University Press, Edinburgh (1978).
15. H. J. Evans, K. E. Buckton, G. E. Hamilton, and A. Carothers, Radiation-induced chromosome aberrations in nuclear dockyard workers, Nature, 277:531-534 (1979).
16. R. A. King, J. I. Belsky, M. Otake, A. A. Awa, and T. Matsui, Chromosome abnormalities in A-bomb survivors, Correlation with findings on examination, Technical Report 15-72 of Atomic Bomb Casualty Commission of USA, Acad. Sci. and Jap. Inst. Hlth.
17. F. Funes-Cravioto, B. Lambert, J. Lindsten, L. Ehrenberg, A. T. Natarajan, and S. Osterman-Golkar, Chromosome aberrations in workers exposed to vinylchloride, Lancet 1:459 (1975).
18. A. T. Natarajan, P. P. W. van Buul, and T. Raposa, An evaluation of the use of peripheral blood lymphocyte systems for assessing cytological effects induced in vivo by chemical mutagens, in: Evans and Lloyd, eds., Mutagen-Induced Chromosome Damage in Man, Edinburgh University Press (1978).
19. D. Anderson, C. R. Richardson, T. M. Weight, I. F. H. Purchase, and W. G. F. Adams, Chromosomal analysis in vinylchloride exposed workers, results from analysis 18 and 42 months after an initial sampling, Mutation Res., 79:151-162 (1980).
20. E. C. Vigliani and G. Saita, Benzene and Leukemia, New York J. Med., 271:872-876 (1964).
21. A. Forni, E. Pacifico, and A. Limonta, Chromosome studies in workers exposed to benzene or toluene or both, Arch. Environm. Hlth., 22:373-378 (1971).
22. I. M. Tough, P. G. Smith, W. M. Court Brown, and D. G. Harnden, Chromosome studies on workers exposed to atmospheric benzene, Eur. J. Cancer, 6:49-55 (1970).
23. T. Meretoja, H. Jarventaus, M. Sorsa, and H. Vainio, Chromosome aberrations in lymphocytes of workers exposed to styrene, Scand. J. Environm. & Hlth., 4:259-264 (1978).
24. T. Meretoja, H. Vainio, and M. Sorsa, Clastogenic activity of styrene in occupational exposure, Mutation Res., 53:229 (1978).

25. M. F. Lyon, Sensitivity of various germ-cell stages of environmental mutagens, ICPEMC working paper 4/1, in press in Mutation Res. and Biol. Zbt.
26. A. J. Natarajan and G. Obe, Screening of human populations for mutations induced by environmental pollutants: use of human lymphocyte system, Ecotoxicol. and Environm. Safety, 4:468-481 (1980).
27. G. Obe, Mutagenic activity of alcohol and tobacco smoke, in: Israel, Glaser, Kalant, Popham, Schmidt, and Smart, eds., Research Advances in Alcohol and Drug Problems, Plenum Press, New York, in press.
28. H. J. Evans, The induction of aberrations in human chromosomes following exposure to mutagens/carcinogens, in: Emmelot and Kriek, eds., Environmental Carcinogenesis, Elsevier/North Holland Biomed. Press, Amsterdam (1979).
29. K. E. Buckton, G. E. Hamilton, L. Paton, and A. D. Langlands, Chromosome aberrations in irradiated Ankylosing Spondylitis patients, in: Evans and Lloyd, eds., Mutagen-Induced Chromosome Damage in Man, Edinburgh University Press (1978).
30. A. Schinzel and W. Schmid, Lymphocyte chromosome studies in humans exposed to chemical mutagens, the validity of the method in 67 patients under cytostatic therapy, Mutation Res., 40: 139-166 (1976).
31. I. F. H. Purchase, Chromosomal Analysis of Exposed Populations: A Review of Industrial Problems, in: Evans and Lloyd, eds., Mutagen-Induced Chromosome Damage in Man, Edinburgh University Press (1978).

MUTAGEN-INDUCED CHROMOSOME DAMAGE IN MAN

Paul E. Perry

MRC Clinical & Population Cytogenetics Unit
Western General Hospital
Edinburgh EH4 2XU
Scotland

INTRODUCTION

Cytologically recognizable chromosome damage includes both structural aberrations, in which a gross change in morphology of the chromosome has occurred, and sister chromatid exchange, which does not result in a change in chromosome morphology. Sister chromatid exchange was the subject of a talk elsewhere in these proceedings and I shall devote this presentation to structural aberrations - their spontaneous and induced incidence in human cells, and the significance of these changes to the cell or the individual.

The importance of chromosomes in human cancer is not a recent finding. In fact Hansemann (1890) postulated over 90 years ago that all carcinomas are characterized by asymmetrical mitosis and in the early years of this century Boveri (1914) theorized from his work on *Ascaris* that the cells of a malignant tumor have an abnormal chromosome constitution and that any event causing such an unbalanced chromosome constitution will result in a malignant tumor. Now, nearly seventy years after Boveri formulated his hypothesis, there is still controversy as to whether chromosome abnormalities precede, or occur as a result of, malignancy.

The first evidence that an inherited chromosome change could predispose to the development of cancer was the observation that individuals with the chromosome constitution 47XXY (Klinefelters syndrome), have an increased risk of breast cancer (Nadel and Koss, 1967) and Down's syndrome individuals (trisomy 21) have an increased risk of leukemia (Stewart et al., 1958). In neither of these cases is the risk dramatic but other inherited chromosome defects involving deletion or translocation have been reported more recently that are associated with a greatly increased risk of malignancy. For example, all cases of sporadic aniridia with mental retardation are characterized by specific deletion on chromosome 11, and one in three of these children develop Wilm's tumor (Riccardi et al., 1978). Retinoblastoma is associated with deletion of part of the long arm of chromosome 13 (e.g., Howard et al., 1974) and renal cell carcinoma has resulted in most of the members of a family in which a translocation between chromosomes 3 and 8 was segregating (Cohen et al., 1979).

In the 1930s it was found that structural aberrations could be induced in germ cells by x-irradiation. Although the types of aberrations induced in somatic cells and germ cells, or their precursors, are identical, the results are quite different. The chromosome changes in somatic cells may be passed on to the daughter cells and transmitted to all descendent cells in the body. Thus although these alterations cannot be inherited they are of great significance to the individual. Structural alterations to the chromosomes of the germ cells, on the other hand, may be transmitted to the products of conception and so on to succeeding generations, and such heritable genetic damage is therefore of great consequence to future generations of that individual.

Before I discuss somatic and germ cell chromosome damage any further I would firstly like to mention the variety of structural aberrations that occur as a result of exposure to chemical or physical mutagens.

Much of our knowledge about chromosomal aberrations stems from the vast amount of information on the effect of ionizing radiation on cells. All aberrations are basically a result of breakage and/or exchange of chromosomal subunits and include breaks, interstitial deletions, inversions, duplications, rings and interchanges between the chromosomes. The type and frequency of these events depends not only upon the properties of the mutagen but also on the stage of the cell cycle at the time of insult. The unit of breakage and exchange is the single chromatid in each case, but if x-irradiation is conducted while the cell is in the pre-replicative G1 phase of the cell cycle, the chromatid must be duplicated during the S phase before the damage can be seen at the following mitosis. Therefore at metaphase both chromatids of the chromosome will be similarly affected and will result in a so-called chromosome-type aberration. If irradiation is conducted during S or G2 stages of the cell cycle all aberrations will be of the chromatid-type because no intervening DNA replication has occurred to duplicate the aberration. In contrast to ionizing radiation, nonionizing radiation and the majority of chemical mutagens cause chromatid-type aberrations if treatment is conducted during G1, but no chromosomal damage results if the insult occurs during the G2 period immediately before cytological ex-

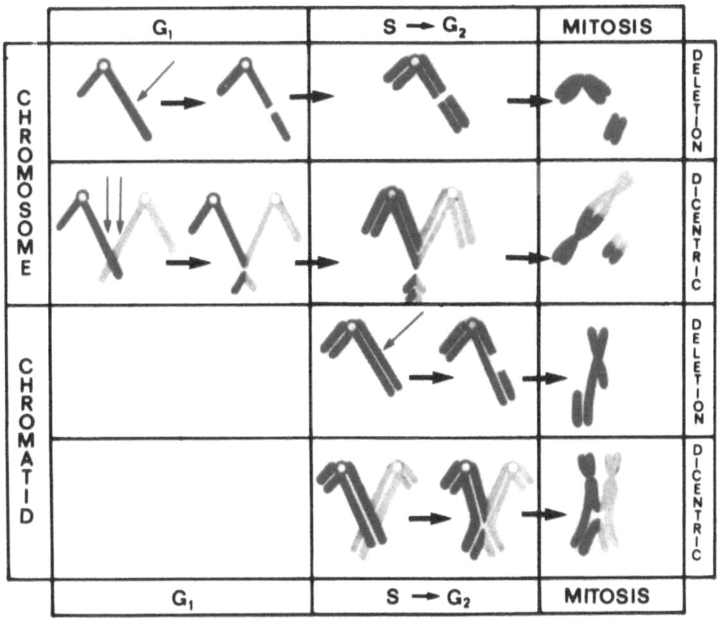

Fig. 1. Chromosome and chromatid-type aberrations and the cell cycle.

amination. The 'S-dependent' chemicals require an intervening round of DNA replication before the aberration is formed. There are also some 'S-independent' chemicals that, like ionizing radiation, can cause aberrations in the G2 period preceding analysis, but for the majority of chemicals, chromatid aberrations only are seen at the metaphase following exposure. Figure 1 shows some examples of chromosome and chromatid-type aberrations that result from exposure to mutagenic agents.

Many kinds of structural aberration lead to mechanical separation problems at mitosis and to genetic duplication or deficiency and consequent cell death of one, or both, daughter cells. Figure 2 illustrates a simple example of breakage and rearrrangement involving two chromosomes at either G1 or G2 stages of the cell cycle. In the case of chromosome dicentric and fragment formation, the acentric fragment is usually excluded from the daughter nuclei at mitosis, while the dicentric chromosome may form a bridge at anaphase with consequent mechanical problems in cell separation. As both daughter nuclei are genetically deficient, cells containing dicentrics are rapidly lost from the cell population. In contrast, reciprocal translocations are not cell lethal as there is no duplication or loss of genetic material, and since they can be transmitted to subsequent cell generations or individuals, these rearrangements therefore have genetic significance.

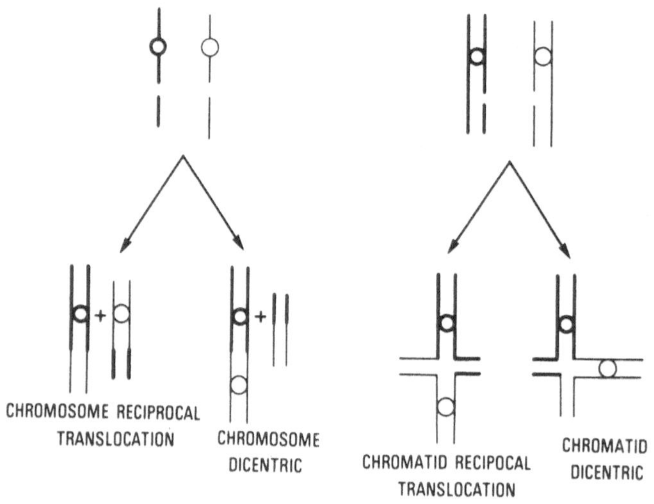

Fig. 2. Diagrammatic representation of the formation of chromosome and chromatid-type translocations and dicentrics.

Chromatid reciprocal translocations result in four possible segregation products when the cell undergoes division. The unexchanged chromatids may segregate together to give a normal cell, the two unchanged chromatids may segregate together to give a stable translocation bearing cell, or a normal chromatid may segregate with an exchange chromatid in two different ways to give duplication or deficiency of genetical material that would probably result in the death of that cell. The probability of recovering the stable reciprocal translocation in the subsequent generation is thus four times greater with chromosome translocations then with chromatid translocations. This is a relatively simple example to illustrate the difference between chromosome and chromatid aberrations, but in general, chromosome-type aberrations will lead to genetic loss and subsequent cell death of one or both daughter cells because both chromatids are affected at the same locus. Chromatid-type aberrations, on the other hand, may result in death of only one of the daughter cells as only one chromatid is affected. From the point of view of the cytogeneticist chromatid-type aberrations are difficult to score and quantify due to their variety and complexity, and for further information on the classification and significance of structural chromosome damage I recommend the review by Savage (1976).

We should note in passing that chromatid type aberrations are converted by duplication into 'derived' or 'secondary' chromosome-type aberrations if they survive the first mitosis, but is it usually not possible to infer the origin of a derived chromosome aberration. Also, not all chemically induced lesions produce aberra-

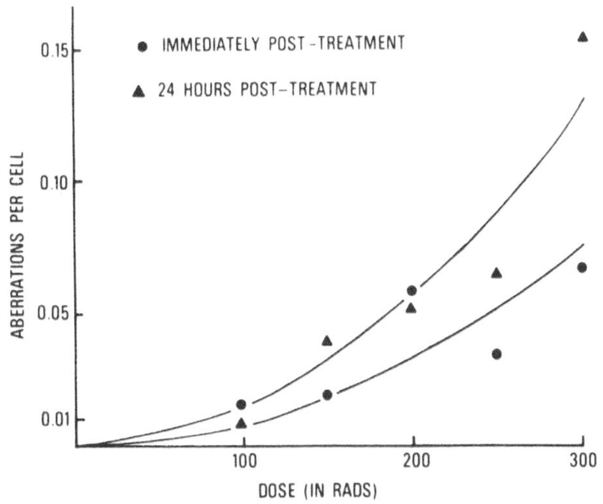

Fig. 3. Incidence of dicentric and ring chromosome aberrations following partial body irradiation in man (from Buckton et al., 1967).

tions at the replication phase immediately following treatment so that new aberrations may be generated in subsequent cell cycles. For the various reasons presented above it is clear that an accurate quantitative analysis of chromosome aberrations can only be performed at the first metaphase following mutagen exposure.

SPONTANEOUS AND INDUCED ABERRATIONS IN SOMATIC CELLS

The most widely used method for studying the cytogentic effects of in vivo exposure to chemical or physical mutagens is short-term culture of peripheral blood lymphocytes. These cells are normally in an arrested Go (like G1) stage of the cell cycle, and the usual culture technique employs a mitogen, such as phytohaemagglutinin, to stimulate the lymphocytes to transform and divide. The cells are harvested for cytogenetic analysis at around 48 h of culture, at which time the vast majority of the dividing cells seen will be in their first mitosis after stimulation. In cultured lymphocytes from a healthy individual there is a very low spontaneous level of chromosomal aberrations, presumably arising as a result of misreplication. In every 1000 cells examined we would expect to find, on average, only one exchange-type aberration, together with 3 or 4 deletions.

It has been firmly established from cytogenetic studies of atom bomb survivors (Awa et al., 1971) and radiotherapy patients (Buckton et al., 1967) that exposure of lymphocytes in vivo to ionizing radiation results in a dose related increase in chromosome-type aber-

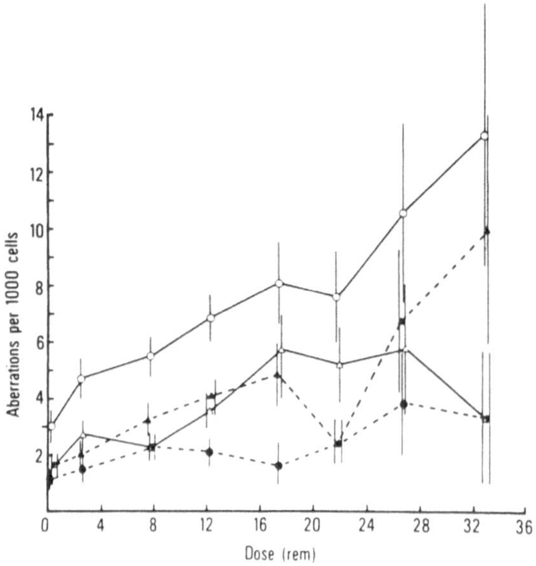

Fig. 4. Relation between accumulated dose (rem) and mean aberration frequencies (± s.e.m.) for dicentrics (Δ), acentric fragments (▲), and for cells containing unstable (○) and stable (●) chromosome aberrations (from Evans et al., 1979).

rations. Figure 3 shows the results of Buckton et al. (1967) who studied the increase in dicentric and ring chromosomes following different doses of partial body irradiation to individuals with ankylosing spondylitis. The yield at these high exposure levels approximates to the square of the dose. Moreover, Buckton et al. (1971) showed that at low doses of irradiation, peripheral blood irradiated _in vitro_ gave essentially the same dose response as blood withdrawn from the same individual following radiotherapy. Because of the similar sensitivity of lymphocyte chromosomes to radiation damage _in vivo_ and _in vitro_, and because of the strict relationship between aberration frequency and radiation dose _in vitro_, it is possible to use lymphocyte aberration frequencies as a biological dosimeter in cases of accidental exposure to radiation (Dolphin and Lloyd, 1974). Aberration incidence can be used in these situations to give an indirect assessment of the risk to the individual because although aberrations _per se_ cannot be related directly to the risk of cancer, there is considerable data available for relating absorbed x-ray dose with cancer risk.

Of equal, if not greater, importance is the risk associated with low levels of ionizing radiation - the sort of level that may be encountered in areas of high natural background radiation, or in occupations in which the workers are subjected to radiation levels that are within the specified maximum chronic exposure level of 5 rem per year. We known from in vitro experiments that we should expect to find a 3- or 4-fold increase in the frequency of dicentric aberrations at this dose, but unfortunately, until recently little direct information on the possible effects of low doses in vivo has been available. Recently Evans et al. (1979) published the results of a long term study on aberration incidence in a population of nuclear submarine refitters who received doses within the maximum permissable limits over periods of up to 10 years. The results, which are summarized in Fig. 4 show that aberration incidence increases with exposure up to a four-fold increase at the highest accumulated dose levels. The estimated rate of increase of dicentric aberrations with dose was 1.4×10^{-4} dicentrics per cell per rem, and the response at these low exposure levels was approximately linear. However, we should note that to detect such small changes in aberration frequency, a very large number of cells must be examined, and in these conditions of exposure, the detection of the estimated effect of 10 rem on the incidence of dicentrics in a single individual would entail cytogenetic analysis of about 10,000 cells!

Unstable aberrations such as dicentric chromosomes are easily identified and so we can be confident that the four-fold increase in dicentrics after 20-30 rem exposure shown in Fig. 4 is a valid reflection of the damage sustained by the cells. However, the stable aberrations, such as translocations, are more difficult to detect and the three-fold increase in individuals who were exposed to more than 25 rem accumulated dose (Fig. 4) is undoubtedly an underestimate. Most of the unstable aberrations are cell lethal whereas the cells containing stable aberrations will be viable. From the point of view of the exposed individual, the persistence of these surviving stable, but chromosomally abnormal, cells must be of considerable significance as each cell will contain some degree of genetic change. Unfortunately, we have no definite evidence that these cells confer any somatic effect and the above data, while proving a useful biological dosimeter, can tell us very little about the possible biological consequences.

There is evidence from other studies that cells with translocations or aneuploid cells that have arisen as a result of nondisjunction can give rise to clones of abnormal cells. Such clones have been reported in lymphocytes of patients treated with the internal emitter, thorotrast, in lymphocytes of ankylosing spondylitis patients treated with x-rays, and in bone marrow cells of atomic bomb survivors and fishermen exposed to radioactive fallout. All these individuals have an increased risk of cancer but there is no direct evidence that the increased cancer incidence in these individuals is connected with these abnormal clones as it has never been demonstrated that the neoplastic cells and clones share the same chromosomal rearrangement.

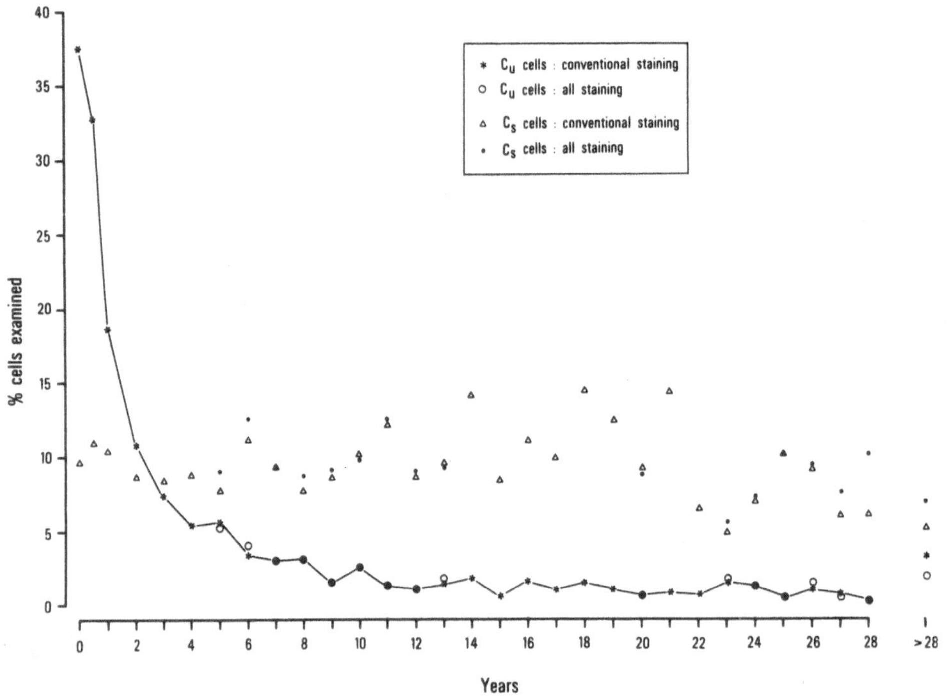

Fig. 5. Frequency cells with unstable (Ca) and stable (s) aberrations, with time in years, in lymphocytes of individuals receiving radiotherapy for ankylosing spondylitis.

Some suggestive evidence of the involvement of chromosomes in neoplasia comes from studies on chronic myeloid leukemia (CML) which is characterized by the presence of the Ph' chromosome - a translocation involving chromosomes 9 and 22. The incidence of CML is greatly increased by radiation and so in this instance it seems that a chromosomal rearrangement of the type that may be induced by radiation may play a significant role in the development of leukemia.

The formation of the clones in the lymphocyte population indicates that a proportion, at least, of the cells are able to proliferate in vivo. However, we also know that a proportion of the small lymphocytes are long lived with a mean Go life span of around 3 years, because aberrations occurring as a result of radiation exposure can still be found several years after exposure has occurred.

It turns out that the incidence of radiation induced exchanges in man decreases over a period of a few weeks (Preston et al., 1974) or months (Buckton et al., 1967, 1978) to about one half of the initial level (see Fig. 5). The reasons for this are not entirely clear but the decrease in exchange yield corresponds roughly to the recovery of the lymphocyte count, and the lymphocytes produced after radiation will obviously be derived from stem cells that contain no cell lethal aberrations. Other factors, such as separation of damaged lymphocytes may also play a part, but the important point to recognize is that retrospective dose estimations made some time after radiation exposure can be unreliable.

With the great interest shown over the last decade in the deleterious biological effect of industrial chemicals, it as inevitable that attention be focused on the induction of chromosome damage in individuals exposed to such chemicals, as a possible method of monitoring past exposure levels. Of course the use of peripheral blood cultures for in vitro mutagen/carcinogen testing is one of a number of important short term assays for the identification of genotoxic substance but I wish to confine my attention in this talk to the induction of chromosome damage in vivo.

Probably the first studies on the induction in vivo of chromosomal damage in lymphocytes were due to Pollini and Colombi (1964) and Vigliani (1964) who found an increased level of aberrations in the lymphocytes of workers exposed to benzene. However, a more comprehensive survey by Tough et al. (1970) high-lighted several problems that are inherent in such surveys. Firstly, the level of unstable chromosomal abnormalities increased with age and presented a confounding factor in the analysis of the results, which in any case, showed only a small increase in treated compared with control individuals. Secondly, the choice of control subjects was shown to be of utmost importance in such a survey, and ideally each exposed subject should be matched for age and sex with an individual exposed to a similar environment but lacking the particular chemical under study, so that the effects of the chemical can be isolated from the multitude of other factors present in the environment. In studies of an atmospheric pollutant such as benzene this is virtually impossible. Unfortunately, the difficulty in selecting and gaining access to suitable control populations has lead to conflicting results between laboratories when comparing the cytogenetic results of benzene exposure.

Other problems in making quantitative in vivo studies of chemically induced chromosome damage include the difficulties in estimating the actual dose received by the target cell and the persistence in the blood stream and possible carry-over of the chemical into culture. The metabolic activation and inactivation of the chemical may vary among individuals and the nature of the lesion in DNA and the extent and efficiency of the repair process will influence the ultimate aberration frequency, as will the period of time elapsed between exposure and blood sampling.

Apart from benzene, the industrial chemical that has been most comprehensively studied for in vivo cytogenetic effects in exposed workers is vinyl chloride monomer (VCM). Epidemiological evidence

Table 1. Incidence of Exchange Aberrations in Lymphocyte Chromosomes in Two Populations (Berlin and Edinburgh) of Inhaling Cigarette Smokers and Matched Nonsmokers

	Berlin	Edinburgh
Control	11.3×10^{-4} (16 in 14,164)	32.5×10^{-4} (14 in 4300)
Smokers	68.0×10^{-4} (26 in 3823)	63.6×10^{-4} (35 in 5500)

demonstrating the carcinogenicity of this chemical to man (Creech and Johnson, 1974) prompted Purchase et al. (1975) to embark on an extensive longitudinal study of workers in the plastic industry. At the first sampling period immediately after exposure to relatively high levels of VCM, they found significantly elevated frequencies of stable and unstable aberrations compared with control samples. Moreover, the increase in chromosome damage was correlated with the length of exposure to the chemical and with the history of exposure during the year prior to sampling. Shortly after this survey was carried out the threshold limit values and plant exposure levels for VCM were reduced and since that time two further surveys have been conducted among the group of workers to determine whether reduced exposure levels would result in reduced in vivo chromosome damage. It was found that after 18 months the chromosome aberration levels were still elevated, but after 42 months the exposed and control populations no longer showed a significant difference. Since considerable overlap was found in the values among various exposure groups in this study, it is clear that the exposure of a single individual cannot be inferred from a single chromosome analysis.

Similar declines in aberration yield following reduction in exposure have been reported by Hansteen et al. (1978) for VCM workers and by Yoder et al. (1973) for agricultural workers who received extensive exposure to pesticides.

Another category of chemicals are those to which man is exposed intentionally either in the course of medical chemotherapy or as a result of "self abuse." Anticancer drugs are often mutagens or carcinogens in any case, and since these chemicals are used in high concentrations (compared, that is, to industrial levels of exposure) it comes as no surprise that many also induce chromosome aberrations in vivo. Small increases in aberration frequency have also been found in inhaling cigarette smokers compared with control levels and the results from two laboratories are shown in Table 1.

In all the examples of chemical exposure cited so far there is an increased risk of malignancy. In the case of benzene and VCM the risks of leukemia and hepatic angiosarcoma respectively are increased. There is a relatively high risk of a secondary neoplasm after cytotoxic chemotherapy and the risks associated with tobacco smoking are well known. In none of these instances is it possible to show any direct connection between mutagenic and chromosome breaking affect and malignant potential. Similarly very little is known about the consequence of increased aberrations in the somatic cells of exposed individuals but we do at least know that damage has been caused to the genetic material of that cell. Of course, if a similar level of chromosome damage were induced in germ cells we should expect the gametes to be genetically abnormal and this would be of considerable consequence to the individual, his offspring and future generations, and this brings me to the effect of chemical and physical mutagens on the chromosomes of cells of the germ line.

In fact there is very little information about either the spontaneous or induced levels of chromosome abnormality in human germ cells. On the other hand a considerable amount of information is available from animal experiments and this data can be translated, with suitable qualifications, into the genetic risk for man. Discussion of these animal results is outside the scope of this talk and I recommend the recent papers by Brewen (1977, 1979) for further information on this subject.

In only one case has direct experimentation been attempted in man and it was found that the rate of induced balanced reciprocal translocations in the spermatogonial stem cells was 7.7×10^{-4} per rad with doses of up to 100 rads (Brewen et al., 1975). Taking embryonic death and various other factors into account, Oftedal and Searle (1980) calculated that about 23 per million severe congenital malformations as a result of unbalanced translocations would occur in the offspring of a man receiving one rad. In the next generation the viable offspring inheriting balanced translocations would produce offspring, half of whom would bear unbalanced rearrangements and the frequency of congenitally malformed liveborn would be reduced to an estimated 6 per million in the second generation. It is interesting to note, however, that extensive studies of offspring conceived after exposure of their parents to irradiation from the atomic bomb have found no increase in the incidence of congenital malformations or chromosomal rearrangements (Awa et al., 1968, 1975).

Finally I would like to briefly mention some work which offers considerable scope for the direct estimation of chromosome damage in human sperm. Rudak et al. (1978) fused human sperm with zona-free hamster eggs and succeeded in reactivating the male nucleus to undergo decondensation thus allowing direct cytological examination of the chromosomes of human sperm after in vitro fertilization.

Of a total of sixty sperm analyzed, three were found to be aneuploid. Clearly this method has considerable potential as a direct means of estimating the effects of irradiation or chemical mutagen exposure on the chromosomes of the gamete.

I think I have shown that in certain situations, particularly in the case of exposure to ionizing radiation, cytogenetics has an important part to play in dosimetry and can therefore make an indirect contribution to the assessment of risk. The situation with exposure to chemical mutagens is much less clear but cytogenetics provides one of the few records of past exposure that are available to us. With the increasing awareness of the relationship between chromosome damage and neoplasia it is perhaps not too optimistic to hope that one day we might learn how better to interpret this information.

REFERENCES

Anderson, D., Richardson, C. R., Weight, T. M., Purchase, I. F. H., and Adams, W. G. F., Chromosomal analyses in vinyl chloride exposed workers. Results from analyses 18 and 42 months after initial sampling, Mutat. Res., 79:151-152 (1980).

Awa, A. A., Neriishi, S., Honda, T., Yoshida, M. C., Sofuni, T., and Matsui, T., Chromosome aberration frequency in cultured blood cells in relation to radiation dose of A-bomb survivors, Lancet, 2:903-905 (1971).

Boveri, T., Zur Frage der Entstehung maligner Tumoren, Gustav Fischer, Jena (1914).

Brewen, J. G., Preston, R. J., and Gengozian, N., Analysis of x-ray induced chromosomal translocations in human and marmoset spermatogonial stem cells, Nature, 253, 468 (1975).

Brewen, J. G., The application of mammalian cytogenetics to mutagenicity studies, in: "Progress in Genetic Toxicology," D. Scott, B. A. Bridges, and F. H. Sobels, eds., Elsevier/North Holland Biomedical Press, Amsterdam (1977).

Brewen, J. G., Cytogenetic studies and risk assessment for chemicals and ionizing radiation, in: "Banbury Report 1. Assessing Chemical Mutagens: The Risk to Humans," V. H. McElheny and S. Abrahamson, eds., Cold Spring Harbor Laboratory (1979).

Buckton, K. E., Langlands, A. O., Smith, P. G., and McLelland, J., Chromosome aberrations following partial and whole body x-irradiation in man, Dose response relationships, in: "Human Radiation Cytogenetics," H. J. Evans, W. M. Court-Brown, and A. S. McLean, eds., North Holland Publishing Co., Amsterdam (1967).

Buckton, K. E., Langlands, A. O., Smith, P. G., Woodcock, G. E., Looby, P. C., and McLelland, J., Further studies on chromosome aberration production after whole body irradiation in man, Int. J.Radiat. Biol., 19:369-378 (1971).

Buckton, K. E., Hamilton, G. E., Paton, L., and Langlands, A. O., Chromosome aberrations in irradiated ankylosing spondylitis patients, in: "Mutagen-Induced Chromosome Damage in Man," H. J. Evans and D. C. Lloyd, eds., Edinburgh University Press, Edinburgh (1978).

Cohen, A. J., Li, F. P., Berg, S., Marchetto, D. J. Shien Tsai, S. M., Jacobs, S. C., and Brown, R. S., Hereditary renal-cell carcinoma associated with a chromosomal translocation, New Engl. J. Med., 301:592-595 (1979).

Creech, J. L., and Johnson, M. N., Angiosarcoma of the liver in the manufacture of polyvinyl chloride, J. Occup. Med., 16: 150-151 (1974).

Dolphin, G. W., and Lloyd, D. C., The significance of radiation-induced chromosome abnormalities in radiological protection, J. Med. Genet., 11:181-190 (1974).

Evans, H. J., Buckton, K. E., Hamilton, G. E., and Carothers, A., Radiation-induced chromosome aberrations in nuclear dockyard workers, Nature, 277:531-534 (1979).

Hansemann, D., Uber asymmetrische Zellteilung in Epithelkrebsen und deren biologische Bedeutung, Virchow's Arch. Path. Anat., 119: 229-326 (1890).

Hansteen, I., Hillstad, L., Thiis-Evensen, E., and Heldaas, S. S., Effects of vinyl chloride in man - A cytogenetic follow-up study, Mutat. Res., 51:271-278 (1978).

Howard, R. O., Breg, W. R., Albert, D. M., and Lesser, R. L., Retinoblastoma and chromosome abnormality: partial deletion of the long arm of chromosome 13, Arch. Ophthalmol., 92:490-493 (1974).

Nadel, M., and Koss, L. G., Klinefelter's syndrome and male breast cancer, Lancet, 2:366 (1967).

Obe, G., and Herha, J., Chromosomal aberrations in heavy smokers, Hum. Genet., 41:259-263 (1978).

Pollini, G., and Colombi, R., Il danno chromosomico midollare nel' anemia aplastica benzolica, Med. Lavoro., 55:241-255 (1964).

Preston, R. J., Brewen, J. G., and Gengozian, N., Persistence of radiation induced chromosome aberrations in Marmoset and Man, Radiat. Res., 60:516-524 (1974).

Purchase, I. F. H., Richardson, C. R., and Anderson, D., Chromosomal and dominant lethal effects of vinyl chloride, Lancet, 2:410-411 (1975).

Purchase, I. F. H., Richardson, C. R., Anderson, D., Paddle, G. M., and Adams, W. G. F., Chromosomal analysis in vinyl chloride-exposed workers, Mutat. Res., 57:325-334 (1978).

Riccardi, V. M., Sujanski, E., Smith, A. C., and Francke, U., Chromosomal imbalance in the aniridia-Wilm's tumor association 11p interstitial deletion, Pediatrics, 61:604-610 (1978).

Rudak, E., Jacobs, P. A., and Yanagimachi, R., Direct analysis of the chromosome constitution of human spermatozoa, Nature, 274: 911-913 (1978).

Savage, J. R. K., Classification and relationships of induced chromosomal structural changes, J. Med. Genet., 13:103-122 (1976).
Stewart, A., Webb, J., and Hewitt, D., A survey of childhood malignancies, Brit. Med. J., 1:1495-1508 (1958).
Tough, I. M., Smith, P. G., Court-Brown, W. M., and Harnden, D. G., Chromosome studied on workers exposed to atmospheric benzene, The possible influence of age, Europ. J. Cancer, 6:49-55 (1970).
Vigliani, E. C., and Saita, G., Benzene and leukemia, New York J. Med., 271:872-876 (1964).
Yoder, J., Watson, M., and Benson, W. W., Lymphocyte chromosome analysis of agricultural workers during extensive occupational exposure to pesticides, Mutat. Res., 21:335-340 (1979).

REPAIR OF RADIATION DAMAGE IN MAMMALIAN CELLS

R. B. Setlow

Biology Department
Brookhaven National Laboratory
Upton, New York 11973
USA

INTRODUCTION

The responses, such as survival, mutation and carcinogenesis, of mammalian cells and tissues to radiation are dependent not only on the magnitude of the damage to macromolecular structures - DNA, RNA, protein and membranes - but on the rates of macromolecular syntheses of cells relative to the half-lives of the damages. Cells possess a number of mechanisms for repairing damage to DNA. If the repair systems are rapid and error free, cells can tolerate much larger doses than if repair is slow or error prone. The general subject of repair of DNA damage has been reviewed extensively [1-4].

It is important to understand the effects of radiation and the repair of radiation damage because there exist reasonable amounts of epidemiological data that permits the construction of dose-response curves for humans. The shapes of such curves or the magnitude of the response will depend on repair. We emphasize in this chapter radiation damage because (a) radiation dosimetry, with all its uncertainties for populations, is excellent compared to chemical dosimetry; (b) a number of cancer-prone diseases are known in which there are defects in DNA repair and radiation results in more chromosomal damage in cells from such individuals [5-7] than in cells from normal individuals; (c) in some cases, specific radiation products in DNA have been correlated with biological effects [1] and, (d) many chemical effects seem to mimic radiation effects [1, 2]. A further reason for emphasizing damage to DNA is the wealth of experimental evidence indicating that damages to DNA can be initiating events in carcinogenesis [8].

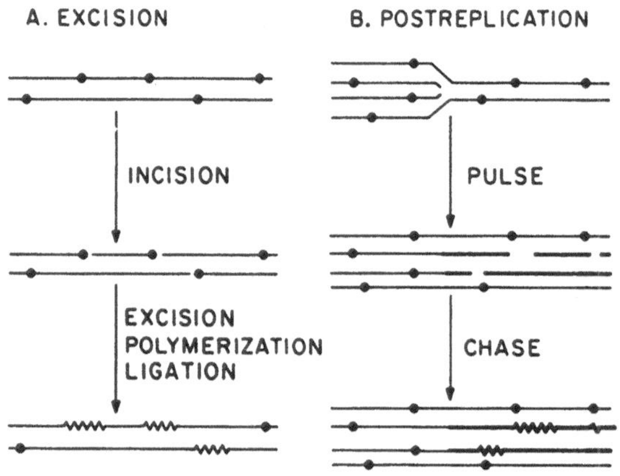

Fig. 1. Schematic diagrams of repair in mammalian cells. (A) Nucleotide excision. (B) Postreplication repair. The solid circles represent damages to DNA, the dark lines, DNA synthesized during a pulse; and the jagged lines repair replication for excision, or gap filling for postreplication repair. The average size of the former is about 100 nucleotides and 200 nucleotides for the latter.

ULTRAVIOLET DAMAGE

In prokaryotic systems, ultraviolet (UV) induced pyrimidine dimers are known to be one of the most important lesions. In higher eukaryotic systems the effects cell killing, mutagenesis and neoplastic transformation of wavelengths less than 313 nm, all follow action spectra - sensitivity versus wavelength - similar to that for making pyrimidine dimers in DNA [9-11]. Moreover, when it has been possible to test it, photoreactivation (see Repair of Ultra-Violet Light Induced Damage in Human Skin) indicates that the important damages are pyrimidine dimers. There are a number of easy experimental ways to measure dimers and their repair [12].

Excision Repair

Figure 1a shows a schematic diagram of the process of nucleotide excision repair. Such repair takes place in cells of all tissues of normal individuals that have been examined (fibroblasts, epithelial cells and lymphocytes). The rate-limiting step in such repair seems to be the initial endonucleolytic incision, and it is this step that is very slow, although not zero (see below), in excision-defective xeroderma pigmentosum cells. The details of action of the endonucleolytic step have not been elucidated for mammalian cells. Thus, it is not clear whether an initial obligatory glycosylase action is needed before incision as is the case for puri-

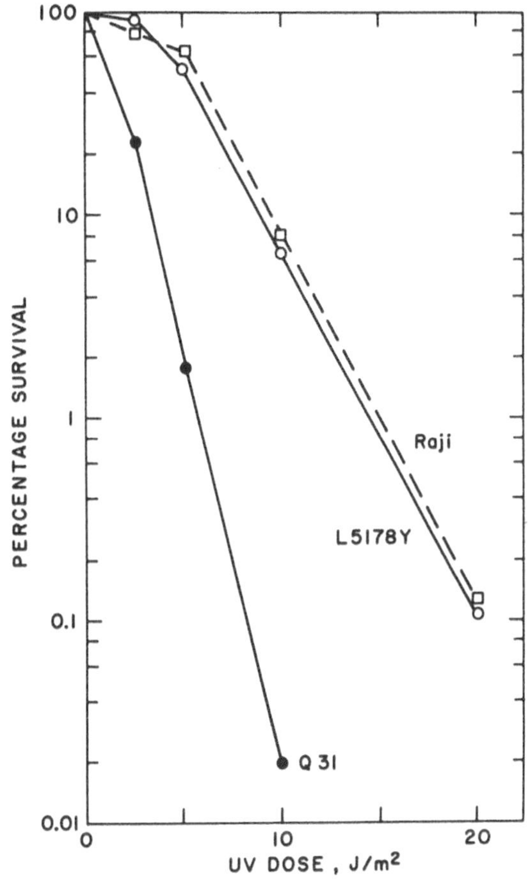

Fig. 2. Survival curves as a function of UV dose for two mouse lymphoma cell lines and a human cell line (adapted from Sato and Setlow [15]). These survival data should be compared with the excision data in Table 1.

Table 1. Excision Repair in Mouse and Human Cell Lines[a] (Sato and Setlow [15])

Cell line	Dimers[b] removed in 24 h (%)
Mouse, L5179y	18
Q31	3
Human, Raji	39

[a]See Fig. 2 for survival curves.
[b]Measured as endonuclease sensitive sites after 10 J/m², 254 nm.

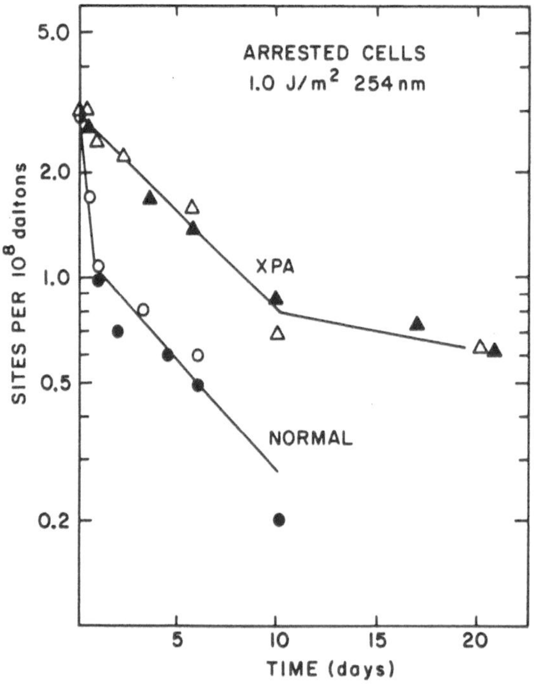

Fig. 3. The excision of pyrimidine dimers, measured as endonuclease sensitive sites, from nondividing normal or xeroderma pigmentosum cells as a function of time (from Kantor and Setlow [16]).

fied prokaryotic enzymes [13, 14]. Xeroderma pigmentosum cells are killed and mutated more readily than are normal cells and there is a rough correlation between the extent of the defect in excision repair, or the defect in the ability to do host cell reactivation of UV irradiated viruses, and the enhancement of the cytotoxicity of UV and the sensitivity of skin to sunlight induced skin cancer. However, such a correlation, although good within one species does not seem to extend across species lines as indicated by the data in Table 1, and the survival curves in Fig. 2 comparing two mouse cell lines and a human cell line.

The extrapolation from cellular repair data to humans is complicated because the cellular data are obtained with acute UV doses and the development of nonmelanoma skin cancer in humans follows from long chronic exposures. At low chronic dose rates, the difference in the magnitude of repair between proficient and deficient cells may not be as marked as shown in Table 1. For example, xeroderma pigmentosum cells are able to do some repair although, for acute doses, with different kinetics than for normal cells (see

Fig. 3). However, even in midday sunlight the low acute doses indicated in Fig. 3 might take times greater than 1 h to deliver to human skin. Thus, there is an urgent need for DNA repair studies at the chronic dose rates found in the environment.

Post Replication Repair

DNA synthesis is inhibited by UV irradiation of cells but the blockage of replication is not complete even in excision repair defective strains. Synthesis returns to normal levels in times compatible with the excision of dimers except for cells from individuals with the light sensitive disease Cockayne's syndrome. DNA synthesis in these cells remains depressed for much longer times, and the cells are killed more readily by UV than are normal ones [17]. Replication takes place on the damaged template in almost all cells before excision repair is complete, and if this replication is faulty, the cell may die, be mutated or transformed.* Replication on a damaged template is often detected experimentally by the changes in molecular weight of newly synthesized, pulse labeled DNA. Hence, the process is called postreplication repair. At short times after irradiation, pulse labeled DNA is small and this small DNA is chased into larger pieces. As Fig. 1b shows, replication seems to leave gaps in the newly synthesized DNA, and the gaps are filled in during a subsequent chase. XP variant cells are proficient in excision but are deficient in postreplication repair [19], and are mutagenized more readily than normal cells at equal levels of survival [20]. Such observations indicate that the postreplication repair process may have an error-prone component to it as do prokaryotic systems. Split UV doses, separated by a number of hours, to normal and especially XP variant cells enhance the rate of post-replication repair following the second dose [21]. Moreover, the rate of fork motion in Chinese hamster cells is enhanced as is the rate of resumption of bulk DNA synthesis in normal cells [22, 23]. The enhancing effects of small ultraviolet doses to cells are also found for the survival and mutagenesis of UV-irradiated viruses plated on such cells [24], although the kinetics of such an enhanced process seem quite different from the kinetics for DNA synthesis.

Inter-Individual Variation

Most skin cancers arise from sunlight exposure and the response seems to be an exponential function of the annual dose [25]. The ultraviolet dose rate changes drastically during the day and during the year. Since habits of sun exposure vary markedly among people, the variation in received dose among individuals can be tremendous

*In nondividing cells, replication is not relevant, but the data indicate that transcription on the damaged template may lead to cell death [18].

Table 2. Variations in Excision Repair among Cells Exposed to 254 nm UV

A. Normal cells-type	No.	Method	Dose (J/m^2)	Std. deviation	Ref.
Fibroblasts	30	BrUra Photolysis	20	17	27
Leukocytes	40	UDS	20	26	28
Leukocytes	90	UDS	20	44	29
		UDS	max	66	29

B. Abnormal cells-type	No.	Method	Repair rel. to normal	Std. deviation	Ref.
XP Fibroblasts	10	BrUra Photolysis	0.1	50	27
Leukocytes from heroin addicts	38	UDS	0.3	100	29

and this large variation might account in part for the exponential shape of the dose response curve. The tremendous (10^3 to 10^4-fold) difference in skin cancer prevalence between normal and XP individuals is explicable in terms of the repair deficiencies of XP cells. On the assumption that defective DNA repair is the explanation for the skin cancer prevalence of XP individuals, one can estimate that proficient DNA repair - photoreactivation, excision and postreplication repair - is able to reduce the effective UV dose to normal individuals by seven- to twenty-fold compared to XP individuals [26]. If such numbers are close to the truth, small changes in repair of UV damage might change the skin cancer susceptibility of individuals by significant factors, although nowhere near the orders of magnitude encountered for XP individuals. What sort of variation is observed among the presumptive non-repair deficient population? Two types of experiments have been done to measure such variations: one used the bromodeoxyuridine photolysis technique to measure excision repair in fibroblast strains from a number of presumptive normal individuals, the other measured unscheduled DNA synthesis (UDS) in terms of cpm/μg of DNA in unstimulated leukocytes from a number of individuals with different lifestyles and ages. The results of such studies are shown in Table 2. Two points of great interest are apparent: lifestyle - heroin addiction - seems to affect the level of DNA repair and, there is a tremendous variation among individuals. The large variation is made

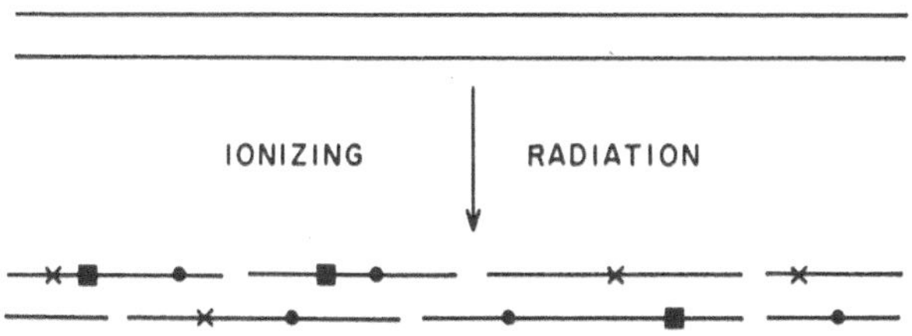

Fig. 4. A schematic diagram illustrating the large numbers of different types of DNA damages, in addition to single and double strand breaks, that arise from ionizing radiation.

up of variances in technique, and real variations from day-to-day for the same individual and variations among individuals. The breakdown of these variations indicates that there is a significant difference among individuals - a difference beyond the experimental or day-to-day variation. The causes for the variations, whether they be genetic or lifestyle related, are not known; nor is there any information on the prognostic value of such findings. However, the lymphocytes of individuals with actinic keratoses, have on the average, less repair than those of normal individuals [30]. The keratoses are felt to be precursor lesions to nonmelanoma skin cancer, and they may indicate that individuals with less repair are more prone to develop actinic keratoses. Skin cancer data are confounded not only by unknown dosimetry but by the fact that individuals have different skin types - types that show relatively large variations in pigmentation and presumably UV transmission. It might be possible by making measurements on the repair capabilities and the skin transmission properties of individuals who have had skin cancer to disentangle these two variables and obtain an estimate of the role of DNA repair capability in skin cancer prevalence among presumably normal individuals.

IONIZING RADIATION

Definitive studies on the molecular mechanisms for the repair of ionizing radiation damage are hampered by our ignorance of which radiation products are responsible for killing, mutation, and transformation (Fig. 4). The easiest damage to measure - single strand breaks in DNA - is repaired at high speed and seems relatively innocuous. No mammalian cell strains have been found that are reproducibly deficient in this type of repair. Cells from individuals with ataxia telangiectasia (AT) are more sensitive to the cytotoxic effects of ionizing radiation than are those from normal individuals (Fig. 5) [6, 31]. However, such cells are very efficient at single strand break repair. Some of the AT fibroblast strains are deficient in repair replication and in the ability to remove endonuclease

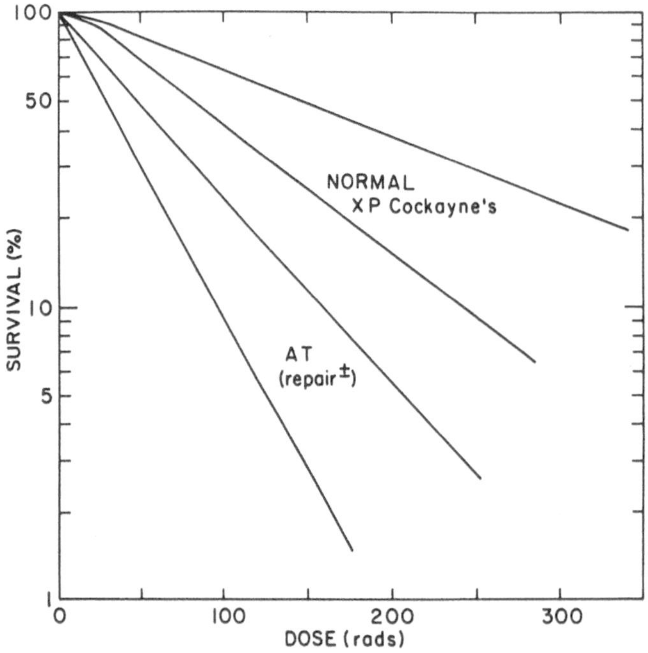

Fig. 5. Survival curves as a function of ionizing radiation dose illustrating the ranges of sensitivities observed (adapted from Arlett and Harcourt [31]). The range of sensitivities for AT cell strains seems to be independent of the abilities to remove endonuclease sensitive to sites or to do repair replication.

sensitive sites from their DNA.* Other AT strains although sensitive to ionizing radiation seem to be as repair proficient as are normal cells. Hence, except for the greater number of chromosome aberrations per unit dose in irradiated AT cells, there seems to be no direct connection between DNA repair defects and cellular sensitivity to ionizing radiation. Moreover, AT cells are hypomutable by ionizing radiation and there is no indication that this type of radiation is the etiologic agent responsible for the increase in cancer risk of AT individuals.

---

*Extracts of M. luteus or E. coli have activities able to nick DNA irradiated by ionizing radiation [32] but the nature of the damage(s) recognized by these enzymes is not known. The numbers of such base damages approximate the number of single strand breaks for anoxic irradiation but is only about half the number of breaks observed for irradiation in air.

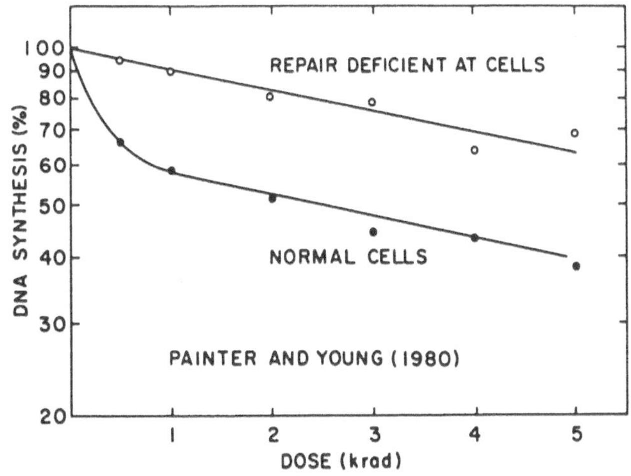

Fig. 6. DNA synthesis as a function of ionizing radiation dose for normal and AT cell strains (adapted from Painter and Young [37]).

There is some epidemiological evidence indicating that AT heterozygotes may be more cancer prone than the average [33], and hence, it would be useful to be able to identify such individuals since they apparently make up close to 1% of the population. Five out of seven heterozygote fibroblast strains are more sensitive to the cytotoxic effect of anoxic radiation [34] and eight out of eight heterozygote lymphoblastoid lines do not proliferate after 80 rads, whereas normal transformed cells proliferate after 100 rads [35].

DNA Synthesis

Low doses to normal human cells result in a rapid decrease in the incorporation of exogenous ^{3}H thymidine and in the appearance of the incorporated label in the high molecular weight component of the DNA sedimented in alkali. These data indicate that ionizing radiation inhibits the initiation of new replicons [36]. Since the effect is observed at low doses - doses that make an initial number of 1000 single strand breaks per 3×10^{12} daltons [5] most of which are repaired in the 30 min before DNA synthesis is measured - there must be a big target, i.e., a cluster of replicons is affected. One could infer that there must have been a big change in the large scale conformation of DNA, a change that does not go to zero for an appreciable time. AT cells, however, show no such inhibition of DNA synthesis (Fig. 6), although one group of investigators [37] observes inhibition in repair proficient AT cells and another does not [38]. Thus, there is the intriguing possibility that AT cells have the capability of winding up the DNA quickly to its preirradiation conformation and so permitting clusters of replicons to initiate synthesis. In any event, the continuation of DNA synthesis in AT cells implies that the growing points will traverse more base damage in DNA than will the growing points in normal cells because base damage is repaired slowly [32]. Hence, the yield of lethal events in AT cells would be expected to be larger than in normal cells. This explanation is consistent with the observation of no defect in AT cells for host-cell reactivation of x-ray irradiated herpes simplex virus [39]. Note, incidentally, that DNA synthesis in Cockayne's syndrome cells was suppressed for a long time by UV irradiation and the suppression was interpreted as giving rise to lethal events. These two different conclusions from the inhibition of DNA synthesis simply indicate that the damage from UV and from ionizing radiations are very different and that the mechanisms of repair of the two types of damage are very different. In the excision repair of UV damage there are long patches; whereas in the repair of ionizing radiation damage there are, on the average, short patches. After long repair times, times comparable to those usually used for UV, some long patch repair is observed [40].

DNA repair activity, repair replication or loss of endonuclease sensitive sites, can only be measured at very high doses - doses near 50 krads, and no distributions of repair activities among normal cells have been obtained as they have for UV.

313 NM RADIATION

The absorption coefficient of DNA decreases rapidly at wavelengths greater than 300 nm and at such wavelengths is much more characteristic of GC residues [41]. Hence one might expect that photoproducts, other than thymine-containing dimers, would be of increasing importance biologically at these longer wavelengths. Such additional photoproducts might be ring saturated thymines [42] or single strand breaks [43]. For 313 nm irradiation, these other products do not seem to be of importance for cytotoxic effects on normal or XP fibroblasts since the relative sensitivity per dimer formed seems to be the same as 313 nm as at shorter wavelengths [9].

Two out of four AT fibroblast strains show enhanced cytotoxic sensitivity to 313 nm (but not to 254 nm) and four out of seven Bloom's syndrome (BS) fibroblasts also show enhanced cytotoxic sensitivity at the long wavelength [44, 45]. There is a rough, but not a complete, correlation between the higher sensitivity of BS cells and the induction of single strand breaks in cells exposed to 313 nm at 37° [46]. However, for irradiation at 0° there is no big increase in single strand breaks [46]. Since gamma irradiation of BS cells makes the same numbers of single strand breaks as in normal fibroblasts, and the repair of such breaks is about the same, it was concluded that the breaks observed after ionizing radiation are different from those observed afer 313 nm irradiation [44]. Moreover, such observations lend force to the argument that the breaks observed as a result of 313 nm irradiation in some of the BS cells result from some alteration in repair capacity - an alteration that is a step beyond the initial endonucleolytic one.

A clastogenic factor in the medium of BS cells could be reduced substantially by superoxide dismutase [47]. This result indicates that reactions at the longer UV wavelength may take place by an active oxygen species and not by a direct action on DNA. As a matter of fact, other than the approximate correlation between the cytotoxicity and single strand break enhancement in irradiated BS cells, there is no good evidence that the enhanced cytotoxicity to 313 nm arises from damage to DNA. Irradiations at this wavelength require large fluxes of light and it is conceivable that other cellular components could be the ultimate targets.

ACKNOWLEDGEMENT

This work was supported by the U.S. Department of Energy.

REFERENCES

1. R. B. Setlow and J. K. Setlow, Effects of Radiation on Polynucleotides, Ann. Rev. Biophys. Bioengineer., 1:293 (1972).
2. J. J. Roberts, The repair of DNA modified by cytotoxic, mutagenic, and carcinogenic chemicals, Adv. Radiat. Biol., 7:211 (1978).
3. P. C. Hanawalt, E. C., Friedberg, and C. F. Fox, "DNA Repair Mechanisms," Academic Press, New York (1978).
4. P. C. Hanawalt, P. K. Cooper, A. K. Ganesan, and C. A. Smith, DNA repair in bacteria and mammalian cells, Ann. Rev. Biochem., 48:783 (1979).
5. R. B. Setlow, Repair deficient human disorders and cancer, Nature, 271:713 (1978).
6. C. F. Arlett and A. R. Lehmann, Human disorders showing increased sensitivity to the induction of genetic damage, Ann. Rev. Genet., 12:95 (1978).
7. E. C. Friedberg, U. K. Ehmann, and J. I. Williams, Human diseases associated with defective DNA repair, Adv. Radiat. Biol., 8:85 (1979).
8. R. B. Setlow, DNA damage and carcinogenesis, in: "Chromosome Damage and DNA Repair," E. Seeberg and K. Kleppe, eds., Plenum Press, New York (1981).
9. G. J. Kantor, J. C. Sutherland, and R. B. Setlow, Action spectra for killing nondividing normal human and xeroderma pigmentosum cells, Photochem. Photobiol., 31:459 (1980).
10. E. D. Jacobson, K. Krell, and M. J. Dempsey, The wavelength dependence of ultraviolet light-induced cell killing and mutagenesis in L5178Y mouse lymphoma cells, Photochem. Photobiol., 33:257 (1981).

11. J. Doniger, E. D. Jacobson, K. Krell, and J. A. DiPaolo, Ultraviolet light action spectra for neoplastic transformation and lethality of Syrian hamster embryo cells correlate with spectrum for pyrimidine dimer formation in cellular DNA, Proc. Natl. Acad. Sci. USA, 78:2378 (1981).
12. E. C. Friedberg and P. C. Hanawalt, eds., "DNA Repair, a Laboratory Manual of Research Procedures," Marcel Dekker, New York (1981).
13. W. A. Haseltine, L. K. Gordon, C. P. Lindau, R. H. Grafstrom, N. L. Shaper, and L. Grossman, Cleavage of pyrimidine dimers in specific DNA sequences by a pyrimidine dimer DNA-glycosylase of M. luteus, Nature, 285:634 (1980).
14. B. Demple and S. Linn, DNA N-glycosylases and DNA repair, Nature, 287:203 (1980).
15. K. Sato and R. B. Setlow, DNA repair in a UV-sensitive mutant of a mouse cell line, Mutat. Res., in press.
16. G. J. Kantor and R. B. Setlow, Rate and extent of DNA repair in nondividing human diploid fibroblasts, Cancer Res., 41:819 (1980).
17. A. R. Lehmann, S. Kirk-Bell, and L. Mayne, Abnormal kinetics of DNA synthesis in ultraviolet light-irradiated cells from patients with Cockayne's syndrome, Cancer Res., 39:4237 (1979).
18. G. J. Kantor and D. R. Hull, An effect of ultraviolet light on RNA and protein synthesis in nondividing human diploid fibroblasts, Biophys. J., 27:359 (1979).
19. A. R. Lehmann, S. Kirk-Bell, C. F. Arlett, M. C. Paterson, P. H. M. Lohman, E. A. deWeerd-Kastelein, and D. Bootsma, Xeroderma pigmentosum cells with normal levels of excision repair have a defect in DNA synthesis after UV-irradiation, Proc. Natl. Acad. Sci. USA, 72:219 (1975).
20. V. M. Maher, L. M. Ouelette, R. D. Curren, and J. J. McCormick, Frequency of ultraviolet light-induced mutations is higher in xeroderma pigmentosum variant cells than in normal human cells, Nature, 261:593 (1976).
21. R. B. Setlow, F. A. Ahmed, and E. Grist, Xeroderma pigmentosum: Damage to DNA is involved in carcinogenesis, in: "Origins of Human Cancer," H. H. Hiatt, J. D. Watson, and J. A. Winsten, eds., Cold Spring Harbor Laboratory, Cold Spring Harbor (1977).
22. J. Doniger, DNA replication in ultraviolet light irradiated Chinese hamster cells: The nature of replicon inhibition and post-replication repair, J. Mol. Biol., 120:433 (1978).
23. E. Moustacchi, U. K. Ehmann, and E. C. Friedberg, Defective recovery of semi-conservative DNA synthesis in xeroderma pigmentosum cells following split-dose ultraviolet irradiation, Mutat. Res., 62:159 (1979).
24. L. E. Bockstahler and C. D. Lytle, Radiation enhanced reactivation of nuclear replicating mammalian viruses, Photochem. Photobiol., 25:477 (1977).

25. E. L. Scott and M. L. Straf, Ultraviolet radiation as a cause of cancer, in: "Origins of Human Cancer," H. H. Hiatt, J. D. Watson, and J. A. Winsten, eds., Cold Spring Harbor Laboratory, Cold Spring Harbor (1977).
26. R. B. Setlow, Different basic mechanisms in DNA repair, Arch. Toxicol. Suppl., 3:217 (1980).
27. R. B. Setlow and J. D. Regan, unpublished results.
28. B. Lambert, U. Ringborg, and L. Skoog, Age-related decrease of ultraviolet light-induced DNA repair synthesis in human peripheral leukocytes, Cancer Res., 39:2792 (1979).
29. J. J. Madden, A. Falek, D. A. Shafer, and J. H. Glick, Effects of opiates and demographic factors on DNA repair synthesis in human leukocytes, Proc. Natl. Acad. Sci. USA, 76:5769 (1979).
30. B. Lambert, U. Ringborg, and G. Swanbeck, Ultraviolet-induced DNA repair synthesis in lymphocytes from patients with actinic keratosis, J. Invest. Dermatol., 67:594 (1976).
31. C. F. Arlett and S. Harcourt, Survey of radiosensitivity in a variety of human cell strains, Cancer Res., 40:926 (1980).
32. M. C. Paterson, Use of purified lesion-recognizing enzymes to monitor DNA repair in vivo, Adv. Radiat. Biol., 7:1 (1978).
33. M. Swift, L. Sholman, M. Perry, and C. Chase, Malignant neoplasms in the families of patients with ataxia telangiectasia, Cancer Res., 36:209 (1976).
34. M. C. Paterson, A. K. Anderson, B. P. Smith, and P. J. Smith, Enhanced radiosensitivity of cultured fibroblasts from ataxia telangiectasia heterozygotes is manifested by defective colony forming ability and reduced repair replication after hypoxic x-irradiation, Cancer Res., 39:3725 (1979).
35. P. Chen, M. F. Lavin, C. Kidson, and D. Moss, Identification of ataxia telangiectasia heterozygotes, a cancer prone population, Nature, 274:484 (1978).
36. R. B. Painter and B. R. Young, X-ray induced inhibition of DNA synthesis in Chinese hamster ovary, human HeLa, and mouse L cells, Radiat. Res., 64:648 (1975).
37. R. B. Painter and B. R. Young, Radiosensitivity in ataxis telangiectasia: A new explanation, Proc. Natl. Acad. Sci. USA, 77:7315 (1980).
38. P. J. Smith and M. C. Paterson, Gamma ray induced inhibition of DNA synthesis in ataxia telangiectasia fibroblasts as a function of excision repair capacity, Biochem. Biophys. Res. Commun., 97:897 (1980).
39. H. Takebe, et al., Genetic aspects of xeroderma pigmentosum and other cancer-prone diseases, in: "Genetic and Environmental Factors in Experimental and Human Cancer," H. V. Gelboin et al., eds., Japan Scientific Societies, Tokyo (1980).
40. R. B. Setlow, F. M. Faulcon, and J. D. Regan, Defective repair of gamma-ray induced DNA damage in xeroderma pigmentosum cells, Int. J. Radiat. Biol., 29:125 (1976).

41. J. C. Sutherland and K. P. Griffin, Absorption spectrum of DNA for wavelengths greater than 3000 nm, Radiat. Res., 86:399 (1981).

42. P. V. Hariharan and P. A. Cerutti, Formation of products of the 5,6-dihydroxydihydrothymine type by ultraviolet light in HeLa cells, Biochemistry, 16:2791 (1977).

43. L. C. Erickson, M. O. Bradley, and K. W. Kohn, Mechanisms for the production of DNA damage in cultured human and hamster cells irradiated with light from fluorescent lamps, sunlamps, and the sun, Biochim. Biophys. Acta, 610:105 (1980).

44. P. J. Smith and M. C. Paterson, Abnormal responses to mid-ultraviolet light of cultured fibroblasts from patients with disorders featuring sunlight sensitivity, Cancer Res., 41:511 (1981).

45. I. Zbinden and P. Cerutti, Near-ultraviolet sensitivity of skin fibroblasts of patients with Bloom's syndrome, Biochem. Biophys. Res. Commun., 98:579 (1981).

46. H. Hirschi, M. S. Netrawali, J. F. Remsen, and P. A. Cerutti, Formation of DNA single-strand breaks by near ultraviolet and x-rays in normal and Bloom's syndrome skin fibroblasts, Cancer Res., 41:2003 (1981).

47. I. Emerit and P. Cerutti, Clastogenic activity from Bloom's syndrome fibroblast cultures, Proc. Natl. Acad. Sci. USA, 78:1868-1872 (1981).

REPAIR AND EXPRESSION OF AFLATOXIN B_1-INDUCED DNA DAMAGE

Steven A. Leadon, Paul A. Amstad
and Peter A. Cerutti

Department of Carcinogenesis
Swiss Institute for Experimental Cancer Research
CH-1066 Epalinges s/Lausanne, Switzerland

SUMMARY

The chemical properties, cellular repair and biological expression of aflatoxin B_1 (AFB_1)-DNA adducts were investigated in mouse embryo fibroblasts 10T1/2, human epithelioid lung cells A549 and human skin fibroblasts (NF). These studies were complicated by the inherent chemical instability of AFB_1-DNA adducts. In order to distinguish enzymatic reactions from spontaneous decomposition it was necessary to compare routinely the reactions occurring intracellularly to those of free AFB_1-DNA in vitro and of AFB_1-DNA in situ in excision repair deficient Xeroderma pigmentosum (XPA) fibroblasts. Following treatment of very actively metabolizing 10T1/2 cells with the procarcinogen AFB_1 or of NF and A549 with microsome activated AFB_1, approximately 90% of the adducts corresponded to 2,3-dihydro-2-(N^7-guanyl)-3-hydroxy-AFB_1 (AFB_1-N^7-Gua). AFB_1-DNA adducts were introduced preferentially in nucleosomal-linker relative to - core DNA both after cellular metabolic activation of AFB_1 and exogenous activation by microsomes. For the determination of the nucleosomal distribution, the primary adducts, AFB_1-N^7-Gua, were transformed into the chemically more stable secondary products 2,3-dihydro-2-(N^5-formyl-2',5',6'-triamino-4'-oxo-N^5-pyrimidyl)-3-hydroxyaflatoxin B_1 (AFB_1-triamino-Py) by a short exposure of the AFB_1-treated cells to pH 9.5 medium.

Adduct removal was studied as a function of post-treatment incubation. The following conclusions were reached using the reactions of free AFB_1-DNA in vitro and AFB_1-DNA in XPA fibroblasts as reference: 1) AFB_1-N^7-Gua is removed spontaneously and enzymatically in 10T1/2, NF and A549 cells. 2) AFB_1-triamino-Py is formed in a spontaneous secondary reaction from AFB_1-N^7-Gua and accumulates in the DNA. It represents the major persistent lesion at prolonged post-treatment incubation.

The major target for the cytotoxic effect of AFB_1 in 10T1/2 cells was identified as DNA. In particular, confluent holding experiments showed that removal of AFB_1-adducts lead to partial recovery of viability. The incompleteness of recovery is probably due to the accumulation of irrepairable AFB_1-triamino-Py adducts in the DNA. The continuous decrease in the concentration of total AFB_1 adducts during confluent holding was not reflected in a corresponding, continuous decrease in malignant transformation of 10T1/2 cells. The number of transformed foci per dish increased during the first 16 h of confluent holding and later decreased below the initial value by 40 h. These results exemplify the complex relationship between the efficiency of transformation, the changes in adduct concentration and the recovery of cell viability as a function of confluent holding.

INTRODUCTION

Aflatoxin B_1 (AFB_1) is a mycotoxin produced by certain strains of Aspergillus flavus. It is hepatotoxic and hepatocarcinogenic in several animal species (Wogan, 1973; Campbell and Hayes, 1976). Epidemiological studies suggest that it may also be an important factor in the etiology of human liver cancer (Shank et al., 1972; Wogan, 1976).

Like many carcinogens, AFB_1 requires metabolic activation to exert its biological effects. It binds covalently to cellular macromolecules both in vivo (Garner and Wright, 1973; Lin et al., 1977; Croy et al., 1978) and after activation in vitro by liver microsomes (Garner et al., 1972; Swenson et al., 1977; Essigmann et al., 1977). The primary AFB_1-DNA adducts (>90%) produced by metabolically active cells or via exogenous activation of AFB_1 with rat liver microsomes possess the structure of 2,3-dihydro-2-(N^7-deoxyguanosyl)-3-hydroxy-AFB_1, which upon mild acid treatment is released as 2,3-dihydro-2-(N^7-guanyl)-3-hydroxy-AFB_1 (AFB_1-N^7-Gua) (Essigmann et al., 1977; Lin et al., 1977; Croy et al., 1978). These primary adducts are chemically unstable and decompose by three major chemical reactions: 1) the release of AFB_1-dhd presumably with concomitant restitution of unaltered guanine residues; 2) the release of AFB_1-N^7-Gua from the DNA backbone upon hydrolytic cleavage of the N-glycosylic bond forming aguaninic sites; 3) the hydrolytic opening of the 5-membered ring of guanine, resulting in the formation of the more chemically stable secondary adduct, the putative 2,3-dihydro-2-(N^5-formyl-2',5',6'-triamino-4'-oxo-N^5-pyrimidyl)-3-hydroxyaflatoxin B_1 (AFB_1-triamino-Py) Lin et al., 1977). The rates of these reactions are extremely sensitive to pH changes in the physiological range (Wang and Cerutti, 1980a). Therefore, it is difficult to know their exact rates in situ in the cell where the local nuclear pH and the interaction with chromosomal proteins may influence the reactions in unpredictable ways. These complicating factors have to be kept in mind when studying the cellular processing and biological expression of AFB_1-DNA adducts and other chemically unstable DNA lesions such as N^7-alkylation and -arylation products of guanine and certain radiation products. Following carcinogen treatment, spontaneous chemical reactions and cellular repair is expected to alter the lesion spectrum continuously. At prolonged post-treatment incubation, more chemically and biologically stable lesions accumulate. Such unremoved, persistent lesions may in many cases represent minor components in the initial adduct spectrum or, as is the case for AFB_1-triamino-Py, they may be formed in secondary reactions.

Even without "pharmacokinetic" analysis, the following general considerations illustrate the degree of complexity which is encountered in attempting to relate the concentrations of individual DNA lesions to the biological effects of a carcinogen, e.g., to its mutagenicity. Fixation of targeted mutation is accomplished by the conversion of potentially mutagenic (or pro-mutagenic) lesions to mutagenic lesions in the course of DNA replication. The following processes may occur before the onset of DNA replication and influence the final mutation frequency: 1) the elimination of potentially mutagenic lesions by repair (either cellular or spontaneous chemical reactions); 2) the introduction of potentially mutagenic lesions or abnormal DNA configurations by constitutive or induced repair processes; 3) the elimination of potentially lethal lesions resulting in the rescue of cells containing high levels of potentially mutagenic lesions; etc. According to this model the relative capacities of a cell to eliminate potentially mutagenic and lethal lesions and/or to introduce mutations by error-prone pathways are expected to determine the overall biological effects of a DNA damaging agent. It should be stressed that potentially mutagenic and lethal lesions may be structurally distinct or result from different modes of expression of structurally identical lesions. Analogous chemical and cellular processes may affect the transforming potency of a carcinogen.

AFB_1-DNA adducts in situ in the cell are removed to a large extent by spontaneous chemical reactions, i.e., "chemical repair." However, in addition, active cellular excision of AFB_1-adducts has been shown to occur in rat liver (Hertzog et al., 1980), mouse embryo fibroblasts 10T1/2 (Wang and Cerutti, 1980b), and more pronounced, in normal human skin fibroblasts (NF) (Leadon et al., 1981) and human lung epithelial cells A549 (Wang and Cerutti, 1979). A linear relationship was observed in 10T1/2 cells between cytotoxicity and total AFB_1-adduct concentration indicating that DNA represents the major cellular target for AFB_1 cytotoxicity. Since cytotoxicity was independent of the exact adduct composition, it appears that structurally distinct lesions, in particular, AFB_1-N^7-Gua and AFB_1-

triamino-Py, possess comparable killing efficiencies. From our discussion in the preceding paragraph it may not be astonishing that no simple relationship was observed in confluent holding experiments between adduct concentration and transformation of 10T1/2 cells, on the other hand. The number of transformed foci per dish first increased and later decreased as a function of confluent holding time while the total DNA adduct concentration decreased and viability increased continuously. Within the frame of our model we suggest that the concentration of "potentially transforming DNA lesions" reaches a maximum during confluent holding while lethal lesions are removed continuously. "Potentially transforming DNA lesions" should be understood in the broadest sense and signifies structurally modified adducts as well as DNA configurations resulting from the processing of primary adducts by repair.

1. Nucleosomal Distribution of AFB_1-DNA Adducts

Ultimate carcinogens introducing bulky substituents preferentially attack nucleosomal linker DNA. For AAAF and BPDE I (Kaneko and Cerutti, 1980, 1981), these initial adduct concentrations were 5-6 times higher in linker- than core-DNA, respectively, and the rates of adduct removal (in μmoles per mole DNA-P removed per unit time) were higher for linker- than core-DNA. It is evident that the nucleosomal structure of chromatin influences adduct excisability. Therefore, we have determined the distribution of AFB_1-DNA adducts between nucleosomal linker- and core-DNA in mouse embryo 10T1/2 cells. The distribution after cellular metabolic activation of AFB_1 for 4 h was compared to that following exogenous activation by rat liver microsomes for 30 min. In both types of experiments 10T1/2 were prelabeled in their DNA with [^{14}C]thymidine and treated with [^{3}H]AFB_1 or microsome activated [^{3}H]AFB_1 in confluency. Immediately following AFB_1-treatment the cells were shortly exposed to pH 9.5 in order to transform the labile AFB_1-N^7-Gua adducts into the chemically more stable AFB_1-triamino-Py adducts. This step is necessary to fix the initial adduct distribution in view of the lengthy purification procedures for nucleosomal core-DNA, and does not cause significant loss of adducts. Initial modification levels for both activation systems were 2.1 to 3.1 μmole AFB_1 per mole DNA-P and analysis by high pressure liquid chromatography (HPLC) showed that more than 80% of the adducts were present in the form of AFB_1-triamino-Py. The protocol for the determination of the adduct concentrations in total nuclear DNA and in highly purified 145 base pair (b.p.) core-DNA and the calculation of the adduct concentration in 45 b.p. linker DNA have been described previously (Kaneko and Cerutti, 1981). Briefly, nuclei are prepared and from an aliquot, total DNA is isolated. The remaining nuclei are mildly digested with micrococcal nuclease followed by the purification of mono- and dinucleosomes by repeated sedimentation on neutral sucrose gradients. Analysis on 6% polyacrylamide gels showed that the mononucleosomes were composed of 145 b.p. and 165 b.p. DNA, while dinucleosomes contained DNA of 335 b.p.

(i.e., 2 × 145 b.p. core plus a 45 b.p. linker, resulting in a nucleosomal repeat length in 10T1/2 of 190 b.p.). The yield of mononucleosomes was 30% of the total nuclear DNA while the yield of dinucleosomes was 11%. The adduct concentrations in the various DNA preparations were calculated from the $[^3H]/[^{14}C]$ratios. Comparable adduct distributions were observed following cellular and exogenous activation of AFB_1. In both cases the initial adduct concentration was much higher in 45 b.p. linker than 145 b.p. core-DNA. The ratios of the adduct concentrations in linker- over core-DNA derived from the concentrations in mononucleosomes and total DNA were 12.7 for cellular activation and 11.1 for exogenous activation; lower ratios of 7.3 for cellular activation and 8.6 for exogenous activation were obtained on the basis of the dinucleosome data. AFB_1 has also been found to be preferentially bound to the linker region compared to core-DNA in trout liver nucleosomes (Bailey et al., 1980).

2. Killing Efficiency of AFB_1-DNA Adducts in Mouse Embryo Fibroblasts 10T1/2

When the logarithm of colony forming ability is plotted against the concentration of total AFB_1-DNA adducts in the range of 1 to 6 μmoles per mole DNA-P, the same linear relationship is obtained when 10T1/2 cells are either treated for a constant length of time (4 h) with increasing AFB_1 concentrations (0.05 to 0.228 μM), treated at a constant AFB_1 concentration (0.2 μM) for various lengths of time (2 to 16 h), or treated at a constant AFB_1 concentration (0.2 μM) for 4 h and replated at low density after different lengths of confluent holding (Fig. 1). The composition of the adduct spectrum differs under these three conditions. After short incubation with AFB_1, AFB_1-N^7-Gua predominates, while after prolonged treatment or prolonged confluent holding, the DNA is enriched in the chemically more stable AFB_1-triamino-Py and minor unidentified adducts which are refractory to excision repair. Under all three conditions approximately 6.7×10^4 AFB_1-DNA adducts kill a 10T1/2 cell. It follows that all (major) AFB_1-adducts possess comparable killing efficiencies and probably kill by a similar or identical mechanism. This may not be astonishing since the structures of the adducts are closely related.

The fact that adduct removal during confluent holding resulted in recovery of viability implicates DNA as a major target for AFB_1 toxicity. Viability recovered by a factor of 4 to 5 regardless of the residual initial viability and the initial adduct concentration. Therefore, the degree of incompleteness of recovery after prolonged confluent holding was larger in experiments with low residual initial viability. The incompleteness of the recovery may be due to the presence of AFB_1-triamino-Py and possibly minor AFB_1-adducts which persist in the DNA.

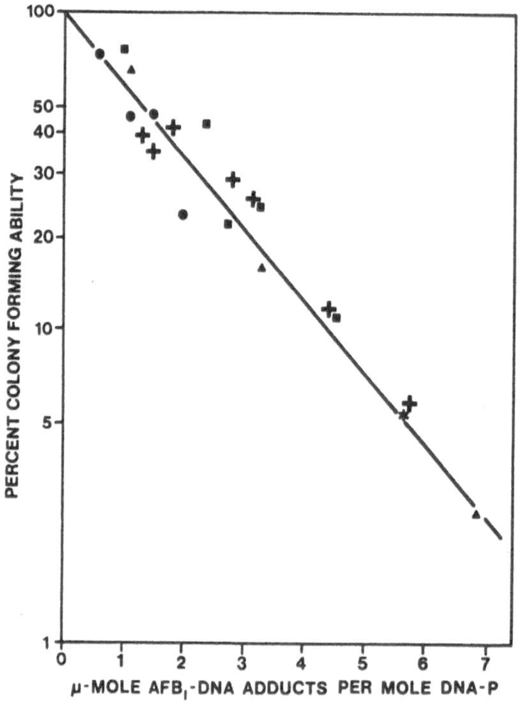

Fig. 1. Killing efficiency of AFB_1-DNA adducts in mouse embryo fibroblasts 10T1/2: relationship between the logarithm of the colony forming ability (CFA) and DNA adduct concentration. Confluent cultures of 10T1/2 cells were treated according to three different protocols and then replated at low densities for the determination of CFA. ●, ▲) Treatment with increasing concentration of AFB_1 from 0.05-0.228 μM for 4 h. ■, *) Treatment with constant AFB_1 concentration of 0.2 μM AFB_1 for increasing length of time from 2-16 h. +) Treatment with 0.2 μM AFB_1 for 4 h followed by confluent holding in conditioned media for 0 to 40 h before replating at low density for CFA determination.

3. Excisability of AFB_1-DNA Adducts

As mentioned in the "Introduction" the extreme lability of AFB_1-DNA adducts complicates the study of their repair. In order to distinguish spontaneous and enzymatic processes we have routinely compared the reactions undergone by AFB_1-DNA *in situ* in the cell to those of free AFB_1-DNA prepared from the same cells but incubated at neutrality in a salt buffer. The latter conditions cannot be considered as truly physiological, however, since the intranuclear pH and the effect of the chromosomal proteins, etc., on the stability

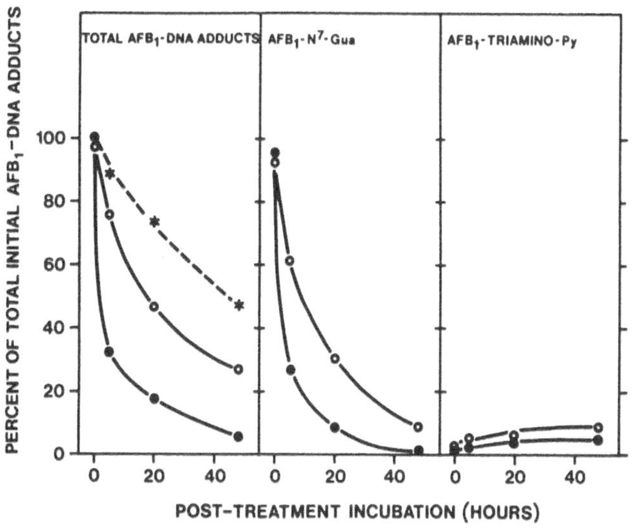

Fig. 2. Kinetics of removal of total AFB_1-DNA adducts, of AFB_1-N^7-Gua and formation of AFB_1-triamino-Py in human epithelioid lung cells A549. Kinetics of the corresponding spontaneous reactions in free AFB_1-DNA prepared from the same cells and incubated at neutrality in vitro as well as of AFB_1-DNA in situ in excision-repair deficient XPA fibroblasts are included as references. A549 cells were pre-labeled with [^{14}C]thymidine and treated for 30 min with 0.25 μM [^{3}H]AFB_1 activated by rat liver microsomes and incubated in conditioned media for 0 to 48 h. The DNA was then isolated and its [^{3}H]- and [^{14}C]-content was determined. In parallel experiments, DNA was incubated in vitro in 0.01 M sodium phosphate - 0.1 M sodium chloride - 0.01 M sodium citrate pH 7.0, at 37°C for 0 to 48 h. The [^{3}H] and [^{14}C]-content of the alcohol precipitable material was determined. The kinetics of the disappearance of AFB_1 adducts are derived from the ratio of the [^{3}H]-content over the total [^{14}C]-content of the sample in relationship to the ratios of samples at 0 h post-treatment incubation. Individual AFB_1 adducts were identified by HPLC. ●) DNA incubated in situ in A549; ○) free DNA incubated in vitro; *) DNA incubated in situ in XPA.

of AFB_1-adducts are not known. Better reference data was obtained by combining the results from free AFB_1-DNA with those of experiments with excision deficient xeroderma pigmentosum group A (XPA) fibroblasts. However, the experiments with XPA also may not yield the exact rates of the spontaneous reactions of intra-cellular AFB_1-DNA. According to present understanding XPA cells are deficient in nucleotide excision repair of bulky DNA lesions but proficient in base excision repair. While our comparative study of XPA and normal human skin fibroblasts (NF) (Leadon et al., 1981) strongly suggest that AFB_1-N^7-Gua is removed (at least in part) by nucleotide excision repair in NF and in analogy also in human epithelioid lung cells A549 (see below), it is conceivable that some adducts are additionally removed via base excision repair. Since repair deficient mutants of mouse embryo fibroblasts 10T1/2 are not available it can only be speculated in analogy to the results with human cells that they also possess the capacity for some enzymatic excision of AFB_1-N^7-Gua. Regardless of the exact contribution of cellular repair it should be stressed that to a large extent the elimination of AFB_1-N^7-Gua was by spontaneous decomposition in all cell types tested.

These conclusions are exemplified in the case of A549 cells in Fig. 2. The kinetics of the disappearance of total AFB_1-adducts and AFB_1-N^7-Gua are shown for cells which had been incubated for 30 min with 0.25 μM AFB_1 in the presence of rat liver microsomes. The experimental conditions have been described previously (Leadon et al., 1981). After different lengths of post-treatment incubation the DNA was prepared by our mild and rapid filter procedure and acid hydrolysates were analyzed by HPLC. In DNA prepared immediately after AFB_1-treatment more than 90% of the adducts consisted of AFB_1-N^7-Gua. Figure 2 also contains the kinetics of the spontaneous reactions undergone by free AFB_1-DNA prepared from the same cells incubated at 37°C in 0.01 M sodium phosphate - 0.1 M sodium chloride - 0.01 M sodium citrate, pH 7.0. For reference purposes the kinetics of the disappearance of total AFB_1-DNA adducts in XPA cells which had been treated and incubated under analogous conditions are included. It is evident that total AFB_1-adducts and AFB_1-N^7-Gua disappear more rapidly from intracellular DNA in A549 implicating cellular repair in the removal process.

The secondary product AFB_1-triamino-Py was formed with similar kinetics in free DNA and *in situ* in A549 cells. Qualitatively similar results were also obtained in NF and 10T1/2 cells. In XPA this adduct was formed more rapidly and to a larger extent presumably because its precursor, AFB_1-N^7-Gua, is removed more slowly in these cells. AFB_1-triamino-Py was chemically and biologically stable in all cell systems tested and persisted in the DNA over prolonged periods of post-treatment incubation.

4. Effect of Confluent Holding on the Transformation of Mouse Embryo Fibroblasts 10T1/2 by AFB_1

In vivo observations suggest that cell proliferation represents an important factor in malignant transformation, e.g., tissues and organs containing rapidly proliferating cells are particularly susceptible to tumor formation (most carcinogens induce cell division and regenerative proliferation in the target tissue as a consequence

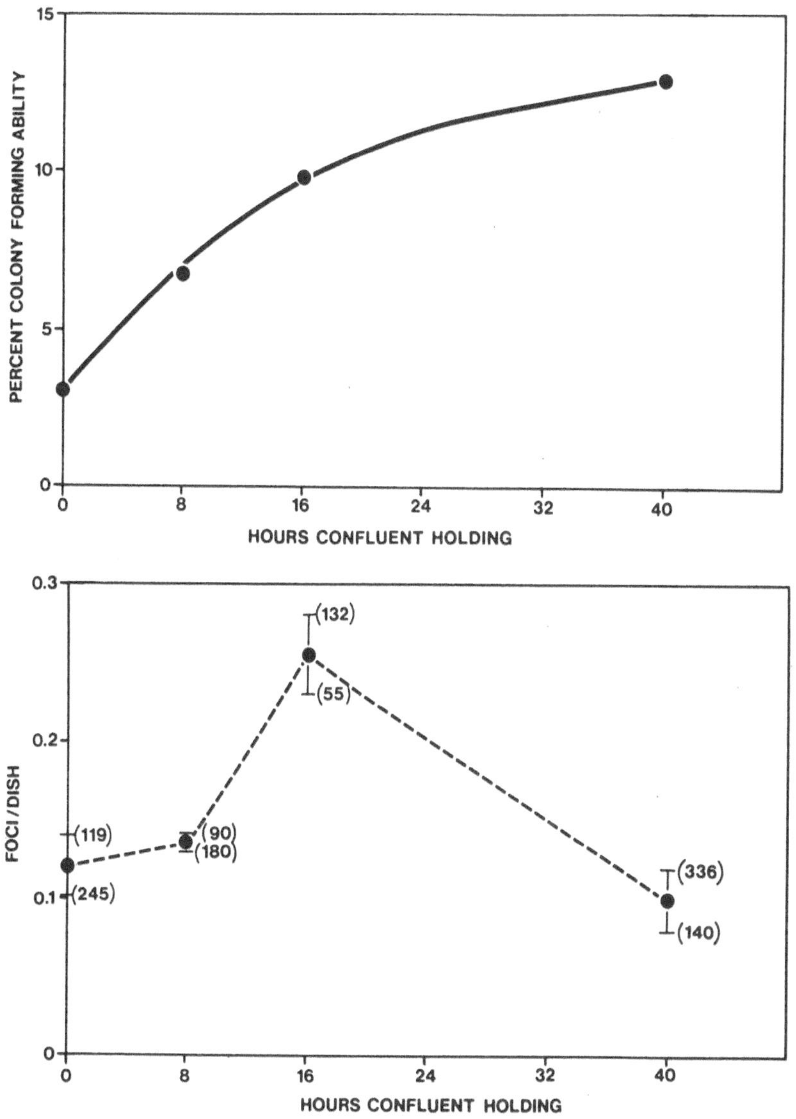

Fig. 3. Effect of confluent holding of AFB_1-treated mouse embryo fibroblasts 10T1/2 cells on colony forming ability (upper half) and formation of transformed foci (lower half). Confluent cultures were treated with 0.3 μM AFB_1 for 16 h and then held in confluency for additional 0 to 40 h before replating at low density for the determination of CFA and the formation of transformed foci. Foci of type II and III per 6 cm Petri dish were scored according to standard procedures (Reznikoff et al., 1973). The values in parenthesis indicate the number of viable cells plated per dish derived from the data for CFA shown in the upper half of the figure.

of their cytotoxic and necrotic effects) (Craddock, 1976; Cayama et al., 1978). Studies with cultured cells also indicate that cell division is a pre-requisite for initiation of transformation following carcinogen treatment (Borek and Sachs, 1974; Kakunaga, 1974). If carcinogen-induced DNA damage represents a trigger in the initiation of transformation, then the elimination or modification of such damage before DNA replication should affect transformation. This concept can be tested in confluent holding experiments. In such experiments cells are treated with the carcinogen in a non-growing, confluent state and replated at low density after differing lengths of post-treatment incubation. Since repair occurs during confluent holding it is expected that the concentration of primary lesions decreases with time. Secondary lesions and particular DNA configurations resulting from repair may increase with confluent holding time, on the other hand. The complexity which may arise for carcinogens inducing a spectrum of structurally distinct lesions has been alluded to in the "Introduction": different lesions produced by the same carcinogen may be processed and biologically expressed with different efficiencies and by different pathways. Therefore, it may be the exception rather than the rule when simple relationships are obtained between the concentration of residual primary DNA lesions at the time of replating from confluency and transformation frequencies as was the case for Balb/3T3 cells treated with 4-nitro-quinoline-N-oxide (Ikenaga and Kakunaga, 1977), 3-methyl-cholanthrene (Kakunaga, 1975) and benzo(a)pyrene (Kakunaga et al., 1980). Results were less straightforward following x-irradiation of 10T1/2 cells (Terzaghi and Little, 1975) and in the present work with AFB_1 (see below).

The aim in our experiments on the effect of confluent holding of AFB_1-treated 10T1/2 cells was to relate the concentration of individual adducts at the time of release from confluency to in vitro transformation. We were particularly interested in the role the persistent lesions AFB_1-triamino-Py play in the transformation process. After confluent holding for 0 to 40 h colony forming ability and potential to form malignant foci were determined according to standard procedures. At the same time DNA was prepared and the concentrations of total AFB_1 adducts, AFB_1-N^7-Gua and AFB_1-triamino-Py were measured by published procedures (Wang and Cerutti, 1980b). At an initial total adduct concentration of 8 µmoles per mole DNA-P the kinetics of adduct removal and formation of AFB_1-triamino-Py were similar to previous results. After 40 h confluent holding 70% of the total adducts and 95% of AFB_1-N^7-Gua had disappeared from the DNA. Approximately half of the remaining adducts now corresponded to AFB_1-triamino-Py. As shown in Fig. 3 (upper half) cell viability recovered by a factor of 4.3 during this time period. The effect of confluent holding on transformation is shown in the lower half of Fig. 3. The number of cells plated for the determination of focus formation after different lengths of confluent holding was adjusted so that the number of viable cells per 6 cm Petri dish stayed in the range of approximately 100-300. The number of transformed foci per dish (foci of type II and III were scored) first increased with confluent holding time, reached a maximum at 16 h and decreased below the initial value after 40 h. (A similar curve is obtained when transformation frequencies, i.e., foci per viable cell, are plotted. However, a strong effect of the number of viable cells plated per dish on the transformation frequencies is now apparent.) It is evident that there exists no simple relationship between the efficiency of transformation, the changes in adduct concentration and the recovery of cell viability as a function of confluent holding. Our results are reminiscent of similar experiments on x-ray-induced transformation of 10T1/2 cells (Terzaghi and Little, 1975). They differ from experiments on transformation of Balb/3T3 cells by 4-nitroquinoline-N-oxide (Ikenaga and Kakunaga, 1977) and 3-methylcholanthrene (Kakunaga, 1975) and benzo(a)pyrene, (Kakunaga et al., 1980) where the decrease in the concentration of the primary carcinogen DNA adducts as a function of confluent holding was paralleled by a corresponding decrease in transformation frequency. It appears that "potentially transforming lesions" are generated during the cellular processing of AFB_1-induced DNA damage which differ from the primary and secondary carcinogen adducts.

ACKNOWLEDGMENT

This work was supported by Grants 3'305.78 and 3'627.80 of the Swiss National Science Foundation.

ABBREVIATIONS

AFB_1: Aflatoxin B_1; AFB_1-N^7-Gua: 2,3-dihydro-2-(N^7-guanyl)-3-hydroxyaflatoxin B_1; AFB_1-triamino-Py: 2,3-dihydro-2-(N^5-formyl-2',5',6'-triamino-4'-oxo-N^5-pyrimidyl)-3-hydroxyaflatoxin B_1; HPLC: high pressure liquid chromatography; NF: normal human skin fibroblasts CRL 1121; XPA: skin fibroblasts strain CRL 1223 from a patient with xeroderma pigmentosum of complementation group A (XP12BE); CFA: colony forming ability; b.p.: base pairs.

REFERENCES

Bailey, G. S., Nixon, J. E., Hendricks, J. D., Sinnhuber, R. O., and Van Holde, K. E., Carcinogen Aflatoxin B_1 is located preferentially in internucleosomal deoxyribonucleic acid following exposure in vivo in rainbow trout, Biochemistry, 19:5836 (1980).

Borek, C., and Sachs, L., The number of cell generations required to fix the transformed state in x-ray induced transformation, Proc. Natl. Acad. Sci. USA, 59:83 (1968).

Campbell, T. C., and Hayes, J. R., The role of aflatoxin metabolism in its toxic lesion, Toxicol. Appl. Pharmacol., 35:199 (1976).

Cayama, E., Tsuda, H., Sarma, D. S. R., and Farber, E., Initiation of chemical carcinogenesis requires cell proliferation, Nature (Lond.), 275:60 (1978).

Craddock, V., in: "Liver Cell Cancer," H. M. Cameron, D. A. Linsell, G. P. Warwick, eds., Elsevier, New York (1976).

Croy, R. G., Essigmann, J. M., Reinhold, V. N., and Wogan, G. N., Identification of the principle aflatoxin B_1-DNA adduct formed in vivo in rat liver, Proc. Natl. Acad. Sci. USA, 75:1745 (1978).

Essigmann, J. M., Croy, R. G., Nadzan, A. M., Busby, W. F., Jr., Reinhold V. N., Büchi, G., and Wogan, G. N., Structural identification of the major DNA adduct formed by aflatoxin B_1 in vitro, Proc. Natl. Acad. Sci. USA, 74:1870 (1977).

Garner, R. C., Miller, E. C., and Miller, J. A., Liver microsomal metabolism of aflatoxin B_1 to a reactive derivative toxic to Salmonella typhimurium TA1530, Cancer Res., 32:2058 (1972).

Garner, R. C., and Wright, C. M., Induction of mutations in DNA-repair deficient bacteria by a liver microsome metabolite of aflatoxin B_1, Br. J. Cancer, 28:544 (1973).

Hertzog, P. J., Smith, J. R. L., and Garner, R. C., A high pressure liquid chromatography study on the removal of DNA-bound aflatoxin B_1 in rat liver and in vitro, Carcinogenesis, 1:787 (1980).

Kakunaga, T., Requirement for cell replication in the fixation and expression of the transformed state in mouse cells treated with 4-nitroquinoline-1-oxide, Int. J. Cancer, 14:736 (1974).

Kakunaga, T., The role of cell division in the malignant transformation of mouse cells treated with 3-methylcholanthrene, Cancer Res., 35:1637 (1975).

Kakunaga, T., Lo, K.-Y., Leavitt, J., and Ikenaga, M., in: "Carcinogenesis: Fundamental Mechanisms and Environmental Effects," B. Pullman, P. Ts'o, and H. Gelboin, eds., D. Reidel, Holland (1980).

Kaneko, M., and Cerutti, P. A., Excision of N-acetoxy-2-acetylaminofluorene-induced DNA adducts from chromatin fractions of human fibroblasts, Cancer Res., 40:4313 (1980).

Kaneko, M., and Cerutti, P. A., Excision of benzo(a)pyrene-diol epoxide I adducts from nucleosomal DNA of confluent normal human fibroblasts, Chem. Biol. Interactions, in press (1981).

Ikenaga, M., and Kakunaga, T., Excision of 4-nitroquinoline 1-oxide damage and transformation in mouse cells, Cancer Res., 37:3672 (1977).

Leadon, S. A., Tyrrell, R. M., and Cerutti, P. A., Excision repair of aflatoxin B_1-DNA adducts in human fibroblasts, Cancer Res., in press (1981).

Lin, J. K., Miller, J. A., and Miller, E. C., 2,3-Dihydro-2(N^7-guanyl)-3-hydroxyaflatoxin B_1, a major acid hydrolysis product of aflatoxin B_1-DNA or -ribosomal RNA adducts formed in hepatic microsome-mediated reactions and in rat liver in vivo, Cancer Res., 37:4430 (1977).

Reznikoff, C. A., Brankow, D. W., and Heidelberger, C., Establishment and characteristics of a cloned line of C3H mouse embryo cells sensitive to postconfluence inhibition of division, Cancer Res., 33:3231 (1973).

Shank, R. C., Gordon, J. E., Wogan, G. N., Nondasuta, A., and Subhamani, B., Dietary aflatoxins and human liver cancer, III., Food Cosmet. Toxicol., 10:71 (1972).
Swenson, D. H., Lin, J. K., Miller, E. C., and Miller, J. A., Aflatoxin B_1-2,3-oxide as a probable intermediate in the covalent binding of aflatoxin B_1 and B_2 to rat liver DNA and ribosomal RNA in vivo, Cancer Res., 37:172 (1977).
Terzaghi, M., and Little, J. B., Repair of potentially lethal radiation damage in mammalian cells is associated with enhancement of maligant transformation, Nature (Lond.), 253:548 (1975).
Wang, T. V., and Cerutti, P. A., Formation and removal of aflatoxin B_1-induced DNA lesions in epithelioid human lung cells, Cancer Res., 39:5165 (1979).
Wang, T. V., and Cerutti, P. A., Spontaneous reactions of aflatoxin B_1-modified DNA in vitro, Biochemistry, 19:1692 (1980a).
Wang, T. V., and Cerutti, P. A., Effect of formation and removal of aflatoxin B_1-DNA adducts in 10T1/2 mouse embryo fibroblasts on cell viability, Cancer Res., 40:2904 (1980b).
Wogan, G. N., Aflatoxin carcinogenesis, Methods Cancer Res., 7:309 (1973).
Wogan, G. N., The induction of liver cell cancer by chemicals, in: "Liver Cell Cancer," H. M. Cameron, D. A. Linsell, and G. P. Warwick, eds., Elsevier, New York (1976).

PARVOVIRAL PROBE FOR ASSESSING THE MUTAGENIC RISK OF LOW DOSES OF RADIATION AND CHEMICALS ADMINISTERED TO HUMAN CELLS

J. J. Cornelis, C. Dinsart, Z. Z. Su, and J. Rommelaere*

Department of Molecular Biology
Université Libre de Bruxelles
B 1640 Rhode Saint Genèse
Belgium

RATIONALE

The marketing of an increasing number of chemicals makes it desirable to dispose of adequate tests for assessing their mutagenic/carcinogenic risk for man. The traditionally used animal tests are often long-lasting and very expensive, especially when the effect of low doses is sought. This led to the development of a battery of semi in vivo and in vitro tests using both prokaryotic and eukaryotic cells, which can be used routinely and serve as a guideline for the in vivo tests [1]. Cells collected from animals, including humans, can be cultured in vitro using appropriate nutritive media. Such cell cultures constitute a relatively well-defined system to analyze the toxic, mutagenic and transforming effect of exposure to environmental compounds. A widely used endpoint is the induction of chromatid and chromosome rearrangements. Visible karyotypic changes, however, do not necessarily accompany mutagenesis and do not provide an absolute indicator of the latter. Selective systems were thus developed, allowing the direct measurement of mutation induction in the genes of mammalian cells [2] or of viruses infecting those cells (see Introduction). The scope of this paper is to validate the use of the Hamster Osteolytic virus H-1, an autonomous parvovirus, for assessing the mutagenic risk associated with the exposure of human cells to low doses of radiations or chemicals.

*To whom correspondence should be addressed.

The genome of parvoviruses is a linear, single-stranded DNA molecule of about 5000 nucleotides [3]. The only known products encoded for by the viral genome are the structural capsid proteins of the virion. The parvovirus H-1 can be propagated in human cells which provide the enzymatic machinery for converting the viral single-strand to a duplex replicative form [4]. The synthesis of parental replicative forms appears to rely entirely on cellular functions. In that respect, parvoviruses are likely to constitute neutral probes of the replication activities displayed by the host cell and can be used to monitor the fidelity of these activities in cells treated with genotoxic agents. In the test to be described below, mutator functions of human cells will thus be identified through their action on the genome of infecting H-1 parvoviruses rather than of the cells themselves.

We feel that parvoviruses offer two unique advantages as a test material for measuring mutagenesis.

(i) Sensitivity

The single-strandedness of the viral genome prevents the occurrence of processes which can antagonize mutation induction. On the one hand, damaged viral single-stranded DNA is not a substrate for the nucleotide excision repair mechanism until converted to a duplex replicative form since the completion of this process requires the presence of a complementary strand. Removal of potentially premutagenic lesions by the pathway of excision repair identified so far in mammalian cells appears essentially error-free [5]. On the other hand, the copy of the viral strand during its conversion to a replicative form is not concomitant with the synthesis of a daughter molecule as is the case when a duplex DNA replicates. In bacteria, the progression of DNA synthesis on a damaged strand has been shown to be helped by the homologous daughter molecule through presumably error-free recombination [6]. In cells infected at a low multiplicity, such a recombinational insertion of preformed segments cannot participate in the conversion of damaged parvoviral DNA which relies instead entirely on de novo synthesis. Therefore, parvoviruses are likely to be especially sensitive to the induction of potentially lethal or mutagenic lesions.

(ii) Rapidity and Convenience

Viral mutagenesis can be measured as viral infectivity under selective conditions preventing the multiplication of nonmutant virus. Parvoviruses are lytic viruses; their infectivity can thus be determined conveniently by their ability to form lysis plaques in monolayers of indicator cells [7]. Using such a plaque assay, parvoviral titers, hence survival and mutagenesis, can be quantitated within a week, all manipulations being confined to the first and last day of the experiment.

Moreover, parvoviruses, like other viral probes, give the opportunity to measure separately two possible mutagenic effects of genotoxic agents. On one hand, direct mutagens can induce the formation of premutagenic DNA lesions which are copied into mutations at the time of replication [8]. On the other hand, work performed with bacteria suggests that some mutagens might also act indirectly by forming lesions whose repair is mutagenic for neighboring sequences [9], and/or by inducing mutator functions which are not expressed by untreated cells [6, 10-12]. The measurement of cell mutagenesis does not allow one to evaluate readily the respective contributions of constitutive and inducible pathways, whereas the use of a viral probe should help by dissociating their effects. On the one hand, a higher mutation frequency in the progeny of virus treated prior to infection of intact cells would be indicative of the operation of constitutive mutagenic process(es), assuming that viral damages are not sufficient to trigger cell mutator activities. On the other hand, the comparison of viral mutagenesis in intact cells and in cultures exposed to a physical or chemical agent prior to infection will indicate whether this treatment activates cellular mutator functions operating on the virus. Therefore, the study of the effects of virus and/or cell treatment on viral mutagenesis should enlighten the relative roles of the direct and indirect routes to mutations in mammalian cells.

SUMMARY

Human and rat cells were exposed to non- or subtoxic doses of UV-light or 2-nitronaphthofuran derivatives prior to infection with intact or UV-irradiated parvovirus H-1. Viral mutagenesis was scored as reversion from the thermosensitive to the wild type phenotype. Cell pretreatment was found to activate the expression or enhance the availability of cellular mutator function(s) responsible for an increased mutation frequency in the progeny of both untreated and UV-damaged H-1 virus. This enhancement of viral mutagenesis appears after a delay following cell treatment and is expressed transiently; it is optimal in cells exposed to non- or subtoxic doses and depends on *de novo* protein synthesis during the interval between cell treatment and virus infection. Viral enhanced mutagenesis is expressed coordinately with an increase in the survival of UV-irradiated virus.

Direct pretreatment of the cells with genotoxic agents is not a prerequisite for the triggering of viral enhanced mutagenesis. Indeed, a similar mutator activity was found to be displayed by undamaged cells provided that they were pre-exposed to extracellularly induced signals. Such exogenous signals include UV-inactivated SV40 or H-1 virus and UV-irradiated DNA from SV40 or calf thymus. These results suggest that DNA lesions *per se* rather than the inactivation of specific cellular genes serve as a signal triggering the expression of viral enhanced mutagenesis. The replication of damaged DNA might not be necessary for the formation of the inducing signal.

Most of the mutations in the progeny of virus exposed to low UV-doses prior to infection of UV-pretreated cells do not result from the formation of premutagenic lesions by virus irradiation; they rather arise from the activation by the cell pretreatment of a mutator function acting upon normal viral DNA. In other words, under those conditions, the majority of viral mutations are apparently generated by an untargeted mutagenesis process stimulated by cell irradiation. Assuming that the viral genome is representative for cellular genes, this observation raises the possibility that a significant fraction of the mutations induced in the genes of cells exposed to low doses of some genotoxic agents might also result from the activation of an untargeted mutator activity. This possibility should be considered when extrapolating the risk at low doses from high doses data.

INTRODUCTION

Viruses have been widely used as probes to identify replication and repair functions of both prokaryotic and eukaryotic cells. This field has been reviewed by Defais et al. [13]. It was first recognized by Weigle [14], back in 1953, that the exposure of bacteria to low fluences of UV-light prior to infection with irradiated bacteriophage increased phage survival and mutagenesis. Further investigation of these phenomena, now known as Weigle reactivation and Weigle mutagenesis, led to the concept of inducible mutator and/or recovery processes as part of a set of different activities, termed SOS functions, whose expression is triggered coordinately in bacteria exposed to various genotoxic agents [10-12]. Although the exact mechanism of Weigle mutagenesis in E. coli is still unknown, it might be associated with the induction of some type of activity allowing to replicate past blocking DNA lesions in the template strand [15, 16].

Phenomena apparently analogous to Weigle reactivation and mutagenesis have been observed in a variety of mammalian, including human cells, using different nuclear-replicating single- and double-stranded DNA viruses as probes [13, 17, 18]. Thus, the survival of these UV-irradiated animal viruses is increased if their host cells are exposed to certain radiations or chemicals prior to infection. This phenomenon, called enhanced virus reactivation [17], is further discussed in an accompanying paper (Rommelaere et al., this volume). Moreover, the treatment of mammalian cells with UV-light [19-25] or certain chemicals [25-27] appears to activate the expression or to enhance the availability of cellular mutator function(s) responsible for an increased mutation frequency in the progeny of both intact [19-23, 25, 26] and UV-irradiated [19, 20, 24, 27] viruses. In some reports however, the mutagenesis of intact [27] or UV-damaged [20-22, 28] virus was found unaltered in cells pre-exposed to these treatments. The reason for this discrepancy is still unclear, although possible parameters have been incriminated [20, 27]. This prompted us to investigate further the phenomenology of enhanced virus mutagenesis, using the single-stranded DNA parvovirus H-1 as a probe of mutagenesis in human and rat cells [23, 26].

The pretreatment of mammalian cells might increase the mutagenesis of infecting viruses (i) by activating or amplifying the expression of cellular mutator functions, or (ii) by enhancing the availability of normally expressed mutator activities, as the result, for instance, of a disturbance of the ongoing cell cycle. Such effects might increase viral as well as cellular mutagenesis. However, a trivial alternative cannot be ruled out, i.e., treated cells are impaired in their competition with the virus for a cellular mutator function. If this were the case, the enhancement of viral mutagenesis would not apply to cellular mutagenesis. Although the data presented in this paper do not rule out the latter possibility, they indicate that a direct cell-deleterious action of the treatment is unlikely to account for their effect on viral mutagenesis. First, undamaged cells display the enhancement of viral mutagenesis upon introduction of an extracellularly induced signal. Second, the inductory ability of closely related derivatives of 2-nitronaphthofuran was found to be correlated with their mutagenicity in a conventional bacterial assay but not with their cytotoxicity. Thus, the possibility should be considered, that the enhanced mutagenesis phenomenon might not be specific to the virus but also relevant to the cell. If so, enhanced virus mutagenesis generates predictions concerning dose-response relationships for mutation induction in mammalian cells. Direct experimental testing of these predictions should challenge the extrapolation of viral mutagenesis to cells.

VIRUS MUTATION ASSAYS

Cell Lines and Virus

The Hamster osteolytic parvovirus (H-1) was propagated in SV40-transformed newborn human kidney cells (NB-E) and Harvey sarcoma virus-transformed rat liver cells (RL5E). Mutagenesis in H-1 virus was studied by determining reversion frequencies of a thermosensitive (ts) mutant to a wild type (wt) phenotype. H-1 ts6 a generous gift of S. L. Rhode, was used routinely. At 39.5°C, H-1 ts6 is deficient in the production of progeny genomes although it is not affected in the formation of double-stranded replicative intermediates. Spontaneous revertant frequencies of the ts6 mutant stocks was about 1×10^{-5}. Conditions of cell maintenance and of virus production and purification have been described previously [23].

Cell Pretreatments

Different treatments were administered to cells prior to H-1 virus infection and tested for their effect on H-1 mutagenesis.

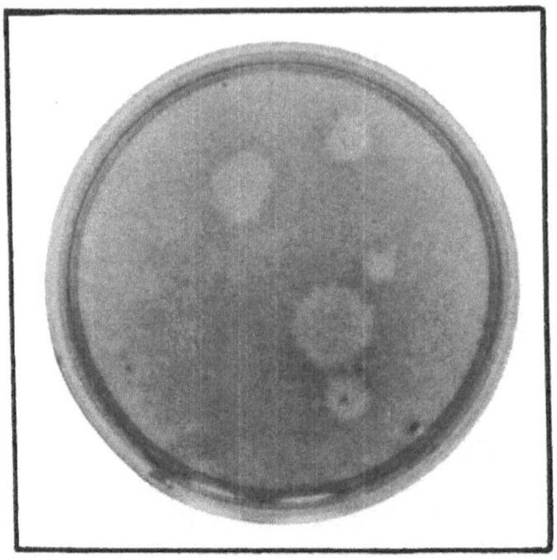

Fig. 1. Plaque formation by H-1 parvovirus in NB-E human indicator cells. Monolayer cultures (8×10^5 cells per 60-mm dish) were infected for 1 h at 37°C with 0.4 ml virus suspension in phosphate buffered saline. Infected cells were overlayed with complete medium containing 0.64% bacto agar. Cultures were stained with neutral red for plaque visualization 6 days after infection.

Direct cell pretreatments were either a short dose of UV-radiation (predominant wavelength = 254-nm) or a one hour-incubation in the presence of 2-nitronaphthofuran derivatives. Two closely related 2-nitronaphthofuran derivatives, termed R 7000 and R 7160, were kindly provided by R. Royer. R 7000 is one of the most potent mutagens in the *Salmonella typhimuorium* reversion assay whereas R 7160 is only a weak mutagen [29].

Indirect cell pretreatments were (i) infection with UV-inactivated H-1 ts6, UV-irradiated MVM (another parvovirus, kindly provided by D. C. Ward) or UV-damaged SV40, or (ii) transfection with UV-irradiated DNA from SV40 or calf thymus. Wild-type SV40 (strain 776) or the early mutant ts A209 [30] (a kind give of R. G. Martin) were used. The ts A SV40 mutant is defective in the initiation of viral DNA replication at 41°C [31]. Supercoiled form I SV40 DNA was isolated by sedimentation in sucrose gradients [32] of total viral DNA extracted from infected cells according to the Hirt procedure [33]; a stock solution (0.1 mg/ml) was prepared in Tris buffer (pH 7.5) and stored at -70°C. Highly polymerized calf thymus DNA type I was obtained from Sigma, purified with repeated chloroform-isoamyl alcohol extractions and ethanol-precipitated; a stock solution (4 mg/ml) was prepared in distilled water and stored at -20°C.

Conditions for cell UV-irradiation, treatment with chemicals and virus infection have been detailed elsewhere [23, 26]. DNA transfection was performed according to either the DEAE-dextran [34] or the calcium phosphate precipitation [35] techniques.

Mutation Assays

Virus revertants were identified by their infectivity at the nonpermissive temperature (39.5°C). Viral infectivity (titer) was quantitated by the formation of lysis plaques in growing monolayers of NB-E indicator cells (Fig. 1).

A single-cycle and two direct-plating assays were used with essentially identical results [23]. Briefly, asynchronous NB-E or RL5E cells were exposed to the above-mentioned inducing pretreatments, incubated for various times at 37°C and infected with H-1 ts6.

For single-cycle assay, the infected cultures were kept at the permissive temperature (33°C) for 30 h under conditions preventing secondary virus infections. The virus produced was harvested and titered at 39.5°C and 33°C, using NB-E as indicators.

The direct-plating assay was either a direct-plaque assay or an infectious-center assay. For the former assay, infected NB-E cultures were used directly as indicators for plaque formation at 33°C and 39.5°C. For the latter assay, primarily infected NB-E or RL5E cells were harvested 4 h after infection, seeded on top of monolayers of untreated NB-E indicator cells and tested for their ability to initiate plaque formation at 33°C and 39.5°C.

The multiplicity of infection (MOI*) varied depending on the assay and conditions. Typical ranges for unirradiated H-1 ts6 were: for the single-cycle assay, 0.7 (PFU/cell); for the direct-plaque assay, 10^{-5}-10^{-4} at 33°C and 1-10 at 39.5°C; for the infectious center assay, 10^{-3} (33°C) and 5-10 (39.5°C). In experiments including UV-irradiated virus, MOIs were: for the single-cycle assay, 5; for the direct plaque assay, 10^{-5}-10^{-2} (33°C) and 1-100 (39.5°C).

Definitions

The mutation frequency is defined as the fraction of infectious particles (plaque-forming units at 33°C) that form plaques at the nonpermissive temperature. Enhanced mutagenesis is expressed by the ratio of the mutation frequency in treated to that in control cells.

*The MOI refers to the number of infectious (plaque-forming) virus particles (PFU) per cell for an equivalent inoculum of unirradiated virus titered by direct-plaque assay at permissive temperature on untreated NB-E cells.

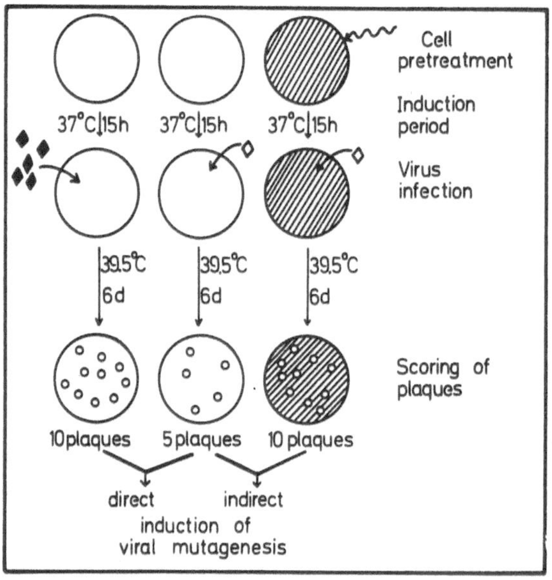

Fig. 2. Direct-plaque assay of enhanced virus mutagenesis. Monolayer cultures of NB-E human cells in 60-mm petri dishes are exposed (hatched circles) or not (open circles) to an inducing treatment, incubated at 37°C for 15 h and infected with intact (◇) or treated (◆) parvovirus H-1 ts6. The higher multiplicity of infection used for treated virus compensates for lethality (as measured at 33°C). After infection, parallel cultures are kept at 33°C (not shown) and 39.5°C for 7 and 6 days respectively, and stained for plaque visualization. An increase in the number of viral revertants forming plaques at nonpermissive temperature can arise directly from the treatment of the virus or indirectly from the pretreatment of the cells. The latter increase defines the enhanced virus mutagenesis phenomenon (provided that a similar effect does not occur at 33°C). Cell pretreatment can also enhance the mutagenesis of damaged parvovirus (not shown).

An increase in the number of revertants (plaques at 39.5°C) in pretreated versus control cells will thus be considered as indicative of enhanced virus mutagenesis, provided that no or a lesser increase is found at 33°C. The most convenient procedure to demonstrate this phenomenon is the direct-plaque assay, as illustrated by Fig. 2. However, the other assays were necessary to rule out that higher virus titers at 39.5°C in pretreated cells, could merely be ascribed to a higher ability of treated indicator cells to reveal the plaques at the nonpermissive temperature or to a greater

Table 1. Indirect Induction of Enhanced Mutagenesis of Intact H-1 ts6

Inducing treatment	Cells	Reversion frequency (× 10^6)	Enhanced mutagenesis
No	NB-E	6.2 ± 0.3	-
	RL5E	6.6 ± 0.2	-
UV-radiation	NB-E	11.9 ± 0.3	1.9 ± 0.5
	RL5E	12.0 ± 0.2	1.8 ± 0.4
R 7000	NB-E	11.8 ± 0.3	1.9 ± 0.4
	RL5E	13.2 ± 0.3	2.0 ± 0.3

NB-E human cells or RL5E rat cells were UV-irradiated (4.5 J m^{-2}) or incubated for 1 h at 37°C with 2-nitro-7-methoxy-naphthofuran (R 7000, 0.1 μg/ml). Treated cultures were incubated for 14 h at 37°C, infected with untreated H-1 ts6 and processed for mutation assay. Enhanced mutagenesis is the ratio of the viral mutation frequency in treated cells versus that in control cultures. Average values and standard deviations of 3 or more experiments.

capacity of treated cells to produce virus under restrictive conditions. The infectious center assay precludes the former pitfall, the single-cycle assay avoids both of them.

RESULTS

Indirect Induction of Enhanced Mutagenesis of Intact Parvovirus H-1 ts6

As shown in Table 1, the reversion frequency of H-1 ts6 is higher if the host human or rat cells are exposed to UV-radiation or to a chemical mutagen prior to infection. This phenomenon is termed enhanced virus mutagenesis. The doses which were administered to the cells in order to activate this response are low and did not induce any cell lethality as measured by colony formation ability [23, 26]. An enhanced viral mutation frequency might arise if the cell pretreatment conferred a selective advantage to the revertants or altered the number of viral DNA replicating rounds. This possibility is not favored by the lack of a detectable effect of the treatment of the cells either on their capacity to plaque H-1 ts6 or revertant virus or on the size and the kinetics of production of the viral bursts [23]. Therefore, it seems more likely that the induction of an enhanced mutagenesis of intact virus arises from the activation of a cellular mutator function responsible for an increased mutation rate during the replication of normal viral DNA.

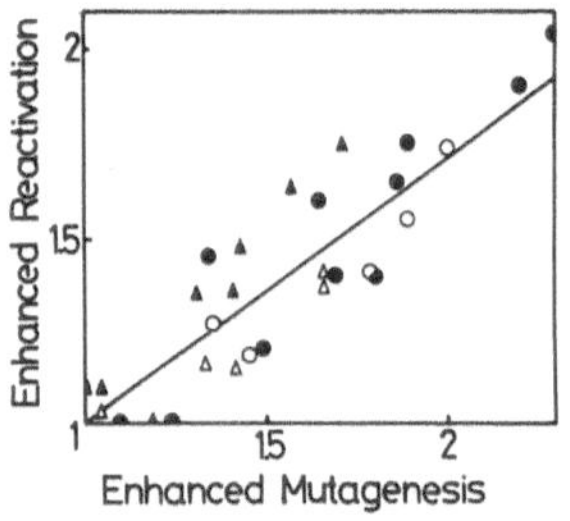

Fig. 3. Correlation between enhanced mutagenesis and enhanced viral reactivation in human and rat cells pretreated with 2-nitronaphthofuran derivatives. NB-E and RL5E cells were incubated for 1 h at 37°C with different concentrations (0.025-4 μg/ml) of the nitronaphthofuran derivatives R 7000 and R 7160. Treated cells were incubated for various times (0-35 h) at 37°C and infected either with unirradiated H-1 ts6 for mutation measurement or with UV-irradiated H-1 wt (85 J m^{-2}; survival = 2×10^{-4}) for survival measurement. Enhanced reactivation is defined by the ratio of the survival of UV-damaged virus in treated versus control cells (see also Rommelaere et al., this volume). Enhanced mutagenesis is defined by the ratio of the mutation frequency of intact virus in treated cultures to that in control cells. Closed symbols, various concentrations of chemicals; open symbols, various incubation times between cell treatment and infection; circles, R 7000; triangles, R 7160. The regression line is drawn.

In an accompanying paper (Rommelaere et al., this volume) we describe another response which is triggered in treated cells, namely the enhanced reactivation of the survival of UV-damaged virus. As shown in Fig. 3, the reactivation of enhanced virus mutagenesis is highly correlated with that of enhanced reactivation in cells exposed to UV-light or to 2-nitronaphthofuran derivatives. Variations in the dose or in the time of administration of the inducer caused similar changes in the amplitude of both phenomena. Enhanced mutagenesis and reactivation are thus expressed coordinately at least with respect to their dose response and time course.

Figure 4a shows the level of enhanced virus mutagenesis in function of the concentration of 2-nitronaphthofuran derivatives (R 7000 and R 7160) administered to the cells prior to infection with intact virus. The amplitude of enhanced mutagenesis increases with the dose up to a maximal value and eventually drops at higher doses. This maximum is higher and is reached at a concentration 25 times lower for R 7000 than for R 7160. R 7000 is thus a much more potent inducer of enhanced virus mutagenesis than R 7160. This property cor-

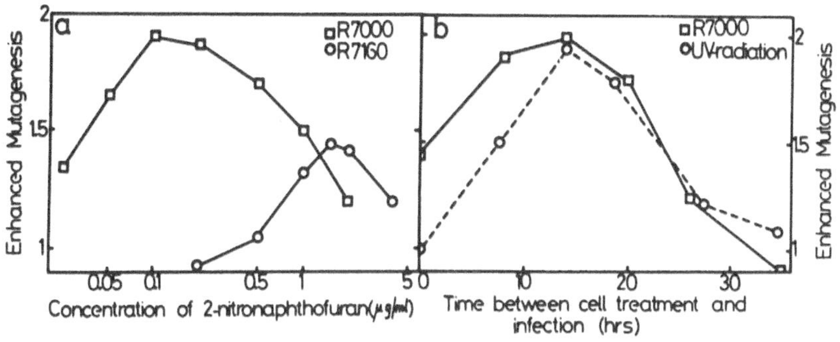

Fig. 4. Dose response (a) and time course (b) of enhanced virus mutagenesis. RL5E cells are exposed to UV-light (4.5 J m^{-2}) or to a 1 h incubation in the presence of various concentrations of R 7000 and R 7160 2-nitronaphthofuran derivatives (a) or 0.1 µg/ml R 7000 (b). Treated cells were incubated at 37°C for 14 h (a), or various times (b) prior to infection with untreated H-1 ts6 and processing for mutation assay. Average values from 2 experiments are presented; standard deviation was less than 20%.

Table 2. Effect of Cycloheximide on Enhanced Mutagenesis of Intact H-1 ts6 in Human or Rat Cells Pretreated with UV-Radiation or R 7000 Nitronaphthofuran Derivative

Treatment	Cells	Enhanced virus mutagenesis without CH	with CH
UV	NB-E	1.9	0.9
UV	RL5E	2.0	1.2
R 7000	RL5E	1.8	1.05

After treatment with UV-light (4.5 J m^{-2}) or R 7000 (0.1 µg/ml, 1 h), cells were incubated for 14 h at 37°C in the presence of 5-7.5 µg/ml cycloheximide (CH). After extensive rinsing, cells were infected with intact H-1 ts6 and processed for mutation assay. Under these conditions, CH did not affect significantly plaque formation in untreated cells. Enhanced mutagenesis is the ratio of the viral reversion frequency in UV- or R 7000-treated cells versus that in control cultures. Data are from 2 experiments; standard deviation was less than 25%.

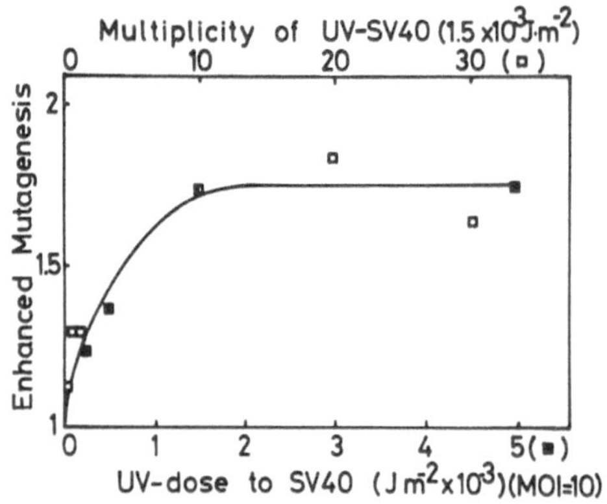

Fig. 5. Dose response of enhanced mutagenesis of intact H-1 ts6 in cells pretreated with UV-damaged wt SV40. RL5E cells were infected with SV40 which had been irradiated either with increasing UV-doses (■, MOI = 10) or with 1.5×10^3 J m^{-2} (□, increasing MOIs). Treated cells were incubated for 12 h at 37°C prior to infection with intact H-1 ts6 and processing for mutation assay. Average values of 2 experiments are shown; standard deviation was less than 25%.

relates with the differential mutagenicity of these compounds in a conventional bacterial mutation test. Indeed, R 7000 is one of the most potent mutagens known in the Salmonella assay whereas R 7160 is a weak mutagen [29]. In contrast, no simple relationship was found between the inducing potency of these derivatives and their cytotoxicity. R 7000 had its highest induction at a nonlethal concentration whereas R 7160 was most efficient at a dose killing 50-80% of the cells [26].

The time-course of enhanced virus mutagenesis is illustrated by Fig. 4b. The expression of this phenomenon is optimal if a 12-15 h delay is allowed between cell treatment with UV-light or R 7000 and virus infection. Moreover, the response is activated transiently and has decayed by 36 h following cell treatment. The induction of enhanced virus mutagenesis requires that active protein synthesis takes place in the cell during the interval between treatment and infection. Indeed, cycloheximide, an inhibitor of de novo protein synthesis, abolished specifically the induction if present during that period (Table 2).

Nature of the Signal-Activating Enhanced Virus Mutagenesis

We posed the question of whether the indirect induction of viral mutagenesis in pretreated cultures required the direct hitting of the cells by the genotoxic agent or whether it could be activated

Table 3. Activation of Enhanced Mutagenesis of Intact H-1 ts6 by Extracellularly Induced Triggers

	Induction treatment	Conditions	Cells	Enhanced mutagenesis
1	UV-H1 ts6	MOI = 10; 200 J m^{-2}	RL5E	2.0 ± 0.4
			NB-E	2.0 ± 0.3
2	UV-MVM	MOI = 40; 200 J m^{-2}	NB-E	1.8 ± 0.3
3	SV40 wt virus	MOI = 10	RL5E	0.9 ± 0.1
4	UV-SV40 wt virus	MOI - 10; 1500 J m^{-2}	RL5E	1.9 ± 0.3
5	SV40 ts A209 virus	MOI = 10; 41°C	RL5E	1.05 ± 0.2
6	UV-SV40 ts A209 virus	MOI = 10; 41°C 1500 J m^{-2}	RL5E	1.8 ± 0.2
7	SV40 wt DNA	14 μg/10^6 cells; DEAE dextran	RL5E	1.2 ± 0.3
		2 μg/10^6 cells; Calcium*	RL5E	1.1
8	UV-SV40 wt DNA	14 μg/10^6 cells; 1500 J m^{-2}; DEAE dextran	RL5E	1.5 ± 0.2
		2 μg/10^6 cells; 1500 J m^{-2}; Calcium*	RL5E	1.85
9	Calf thymus DNA	10 μg/10^6 cells; DEAE dextran	RL5E	1.0 ± 0.2
		15 μg/10^6 cells; DEAE dextran	NB-E	1.05 ± 0.2
10	UV-calf thymus DNA	10 μg/10^6 cells; 1500 J m^{-2}; DEAE dextran	RL5E	1.4 ± 0.3
		15 μg/10^6 cells; 1500 J m^{-2}; DEAE dextran	NB-E	1.5 ± 0.3

RL5E or NB-E cells were either infected with UV-inactivated parvovirus H-1 ts6 or MVM or with intact or UV-damaged SV40 virus, or they were transfected with intact or UV-irradiated DNA from SV40 or calf thymus. After treatment cells were incubated for 14 h at 41°C (cultures treated with SV40 ts A) or 37°C (all other cultures), they were infected with intact H-1 ts6 and processed for mutation assay (infectious center procedure). Enhanced mutagenesis is the ratio of the reversion frequency of intact H-1 ts6 in cells exposed to exogenous inducers to that in control cultures. Results from a single (*) or at least 2 experiments (average values and standard deviations).

by extracellularly induced signals introduced into undamaged cells. The latter possibility is supported by the data shown in Table 3. An enhanced mutagenesis of intact H-1 ts6 could be induced with the same amplitude as in UV-pretreated cells, by preinfecting intact cells with UV-irradiated single-stranded (lines 1, 2) or double-stranded (line 4) DNA viruses. In order to exert its activity, the "signalling" virus has to be irradiated (lines 3, 4), suggesting that UV-lesions confer an inducing ability which is not normally expressed by undamaged virus. As shown in Fig. 5, the level of enhanced mutagenesis is determined by the total number of lesions introduced into the cell by the viral carrier, irrespectively of whether this number is varied by changing the UV-dose to the virus or the multiplicity of infection. Although it was not measured directly, one can estimate from the particle to infectivity ratio of the viruses used as signal, that in the conditions of Table 3 (lines 1-4), UV-irradiated H-1, MVM and SV40 introduced similar numbers of lesions per cell [23]. These viruses also induced the same amplitude of enhanced mutagenesis of intact H-1 ts6, suggesting that this phenomenon does not depend on the homology between the signalling and probe viruses. The time course of enhanced virus mutagenesis in cells preinfected with UV-damaged virus is similar to that shown in Fig. 4b for UV-preirradiated cells [23].

The data presented in Table 3, lines 7-10, strongly suggest that the lesions involved in the activation of the cellular mutator function reside in DNA. Indeed, extracellularly irradiated DNA from SV40 or calf thymus enhances viral mutagenesis upon transfection of undamaged cells. Similarly to intact virus, unirradiated DNA has no or little signalling capacity. An intriguing possibility is that replication forks blocked in the vicinity of lesions in parental DNA mediate the induction process [36, 37]. We challenged this possibility by testing whether the inhibition of the replication of SV40 DNA affected its signalling capacity. Although the rat cells used were nonpermissive to SV40, an abortive initiation of SV40 DNA replication cannot be ruled out. Therefore, we used a thermosensitive SV40 mutant belonging to the A complementation group. At the restrictive temperature, SV40 tsA is unable to initiate DNA replication, although a low frequency of aberrant initiation from secondary origins might occur [38]. As shown in Table 3 (lines 5, 6) this deficiency did not impede induction by UV-irradiated SV40, suggesting that the blockage of normal DNA replication might not be necessary for the generation of the signal from damaged DNA.

Effect of Virus UV-Irradiation on Its Mutagenesis in Control and UV-Pretreated Cells

The data presented in the previous section emphasize a possible pitfall of the use of UV-damaged virus as a probe of the enhanced mutagenesis process. Indeed, irradiated virus itself may provide the cells with an inducing signal. If this selftriggering satur-

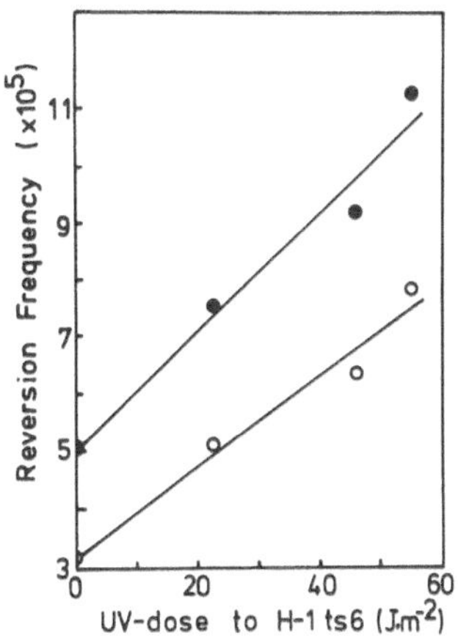

Fig. 6. Effect of UV-irradiation of H-1 ts6 on its mutagenesis in control and UV-irradiated human cells. NB-E cells were UV-irradiated (4.5 J m^{-2}) or not, incubated for 14 h at 37°C and infected with H-1 ts6 (MOI = 5) which had been irradiated with increasing UV-doses. Cultures were then processed for single-cycle mutation assay. o) Unirradiated cells; •) UV-irradiated cells. Average values of 4 experiments are shown; standard deviations were less than 25%.

ated the inducibility of the culture, it would mask the effect of the pretreatment of the cells. Dose and infection conditions were thus sought, minimizing the signalling action of UV-irradiated parvovirus. At a multiplicity of infection of 5, UV-damaged parvovirus MVM has little effect on the mutagenesis of coinfecting intact H-1 ts6 up to a dose of 60 J m^{-2} (not shown). These conditions were selected to analyze the mutagenesis of UV-irradiated H-1 ts6 in control and UV-pretreated cells.

Figure 6 shows that the reversion frequency in H-1 ts6 increases with the UV-dose administered to the virus, in both intact and UV-preirradiated cells. Control and treated cultures differ however, in two respects: (i) at the zero dose, the viral mutation frequency is higher in irradiated cells; this enhanced "untargeted" mutagenesis has been described in previous sections; (ii) if the results obtained so far are fitted to linear dose responses, the slope of the mutation induction curve is steeper for UV-pretreated cells. As the dose to the virus increases, the level of induction due to cell preirradiation progressively shifts from enhanced untargeted mutagenesis to the ratio of the slopes for treated versus control cells. It is apparent from Fig. 6 that this ratio is greater than 1.0 in our system, although the induction is small and should be validated by further experiments. If confirmed, these results would indicate that in addition to its effect on the mutagenesis of normal DNA, the cell pretreatment increases specifically the risk of mutation at (some) UV-induced DNA sites. It should be noted however, that for UV-doses to H-1 ts6 similar to the inducing treatment given to the cells (less than 5 J m^{-2}), the majority of the viral mutations induced in preirradiated cells arises from enhanced untargeted mutagenesis, irrespective of the presence of premutagenic lesions in viral DNA.

DISCUSSION

1. The Enhanced Virus Mutagenesis Phenomenon

The evidence presented in this paper (Tables 1 and 3) and from the literature [19-27] suggests that intracellular endogeneous or exogeneous DNA damaged by various physical or chemical agents, generates conditions promoting the mutagenesis of infecting viruses. Enhanced virus mutagenesis can be activated by treatments devoid of any detectable cell-killing effect. Moreover, equitoxic compounds can differ drastically in their inducing potency (Fig. 4a). The enhancement of viral mutagenesis is therefore unlikely to be accounted for by a non-specific impairment of treated cells in their competition with the virus for shared cellular factors. An attractive alternative would thus be that tolerable amounts of certain DNA lesions within the cells generate, activate or enhance the availability of cellular factors stimulating mutagenesis.

2. Mechanism of Mutagenesis

The pretreatment of the cells might enhance viral mutagenesis by decreasing the fidelity of the DNA replication machinery and/or its ability to tolerate lesions in parental strands. Other candidate mechanisms which might be induced in treated cells include (i) mutagenic repair or modification of primary or secondary DNA lesions, and (ii) generation of non-lethal but premutagenic DNA lesions. The pretreatment of the cells appears to increase the probability of mutagenesis both at normal [19-23, 25, 26] and UV-damaged [19, 20, 24, 27] viral DNA sites (Fig. 6b). This result is consistent with an effect of the treatment on the properties of the DNA replication machinery. However, a role of repair or modification of lesions cannot be ruled out since the so-called intact parvovirus might comprise a significant number of spontaneous lesions, such as depurination sites [39].

The expression of the enhancement of viral mutagenesis is tightly coupled to that of an enhanced reactivation of virus survival [19-22, 24-27] (Fig. 3). A single mechanism might give rise to both phenomena by rendering (some) lesions more mutagenic but also more tolerable. Alternatively, the mechanisms of reactivation and mutagenesis might be different but expressed coordinately as part of a set of activities under common regulation like the SOS functions in bacteria [10-12]. Actually, parvovirus reactivation was shown to be enhanced concomitantly with the cell capacity to replicate intact virus, but the triggering of both responses could be dissociated in certain cell lines [40]. Whether the same relationship applies to enhanced mutagenesis, is an open question.

Exposure to bacteria to SOS conditions has been shown to alleviate the inhibition of replication of damaged phage DNA. The tolerance of lesions such as pyrimidine dimers [15] or apurinic sites [16] might lead to increased misincorporation. It is not known whether induced mutagenesis operates via a similar route in mammalian cells, although data consistent with this possibility have been presented [27].

3. Process of Induction

Damaged DNA apparently provides the primary signal triggering enhanced viral mutagenesis (Table 3). The active effector which lies in or is generated from damaged DNA is not known. A good correlation was found between the ability of various compounds to induce enhanced virus reactivation and to arrest DNA replication, suggesting that blocked replication forks are a direct or indirect signal of induction [36, 37]. Yet, the evidence presented in Table 3, using SV40 ts A as a trigger, suggests that the inhibition of the replication of damaged DNA does not impede its signalling activity. Blockage of DNA replication might thus not be an absolute prerequisite for induction. Secondary DNA gaps or degradation products could possibly serve as intermediates. In bacteria, specific oligodeoxynucleotides have been shown to possess an inducing potency [41].

The expression of enhanced mutagenesis is delayed following cell treatment [19, 21-23, 25, 26] and requires active cellular protein synthesis during this interval [23, 26] (Fig. 4b; Table 2). The inhibition of protein synthesis during the induction period specifically abolishes the enhancement of viral mutagenesis without affecting significantly its spontaneous level. These properties are consistent with the induction of the synthesis of new or amplified proteins directly or indirectly responsible for increased mutagenesis. However, ongoing constitutive processes involving short-lived or cell cycle-dependent protein might also account for these results.

The magnitude of enhanced virus mutagenesis increases with the dose given to cells, then saturates and eventually drops at higher doses [23-27] (Fig. 4a). This response might be inherent in the induction process. Alternatively, it might result from a competition between the inducing action of the treatment and its inactivating effect, which would be in favor of the former at low doses and of the latter at high dose.

4. Applicability of the Viral Mutation Assay

The dose administered to cells for inducing maximal enhancement of viral mutagenesis is low and devoid of any killing effect, at least for potent inducers such as UV-light [23] or the R 7000 2-nitronaphthofuran derivatives [26]. In this respect, the enhanced virus mutagenesis assay provides a sensitive screening test for indirect mutagens. The UV-dose eliciting maximal enhanced reactivation and mutagenesis was around 3 J m^{-2} for parvovirus H-1 in human NB-E cells. The use of excision-deficient human fibroblasts from Xeroderma pigmentosum patients increased the sensitivity of the reactivation assay to 0.1 J m^{-2} [42]. Such doses are similar to those required for a significant induction of cell mutations in in vitro cultures [43]. It should be noted that the enhancement factor is small (of the order of two-fold), yet the viral mutation assay is most reliable (standard deviation for independent measurements of enhanced parvorvirus mutagenesis was less than 20%). The wide host range of parvovirus gives also the hope of increasing the applicability of the assay by selecting human cells in which the enzymatic activating system necessary for many carcinogens is present.

For the series of 2-nitronaphthofuran derivatives studied, a good correlation was found between the activity in a conventional mutation assay [29] and the ability to trigger enhanced virus reactivation [26, 37] or mutagenesis [26] (Fig. 4a). These responses thus appear to be good indicators of the mutagenicity of such chemicals. However, other compounds might conceivably be poor inducers of enhanced virus mutagenesis but still be potent direct mutagens [8]. In order to be used as a screening test, the viral mutation assay should thus include a measurement of the direct induction of mutations by treatment of the virus prior to infection of intact cells (Fig. 6). As discussed previously, parvoviruses are likely to be a sensitive probe for this type of measurement too.

5. Implication for Cell Mutagenesis: Dose Response Relationship

Let us consider the routes of mutation induction in the progeny of H-1 ts6 exposed to a UV-dose of 4 J m^{-2} prior to infection of cells preirradiated with the same dose. It is apparent from Fig. 6 that under these conditions, most of viral mutations would arise from the activation of untargeted mutagenesis rather than from the formation of premutagenic lesions in viral DNA. If the dose to the virus was increased, the untargeted component induced by the pretreatment of the cells, would get progressively masked by targeted mutagenesis.

If the same routes led to cell mutagenesis, the majority of mutations induced in cells exposed to low doses of UV-light or UV-mimicking chemicals might also result from the activation of a mutator function misreplicating undamaged DNA. However, the validity of generalizing the mutagenesis of parvovirus to that of the host cell remains to be demonstrated. It should be indeed be considered that (i) the parvoviral genome is devoid of part of the structural complexity of a cellular gene; (ii) the number of DNA replication rounds during the period of expression of enhanced mutagenesis, is much higher for virus than for cells, and (iii) the specific interdependence of the virus and its host might bias viral mutagenesis.

Bearing these restrictions in mind, the enhanced virus mutagenesis phenomenon questions the prediction of the cell mutation risk at low doses from high-dose data. Indeed, an induced saturable mutator function operating, in particular, upon intact portions of DNA, might increase unexpectedly the mutation risk at low doses and give rise to nonlinear dose responses. The analysis of cell mutation induction curves does not readily reveal such characteristics and has not so far provided any conclusive evidence to support the activation of a mutator function in mammalian cells [44]. However, experimental fluctuations inherent to the cell mutation assays obscure the study of the effect of low doses. Recent improvements in the sensitivity of these assays will hopefully allow one to challenge the possibility that the cellular process enhancing viral mutagenesis is also active on the DNA of the cells themselves.

ACKNOWLEDGMENTS

We thank very much Prof. D. C. Ward in whose laboratory this work was initiated and Prof. M. Errera for his interest and support. We acknowledge Dr. S. L. Rhode III for his gift of the H-1 mutant and Dr. R. Royer for providing 2-nitronaphthofurans. We are indebted to D. Rommelaere for editorial assistance. This work was supported by the European Communities (Contract ENV/355/B), the Ministère de la Santé Publique (Contract 0392/1980) and the Fonds National de la Recherche Médicale (Contract 3.4514.80). J. Rommelaere is Chercheur Qualifié du Fonds National Belge de la Recherche Scientifique.

REFERENCES

1. M. Hollstein and J. McCann, Short term tests for carcinogens and mutagens, Mutation Res., 65:133 (1979).
2. R. S. Gupta and L. Siminovitch, Genetic markers for quantitative mutagenesis studies in Chinese hamster ovary cells, Mutation Res., 69:113 (1980).
3. P. Tattersall and D. C. Ward, The parvoviruses: an introduction, in: "Replication of Mammalian Parvoviruses," D. C. Ward and P. Tattersall, eds., p. 3 Cold Spring Harbor Laboratory, New York (1978).

4. S. L. Rhode, H-1 DNA synthesis, in: "Replication of Mammalian Parvoviruses," D. C. Ward and P. Tattersall, eds., p. 279, Cold Spring Harbor Laboratory, New York (1978).
5. T. W. Glover, C. C. Chang, J. E. Trosko, and S. L. Li, Ultraviolet light induction of diphteria toxin-resistant mutants in normal and Xeroderma pigmentosum human fibroblasts, Proc. Natl. Acad. Sci. USA, 76:3982 (1979).
6. J. D. Hall and D. W. Mount, Mechanisms of DNA replication and mutagenesis in ultraviolet-irradiated bacteria and mammalian cells, Progress in Nucleic Acid Res., 25:53 (1981).
7. S. L. Rhode, Replication process of the parvovirus H-1, J. Virol., 17:659 (1976).
8. J. W. Drake and R. H. Baltz, The biochemistry of mutagenesis, Ann. Rev. Biochem., 45:11 (1976).
9. B. A. Bridges, Ultraviolet light mutagenesis in bacteria: a result of the failure of normal error-correcting mechanisms?, in: "Progress in Environmental Mutagenesis," M. Alacevic, ed., p. 131, Elsevier, Amsterdam (1980).
10. M. Radman, SOS repair hypothesis: phenomenology of an inducible DNA repair which is accompanied by mutagenesis, in: "Molecular Mechanisms for Repair of DNA," P. C. Hanawalt and R. B. Setlow, eds., p. 355, Plenum, New York (1975).
11. E. M. Witkin, Ultraviolet mutagenesis and inducible DNA repair in Escherichia coli, Bacteriol. Rev., 40:869 (1976).
12. S. Gottesman, Genetic control of the SOS system in Escherichia coli, Cell, 23:1 (1981).
13. M. J. Defais, P. C. Hanawalt, and A. R. Sarasin, Viral probes for DNA repair, Adv. in Radiat. Biol., 10:in press (1981).
14. J. J. Weigle, Induction of mutations in a bacterial virus, Proc. Natl. Acad. Sci. USA, 39:628 (1953).
15. P. Caillet-Fauquet, M. J. Defais, and M. Radman, Molecular mechanisms of induced mutagenesis: replication in vivo of bacteriophage ϕX174 single-stranded, ultraviolet light-irradiated DNA in intact and irradiated host cells, J. Mol. Biol., 117:95 (1977).
16. R. M. Schaaper and L. A. Loeb, Depurination causes mutations in SOS-induced cells, Proc. Natl. Acad. Sci. USA, 78:1773 (1981).
17. C. D. Lytle, Radiation-enhanced virus reactivation in mammalian cells, J. Natl. Cancer Inst. Monogr., 50:145 (1978).
18. M. Radman, Is there SOS induction in mammalian cells?, Photochem. Photobiol., 32:823 (1980).
19. U. Das Gupta and W. C. Summers, Ultraviolet reactivation of herpes simplex virus is mutagenic and inducible in mammalian cells, Proc. Natl. Acad. Sci. USA, 75:2378 (1978).
20. C. D. Lytle, J. G. Goddard, and C. H. Lin, Repair and mutagenesis of herpes simplex virus in UV-irradiated monkey cells, Mutation Res., 70:139 (1980).

21. J. J. Cornelis, J. H. Lupker, and A. J. van der Eb, UV-reactivation, virus production and mutagenesis of SV40 in UV-irradiated monkey kidney cells, Mutation Res., 71:139 (1980).
22. J. J. Cornelis, J. H. Lupker, B. Klein, and A. J. van der Eb, The effect of cell irradiation on mutation in ultraviolet-irradiated and intact simian virus 40, Mutation Res., 82:1 (1981).
23. J. J. Cornelis, Z. Z. Su, D. C. Ward, and J. Rommelaere, Indirect induction of mutagenesis of intact parvovirus H-1 in mammalian cells treated with UV-light or with UV-irradiated H-1 or simian virus 40, Proc. Natl. Acad. Sci. USA, 78:in press (1981).
24. A. Sarasin and A. Benoit, Induction of an error-prone mode of DNA repair in UV-irradiated monkey kidney cells, Mutation Res., 70:71 (1980).
25. J. J. Cornelis, B. Klein, J. H. Lupker, P. J. Abrahams, R. A. M. Hooft van Huysduynen, and A. J. van der Eb, The use of viruses to study DNA repair and induced mutagenesis in mammalian cells, Progress in Mutation Res., 4:in press (1981).
26. Z. Z. Su, J. J. Cornelis, and J. Rommelaere, Mutagenesis of intact parvovirus H-1 is expressed coordinately with enhanced reactivation of ultraviolet irradiated virus in human and rat cells treated with 2-nitronaphthofurans, Carcinogenesis, 10: in press (1981).
27. A. Sarasin, C. Gaillard, and J. Feunteun, Induced mutagenesis of simian virus 40 in carcinogen-treated monkey cells, in: "Induced Mutagenesis-Molecular Mechanisms and Their Implications for Environmental Protection," C. W. Lawrence, ed., in press, Plenum, New York (1982).
28. R. S. Day and C. Ziolkowski, Studies on UV-induced viral reversion, Cockayne's syndrome, and MNNG damage using adenovirus 5, in: "DNA Repair Mechanisms," P. C. Hanawalt, E. C. Friedberg, and C. F. Fox, eds., p. 535, Academic Press, New York (1978).
29. N. Weill-Thevenet, J. P. Buisson, R. Royer, and M. Hofnung, Mutagenic activity of benzofurans and naphthofurans in the Salmonella/microsome assay: 2-nitro- 7-methoxy- naphtho (2.1-b) furan (R 7000), a new highly potent mutagenic agent, Mutation Res., 88:355 (1981).
30. J. Y. Chou and R. G. Martin, DNA infectivity and the induction of host DNA synthesis with temperature-sensitive mutants of simian virus 40, J. Virol., 15:145 (1975).
31. J. Tooze, DNA Tumor Viruses, Part 2, Cold Spring Harbor Laboratory, New York (1980).
32. E. D. Sebring, T. J. Kelly, M. M. Thoren, and N. P. Salzman, Structure of replicating simian virus 40 deoxyribonucleic acid molecules, J. Virol., 8:478 (1971).
33. B. Hirt, Selective extraction of polyoma DNA from infected mouse cell cultures, J. Mol. Biol., 26:365 (1967).

34. P. J. Abrahams and A. J. van der Eb, Host-cell reactivation of ultraviolet-irradiated SV40 DNA in five complementation groups of xeroderma pigmentosum, Mutation Res., 35:13 (1976).
35. F. L. Graham and A. J. van der Eb, A new technique for the assay of infectivity of human adenovirus 5 DNA, Virology, 52:456 (1973).
36. A. R. Sarasin and P. C. Hanawalt, Carcinogens enhance survival of UV-irradiated simian virus 40 in treated monkey kidney cells: induction of a recovery pathway? Proc. Natl. Acad. Sci. USA, 75:346 (1978).
37. S. Nocentini, J. Coppey, J. P. Buisson, and R. Royer, Inhibition of DNA synthesis in relation to induced herpes virus reactivation in monkey cells treated by a variety of 2-nitronaphthofurans, Mutation Res., in press (1981).
38. R. G. Martin and V. P. Setlow, The initiation of SV40 DNA synthesis is not unique to the replication origin, Cell, 20:381 (1980).
39. T. Lindahl and B. Nyberg, Rate of depurination of native deoxyribonucleic acid, Biochemistry, 11:3610 (1972).
40. J. M. Vos, J. J. Cornelis, S. Limbosch, F. Zampetti-Bosseler, and J. Rommelaere, UV-irradiation of related mouse hybrid cells: similar increase in capacity to replicate intact Minute-Virus-of-Mice but differential enhancement of survival of UV-irradiated virus, Mutation Res., in press (1981).
41. R. M. Irbe, L. M. E. Morin, and M. Oishi, Prophage (ϕ80) induction in Escherichia coli K-12 by specific deoxyoligonucleotides, Proc. Natl. Acad. Sci. USA, 78:138 (1981).
42. J. Coppey and S. Menezes, Enhanced reactivation of ultraviolet damaged herpes virus in ultraviolet pretreated skin fibroblasts of cancer prone donors, Carcinogenesis, in press (1981).
43. J. J. Mc Cormick and V. M. Maher, Mammalian cell mutagenesis as a biological consequence of DNA damage, in: "DNA Repair Mechanisms," P. C. Hanawalt, E. C. Friedberg, and C. F. Fox, eds., p. 739, Academic Press, New York (1978).
44. C. C. Chang, S. M. D'Ambrosio, R. Schultz, J. E. Trosko, and R. B. Setlow, Modifications of UV-induced mutation frequencies in Chinese hamster cells by dose fractionation, cycloheximide and caffeine treatments, Mutation Res., 52:231 (1978).

ASSESSMENT OF HUMAN LYMPHOID CELL DAMAGE INDUCED BY THERAPEUTIC LEVELS OF 8-METHOXYPSORALEN AND LONG WAVELENGTH ULTRAVIOLET RADIATION *IN VITRO*

Kenneth H. Kraemer

Laboratory of Molecular Carcinogenesis
National Cancer Institute
Bethesda, Maryland 20205

INTRODUCTION

An earlier presentation to this conference dealt with general properties of human lymphoblastoic cell lines and their possible role in risk assessment. This paper will present a specific example of the use of lymphoblastoid cell lines to evaluate risk in patients receiving oral 8-methoxypsoralen (8-MOP) plus longwave ultraviolet radiation (UV-A) photochemotherapy. This experimental therapy has been given the acronym "PUVA."

PUVA PHOTOCHEMOTHERAPY

PUVA photochemotherapy is a new form of treatment, explicitly combining photoactive drugs with ultraviolet radiation. This procedure is presently under investigation for treatment of human diseases. The combination of oral 8-MOP plus UV-A has been found to be effective in attaining clinical remissions in psoriasis and in the cutaneous lymphoma, mycosis fungoides [1-4].

8-MOP is a naturally occurring tricyclic furocoumarin. Furocoumarins are found in parsnips, celery, figs, limes, and other plants of the families Umbelliferae, Moraceae, and Rutaceae [5, 6]. 8-MOP intercalates non-covalently in DNA. In the presence of UV-A, covalent cyclobutane type addition products may be formed linking the 8-MOP to pyrimidines in DNA. Mono-adducts or interstrand diadducts (crosslinks) may be formed. Therapeutic efficacy is thought to be related to the adduct-induced alteration in DNA synthesis. However, photoactivated 8-MOP has been shown to be cytotoxic and mutagenic in bacteria and cultured mammalian cells, and carcinogenic in mice and humans [6-8].

Psoriasis is a common disorder affecting about 1-3% of the population in the United States [9]. In about half of the patients, there is a family history of psoriasis, thus there is thought to be a genetic component to the disease. Psoriasis commonly is manifested by localized plaques with silvery scales involving the elbows, knees and scalp although the entire body may be involved in severe cases. A small proportion of the patients have associated psoriatic arthritis. In psoriasis, there is a benign hyperproliferation of the epidermal cells. Epidermal cell transit time may be reduced to as low as 2 days from the normal rate of 28 days. Histologically, the epidermis is thickened with elongated rete and hyperkeratosis. The basal cell layer is increased from the usual one cell thickness to two or three cell layers thickness. The dermal blood vessels are enlarged and an inflammatory infiltrate may be present.

In oral 8-MOP photochemotherapy, the proliferating cells in the skin are thought to be the primary treatment target but circulating lymphoid cells may also be affected. Since the 8-MOP is taken orally, the drug is present in the blood and there is a substantial circulation of blood through the dermis. In disease states the circulation may be increased and, in addition, leukocytes may leave the skin in considerable numbers and accumulate in the dermis. Short wavelength ultraviolet radiation is absorbed by the epidermis, but long wavelength ultraviolet radiation may penetrate through to the dermis and thus potentially interact with psoralen-bathed lymphoid cells.

Oral 8-MOP photochemotherapy treatment has been reported to induce immunological abnormalities. These include diminished cutaneous sensitization with dinitrochlorobenzene [10], decreased leukocyte thymidine incorporation [11, 12], diminished leukocyte responsiveness to phytohemagglutinin (PHA) [12], or $HgCl_2$ [13], decreased circulating E-rosette forming T lymphocytes [14-15]. Increased frequency of circulating thioguanine resistant (possible mutated) lymphocytes have been found in patients [16] (see also contribution by G. Strauss in this volume). _In vitro_ UV-A exposure of human leukocytes pre-treated with 8-MOP [12, 17-22] or obtained from patients who received oral 8-MOP [23] resulted in decreased cell turnover, decreased thymidine incorporation, diminished PHA-responsiveness and reduced mixed leukocyte culture reactivity.

The _in vitro_ assay system to be described [18, 19] reproduces some of the features of _in vivo_ 8-MOP photochemotherapy with respect to lymphoid cell PUVA exposure. The assay system permits quantitation and simultaneous correlation of multiple biological and physical effects of photochemotherapy on human lymphoid cells. It may be useful in defining the direct actions of drug and radiation and in predicting possible effects in humans under therapy.

CUTANEOUS OPTICS AND CIRCULATORY PHYSIOLOGY

Human skin serves as a filter of ultraviolet radiation [24-26]. The shorter the wavelength of radiation, the greater the filtration. This is readily demonstrated by holding a flashlight against one's hand in a darkened room. The shorter wavelength radiation is blocked but red light, of wavelength about 700 nm, can be seen passing through the entire skin thickness. This phenomenon is utilized in medicine by pediatricians who transilluminate the cranium of infants to diagnose nervous system abnormalities and by otolaryngologists looking for evidence of sinus inflammation.

The stratum corneum, or outer layer of skin, is the primary barrier to short wavelength ultraviolet radiation. It transmits less than 20% of the radiation below 300 nm [24]. The entire epidermis, however, transmits about 45% of incident radiation in the UV-A region (from 320 to 400 nm) [24-26]. This UV-A radiation may exert direct photobiological effects on dermal structures including blood within capillaries and lymphoid cells [25].

Blood flow through the skin has been measured to be about 500 ml/min [27]. Since the total blood volume is approximately 5500 ml, the equivalent of the entire total blood volume circulates through the skin every 11 min at rest. One can formulate a crude estimate of the average dose of UV-A a circulating leukocyte would receive (D_L) from skin surface UV-A exposure by considering the fraction of radiation transmitted by the epidermis (A_e), the treatment time (T), the rate of cutaneous blood flow (R), the number of circuits (n) a cell would make during the treatment time, the volume of blood in the body (V_b), and the volume of blood in the dermis (V_d).

Let p represent the fraction of the surface dose received by a leukocyte. Then:

1) $D_L = p\ D_S$.

Now:

2) $D_S = F_S \times T$,

where F_S is the fluence at the skin surface.

If F_d is the fluence in the dermis and t_L is the time a leukocyte spends in the dermis per circuit, then:

3) $D_L = F_D \times t_L \times n$.

Now:

4) $R = V_d/t_L = V_b/t_b$,

where t_b is the time for the total blood volume to pass through the dermis. This may be rearranged to:

4a) $t_1/t_b = V_d/V_b$.

But:

5) $n = T/t_b$.

Also,

6) $F_d = A_e \times F_s$.

Thus,

$$p = \frac{D_1}{D_s} = \frac{F_d \times t_1 \times n}{F_s \times T} = \frac{A_e \times F_s \times t_1}{F_s \times T} \times \frac{T}{t_b} = \frac{A_e \times t_1}{t_b}$$

Hence:

7) $p = A_e \times V_d/V_b$.

Equation 7 indicates that the fraction of the surface dose received by a circulating leukocyte is equal to the fraction of radiation transmitted by the epidermis times the ratio of the dermal blood volume to the total body blood volume. The epidermis transmits about 45% of the UV-A (A_e) [24-26] and the total blood volume (V_b) is about 5500 ml [6, 17, 27]. From these considerations it is apparent that the crucial unmeasured component in determining the extent of UV-A exposure to leukocytes is the cutaneous blood volume. The flow rate is of secondary importance since increases in flow rate resulting in less exposure per circuit are compensated for by more circuits during the period of exposure. I have been unable to find reliable estimates of human cutaneous blood volume. Data has been published for rodents and range from 20 to 70 µl blood per gram of skin [17]. If one assumes a human cutaneous blood volume of 100 to 500 ml (representing 50 to 250 µl/g skin), then circulating leukocytes would receive approximately

$$p = 0.45 \times \frac{100\text{-}500 \text{ ml}}{5500 \text{ ml}} = 0.8 \text{ to } 4\%$$

of the skin surface dose. Thus, with a typical human skin exposure of 10,000 J/m^2 during photochemotherapy from a source delivering 100 $J/m^2/sec$, each lymphocyte would be estimated to receive 800 to 4000 J/m^2 UV-A.

SERUM PSORALEN CONCENTRATIONS

Several methods have been described to measure serum 8-MOP concentrations. These include thin layer chromatography, high pressure liquid chromatography, and bacterial bioassay [28-40]. The standard dosage of oral 8-MOP in photochemotherapy is about 0.6 mg/kg. Peak levels have generally been found at 2 h after ingestion, however, there is considerable variation among patients. Detectable peak levels have been reported to vary widely among patients ranging from a low of 0.002 μg/ml to a high value of 4 μg/ml. Some of this variation may be due to variations in drug composition or absorption [33, 38]. However, even a single laboratory reports 100-fold differences in peak values among patients. Most laboratories found peak values between 0.1 and 1.0 μg/ml. Since 8-MOP is metabolized by hepatic enzymes, some of the reported values may include circulating metabolites. The possibilities of these metabolites have not been thoroughly investigated.

IN VITRO ASSAY SYSTEM

Human lymphoid cells were chosen for use in the *in vitro* assay [18-22]. Primary cultures containing large numbers of lymphocytes were obtained by leukophoresis of normal donors and further purified by flotation in lymphocyte separation medium. They could be maintained in short term culture in RPMI 1640 medium supplemented with 17% fetal calf serum. This procedure resulted in a mild blastogenic response to the calf serum. These cells were used for short term assessment of DNA synthesis [18, 19]. Smaller numbers of fresh leukocytes obtained by differential centrifugation of heparinized blood were used to examine immune reactivity [22].

Long term cultures utilized Epstein-Barr virus-transformed lymphoblastoid cells from normal donors. These cells grow indefinitely in suspension in the culture medium. Their use permits assessment of long term cellular effects such as survival following treatment. Large numbers of the lymphoblastoid cells can be rapidly grown to facilitate measures of physical parameters such as DNA cross-linking [21].

The cells were exposed to radiation from the same type of lamp as that used in photochemotherapy. The peak energy of the unfiltered lamp was at 355-365 nm. Ninety-eight percent of the measured ultraviolet output was in the UV-A region between 320 and 400 nm. Approximately 2% of the radiation from the unfiltered lamp was between 280 and 320 nm, in the UV-B region. This UV-B radiation is known to be more active biologically than UV-A radiation but it is filtered out by the epidermis [24-26]. Thus, we utilized a 6 mm thickness of plate glass to filter out the UV-B radiation. With the plate glass filter, there was virtually no emission below 320 nm. The plate glass also partially mimics the filtering effect of epidermis.

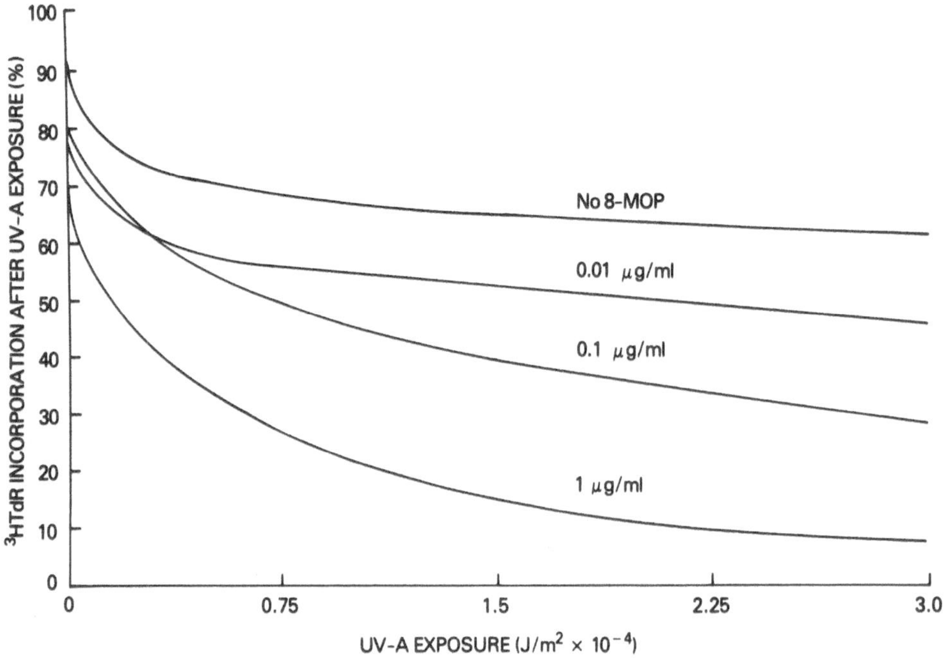

Fig. 1. DNA synthesis in a human lymphoblastoid cell line after 8-MOP plus UV-A *in vitro*. Relative effect of *in vitro* exposure to UV-A and UV-A plus 8-MOP (1.0, 0.1, and 0.01 μg/ml) on ^{3}HTdR incorporation in lymphoblastoid cell line E-1 (modified from references 18, 19).

Cells were irradiated at 37° from beneath the flasks. They were suspended in a UV-A transmitting salt solution to minimize possible UV interactions with medium components and thereby to measure direct photochemical effects. The cells were kept in suspension and exposed to different portions of the field during the time of irradiation by shaking the plate glass at approximately 40 revolutions per minute.

8-MOP was added to the cells prior to UV-A exposure. All manipulations were performed with gold fluorescent lamp illumination.

MEASUREMENTS OF DNA SYNTHESIS FOLLOWING 8-MOP PLUS UV-A

DNA synthesis was assessed by measuring tritiated thymidine (^{3}HTdR) incorporation into the lymphoid cells during the first two hours after treatment using a filter assay. A dose dependent decrease in DNA synthesis was apparent in primary lymphocyte cultures after exposure to UV-A in the absence of 8-MOP. Pretreatment with 8-MOP before UV-A exposure resulted in additional decrease in DNA synthesis.

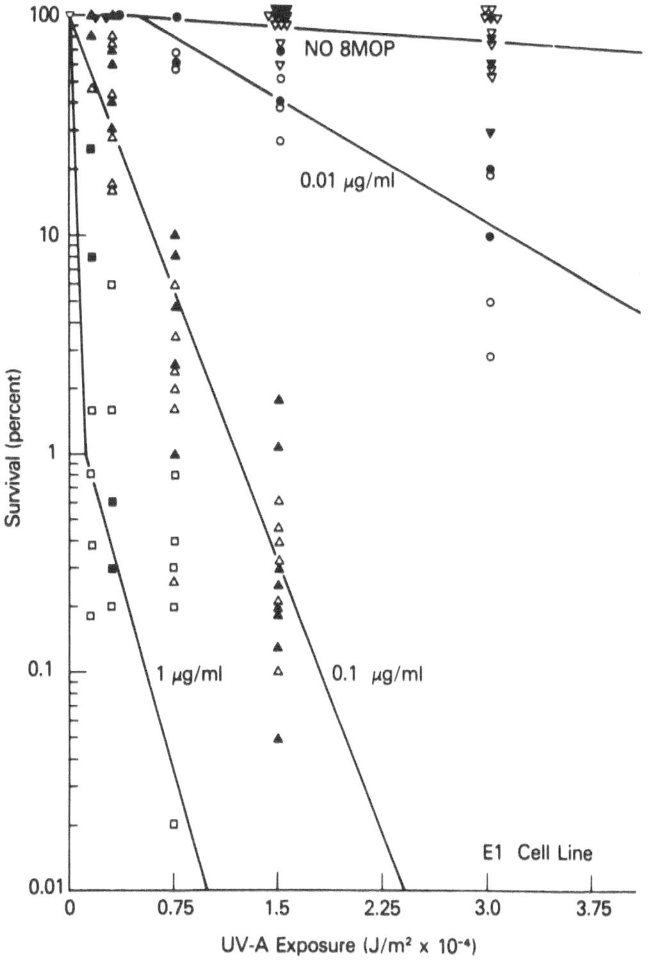

Fig. 2. Survival of human lymphoblastoid cells after 8-MOP plus UV-A _in vitro_. Log phase cells were treated with 0, 0.01, 0.1, or 1.0 μg/ml 8-MOP and exposed to UV-A. Survival was measured by extrapolation from growth curves (closed symbols) and by growth in microtiter wells (open symbols) (modified from reference 19).

We have previously studied DNA synthesis in leukocytes of psoriasis patients receiving photochemotherapy [11] by measuring ^{3}HTdR incorporation in unstimulated leukocytes obtained immediately before and after the UV-A treatment. The extent of the decrease in leukocyte DNA synthesis observed _in vitro_ following 8-MOP plus UV-A was 60% inhibition in ^{3}HTdR incorporation. This finding is consistent with the thesis that the decreased DNA synthesis observed _in vivo_ is a direct effect of the 8-MOP plus UV-A treatment. Further, the

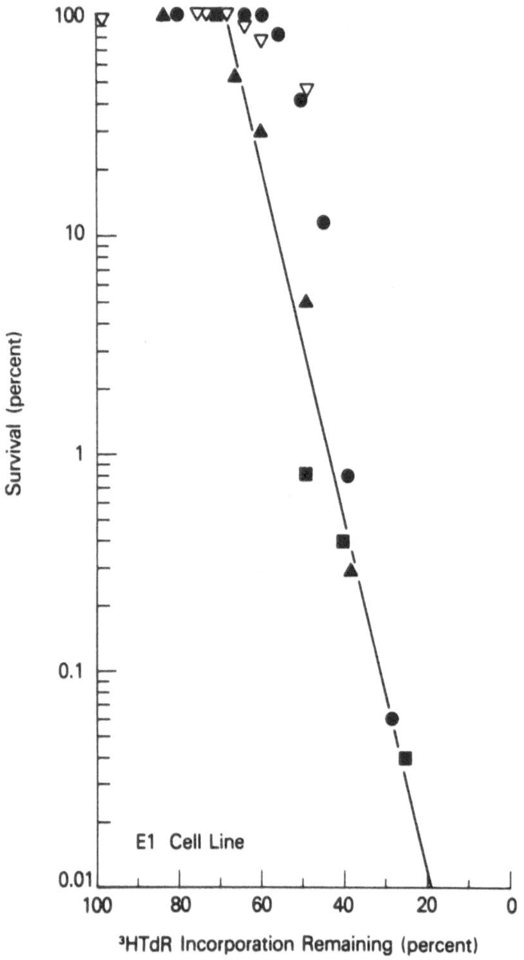

Fig. 3. Relation of lymphoblastoid cell survival to DNA synthesis inhibition after 8-MOP plus UV-A. The mean survival after treatment with 0.01 μg/ml (●), 0.1 μg/ml (▲), 1.0 μg/ml (■), or no (∇) 8-MOP plus UV-A was calculated from Fig. 2 and compared to the mean determinations of ^{3}HTdR incorporation remaining as shown in Fig. 1 (reproduced from reference 9).

crude assumptions made in predicting leukocyte UV-A exposure (see above), yield approximately congruent results: Thus 1000 to 1500 J/m^2 UV-A exposure following 8-MOP sensitization in vitro resulted in 40 to 60% inhibition of DNA synthesis; these values are similar to those observed following skin exposure of 50,000 to 300,000 J/m^2 in vivo [11].

DNA synthesis was also inhibited in the lymphoblastoid cells following UV-A exposure and was further decreased by pre-treatment with 8-MOP (Fig. 1). Within the range of doses studied a 10-fold increase in 8-MOP concentration resulted in an increase of approximately 20% in the extent of inhibition of ^{3}HTdR incorporation, while a 10-fold increase in UV-A exposure resulted in an approximately 30% increase in the extent of inhibition of ^{3}HTdR incorporation. Thus changes in UV-A exposure had a greater effect on DNA synthesis than changes in 8-MOP concentration.

EFFECT OF 8-MOP PLUS UV-A TREATMENT ON LYMPHOID CELL SURVIVAL

Cell proliferation could be evaluated in the lymphoblastoid cells following 8-MOP plus UV-A treatment. Proliferation was measured by two methods (Fig. 2): 1) daily hemocytometer counts of trypan-blue dye excluding cells and 2) by growth of small numbers of cells in microtiter wells [20]. Untreated cells grew exponentially in culture. Survival was not altered by treatment with 1 μg/ml 8-MOP alone or with 30,000 J/m^2 UV-A alone. Combined treatment with 8-MOP followed by UV-A resulted in a dose-dependent decrease in proliferation. Thus, UV-A exposure of 7500 J/m^2 following pretreatment with 1.0 μg/ml, 0.1 μg/ml, or 0.01 μg/ml 8-MOP resulted in survivals of 0.03%, 6%, and 80%, respectively. Neither 8-MOP treatment alone or UV-A exposure alone significantly reduced cell survival. The survival assay also indicates a greater effect of changes in UV-A exposure than in changes in 8-MOP concentration.

The in vitro assay permits correlation of decreased DNA synthesis immediately after 8-MOP plus UV-A treatment with subsequent cell survival (Fig. 3). Survival was not altered by treatment resulting in 60 to 70% of control ^{3}HTdR incorporation remaining. However, treatment-induced reduction in ^{3}HTdR incorporation to 50% of control was associated with approximately 0.5% survival. Similar survival was observed at a similar extent of ^{3}HTdR incorporation inhibition obtained by different combinations of 8-MOP plus UV-A. Some psoriasis patients receiving photochemotherapy had 50% reduction in leukocyte DNA synthesis immediately after treatment [11]. This in vitro assay would predict that the proliferative ability of these cells would be impaired.

INDUCTION OF DNA CROSSLINKS BY 8-MOP PLUS UV-A

DNA crosslink induction in vitro was measured by a very sensitive technique known as alkaline elution [19, 21, 41, 42]. Cells with their DNA labeled with radioactive thymidine were irradiated with 300R x-ray to break the DNA into small fragments. The cells were layered on top of polyvinylchloride filters with large (2 μm) pores and then lysed. The DNA was slowly eluted with an alkaline solution at pH 12.1. The fragmented DNA eluted through the filter

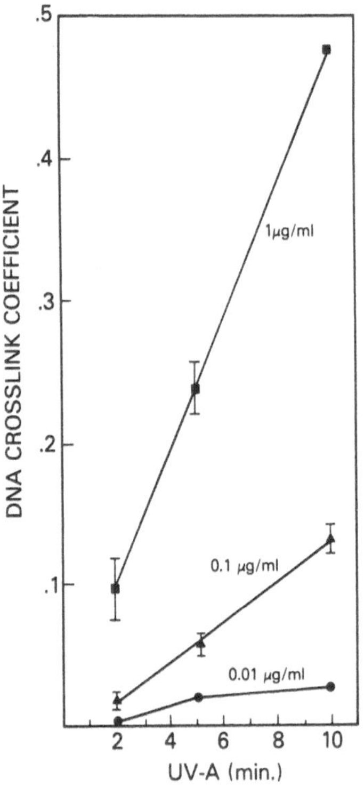

Fig. 4. DNA crosslink coefficient as a function of 8-MOP concentration and UV-A exposure. Human lymphoblastoid cells were treated with 0, 0.01, 0.1, or 1.0 μg/ml 8-MOP and then exposed to 15,000 J/m^2 (10 min), 7500 J/m^2 (5 min), or 3000 J/m^2 (2 min) UV-A. DNA crosslinking was measured by alkaline elution and the DNA crosslink coefficient was calculated for each combination of 8-MOP with UV-A. There was an increase in the DNA crosslink coefficient with increasing 8-MOP concentration at each UV-A exposure level (modified from reference 19).

relatively rapidly. DNA fragments that are crosslinked are retarded in their passage through the filter and elute more slowly. This difference in elution rates may be used to measure DNA crosslinks. Treatment of cells with 8-MOP plus UV-A retards the elution of fragmented DNA. The extent of crosslink formation is related to both the 8-MOP concentration and the UV-A exposure (Fig. 4) but is more sensitive to changes in UV-A exposure than to changes in 8-MOP concentration.

The extent of DNA crosslinking may be correlated with the inhibition of ^{3}HTdR incorporation (Fig. 1) measured immediately after treatment. When DNA synthesis was less than 50% of control, there was a dose dependent increase in 8-MOP-DNA crosslinking detected. Similarly, these was a linear relationship between cell survival and DNA crosslinks induced [21]. This suggests that the cytotoxic effects of photoactivated 8-MOP in human lymphoid cells may depend on DNA interstrand crosslinks.

OTHER EFFECTS OF 8-MOP PLUS UV-A ON LYMPHOID CELLS IN VITRO

The in vitro assay described was used to measure the effect of 8-MOP plus UV-A on immune reactivity [22]. Treatment with 8-MOP plus UV-A could completely abrogate the two-way mixed leukocyte reaction. One-way mixed leukocyte reactions demonstrated dose-dependent reductions in both stimulating ability and mixed leukocyte culture reaction induced proliferation of peripheral blood leukocytes following in vitro PUVA treatment.

Sister chromatid exchange induction was measured following in vitro exposure to 8-MOP plus UV-A [19]. Dose dependent increases in sister chromatid exchanges were observed in both lymphocytes and lymphoblastoid cell lines.

SUMMARY

An in vitro assay system that mimics some of the features of in vivo photochemotherapy in relationship to human lymphoid cells is described. The assay subjects suspension cultures of human lymphocytes or lymphoblastoid cells to therapeutic concentrations of 8-MOP and to a UV-A spectrum modified to approximate dermal exposure. The assay permits correlation and quantitation of multiple 8-MOP plus UV-A induced biological and physical alterations in the same assay system. The assay demonstrated inhibition of DNA synthesis, reduction of cell survival, production of DNA cross links, and loss of mixed leukocyte reactivity induced by combinations of 8-MOP and UV-A in or near the presumed therapeutic range. This assay may be useful for predicting lymphoid cellular toxicity of other photoactive agents as well as for examining the molecular effects of these agents.

REFERENCES

1. Parrish, J. A., Fitzpatrick, T. B., Tanenbaum, L., and Pathak, M. A., Photochemotherapy of psoriasis with oral methoxsalen and longwave ultraviolet light, N. Engl. J. Med., 291:1207-1222 (1974).
2. Melski, J. W., Tanenbaum, L., Parrish, J. A., Fitzpatrick, T. B., and Bleich, H. L., Oral methoxsalen photochemotherapy for the treatment of psoriasis, A cooperative clinical trial, J. Invest. Dermatol., 68:328-335 (1977).

3. Gilchrest, B. A., Parrish, J. A., Tanenbaum, L., Haynes, H. A., and Fitzpatrick, T. B., Oral methoxsalen photochemotherapy of mycosis fungoides, Cancer, 38:683-689 (1976).
4. Roenigk, H. H., Photochemotherapy for mycosis fungoides, Arch. Dermatol., 113:1047-1051 (1977).
5. Pathak, M. A., Daniels, F., and Fitzpatrick, T. B., The presently known distribution of furocoumarins (psoralens) in plants, J. Invest. Dermatol., 39:225-239 (1962).
6. Scott, B. R., Pathak, M. A., and Mohn, G. R., Molecular and genetic basis of furocoumarin reactions, Mutat. Res., 39:29-74 (1976).
7. Burger, P. M., and Simons, J., Mutagenicity of 8-methoxypsoralen and long-wave ultraviolet irradiation in diploid human skin fibroblasts, An improved risk estimate in photochemotherapy, Mutat. Res., 63:371-389 (1979).
8. Stern, R. S., Thibodeau, L. A., Kleinerman, R. A., Parrish, J. A., and Fitzpatrick, T. B., Risk of cutaneous carcinoma in patients treated with oral methoxsalen photochemotherapy for psoriasis, N. Engl. J. Med., 300:809-813 (1979).
9. Farber, E. M., and Van Scott, E. J., Psoriasis, in: T. B. Fitzpatrick, A. Z. Eisen, K. Wolff, I. M. Freedberg, and K. F. Austen, eds., "Dermatology in General Medicine," New York, McGraw-Hill (1979), pp. 233-247.
10. Strauss, G. H., Bridges, B. A., Greaves, M., Hall-Smith, P., Price, M., and Vella-Briffa, D., Inhibition of delayed hypersensitivity reaction in skin (DNCB test) by 8-methoxypsoralen photochemotherapy, Lancet, 2:556-559 (1980).
11. Kraemer, K. H., and Weinstein, G. D., Decreased thymidine incorporation in circulating leukocytes after treatment of psoriasis with psoralen and long-wave ultraviolet light, J. Invest. Dermatol., 69:211-214 (1977).
12. Friedman, P. S., and Rogers, S., Photochemotherapy of psoriasis, DNA damage in blood lymphocytes, J. Invest. Dermatol., 74:440-443 (1980).
13. Lischka, G., Bohnert, E., Bachtold, G., and Jung, E. G., Effects of 8-methoxypsoralen and UV-A on human lymphocytes, Arch. Derm. Res., 259:293-298 (1977).
14. Ortonne, J. P., Claudy, A. L., Alario, A., and Thivolet, J., Decreased circulating E rosette forming cells in psoralen UV-A treated patients, Arch. Derm. Res., 258:305-306 (1977).
15. Haftek, M., Glinski, W., Jablonska, S., and Obalek, S., T lymphocyte E rosette function during photochemotherapy (PUVA) of psoriasis, J. Invest. Dermatol., 72:214-218 (1979).
16. Strauss, G. H., Albertini, R. J., Krusinski, P. A., and Baughman, R. D., 6-thioguanine resistant peripheral blood lymphocytes in humans following psoralen, longwave ultraviolet light (PUVA) therapy, J. Invest. Dermatol., 73:211-216 (1979).
17. Wulf, H. C., and Wettermark, G., Toxic effects of 8-methoxypsoralen on lymphocyte division, Arch. Derm. Res., 260:87-92 (1977).

18. Kraemer, K. H., Waters, H. L., Ellingson, O. L., and Tarone, R. E., Psoralen plus ultraviolet radiation-induced inhibition of DNA synthesis and viability in human lymphoid cells in vitro. Photochem. Photobiol., 30:263-270 (1979).
19. Kraemer, K. H., Waters, H. L., Cohen, L. F., Popescu, N. C., Amsbaugh, S. C., DiPaolo, J. A., Glaubiger, D., Ellingson, O. L., and Tarone, R. E., Effects of 8-methoxypsoralen and ultraviolet radiation on human lymphoid cells in vitro. J. Invest. Dermatol., 76:80-87 (1981).
20. Kraemer, K. H., Waters, H. L., and Buchanan, J. K., Survival of human lymphoblastoid cells after DNA damage measured by growth in microtiter wells, Mutat. Res., 72:285-294 (1980).
21. Cohen, L. F., Kraemer, K. H., Waters, H. L., Kohn, K. W., and Glaubiger, D. L., DNA crosslinking and cell survival in human lymphoid cells treated with 8-methoxypsoralen and long wavelength ultraviolet radiation, Mutat. Res., 80:347-356 (1981).
22. Kraemer, K. H., Levis, W. R., Cason, J. C., and Tarone, R. E., Inhibition of mixed leukocyte culture reaction by 8-methoxypsoralen and long wavelength ultraviolet radiation, J. Invest. Dermatol., 77:235-239 (1981).
23. Scherer, R., Kern, B., and Braun-Falco, O., UV-A induced inhibition of proliferation of PHA-stimulated lymphocytes from humans treated with 8-methoxypsoralen, Brit. J. Dermatol., 97: 519-528 (1977).
24. Everett, M. A.,Yeargers, E., Sayre, R., and Olson, R. L., Penetration of the epidermis by ultraviolet rays, Photochem. Photobiol., 5:553-542 (1966).
25. Parrish, J. A., Anderson, R. R., Urback, F., and Pitts, D., "UV-A Biological Effects of Ultraviolet Radiation with Emphasis on Human Responses to Longwave Ultraviolet," New York, Plenum Press (1978).
26. Kaidbey, K. H., Agin, P. P., Sayre, R. M., and Kligman, A. M., Photoprotection by melanina comparison of Black and Caucasian skin, J. Am. Acad. Derm., 1:249-260 (1979).
27. Wade, O. L., and Bishop, J. M., "Cardiac Output and Regional Blood Flow," Oxford, Blackwell (1962), pp. 92-93.
28. Steiner, I., Prey, T., Gschnait, F., Washuttl, J., and Greiter, F., Serum level profiles of 8-methoxypsoralen after oral administration, Arch. Derm. Res., 259:299-301 (1977).
29. Herbst, M. J., Koot-Gronsveld, E. A. M., and deWolff, F. A., Serum levels of 8-methoxypsoralen in psoriasis patients using a new fluorodensitometric method, Arch. Derm. Res., 262:1-6 (1978).
30. Chakrabarti, S. G., Gooray, D. A., and Kenney, Jr., J. A., Determination of 8-methoxypsoralen in plasma by scanning fluorometry after thin layer chromatography, Clin. Chem., 24:1155-1157 (1978).
31. Busch, U., Schmid, J., Koss, F. W., Zipp, H., and Zimmer, A., Pharmacokinetics and metabolite-pattern of 8-methoxypsoralen in man following oral administration as compared to the pharmacokinetics in rat and dog, Arch. Dermatol. Res., 262:255-265 (1978).

32. Gazith, J., Schalla, W., and Schaefer, H., 8-methoxypsoralen-gas chromatographic determinations and serum kinetics, Arch. Dermatol. Res., 263:215-222 (1978).
33. Ehrsson, H., Nilsson, S. O., Ehrnebo, M., Wallin, I., and Wennersten, G., Effect of food on kinetics of 8-methoxypsoralen, Clin. Pharmacol. Ther., 25:167-171 (1979).
34. Schmid, J., and Koss, F. W., Rapid sensitive gas chromatographic analysis of 8-methoxypsoralen in human plasma, J. Chromatog., 146:498-502 (1978).
35. Wilkinson, D. I., and Farber, E. M., Gas-liquid chromatographic determination of 8-methoxypsoralen in serum, in: "Psoriasis: Proceeding of the Second International Symposium," E. M. Farber, A. J. Cos, P. H. Jacobs, and M. L. Nall, eds., New York Medical Books (1977), pp. 480-482.
36. Hensby, C. P., The qualitative and quantitative analysis of 8-methoxypsoralen by HPLC-UV and GLC-MS, Clin. Exp. Dermatol., 3:355-366 (1978).
37. Puglisi, C. V., Arthur, J., deSilva, F., and Meyer, J. C., Determination of 8-methoxypsoralen, a photoactive compound, in blood by high pressure liquid chromatography, Analyt. Lett., 10:39-50 (1977).
38. Ljunggren, B., Carter, D. M., Albert, J., and Reid, T., Plasma levels of 8-methoxypsoralen determined by high pressure liquid chromatography in psoriatic patients ingesting drug from two manufacturers, J. Invest. Dermatol., 74:59-62 (1980).
39. Ljunggren, B., Bjellerup, M., and Carter, D. M., Dose-response relations in phototoxicity due to 8-methoxypsoralen and UV-A in man, J. Invest. Dermatol., 76:73-75 (1981).
40. Glew, W. B., Roberts, B. S., Malinin, G. I., and Nigra, T. P., Quantitative determination by bioassay of photoactive 8-methoxypsoralen in serum, J. Invest. Dermatol., 75:230-234 (1980).
41. Ewig, R. A. G., and Kohn, K. W., DNA protein cross-linking and DNA interstrand cross-linking, Cancer Res., 38:3197-3203 (1978).
42. Kohn, K. W., Ewig, R. A. G., Erickson, L. C., and Zwelling, L. A., Measurements of strand breaks and cross-links in DNA by alkaline elution, in: "DNA Repair: A Laboratory Manual of Research Procedures," E. Friedberg and P. Hanawalt, eds., Vol. 1, Part B, New York, Marcel Dekker (1981), pp. 379-401.

THE MUTAGEN SENSITIVITY RESPONSE OF CELLS FROM INDIVIDUALS HETEROZYGOUS FOR DNA REPAIR DEFICIENCY GENES

Colin F. Arlett and Susan A. Harcourt

MRC Cell Mutation Unit
University of Sussex
Falmer, Brighton
England

THE DISEASES OF INTEREST

A number of rare, recessive human syndromes have been described as both cancer prone and to exhibit defects in the repair of DNA damage. These include xeroderma pigmentosum (XP), ataxia-telangiectasia (A-T), Fanconi's anaemia (FA) and Bloom's syndrome (BS) [1].

The evidence for this statement is particularly strong [2] for XP where the startling incidence of skin cancer is seen in virtually all patients whose cells exhibit defects in either excision repair [3] or daughter strand repair [4] following treatment with 254 nm UV light. The enzymological nature of the defect is far from being understood since extracts of XP cells appear to be able to overcome the apparent defect in the endonuclease step when applied to naked DNA but not to chromatin [5]. The genetics of the defect in excision repair are very complicated; a minimum of seven (A-G) complementation groups have been recognized so far [6]. It is not known whether this implies the existence of a large gene complex or a number of single genes all differing in some subtle way in the same process since the defect in all complementation groups lies in the incision step. This observation together with the geographical differences in the distribution of the various complementation groups [7] show that XP is a disease of relatively uniform clinical description but diverse genetic origin.

With A-T the incidence of cancer of the reticulo-endothelial system is high. There are 108 cases of A-T with cancer in the Immonodeficiency Cancer Registry [8] which indicates that approximately 10% of all A-T cases get cancer. This does not appear dramatic when set against the fact that approximately 20% of all normal people get cancer on the basis of a lifetime incidence. However, the data represent a large increase in age-specific cancer incidence because A-T individuals present with childhood cancers. The pattern of incidence is not like the pattern of childhood cancers in general nor is it like that of radiation-induced cancer in children [9].

The evidence for DNA repair defects in A-T is less secure. The original observations by Paterson et al. [10] that A-T cells fail to remove sites sensitive to *Micrococcus luteus* endonuclease have not been confirmed [11]. The reported [12] defect in A-T cells of a primer activity which makes damaged DNA a suitable substrate for the action of DNA polymerases has been confirmed by one group [13] but not by others [14].

Despite the fragile nature of the repair studies at least two complementation groups have been claimed [15-17]. This implies that, like XP, there is a considerable degree of genetic heterogeneity in A-T as indeed is reflected in the problems of diagnosis.

With Fanconi's anaemia the information available suggests that cancer occurs more commonly in this syndrome than in the general population of children and young adults. However, some caution must be exercised when reviewing the data [18] since there are a number of alternative explanations which may make the association between FA and cancer fortuitous. The most important of these explanations is that the cancer itself is a consequence of the androgen administration employed since 1959. Nevertheless, the generally accepted explanation [18] is that cancer predisposition is a feature of the syndrome and that the modern medical management delays death from bone marrow failure thus permitting time for the predisposition to be manifest.

Studies of DNA repair in this syndrome indicate that the cells are defective in a repair process which can ameliorate the effects of DNA-DNA crosslinks.

For Bloom's syndrome the registry data [18] distinguish individuals suffering from this condition from the normal population in showing that there is a greater than normal incidence of some classes of acute leukaemia during childhood and a premature onset of carcinoma in young adults. To date, with BS, there has been no demonstration of a DNA repair defect although the existence of such defects have been invoked [1, 19].

EPIDEMIOLOGICAL STUDIES ON HETEROZYGOTES

The question as to whether persons heterozygous for the recessive genes determining these rare conditions are themselves subject to an increased risk of developing cancer is, clearly, an important subject [21, 22].

Although the homozygotes themselves are rare the frequency of heterozygotes can be relatively high. For XP the frequency of heterozygotes has been variously described as being approximately 1 in 250,000 in the USA and Western Europe but 1 in 40,000 in Japan [2]. Application of the Hardy-Weinberg relationship means that heterozygotes for each of the XP genes consititute 0.1% of the population [20, 21]. In an epidemiological study [20], 31 families were studied in 18 states of the USA and the data show that there were significantly more blood relatives (30/1046) than spouse controls (11/855) who presented with a nonmelanoma skin cancer. The difference between blood relatives and spouse controls was most marked for persons living in the southern states and with outdoor occupations consistent with a need for exposure to the inducing agent, sunlight.

Since this study of cancer in XP heterozygotes was retrospective and, therefore, subject to all the problems of ascertainment and verification of information on medical records there is clearly a need for this study to be repeated or extended perhaps in a country like Japan where both the frequency of the gene and genetic isolation are high even though the incidence of skin cancer may be low (M. Swift, personal communication). A prospective study using computerized health service records should provide an unequivocal confirmation in a relatively short period.

The frequency of A-T homozygotes has been estimated as 1 in 40,000 leading to the incidence of heterozygotes as 1 in 100 [21]. Swift [22] has estimated that as much as 5% of all cases of cancer below the age of 45 years may be A-T gene carriers. While it is clear that the incidence of A-T varies from area to area and Harnden and Bridges [9] suggest that the incidence in the UK is ten fold less, the frequency of heterozygotes is still around 1 in 300. If we accept the validity of the assignment of a minimum of two complementation groups in A-T then the frequency of heterozygotes increases by $1/\sqrt{N}$, where n is the number of complementation groups of equal frequency.

Swift [23] has provided evidence to show that A-T heterozygotes may be predisposed to diabetes, severe scoliosis and possibly neural tube defects in addition to cancer. The most striking finding in the A-T families was that the number of deaths from cancer significantly exceeded the expected number particularly at the younger ages. This is especially clear when set against the observed and expected cancer deaths from XP and FA. An attempt is being made in the UK to confirm these observations in view of their importance (Acheson and Bridges, personal communication).

Fanconi's anaemia has been estimated to occur at a frequency of 1 in 360,000 in North America [21] and 1 in 70,000 in mid-Europe [24], the former value leading to an estimated heterozygote frequency of 0.003. In a first study [21] of the syndrome heterozygotes appeared to be more cancer-prone than normal individuals. A larger and more complete investigation has led to the conclusion that there were fewer observed than expected cancer deaths in FA families even though there are some associations of individual neoplasms with the FA gene in heterozygotes [25].

Bloom's syndrome is almost entirely restricted to Ashkenazi Jews where Swift [21] has estimated the heterozygote frequency as approximately 0.005. As far as we are aware no studies of cancer incidence in BS heterozygotes have been made available.

EXISTING CELLULAR STUDIES

If the epidemiological data can be transferred to and confirmed by cellular studies in the laboratory then a number of possibilities follow. First there would become available methods for detecting heterozygotes and thereby individuals at risk; such information could be used to protect such individuals and be of value in genetic counselling. Secondary, such studies would make available means whereby the molecular origin of cancer might be investigated.

Information on the cellular response of heterozygotes is already available. For XP there have been no reports of increased sensitivity to the lethal effects of UV or defects in excision repair although one report [26] indicates that some heterozygotes might be less rapid than normals in mobilizing the excision repair process as measured by unscheduled DNA synthesis. XP heterozygotes show a response intermediate between homozygotes and normals for an assay which measures the ability of cells to permit recovery of functions in irradiated virus [27].

Ataxia-telangiectasia is the disease where the heterozygotic frequency is the greatest and most studies have been concerned with such material. A-T heterozygotes have been shown to have increased radiosensitivity using both chromosomal and cell survival techniques [28, 29]. Thus in lymphoblastoid cell lines the D_0 for normals is 110 ± 6 rads (14 subjects, for A-T homozygotes it is 38 ± 5 (6 subjects) and for heterozygotes it is 78 ± 6 (9 subjects). For gamma irradiation the total induced chromosome aberration frequency per cell in lymphoblastoid cell lines was controls, 0.38 ± 0.08 (7 subjects); A-T homozygotes, 1.19 ± 0.36 (7 subjects); and heterozygotes, 0.86 ± 0.09 (9 subjects). These observations hold out some prospect for the detection of A-T heterozygotes.

The data for untransformed fibroblasts is more controversial. Kidson et al. [29] have found that some but not all fibroblast strains from obligate heterozygotes are sensitive to gamma irradiation. Similar results have been recorded by Arlett and Harcourt [30]. Paterson et al. [31] have detected increased radiosensitivity in some obligate heterozygotes using cell survival techniques under

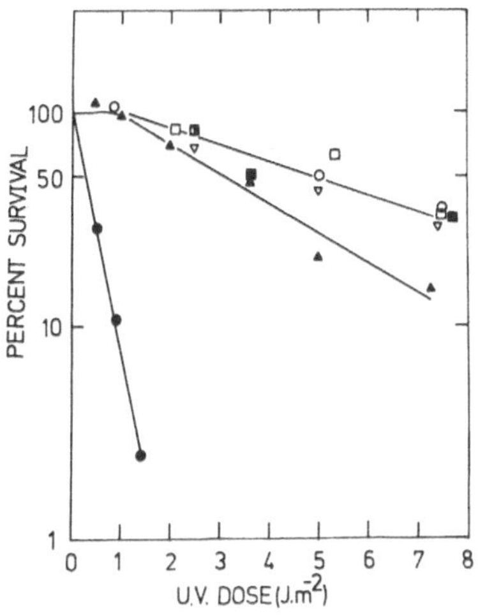

Fig. 1. The lethal effects of ultraviolet light on normal, XP, and XP heterozygote cell strains. Normal cell strains; ○) GM730, 6 experiments; □) 1BR, 8 experiments; ■) 54BR, 9 experiments. ●) XP4LO, 1 experiment. XP heterozygotes; ▽) XPHM4LO (mother) 3 experiments; ▲) XPHF4LO (father) 5 experiments.

hypoxic conditions and suggest that the differences are lost under oxic conditions. This result was confirmed by a second series of experiments in a different laboratory [9]. A correlated defect in Gamma-ray induced DNA repair replication has been observed in those heterozygotes with enhanced sensitivity to the lethal effects of gamma-irradiation under anoxic conditions [31]. For the present it would seem that the cell survival technique is too crude a tool to serve to detect heterozygotes unless methods can be found to maximize the differences between heterozygotes and normals. Experiments based upon modifying the repair of potentially lethal damage [32] when differences between A-T homozygotes and normals may be magnified to 40-fold hold out some prospects here. It remains to be seen whether A-T heterozygotes will behave more like homozygous A-T or normals under these conditions or whether the heterozygote response is maintained.

For FA, fibroblast cultures of heterozygotes can be distinguished from normal fibroblasts by their increased sensitivity to chromosomal damage on exposure to diexpoxybutane [33].

NEW STUDIES ON FIBROBLAST CELL STRAINS

In the light of the preceding information we initiated a program of study of heterozygotes of both XP and A-T and have attempted to integrate biochemical investigations of repair with the cell survival and mutation end points.

Table 1. Spontaneous Mutation Frequencies in Human Fibroblast Cell Strains

Cell strain	Phenotype of individual	Mutation frequency × 10^{-6}		
		Mean	± Standard error	Number of observations
1. 1BR	Normal	3.8	0.9	30
2. 48BR		8.0	-	2
3. 54BR		1.3	0.9	4
4. 2BI		1.5	0.4	18
5. GM730		7.3	1.8	8
6. XP4LO	xeroderma pigmentosum	9.2	2.3	3
7. XPHM4LO	XP heterozygotes parents of XP4LO	0.7	0.3	4
8. XPHF4LO		3.2	0.7	7
9. AT4BI	ataxia-telangiectasia	4.0	-	2
10. ATHM4BI	A-T heterozygote mother of AT4BI	4.1	1.5	4
11. ATH96TO	A-T heterozygote	1.9	1.0	4

Xeroderma Pigmentosum

The response to the lethal effects of 254 nm UV light is shown for XP4LO and the two parental cell strains XPHF4LO and XPHM4LO together with data for three normal cell strains in Fig. 1. All the results were collected in the same period of time and the heterozygotes were paired with normal cell strains in particular experiments. It is clear from these data that the cell strains from the father, XPHF4LO, shows some, albeit limited, hypersensitivity to UV.

Mutation data for resistance to 6-thioguanine at 2.5 μg/ml (TG) [34, 35] is shown in Table 1 and Fig. 2. The mutation frequencies observed (Table 1) indicate that spontaneous mutation is not ele-

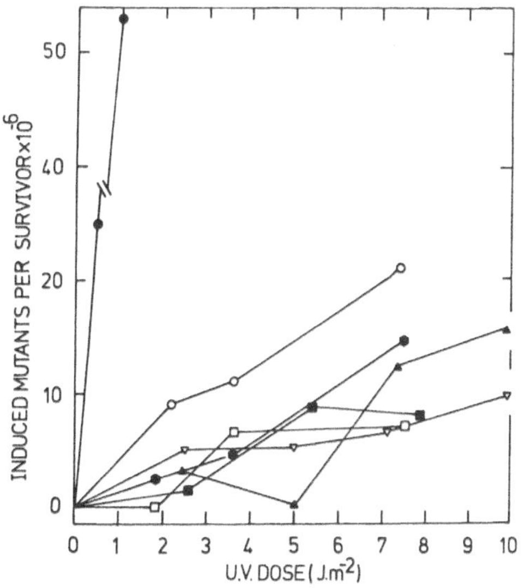

Fig. 2. The induction of 6-thioguanine resistant mutants by ultraviolet light in normal, XP, and XP heterozygote cell strains. Normal cell strains: ○) GM730, 1 experiment; □) 1BR, 3 experiments; ■) 54BR, 1 experiment; ⬢) 2BI, 2 experiments. ●) XP4LO, 1 experiment. XP heterozygotes: ▽) XPHM4LO (mother), 2 experiments; ▲) XPHF4LO (father), 2 experiments.

vated in heterozygotes. Similarly there is no evidence from our data of elevated induced mutation frequencies in the two heterozygotes compared with four normal cell strains.

Repair studies by Dr. A. R. Lehmann in our laboratory on unscheduled DNA synthesis, daughter strand repair and recovery of DNA synthesis following UV treatment on XPHF4LO showed this cell strain to be indistinguishable from normal unlike the proband XP4LO which shows defects in all these characteristics. Dr. R. Waters at the University College of Wales, Swansea, has undertaken a study of the kinetics of excision repair using the "ara-C technique" which permits an assessment of strand breaks resulting from ara-C incorporation during excision [36]. He has also measured the amount of DNA replication after UV. Two normal cell strains, HSBP and 1BR, two XP's from complementation group A, XP101LO and XP4LO and a single XP from complementation group C, XP106LO were compared with the relevant heterozygotes, XPHM101LO, XPHM4LO, XPHF4LO, and XPHF106LO. Regardless of the parameter measured none of the heterozygotes tested gave a response that was significantly different from normal cells.

The results to date indicate with the exception of the lethal response of XPHF4LO there is no indication of any heterozygote

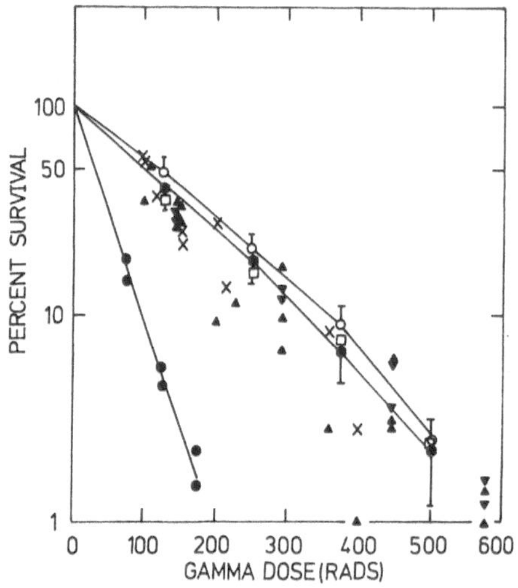

Fig. 3. The lethal effectsof gamma-irradiation on normal, A-T and A-T heterozygote cell strains. Normal cell strains: ○) GM730, 3 experiments; □) 1BR, 2 experiments; ⬢) 54BR, 3 experiments; ●) AT4BI, 2 experiments - data shown as individual points. A-T heterozygotes: ▲) ATHM4BI (mother), 6 experiments; ▼) ATHF4BI (father), 2 experiments; ×) ATH96TO, 3 experiments. The data for the A-T heterozygotes illustrated as separate points.

effect at the cellular level in XP. Clearly we need to study more heterozygotes including representatives of complementation groups other than A.

Ataxia-Telangiectasia

The lethal response to gamma-irradiation, in air, of three normal cell strains (GM730, 1BR, and 54BR) and A-T homozygote AT4BI, his parents ATHM4BI and ATHF4BI and third heterozygote ATH96TO is illustrated in Fig. 3. We are not able to claim any consistent hypersensitivity for any of these heterozygotes.

The spontaneous and induced mutation frequencies for TG resistance for the A-T heterozygotes are indistinguishable from normal (Table 1 and Fig. 4). The proband AT4BI has proved hypomutable in our hands [35, 37]. To date it has not seemed appropriate to commission any studies of repair in A-T heterozygotes.

DISCUSSION AND CONCLUSIONS

Despite the existence of a convincing body of data both epidemiological and experimental which shows that the heterozygotes of

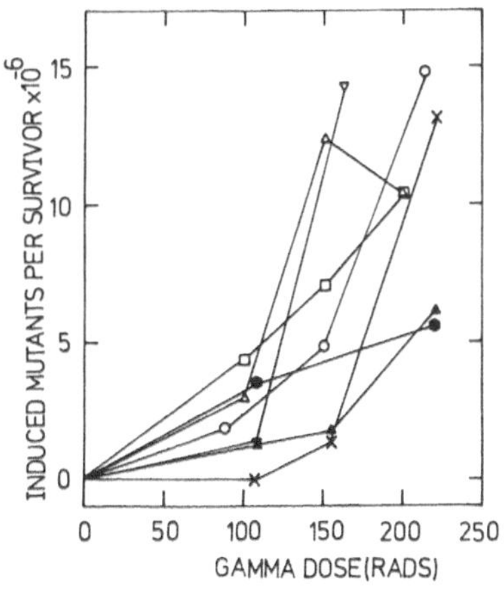

Fig. 4. The induction of 6-thioguanine resistant mutants by gamma irradiation in normal and A-T heterozygote cell strains. Normal cell strains: ○) GM730, 1 experiment; □) 1BR, 3 experiments; ▽) 48BR, 1 experiment; ●) 54BR, 1 experiment; and △) 2BI, 2 experiments. A-T heterozygotes: ▲) ATHM4BI, 2 experiments; ×) ATH96TO, 1 experiment.

A-T and XP can be distinguished from normals we have produced no convincing evidence of any differences with the single exception of the sensitivity of XPHF4LO to the lethal effects of UV. The level of hypersensitivity here was approximately that of an XP variant [38]. While the response of this individual's cell was clearly different from the other normal cell strains used in our study it is not clear that it may necessarily be discriminated from a larger population of normals or that the sensitivity was, in any way, a consequence of the presence of the recessive XP gene.

XP homozygotes are clearly hypermutable (Fig. 2) [35, 37, 39], but the heterozygotes could not be discriminated from normals. This is surprising in the light of the epidemiological data [20] which suggests that the greatest differentiation between XP heterozygotes and normals is achieved where maximum insolation is received, a situation which should easily be modelled in the laboratory. More XP heterozygotes will require study to confirm this observation but we have to accept, for the moment, that the experimental induction of TG resistant mutants by UV does not parallel the epidemiological data for cancer incidence.

The data for increased cancer in A-T heterozygotes is, perhaps, more convincing since it does not depend upon dose of carcinogen and the frequency of heterozygotes is higher. The dilemma here, in contrast to XP, is that the A-T homozygotes are not more mutable than normals [40], indeed we suggest that they may even be hypomutable

[35, 37]. It is difficult to envisage, therefore, that the increased cancer frequency in the homozygotes is a direct consequence of either the radiation hypersensitivity or any repair defect, rather that it is related to the impaired immune status of the individuals leading to a reduction in immune surveillance. Increased cancer incidence in heterozygotes would follow from a similar impairment and we should not be surprised by a lack of correlation between cancer and mutation induction in this syndrome.

ACKNOWLEDGMENTS

We are indebted to Prof. B. A. Bridges for many helpful comments. The study was supported in part by Euratom Contract No. 166-76-1-BIO.

REFERENCES

1. C. F. Arlett and A. R. Lehmann, Human disorders showing increased sensitivity to the induction of genetic damage, Ann. Rev. Genet., 12:95 (1978).
2. K. H. Kraemer, Xeroderma pigmentosum, in: "Clinical Dermatology," D. J. Dennis, R. L. Dobson, and J. McGuire, eds. (Unit 19.7:Vol. 4), Harper and Row, Hagerstown (1980).
3. J. E. Cleaver, Defective repair replication of DNA in xeroderma pigmentosum, Nature, 218:652 (1968).
4. A. R. Lehmann, S. Kirk-Bell, C. F. Arlett, M. C. Paterson, P. H. M. Lohman, E. A. de Weerd-Kastelein, and D. Bootsma, Xeroderma pigmentosum cells with normal levels of excision repair have a defect in DNA synthesis after UV irradiation, Proc. Natl. Acad. Sci. USA, 72:219 (1975).
5. K. Mortelmanns, E. C. Friedberg, H. Slor, T. Thomas, and J. E. Cleaver, Defective thymine dimer excision by cell-free extracts of xeroderma pigmentosum cells, Proc. Natl. Acad. Sci. USA, 73: 2757 (1976).
6. W. Keijzer, N. G. J. Jaspers, P. J. Abrahams, A. M. R. Taylor, C. F. Arlett, B. Zelle, H. Takebe, P. D. S. Kinmont, and D. Bootsma, A seventh complementation group in excision-deficient xeroderma pigmentosum, Mutation Res., 62:183 (1979).
7. H. Takebe, Y. Miki, T. Kozuka, J.-I. Furuyama, K. Tanaka, M. S. Sasaki, Y. Fujiwara, and H. Akiba, DNA repair characteristics and skin cancers of xeroderma pigmentosum patients in Japan, Cancer Res., 37:490 (1977).
8. B. D. Spector, A. H. Filipovich, G. S. Perry, III, and J. H. Kersey, Epidemiology of cancer in ataxia-telangiectasia, in: "Ataxia-Telangiectasia - A Cellular and Molecular Link between Cancer, Neuropathology and Immune Deficiency," B. A. Bridges and D. G. Harnden, eds., John Wiley and Sons, London (1981).
9. D. G. Harnden and B. A. Bridges, Ataxia-Telangiectasia (A-T) - A model of cancer susceptibility, in: "Ataxia-Telangiectasia - A Cellular and Molecular Link between Cancer, Neuropathology, and Immune Deficiency," B. A. Bridges and D. G. Harnden, eds., John Wiley and Sons, London (1981).

10. M. C. Paterson and P. J. Smith, Ataxia-Telangiectasia: An inherited human disorder involving hypersensitivity to ionizing radiation and related DNA-damaging chemicals, Ann. Rev. Genet., 13:291 (1979).
11. G. P. van der Schans, H. B. Centen, and P. H. M. Lohman, Studies on the repair defects in ataxia-telangiectasia, in: "Chromosome Damage and Repair," E. Seeberg and K. Kleppe, eds., Plenum Press, New York (1982).
12. T. Inoue, K. Hirano, A. Yokoiyama, T. Kada, and H. Kato, DNA repair enzymes in ataxia-telangiectasia and Bloom's syndrome fibroblasts, Biochim. Biophys. Acta, 479:497 (1977).
13. M. J. Edwards, A. M. R. Taylor, and G. Duckworth, An enzyme activity in normal and ataxia-telangiectasia cell lines which is involved in the repair of gamma-irradiation induced DNA damage, Biochem. J., 188:677 (1980).
14. A. R. Lehmann and P. Karran, quoted in reference 9.
15. M. C. Paterson, B. P. Smith, P. H. M. Lohman, A. K. Anderson, and L. Fishman, Defective excision repair of gamma-ray-damaged DNA in human (ataxia-telangiectasia) fibroblasts, Nature, 260: 444 (1976).
16. T. Inoue, M. S. Sasaki, A. Yokoiyama, and T. Kada, Primer activating enzyme deficiency and *in vitro* complementation of the enzyme activity in cell-free extracts from ataxia-telangiectasia fibroblasts, in: "Ataxia-Telangiectasia - A Cellular and Molecular Link between Cancer, Neuropathology, and Immune Deficiency," B. A. Bridges and D. G. Harnden, eds., John Wiley and Sons, London (1981).
17. N. G. J. Jaspers, J. de Wit, and D. Bootsma, The rate of DNA synthesis in ataxia-telangiectasia fibroblasts after exposure to DNA damaging agents, in: "Ataxia-Telangiectasia - A Cellular and Molecular Link between Cancer, Neuropathology, and Immune Deficiency," B. A. Bridges and D. B. Harnden, eds., John Wiley and Sons, London (1981).
18. J. German, Chromosome-breakage syndromes: Different genes, different treatments, different cancers, in: "DNA Repair and Mutagenesis in Eukaryotes," W. M. Generoso, M. D. Shelby, and F. J. de Serres, eds., Plenum Press, New York (1980).
19. F. Giannelli, P. F. Benson, S. A. Pawsey, and P. E. Polani, Ultraviolet light sensitivity and delayed DNA-chain maturation in Bloom's syndrome fibroblasts, Nature, 256:466 (1977).
20. M. Swift and C. Chase, Cancer in xeroderma pigmentosum families, J. Natl. Cancer Inst., 62:1415 (1979).
21. M. Swift, Malignant disease in heterozygous carriers, Birth Defects, Orig. Artic. Ser. XII:33 (1976).
22. M. Swift, L. Sholman, M. Perry, and C. Chase, Malignant neoplasms in the families of patients with ataxia-telangiectasia, Cancer Res., 36:209 (1976).
23. M. Swift, Disease predisposition of ataxia-telangiectasia heterozygotes, in: "Ataxia-Telangiectasia - A Cellular and Molecular Link between Cancer, Neuropathology, and Immune Deficiency," B. A. Bridges and D. G. Harnden, eds., John Wiley and Sons, London (1981).

24. E. Wunder, personal communication.
25. M. Swift, R. J. Caldwell, and C. Chase, Reassessment of cancer predisposition of Fanconi anaemia heterozygotes, J. Natl. Cancer Inst., 65:863 (1980).
26. F. Giannelli and S. A. Pawsey, DNA repair synthesis in human heterokaryons: II. A test for heterozygosity in xeroderma pigmentosum and some insight into the structure of the defective enzyme, J. Cell Sci., 15:63 (1974).
27. A. J. Rainbow, Reduced capacity to repair irradiated adenovirus in fibroblasts from xeroderma pigmentosum heterozygotes, Cancer Res., 40:3945 (1980).
28. P. Chen, M. F. Lavin, C. Kidson, and D. Moss, Identification of ataxia-telangiectasia heterozygotes, a cancer prone population, Nature, 274:484 (1978).
29. C. Kidson, P. Chen, and P. Imray, Ataxia-telangiectasia heterozygotes: Dominant expression of ionizing radiation-sensitive mutants, in: "Ataxia-Telangiectasia - A Cellular and Molecular Link between Cancer, Neuropathology, and Immune Deficiency," B. A. Bridges and D. G. Harnden, eds., John Wiley and Sons, London (1981).
30. C. F. Arlett and S. A. Harcourt, Survey of radiosensitivity in a variety of human cell strains, Cancer Res., 40:926 (1980).
31. M. C. Paterson, A. K. Anderson, B. P. Smith, and P. J. Smith, Enhanced radiosensitivity of cultured fibroblasts from ataxia-telangiectasia heterozygotes manifested by defective colony-forming ability and reduced DNA repair replication after hypoxic gamma irradiation, Cancer Res., 39:3725 (1979).
32. R. Cox, A cellular description of the repair defect in ataxia telangiectasia, in: "Ataxia-Telangiectasia - A Cellular and Molecular Link between Cancer, Neuropathology, and Immune Deficiency," B. A. Bridges and D. G. Harnden, eds., John Wiley and Sons, London (1981).
33. A. D. Auerbach and S. R. Wolman, Carcinogen-induced chromosome breakage in Fanconi's anaemia heterozygous cells, Nature, 271: 69 (1977).
34. R. Cox and W. K. Masson, X-ray induced mutation to 6-thioguanine resistance in cultured human fibroblasts, Mutation Res., 37:125 (1976).
35. C. F. Arlett, Mutagenesis in repair-deficient human cell strains, in: "Progress in Environmental Mutagenesis," M. Alacevic, ed., Elsevier, Amsterdam (1980).
36. E. A. Hiss and R. J. Preston, The effect of cytosine arabinoside on the frequency of single-strand breaks in DNA of mammalian cells following irradiation or chemical treatment, Biochim. Biophys. Acta, 478:1 (1977).
37. C. F. Arlett and S. A. Harcourt, Variation in response to mutagens amongst normal and repair-defective human cells, in: "Indeed Mutagenesis: Molecular Mechanisms and Their Implication for Environmental Protection," C. W. Lawrence, L. Prakash, and F. Sherman, eds., 14th Rochester International Conference on Environmental Toxicity, Plenum Press, New York (in press).

38. C. F. Arlett, S. A. Harcourt, and B. C. Broughton, The influence of caffeine on cell survival in excision-proficient and excision-deficient xeroderma pigmentosum and normal human cell strains following ultraviolet irradiation, Mutation Res., 33: 341 (1975).
39. V. M. Maher, R. D. Curren, L. M. Ouellette, and J. J. McCormick, Effect of DNA repair on the frequency of mutations induced in human cells by ultraviolet irradiation and by chemical carcinogens, in: "Fundamental in Cancer Prevention," P. N. Magee, S. Takayama, T. Sugimura, and T. Matsushima, eds., Tokyo Univ. Press, Tokyo (1976).
40. J. W. I. M. Simons, Studies on survival and mutation in ataxia-telangiectasia cells after x-irradiation under oxic and anoxic conditions, in: "Ataxia-Telangiectasia - A Cellular and Molecular Link between Cancer, Neuropathology, and Immune Deficiency," B. A. Bridges and D. G. Harnden, eds., John Wiley and Sons, London (1981).

REPAIR OF CHEMICAL DAMAGE IN MAMMALIAN CELLS

R. B. Setlow

Biology Department
Brookhaven National Laboratory
Upton, New York 11973
USA

INTRODUCTION

The repair of chemical damage to DNA differs in many ways from the repair of radiation damage and its interpretation is often more complicated. For example, most chemicals of environmental concern do not react directly with cellular macromolecules but must first be activated to nucleophiles [1]. Hence the dosimetry of chemicals is complicated and may vary markedly from tissue to tissue, organelle to organelle [2] or from linker to the core region of DNA [3]. The different reactivities between agents reacting directly and those that react indirectly may give rise to products whose yields as a function of dose are completely different even though the products themselves may be the same. Thus Fig. 1 [4] shows a way of estimating chemical doses in vivo from alkylating agents in terms of the level of specific alkylation of hemoglobin. The direct acting agent methylmethanesulfonate (MMS) yields a linear response curve but alkylation from dimethylnitrosamine (DMN), which needs activation, shows a much lower response and the response increases as some higher power of injected dose measured in mg/kg body weight. On the other hand the development of immunological probes for specific DNA damages offers the possibility of measuring such damages at levels of fmoles [5, 6].

Although one can make a strong argument that damages to DNA are initiating events in carcinogenesis [7, 8] many other factors are important in the carcinogenic process and there is not necessarily a one to one relationship between mutation (damage to DNA) and neoplastic transformation. Moreover because of the multitude of products resulting from chemical treatment it is not easy to decide

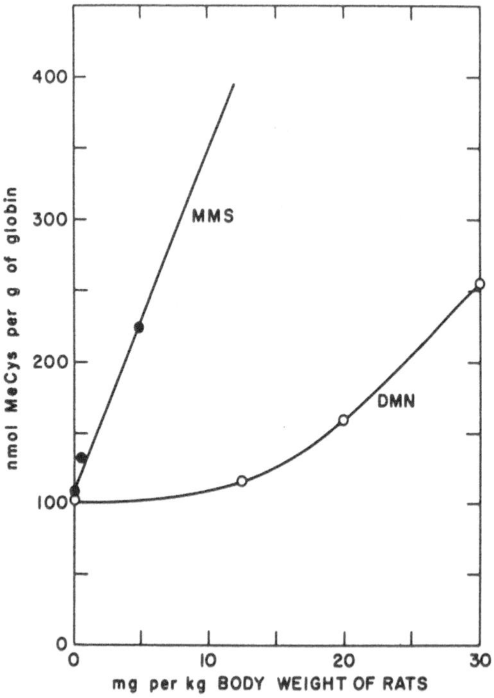

Fig. 1. Dose response curves for the appearance of methylcysteine in the hemoglobin of rats injected either with a direct acting agent MMS or an alkylating agent that first needs activation, DMN. Note at zero dose the existence of a high background of methylcysteine, the origin of which is not understood (adapted from 4).

which product is important for a biological endpoint and, indeed, the most plentiful product is not necessarily the one to worry about. One product may be more associated with cell cytoxicity and another with mutagenesis [9].

Nucleotide excision measurements of DNA repair are used extensively to detect agents that react with DNA and such measurements help identify DNA adducts that are dangerous [7, 8, 10-12]. A number of chemical agents mimic ultraviolet (UV) in the following ways [8, 13]. 1) Xeroderma pigmentosum (XP) cells are more sensitive to the cytotoxic effect of UV and to the chemical than are normal cells. 2) Chemically treated viruses show a higher survival on normal cells than on XP cells. 3) XP cells deficient in repair of UV damage are also deficient in the excision of chemical damage. 4) Excision repair of UV and of chemical damage involves long patches. 5) XP complementation groups observed for the repair of

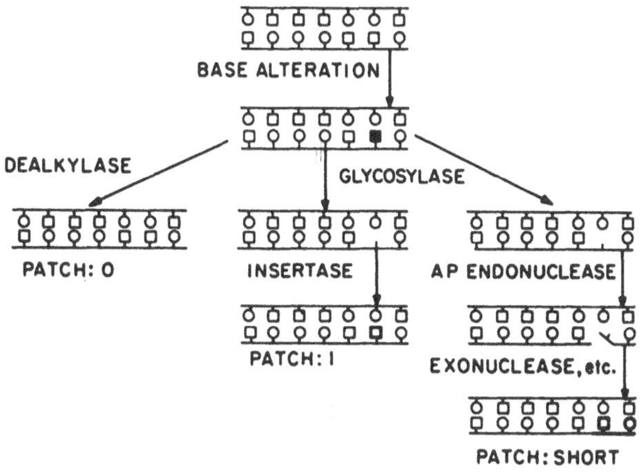

Fig. 2. Schematic diagrams showing three possible pathways of base excision repair. ■) An altered base; heavy lines, repair incorporation.

chemical damage are the same as those for UV damage. Moreover, the complementation groups for UV sensitive Chinese hamster cells are the same for UV and for chemical damage [14]. The chemical damages that mimic UV are repaired by nucleotide excision (see Repair of Radiation Damage in Mammalian Cells), and the chemicals are those that give rise to bulky adducts [15]. Thus the repair of 7β,8α-dihydroxy-9α,10α-epoxy-7,8,9,10-tetrahydrobenzo[a]pyrene is by a long patch mode [16] and its damage - mostly N^2-deoxyguanosine - is not repaired in XP cells but its repair by confluent cultures of normal cells is paralleled by an increase in survival and a decrease in mutagenesis indicating that this excision repair is error free [17]. Although the excision repair of bulky DNA adducts mimics the repair of UV damage in many ways, the identity of the repair pathways is a subject of controversy [18, 19].

REPAIR BY BASE EXCISION

Many chemical alterations to DNA, for example, simple alkylations are repaired by removal of the altered base without any initial attack on the polynucleotide backbone. Figure 2 shows some of the possible repair pathways involved in base excision [20]. One of the more important repair pathways that works on O^6-alkylguanine takes place by a dealkylation reaction that removes that alkyl group and transfers it to a cysteine of an acceptor protein [21] by a mechanism that seems analogous to that identified earlier in E. coli [22]. Such a repair reaction can not be detected by the conventional means, such as, repair replication or unscheduled DNA synthesis that are used to measure nucleotide excision, since as illustrated, the patch size in dealkylation is zero. The other possible pathways involve the initial action of a glycosylase [23] to remove the altered base from the poly-nucleotide. The removal may be followed either by a direct insertion of the proper base yielding a patch size of one or by the action of an apurinic/apyrimidinic endonuclease [23] as a result of which a short batch of several nucleotides may result [15]. The former pathway would not be measured if the altered base removed was a purine since the conventional measurements of unscheduled synthesis use radioactive thymidine or analogs of thymidine. The endonucleolytic pathway could also follow the chemical depurination of alterations such as 7-alkylguanine. Since the latter is the major product formed by simple alkylating agents [24], but is not as important biologically as the O^6 product, unscheduled synthesis measurements on cells treated with alkylating agents may be measuring the wrong repair and hence, although indicating the presence of DNA damage, may have little quantitative relevance to repair of biological significance.

The short patch repair observed in cells irradiated with ionizing radiation is also observed in cells treated by a number of chemicals [15] and indeed ataxia telangiectasia (AT) cells are not only more sensitive that normal ones to ionizing radiation (see Repair of Radiation Damage in Mammalian Cells), but are also killed more readily by chemicals such as N-methyl-N-nitroguanidine (MNNG) [25] and bleomycin [26]. The analogy between chemical damage and damage from ionizing radiation is not complete however since the latter compound inhibits the initiation of clusters of replicons as does ionizing radiation but the former does not [27].

REMOVAL OF O^6-ALKYLGUANINE

The experimental evidence indicating the important role played by O^6-alkylguanine in mutagenesis and carcinogenesis [24] involves numerous animal experiments on the production and repair of various alkylation products in DNA in different tissues as a result of acute and chronic administration of alkylating agents. For example, chronic treatment of rats with DMN results in an increase in the activity that removes the O^6-product from liver [28] (but no changes in 3-methyladenine or 7-methylguanine) and no liver tumors are observed after such treatment.

Experiments dealing with human cells in culture indicate that they may be classified as either proficient in the repair of methyl damage (Mer^+) or deficient (Mer^-) in its repair. Not only does adeno 5 virus treated with methylating agents show higher survival on Mer^+ cell strains but Mer^+ strains themselves survive treatment with alkylating agents better than do Mer^- ones (Fig. 3) [29]. Moreover, Mer^- cells are defective in the ability to remove O^6-methylguanine [30].

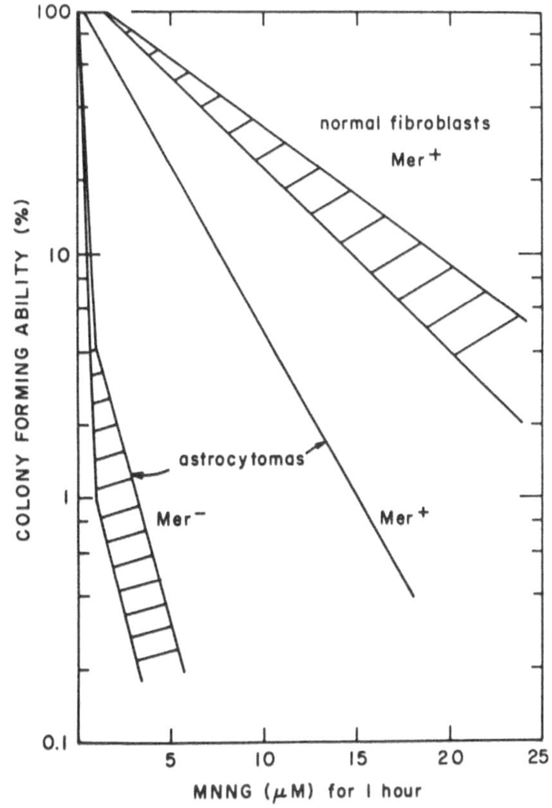

Fig. 3. Survival curves for human cell strains treated with MNNG for one hour (adapted from 29).

Many, but not all, of the Mer$^-$ strains originate from human tumors or from virally transformed cells [30, 31]. However, fibroblasts from individuals from which the tumor strains were derived are Mer$^+$. These observations put in perspective the finding that SV40 transformed XP cells were defective in the repair of alkylation damage [32]. The defect is presumably a result of the transformation and not of the XP genotype. At high doses the repair system working on O^6-methylguanine is readily saturated [33] as would be expected from a stoichiometric reaction [21, 22]. Hence one would not expect the dose response relations for the presence of products after alkylation treatment, or for some biological effects, to be linear ones. The repair of other products, such as 3-methyladenine and 7-methylguanine is not saturated readily.

It is clear from Fig. 3 that there is a range of cellular sensitivities to alkylating agents. Repair synthesis after treatment of

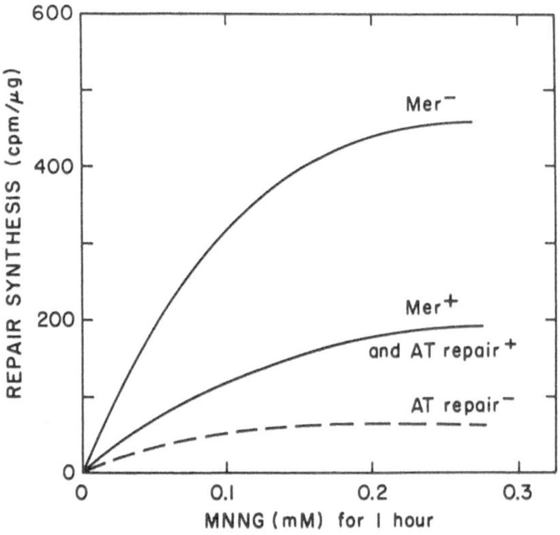

Fig. 4. Repair synthesis as a function of MNNG concentration. ^{3}H-thymidine was present for the one hour during treatment with the alkylating agent. (This figure is adapted from data in 25, 29.)

various cell strains with MNNG has been measured [25, 29] and indicates that AT cells are deficient compared to normal ones, but that Mer$^-$ cells show an enhanced repair (Fig. 4).

The explanation for these seemingly anomalous repair findings may be that dealkylation, with a patch size of zero, represents the major repair pathway and the observed repair synthesis represents only a minor component (Fig. 2). More cells may utilize the minor pathway when the major one is inoperative. Figure 4 seems to be an extreme case of a lack of correlation of repair synthesis with the repair of an important DNA repair adduct. Although the references from which Fig. 4 is adapted are not guilty of any unwarranted interpretation, these findings should be taken as a warning against using indiscriminate repair measurements as quantitative risk estimators.

ACKNOWLEDGMENT

This work was supported by the U.S. Department of Energy.

REFERENCES

1. E. C. Miller, Some Current perspectives on chemical carcinogenesis in humans and experimental animals, Cancer Res., 38: 1479 (1978).

2. J. M. Backer and I. B. Weinstein, Mitochondrial DNA is a major target for a dihydrodiol-epoxide derivative of benzo[a]pyrene, Science, 209:297 (1980).
3. C. J. Jahn and G. W. Litman, Accessibility of deoxyribonucleic acid in chromatin to the covalent binding of the chemical carcinogen benzo[a]pyrene, Biochemistry, 18:1442 (1972).
4. E. Bailey, T. A. Connors, P. B. Fermer, S. M. Gorf, and J. Rickard, Methylation of cysteine in hemoglobin following exposure to methylating agents, Cancer Res., 41:2514 (1981).
5. R. Mueller and M. F. Rajewsky, Sensitive radioimmunassay for the detection of O^6-ethyldeoxyguanosine in DNA exposed to the carcinogen ethylnitrosourea in vivo or in vitro, Zeit f. Naturforsch., 33C:897 (1978).
6. I. C. Hsu, M. C. Poirier, S. H. Yuspa, D. Grunberger, I. B. Weinstein, R. H. Yolken, and C. C. Harris, Cancer Res., 41:1091 (1981).
7. R. B. Setlow, DNA damage and carcinogenesis, in: "Chromosome Damage and DNA Repair," E. Seeberg and K. Kleppe, eds., Plenum Press, New York (1981).
8. R. B. Setlow, Repair deficient human disorders and cancer, Nature, 271:713 (1978).
9. L. C. Erickson, M. O. Bradley, and K. W. Kohn, Measurements of DNA damage in Chinese hamster cells treated with equitoxic and equimutagenic doses of nitrosoureas, Cancer Res., 38:3379 (1978).
10. J. J. Roberts, The repair of DNA modified by cytotoxic mutagenic, and carcinogenic chemicals, Adv. Radiat. Biol., 7:211 (1978).
11. P. C. Hanawalt, E. C. Friedberg, and C. F. Fox, "DNA Repair Mechanisms," Academic Press, New York (1978).
12. E. C. Friedberg, U. K. Ehmann, and J. I. Williams, Human diseases associated with defective DNA repair, Adv. Radiat. Biol., 8:85 (1979).
13. R. B. Setlow, Excision repair of bulky lesions in the DNA of mammalian cells, in: "Chromosome Damage and DNA Repair," E. Seeberg and K. Kleppe, eds., Plenum Press, New York (1981).
14. L. H. Thompson, D. B. Busch, K. Brookman, C. L. Mooney, and D. A. Glaser, Genetic diversity of UV-sensitive DNA repair mutants of Chinese hamster ovary cells, Proc. Natl. Acad. Sci. USA, 78:3734 (1981).
15. J. D. Regan and R. B. Setlow, Two forms of repair in the DNA of human cells damaged by chemical carcinogens and mutagens, Cancer Res., 34:3318 (1974).
16. J. D. Regan, A. A. Francis, W. C. Dunn, O. Hernandez, and D. M. Jerina, Repair of DNA damaged by mutagenic metabolites of benzo[a]pyrene in human cells, Chem. Biol. Interact., 20:279 (1978).
17. L. L. Yang, V. M. Maher, and J. J. McCormick, Error-free excision of the cytotoxic, mutagenic N^2-deoxyguanosine DNA adduct formed in human fibroblasts by (±)-7β,8α-dihydroxy-9α,10α-epoxy-7,8,9,10-tetrahydro-benzo[a]pyrene, Proc. Natl. Acad. Sci. USA, 77:5933 (1980).

18. F. E. Ahmed and R. B. Setlow, DNA repair in xeroderma pigmentosum cells treated with combinations of ultraviolet radiation and N-acetoxy-2-acetylaminofluorene, Cancer Res., 39:471 (1979).
19. A. J. Brown, T. H. Fickel, J. E. Cleaver, P. H. M. Lohman, M. H. Wade, and R. Waters, Overlapping pathways for repair carcinogens in human fibroblasts, Cancer Res., 39:2522 (1979).
20. R. B. Setlow, DNA repair pathways, in: "DNA Repair and Mutagenesis in Eukaryotes," W. M. Generoso, M. D. Shelby, and F. J. de Serres, eds., Plenum Press, New York (1980).
21. J. R. Mehta, D. B. Ludlum, A. Renard, and W. G. Verly, Repair of O^6-ethylguanine in DNA by a chromatin fraction from rat liver: Transfer of the ethyl group to the acceptor protein, Proc. Natl. Acad. Sci. USA, in press (1981).
22. M. Olsson and T. Lindahl, Repair of alkylated DNA in Escherichia coli: Methyl group transfer from O^6-methylguanine to a protein cysteine residue, J. Biol. Chem., 255:10569 (1980).
23. T. Lindahl, DNA glycosylases, endonucleases for apurinic/apyrimidinic sites, and base excision repair, Prog. Nucl. Acid. Res. Mol. Biol., 22:135 (1979).
24. B. Singer, N-nitrosoalkylating agents: Formation and persistence of alkyl derivatives in mammalian nucleic acids as contributing factors in carcinogenesis, J. Natl. Cancer Inst., 62: 1329 (1979).
25. D. A. Scudiero, Decreased repair synthesis and defective colony-forming ability of ataxia telangiectasia fibroblast cell strains treated with N-methyl-N'-nitro-N-guanidine, Cancer Res., 40:984 (1980).
26. A. M. R. Taylor, C. M. Rosney, and J. B. Campbell, Unusual sensitivity of ataxia-telangiectasia cells to bleomycin, Cancer Res., 39:1046 (1979).
27. P. Cramer and R. B. Painter, Bleomycin-resistant DNA synthesis in ataxia telangiectasia cells, Nature, 291:671 (1981).
28. R. Montesano, H. Bresil, G. Planche-Martel, G. P. Margison, and A. E. Pegg, Effect of chronic treatment of rats with dimethylnitrosamine on the removal of O^6-methylguanine from DNA, Cancer Res., 40:452 (1980).
29. R. S. Day III, C. H. J. Ziolkowski, D. A. Scudiero, S. A. Meyers, M. R. Mattern, Human tumor cell strains defective in the repair of alkylation damage, Carcinogenesis, 1:21 (1980).
30. R. S. Day III, C. H. J. Ziolkowski, D. A. Scudiero, S. A. Meyer, A. S. Lubiniecki, A. J. Girardi, S. M. Galloway, and G. D. Bynum, Defective repair of alkylated DNA by human tumor and SV40-transformed human cell strains, Nature, 288:724 (1980).
31. R. Sklar and B. Strauss, Removal of O^6-methylguanine from DNA of normal and xeroderma pigmentosum-derived lymphoblastoid lines, Nature, 289:417 (1981).
32. R. Goth-Goldstein, Repair of DNA damaged by alkylating carcinogens is defective in xeroderma pigmentosum-derived fibroblasts, Nature, 267:81 (1977).

33. A. S. C. Medcalf and P. D. Lawley, Time course of O^6-methylguanine removal from DNA of N-methyl-N-nitrosourea-treated human fibroblasts, Nature, 289:796 (1981).

EFFECTS OF VARIOUS PROMOTERS ON CELL TRANSFORMATION BY SIMIAN VIRUS 40 MUTANTS

L. Daya-Grosjean, R. Monier, and A. Sarasin

Instiut de Recherches Scientifiques sur le Cancer
CNRS, Laboratoire de Chimie des Acides Nucléiques
B.P. NO. 8, 94802 Villejuif Cedex
France

INTRODUCTION

It is widely admitted that tumor induction occurs through a multistep process, the two first steps of which should be initiation and promotion (see Berenblum, 1975). Most carcinogens interact directly or indirectly with DNA to give rise to lesions on DNA which generally need to be repaired in order to permit the cell survival (Miller, 1978). The relationships between DNA repair and carcinogenesis become evident when studying some human syndromes such as xeroderma pigmentosum (XP), where patients develop skin cancer with a very high incidence after exposure to sun-light (Cleaver, 1968). The cells isolated from XP patients are unable to repair *in vitro* the DNA lesions, essentially pyrimidine dimers, made by UV-light. This result clearly indicates that unrepaired DNA lesions represent one of the first steps of carcinogenesis probably by giving rise to mutations due to incorrect base-pairing with the damaged base. Another way to get mutations is to use an error-prone repair pathway to repair lesions on DNA. Such an error-prone repair process has been well established in bacteria where it has been called the SOS repair pathway (Radman, 1975; Witkin, 1976; Devoret et al., 1977). Treatment of bacteria by various physical or chemical carcinogens, which inhibit DNA replication, induces the SOS repair pathway which will repair DNA lesions more efficiently but with a high rate of errors (Sarasin et al., 1977). A similar SOS repair pathway has been described in eucaryotic cells when one uses DNA viruses as a biological probe: repair of UV-irradiated SV40 is highly mutagenic in monkey cells in which the SOS repair process has been turned on by carcinogens (Sarasin and Hanawalt, 1978; Sarasin and Benoit, 1980). Only after the initiation step has been carried out, the partially reversible promotion step can occur as shown by the pioneer work of Berenblum (Berenblum, 1954; 1975) using polycyclic aromatic hydrocarbons and croton oil on mouse skin. Later, the isolation and characterization of the 12-O-tetradecanoyl-phorbol-13-acetate (TPA) as the active compound of croton oil provided a major step to analyze at the molecular level the mechanism of tumor promotion (Hecker, 1971). TPA shows numerous effects at various cellular levels such as membranes, lysosomes, chromosomes, ... (see Diamond et al., 1980). However, the most important target of TPA in cells is not yet understood.

The two-step process, initiation and promotion, has been reproduced in vitro by using a cell transformation assay (Lasne et al., 1974; Heidelberger et al., 1978). This system represents a good approach for analyzing promotion under reproducible conditions. Moreover, a combination of carcinogens and viruses or viruses and promoters allows us to use the considerable molecular biology data available about viruses to carefully analyze in vitro, the mechanisms of initiation and promotion. It has been reported that viral transformation by adenovirus or Simian Virus 40 (SV40) is stimulated by treating cells with carcinogens prior to infection (Casto et al., 1976; Fisher et al., 1978; Diamond et al., 1974; Hirai et al., 1974). It is also known that TPA increases the anchorage-independent growth of cells previously transformed by adenovirus or SV40 (Fisher et al., 1979a; Fisher et al., 1979b; Sivak and Van Duuren, 1967). We have taken advantage of the availability of various SV40 mutants to analyze in greater detail the interaction between a transforming DNA virus, carcinogens and promoters. In this report we clearly show that the efficiency of transformation of Swiss 3T3 cells by wild type SV40 is greatly enhanced after cell treatment by carcinogens such as UV-light or acetoxy-acetylaminofluorene. We also describe unique experiments which show that in the presence of tumor promoters, colonies of cells growing in soft-agar can be obtained at the restrictive temperature of 39°C from SV40 tsA infected Swiss mouse 3T3 cells. Studies with the dl54-59 early mutants are also described.

The Use of Simian Virus 40 as a Biological Probe

Simian Virus 40 is a small oncogenic papovavirus whose natural host is the African green monkey. The viral particle is composed of a circular, double-stranded supercoiled DNA having a molecular weight of 3.5×10^6 daltons contained in a icosahedral capsid composed of three viral proteins VP1, VP2, and VP3 (see Tooze, 1980).

In vitro infection by SV40 can result in either a lytic (productive) or incomplete (abortive) infection depending on the species of origin, genetic properties, and physiological state of the cells as well as the genetic characteristics of the infecting virus. During infection of the permissive cell (African green monkey kidney cells) two distinct phases of infection are observed: the early phase during which the early proteins composed of the large (T) and small (t) tumor antigens are synthesized, and the late phase when the capsid proteins are synthesized. The replication of the viral DNA begins before the second phase of infection and is known to be bidirectional and under the control of cellular host proteins as well as the viral early large T-antigen. During viral infection of nonpermissive cells, viral DNA replication is very inefficient and only early functions appear to be expressed at a significant level while a very small percentage of the infected population eventually becoming transformed by retaining some viral sequences integrated into the host chromosome (Tooze, 1980).

The early mutants of SV40 have been very valuable tools for identifying and analyzing functions of SV40 expressed in lytically infected and transformed cells (Fig. 1). Viable deletions located in the SV40 genome betweem map positions 0.54 and 0.59 (dl54-59) alter or completely suppress the synthesis of small t (Shenk et al., 1976) and this SV40 small t seems entirely dispensable under *in vitro* conditions of viral growth (Feunteun et al., 1978). The dl54-59 mutants are, however, impaired in their ability to transform established cells lines. Transformants obtained by infection of rat embryo fibroblasts have fewer of the characteristics of a fully transformed phenotype (for example, growth in low serum, increased saturation density, growth in semisolid medium) than those transformed by wild type virus (Sleigh et al., 1978).

The tsA class of early SV40 mutants are known to affect the thermal stability of the large tumor antigen (T). At the restrictive temperature, such mutants are blocked in viral DNA replication at the level of initiation. They cannot induce permanent *in vitro* transformation at the restrictive temperature, probably because their genome cannot integrate in the cellular genome (Fluck and Benjamin, 1979).

The characterization of these early mutants has been very important in the understanding of the viral functions required for establishment and maintenance of transformation. However, at the present time, there is no unique rational definition of the "transformed" cell which is distinguished from the "normal" cell, by comparing a number of properties, such as growth control, morphology, cell surface structure and expression of enzyme activities.

Fully transformed cells are characterized by the following properties:

1. Ability to form clones when seeded at low densities;

2. ability to growth continuously upon successive prolonged passage in culture (immortality);

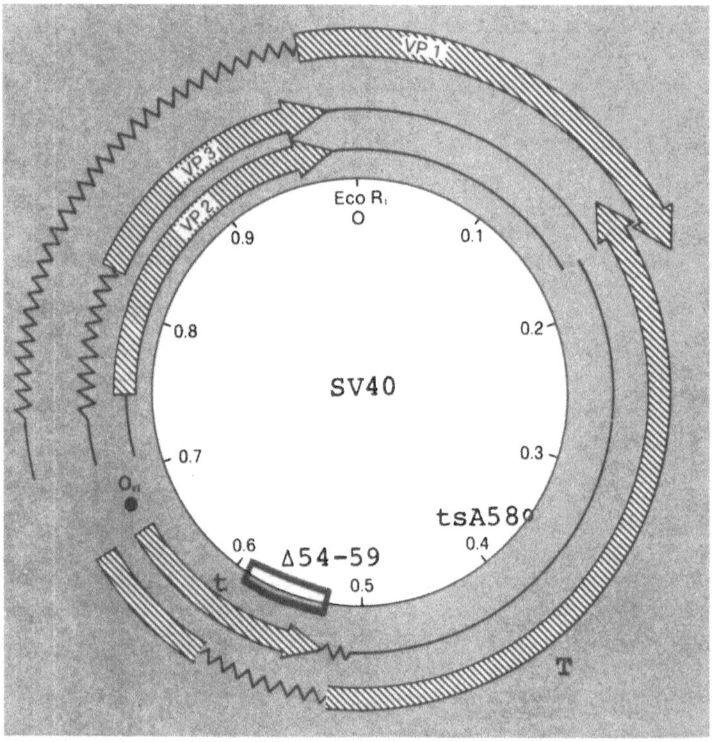

Fig. 1. Genetic map of sv40 genome. Ori represents the unique site of SV40 in DNA replication; t is the early gene coding for the small t antigen where Δ54-59 corresponds to deletion mutants in the expression of small t antigen; T is the early gene coding for the large T antigen where the tsA58 and the other tsA mutants we have used are mapped (Tegtmeyer, 1972); VP1, VP2, VP3 are the late genes coding for the capsid proteins; ⇨ symbolizes the coding messenger RNA; ⩘⩘ symbolizes the splicing region; —— symbolizes the noncoding messenger RNA. The map units start at the position of the Eco RI restriction enzyme site.

3. low requirements for serum growth factors;

4. ability to overgrow continuous layers of cells - dense foci on monolayers;

5. ability to grow in semisolid medium - anchorage-independent growth;

6. ability to form tumors after injection in newborn animals.

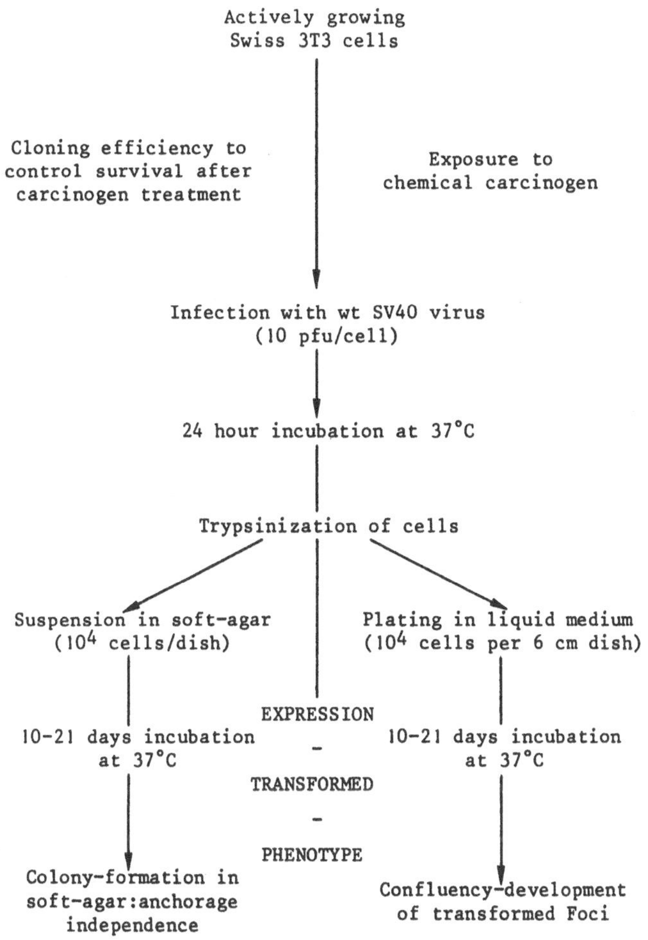

Fig. 2

Other characteristics of transformation include changes in the distribution of cytoskeleton elements (Pollack et al., 1975), membrane structure modifications (Vlodavsky et al., 1973), increased rate of hexose transport and plasminogen activator production (Pollack et al., 1974), and decreased fibronectin (Hynes, 1973). It should be noted that two of the growth properties (ability to clone on plastic and immortality) are already displayed by all continuous cell lines.

Enhancement of Virial Transformation by Pretreatment of Cells with Physical or Chemical Agents

We have studied two established mouse lines, the Swiss 3T3 mouse fibroblast line from American Type Culture Collection, and the C3H mouse embryo fibroblast derived line - 10 T 1/2 clone 8 which was isolated by Reznikoff et al. (1973). Actively growing cell cultures were exposed to the appropriate agent and then infected with wild type SV40 virus at 10 pfu/cell. Cells were then incubated in normal medium for 24 h at 37°C and then plated out at 10^4 cells per 6 cm Petri dish as shown in Fig. 2. After ten to 21 days, depending on the cell line and selection method used, cell proliferation leads to the formation of transformed foci (Fig. 3) on confluent monolayer cell cultures or the formation of anchorage-independent clones in soft agar. Table 1 shows the results obtained when Swiss 3T3 cells were exposed to UV-irradiation before virus infection, and Table 2 shows the effects of exposure of C3H 10 T 1/2 cells to acetoxy-acetylaminofluorene before viral infection.

As can be seen from these results, transformation frequency increases with pretreatment of cells by the carcinogenic agents used and it should also be noted that there is a dose response in the enhancement of the transformation frequency. As previously suggested the effects we have observed are probably due to the increased number of sites of integration available for the SV40 genome in the treated cell. However, it is also possible that carcinogen treatment turns on some specific genetic program which will permit the cell to become more permissive to the virus and to allow more DNA replication cycles leading to more change to integrate viral sequences. It is generally agreed that the chemical oncogen plus virus directly cotransforms nonmalignant cells and there is not a selection for preexisting malignant cells. This type of cellular system has been successfully used as a screening method for testing oncogenic activity of a large number of substances (Casto et al., 1976; Diamond et al., 1974; Hirai et al., 1974).

Table 1. Effect of UV-Irradiation on the Efficiency of SV40 Transformation of Swiss 3T3 Cells

UV-dose J/m^2	Cloning efficiency (%)	Transformation frequency*		
		uninfected cells	infected cells (10 pfu/cell)	
			foci $\times 10^{-2}$	agar colonies $\times 10^{-2}$
0	25	$<10^{-5}$	1.2	1.2
2.5	22	$<10^{-5}$	5.4	5.0
5.0	20	$<10^{-5}$	7.5	6.5

*Results corrected for cloning efficiency after each treatment. Twenty-four hour cultures of Swiss 3T3 cells (from ATCC, ref. No. CCL92) were washed with PBS, irradiated with a germicidal lamp and infected with wild-type virus at 10 pfu/cell. The transformation assays are carried out as in Fig. 2.

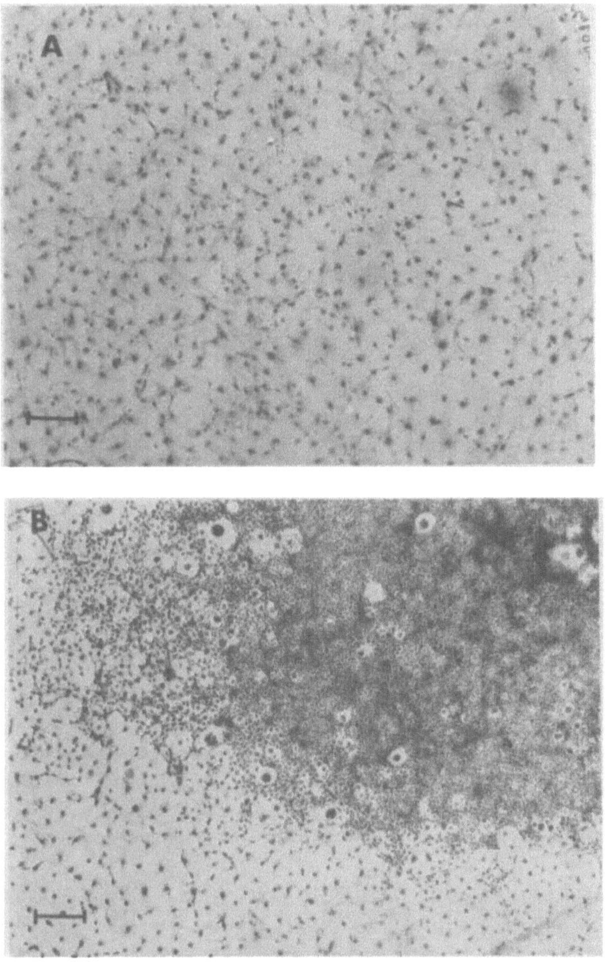

Fig. 3. Photomicrographs of fixed stained cultures of Swiss 3T3 cells. A) Control untreated cells forming a well-defined monolayer; B) transformed colony showing crisscross piling up of phenotypically transformed cells after treatment with UV and wt SV40. Bar represents 0.2 mm.

The Effect of TPA on Cell Transformation by SV40 Mutants

Promotion of in vitro transformation of fibroblast cell cultures previously exposed to chemical carcinogens, ultraviolet light or x-rays has already been demonstrated (Lasne et al., 1974; Kennedy et al., 1978). It has already been shown that the potent tumor promoter TPA increases the yield of transformed foci from adenovirus infected secondary rat embryo cells (Fisher et al., 1978). TPA also

Table 2. Effect of AAAF-Treatment on the Efficiency of Transformation of C3H 10 T 1/2 Cells by wt SV40

Dose AAAF μM	Cloning efficiency (%)	Transformation frequency*		
		uninfected cells	infected cells (10 ptf/cell)	
			foci $\times 10^{-2}$	agar colonies $\times 10^{-2}$
0	20	10^{-5}	1.0	0.5
0.5	28	10^{-5}	4.4	2.2
2	13	10^{-5}	7.7	15
4	5	10^{-5}	20	20

*Results corrected for cloning efficiency after each treatment. C3H 10 T 1/2 cells (a gift from Dr. J. Little, Harvard University) were washed with PBS, treated with AAAF (a gift from Dr. J. A. Miller, University of Wisconsin) and infected with wild-type SV40. Experimental procedure is described in Table 1 and Fig. 2.

has an effect on the anchorage-independent growth of cells previously transformed by adenovirus 5 (Fisher et al., 1979a; Fisher et al., 1979b) and on the behavior of SV40-transformed cells (Sivak and Van Duuren, 1967).

The availability of SV40 mutants, in which the transforming early region of the genome has been mutated, has provided an ideal tool for the analysis of interactions between promoters and the various genes of a transforming DNA virus.

The greater part of our work was carried out using the tsA mutants which are capable of abortive transformation at the restrictive temperature of 39°C but do not form stable transformants at the nonpermissive temperature. Actively growing Swiss 3T3 cells were infected by the tsA virus (10 pfu/cell) and incubated for 24 h at 33°C. The cells were then resuspended in soft-agar according to MacPherson and Montagnier (1964). The tumor promoter TPA and the other substances tested in our experiments were incorporated into the soft agar at the concentration required. The soft-agar cultures (10^4 cells per 6 cm Petri dish) were then incubated at 33°C or 39°C and the number of colonies formed were scored after two (39°C) and three (33°C) weeks of incubation (Fig. 4).

In Table 3 are summarized the results obtained using four different SV40 tsA mutants: 7, 30, 58, and 209. It can be seen that

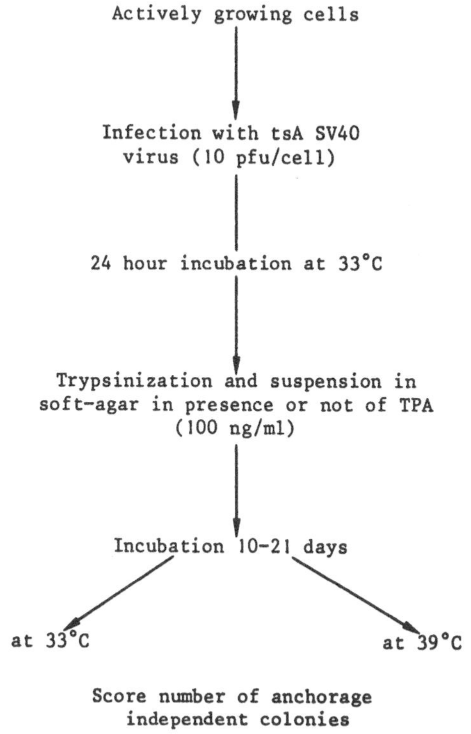

Fig. 4. Protocol to look at the effects of tumor promoters on the formation of soft-agar colonies by Swiss 3T3 cells infected with SV40 tsA mutants.

the inclusion of TPA in the soft agar allows the appearance of macroscopic colonies (Fig. 5) at 39°C in cells previously infected with the various tsA mutants. In the absence of promoters, no colonies were present. At 33°C, colony formation occurs after tsA infection, in the absence of TPA, but the efficiency of transformation is increased 4-fold in the presence of TPA. Under our experimental conditions, no colonies were observed when virus infection was omitted. Moreover, we observed this dramatic effect with various different tsA mutants which indicated that we are not looking at a specific effect of one particular SV40 mutant. Furthermore, UV-irradiated virus could not replace viable virus in our assay, indicating that expression of viral genes are necessary to induce growth in soft agar (Table 3).

A simple explanation for these observations could be that the TPA stimulates the expression of the early viral functions, thereby increasing the residual activity of the gene affected by the tsA mutations, which results in transformation by normal mechanisms. We

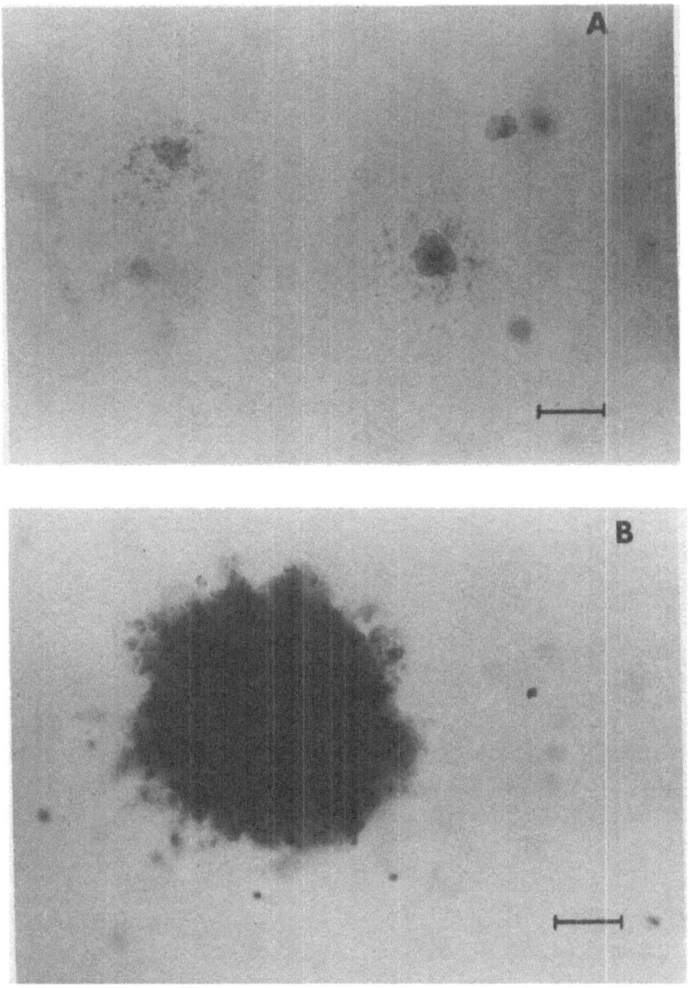

Fig. 5. A) tsA infected Swiss 3T3 cells in soft-agar suspension incubated at 39°C. B) tsA infected Swiss 3T3 cells in soft-agar suspension including TPA (100 ng/ml). Photographs were taken with a Leitz-Orthoplan microscope fitted with the Orthomat photographing equipment. Bar represents 100 microns.

tested this hypothesis by measuring the level of T antigen synthesis at 33°C and 39°C, in Swiss 3T3 cells infected by the tsA58 mutant in the presence or absence of TPA. Cells were analyzed at various times after infection by radioimmunoprecipitation assay (May et al., 1981) or indirect immunofluorescence. As no difference in the level of T antigen was observed in cultures treated with TPA when compared

Table 3. Effect of TPA on the Formation of Soft-Agar Colonies by Swiss 3T3 Cells Infected with SV40 tsA Mutants at 33°C and 39°C

SV40 mutant	33°C		39°C	
	TPA ng/ml		TPA ng/ml	
	0	100	0	100
-	$<10^{-5}$	$<10^{-5}$	$<10^{-5}$	$<10^{-5}$
tsA7	3.0×10^{-3}	1.2×10^{-2}	$<10^{-5}$	2.5×10^{-3}
tsA30	3.8×10^{-3}	1.3×10^{-2}	$<10^{-5}$	4.0×10^{-3}
tsA58	4.2×10^{-3}	1.3×10^{-2}	$<10^{-5}$	5.0×10^{-3}
tsA209	2.8×10^{-3}	1.1×10^{-2}	$<10^{-5}$	3.0×10^{-3}
UV-irradiated tsA58	nd	nd	$<10^{-5}$	$<10^{-5}$
			4-α-PDD ng/ml	
			0	100
tsA58	-	-	$<10^{-5}$	$<10^{-5}$

The active tumor promoting agent, 12-O-tetradecanoyl-phorbol-13-acetate (TPA) and the inactive phorbol ester 4-α-phorbol-12-13-didecanoate (4-α-PDD) were obtained from Dr. P. Borchert (University of Minnesota). Stock solutions of these compounds were made in acetone and stored at -20°C in the dark. The Swiss 3T3 cells were plated at 33°C in 35 mm plastic Petri dishes at 2×10^5 cells per dish. They were infected 24 h later, at subconfluence (10 pfu/cell) and further incubated at 33°C for 24 h. The cells were trypsinized and plated in soft-agar (10^4 cells per 6 cm Petri dish) according to MacPherson and Montagnier (1964). TPA or 4-α-PDD were added to the soft agar (100 ng/ml) as required. Further incubation was carried out at either 33°C or 39°C. Cell cultures were refed weekly with soft-agar medium eventually containing TPA or 4-α-PDD. Colonies were scored after 3 weeks incubation at 33°C and after 2 weeks at 39°C.

with control cultures (Fig. 6), it was concluded that effect of the promoter was not due to a detectable simple stimulation of early viral genes.

Another interesting hypothesis to explain the effects of TPA we observed would be that TPA provides an integration pathway independent of the large T antigen. In order to test this hypothesis several cell lines were established from the soft-agar colonies ob-

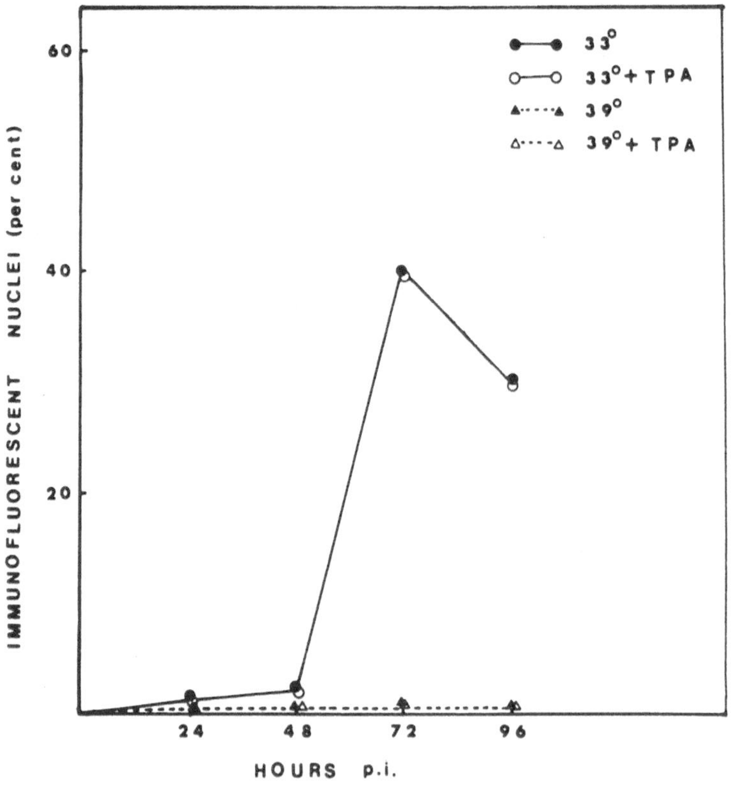

Fig. 6. Effect of TPA on the level of T antigen synthesis at 33°C and 39°C in Swiss 3T3 cells infected by tsA58. Infected cover-slip cultures were treated with hamster anti-SV40 tumor serum followed by antihamster fluorescent serum. T antigen specific fluorescent nuclei were scored.

tained at the restrictive temperature by the combined effect of ts-A58 viral infection and TPA. All cell lines showed a typical transformed cell morphology but did not clone efficiently in agar. Also no viral information could be detected in these cell lines, neither when assayed for specific T antigen (indirect immunofluorescence or radioimmunoprecipitation assay) nor when analyzed for integrated viral DNA by the Southern hybridization technique (Southern, 1975). Therefore the mode of action of the TPA is still to be resolved. TPA is known to have numerous effects on cell cultures in vitro. These include membrane and cytoskeleton modifications which are probably responsible for the "transformed cell" characteristics remarked in cell cultures grown in the presence of TPA. Nevertheless, these local effects of TPA could not be responsible for our observations as control uninfected cells in the presence of TPA did not form soft-agar colonies. Therefore the viral infection is an es-

Table 4. Effect of Different Tumor Promoters on the Formation of Soft-Agar Colonies by Swiss 3T3 Cells Infected with SV40 tsA58 Mutant at 39°C

Tumor promoter	Fraction of infected cells ($\times 10^{-3}$) which form soft-agar colonies at final drug concentration (ng/ml)						
	0.1	1	10	100	5×10^4	10^5	5×10^5
TPA	2.2	3.5	2.8	4.2	nd	nd	nd
Phorbol didecanoate	nd	1.5	2.2	3.5	nd	nd	nd
Phorbol dibenzoate	nd	1.4	1.8	2.2	nd	nd	nd
Phorbol dibutyrate	nd	1.7	1.5	2.0	nd	nd	nd
Teleocidin B	nd	2.0	4.1	2.9	nd	nd	nd
Saccharin	nd	nd	nd	$<10^{-5}$	2.6	3.4	1.8
Anthralin*	nd	nd	1.2	1.8	1.6	nd	nd

*For anthralin, concentrations are respectively: 23, 230, and 2300 ng/ml. Phorbol-12-13-didecanoate (PDD), phorbol-12-13-dibenzoate (PDB) and phorbol-12-13-dibutyrate (PDBr) were obtained from Dr. P. Borchert. Stock solutions in acetone were stored at -20°C in the dark. Teleocidin B, a gift from Dr. Sugimura, was kept as a solution in acetone at -20°C in the dark. Saccharin obtained from Sigma was used as a concentrated solution in distilled water. Anthralin, a gift from Dr. M. Castagna, was stored in acetone solution at -20°C in the dark. The compounds tested were included in the soft-agar at the concentrations shown. nd: not done.

sential step in the phenomenon observed as irradiated virus did not allow soft-agar colony formation. A reasonable explanation could be that the promoter increases in a small fraction of the cell population the number of cell divisions which take place after infection by a tsA mutant at the restrictive temperature to continue, producing a "prolonged abortive transformation."

Besides its effect on transformation, TPA is also known to affect the properties of already transformed cells (Fisher et al., 1978; Sivak and Van Duuren, 1967). We have confirmed these observations using a mouse embryo cell line Δ121 obtained by transformation with a dl54-59 mutant of SV40 (dl2112: Feunteun et al., 1978), which does not produce any small t antigen while the large T antigen is normal.

This cell line is a minimal transformant, behaving like a 3T3 continuous cell line, and is unable to form colonies in soft agar. In the presence of TPA, macrocolonies growing in soft agar were obtained. The tumor promoter thus apparently complements for the small t antigen and permits conversion to maximal transformants.

The Effect of Other Tumor Promoters on Cell Transformation by SV40 Mutants

Since TPA, which is a very active tumor promoter, allows the formation of soft-agar colonies of tsA infected 3T3 cells at 39°C, it was of interest to test other compounds under the same experimental conditions. Other phorbol esters which are known to have various levels of promoting activity (Diamond et al., 1980) are also able, at very low concentrations, to allow soft-agar colony formation (Table 4). The results obtained with teleocidin B and anthralin, show that other chemical classes of tumor promoters are also active in our assay at low concentrations. Saccharin, which has been described as a weak promoter, can allow soft-agar colony growth but at much higher concentrations than the other promoters tested (Table 4). However, our assay allows the detection of tumor promoters at much lower concentrations than other previously described assays (Trosko et al., 1980). It is indispensable to note that the phorbol ester (4-α-phorbol-12-13-didecanoate) which does not possess any promoting activity, did not allow the formation of soft-agar colonies under the same conditions (Table 3).

Recently, Seif (1980) speculated that tumor promoters act by inducing a partial disorganization of the mitotic spindle, causing chromosome aberrations. He tested a number of agents, known to affect the mitotic spindle and/or the cytoskeleton, including some antitumor, and antimitotic drugs. All these agents enhanced the frequency of cell transformation by polyoma virus. Preliminary experiments in our laboratory have shown that vinblastine, colcemide and colchicine did not behave like TPA in the formation of soft-agar colonies under our experimental conditions, in contrast to the results obtained by Seif (1980).

CONCLUSIONS

The mechanism of action of the tumor promoters in general is not understood mainly due to the very many different often contradictory effects they produce *in vivo* and *in vitro*. A recent proposal considers promotion to be the expression of a recessive mutation by abnormal genetic segregation during cell division (Kinsella and Radman, 1978). It could be imagined that in the phenomenon we have observed, the viral infection "initiates" the cell, but is not sufficient by itself to give rise to transformants due to restrictive conditions and the promoter causes loss of growth control, thereby allowing colony formation in soft agar.

The use of in vivo assays for promoters is a lengthy and costly method for assessing the promoting activity of substances. Our observations testing tumor promoters in vitro, seems a far more sensitive and rapid method for screening new substances. The results with saccharin also show that we can detect promoting activity at concentrations much lower than those previously described by Trosko et al. (1980) who used an in vitro metabolic cooperation assay.

We are at present developing our methodology in order to establish a new relatively rapid and sensitive assay for promoter.

REFERENCES

Berenblum, I., The probable nature of promoting action and its significance in the understanding of the mechanism of carcinogenesis, Cancer Res., 14:471 (1954).

Berenblum, I., Origin of the concept of sequential stages of skin carcinogenesis, in: "Cancer: A comprehensive treatise," Becker, ed., Plenum Press, New York (1975).

Casto, B. C., Pieczynski, W. J., Janowsko, N., and Di Paolo, J. A., Significance of treatment interval and DNA repair in the enhancement of viral transformation by chemical carcinogens and mutagens, Chem. Biol. Interactions, 13:105 (1976).

Cleaver, J. E., Defective repair replication of DNA in Xeroderma pigmentosum, Nature, 218:652 (1968).

Devoret, R., Goze, A. Moulé, Y., and Sarasin, A., Lysogenic induction and induced phage reactivation by aflatoxin B_1 metabolites, in: "Mécanismes d'alteration et de réparation du DNA: relation avec la mutagénèse et al cancérogénèse chimique," R. Daudel, Y. Moulé, F. Zajdela, eds., C.N.R.S., Paris (1977).

Diamond, L., Knorr, R., and Shimizu, Y., Enhancement of simian virus 40-induced transformation of Chinese hamster embryo cells by 4-nitroquinoline-1-oxide, Cancer Res., 34:2599 (1974).

Diamond, L., O'Brien, T. G., and Baird, W. B., Tumor promoters and the mechanism of tumor promotion, Adv. Cancer Res., 32:1 (1980).

Feunteun, J., Kress, M., Gardes, M., and Monier, R., Viable deletion mutants in the simian virus 40 early region, Proc. Natl. Acad. Sci. USA, 75:4455 (1978).

Fisher, P. B., Bozzone, J. H., and Weinstein, I. B., Tumor promoters and epidermal growth factor stimulate anchorage-independent growth of adenovirus transformed rat embryo cells, Cell, 18:695 (1979a).

Fisher, P. B., Dorsch-Häsler, K., Weinstein, I. B., and Ginsberg, H. S., Tumor promoters enhance anchorage-independent growth of adenovirus-transformed cells without altering the integration pattern of viral sequences, Nature, 281:591 (1979b).

Fisher, P. B., Weinstein, I. B., Eisenberg, D., and Ginsberg, H. S., Interactions between adenovirus, a tumor promoter, and chemical carcinogens in transformation of rat embryo cell cultures, Proc. Natl. Acad. Sci. USA, 75:2311 (1978).

Fluck, M. M., and Benjamin, T., Comparisons of two early gene functions essential for transformation in polyoma virus and SV40, Virology, 96:205 (1979).

Hecker, E., Isolation and characterization of the co-carcinogenic principles from croton oil, Meth. Cancer Res., 6:439 (1971).

Heidelberger, C., Mondal, S., and Peterson, A. R., Initiation and promotion in cell cultures, in: "Mechanisms of tumor promotion and cocarcinogenesis," T. Slaga, A. Sivak, R. Boutwell, eds., Raven Press, New York (1978),

Hirai, K., Defendi, V., and Diamond, L., Enhancement of simian virus 40 transformation and integration by 4-nitroquinoline-1-oxide, Cancer Res., 34:3497 (1974).

Hynes, R. O., Alteration of cell-surface proteins by viral transformation and by proteolysis, Proc. Natl. Acad. Sci. USA, 70: 3170 (1973).

Kennedy, A. R., Mondal, S., Heidelberger, C., and Little, J. B., Enhancement of x-radiation transformation by a phorbol ester using C3H 10 T 1/2 cl 8 mouse embryo fibroblasts, Cancer Res., 38:439 (1978).

Kinsella, A. R., and Radman, M., Tumor promoter induces sister chromatid exchanges: relevance to mechanisms of carcinogenesis, Proc. Natl. Acad. Sci. USA, 75:6149 (1978).

Lasne, C., Gentil, A., and Chouroulinkov, I., Two-stage malignant transformation of rat fibroblasts in tissue culture, Nature, 247:490 (1974).

MacPherson, I., and Montagnier, L., Agar suspension culture for the selective assay of cells transformed by polyoma virus, Virology, 23:291 (1964).

May, E., Kress, M., Daya-Grosjean, L., Monier, R., and May, P., Mapping of the viral mRNA encoding a super-T antigen of 115,000 daltons expressed in simian virus 40-transformed rat cell lines, J. Virol., 37:24 (1981).

Miller, E. C., Some current perspectives on chemical carcinogenesis in humans and experimental animals, Cancer Res., 38:1479 (1978).

Pollack, R., Osborn, M., and Weber, K., Patterns of organization of Actin and Myosin in normal and transformed cultured cells, Proc. Natl. Acad. Sci. USA, 72:994 (1975).

Pollack, R., Risser, R., Conlon, S., and Rifkin, D., Plasminogen activator production accompanies loss of anchorage regulation in transformation of primary rat embryo cells by simian virus 40, Proc. Natl. Acad. Sci. USA, 71:4792 (1974).

Radman, M., SOS repair hypothesis: phenomenology of an inducible DNA repair which is accompanied by mutagenesis, in: "Molecular Mechanism for Repair of DNA," P. C. Hanawalt, R. B. Setlow, eds., Plenum Press, New York (1975).

Reznikoff, C. A., Bronkow, D. W., and Heidelberger, C., Establishment and characterization of a cloned line of C3H mouse embryo cells sensitive to postconfluence inhibition of cell division, Cancer Res., 33:3231 (1973).

Sarasin, A., and Benoit, A., Induction of an error-prone mode of DNA repair in UV-irradiated monkey kidney cells, Mutation Res., 70:71 (1980).

Sarasin, A., and Hanawalt, P. C., Carcinogens enhance survival of UV-irradiated simian virus 40 in treated monkey kidney cells: induction of a recovery pathway? Proc. Natl. Acad. Sci. USA, 75:346 (1978).

Sarasin, A., Goze, A., Devoret, R., and Moulé, Y., Induced reactivation of UV-damaged phage λ in E. coli K_{12} host cells treated with aflatoxin B_1 metabolites, Mutation Res., 42:205 (1977).

Seif, R., Factors which disorganize microtubules of microfilaments increase the frequency of cell transformation by polyoma virua, J. Virol., 36:421 (1980).

Shenk, T. E., Carbon, J., and Berg, P., Construction of analysis of viable deletion mutants of simian virus 40, J. Virol., 18:664 (1976).

Sivak, A., and Van Duuren, B. L., Phenotypic expression of transformation: induction in cell culture by a phorbol ester, Science, 157:1443 (1967).

Sleigh, M. J., Topp, W. C., Hanich, R., and Sambrook, J. F., Mutants of SV40 with an altered small t protein are reduced in their ability to transform cells, Cell, 14:79 (1978).

Southern, G., Detection of specific sequences among DNA fragments separated by gel electrophoresis, J. Mol. Biol., 98:503 (1975).

Tegtmeyer, P., Simian virus 40 DNA synthesis: the viral replicon, J. Virol., 10:591 (1972).

Tooze, J., "DNA tumor viruses, molecular biology of tumor viruses (Part II)," Cold Spring Harbor Laboratory (1980).

Trosko, E., Dawson, B., Yotti, L. P., and Chang, C. C., Saccharin may act as a tumor promoter by inhibiting metabolic cooperation between cells, Nature, 285:109 (1980).

Vlodavsky, I., Inbar, M., and Sachs, L., Membrane changes and adenosine triphosphate content in normal and malignant transformed cells, Proc. Natl. Acad. Sci. USA, 70:1780 (1973).

Witkin, E. M., Ultraviolet mutagenesis and inducible DNA repair in Escherichia coli, Bacteriol. Res., 40:869 (1976).

REPAIR OF ULTRAVIOLET-LIGHT-INDUCED DAMAGE IN HUMAN SKIN

Betsy M. Sutherland

Biology Department
Brookhaven National Laboratory
Upton, New York 11973

Sunlight exposure induces skin thickening, hyper- and hypopigmentation, and skin cancer in man (see Epstein, 1970). Several lines of evidence indict the ultraviolet components (290-400 nm) of sunlight as the causative agent of both basal and squamous cell carcinomas: 1) the predominance of the cancers on sunlight-exposed skin areas (see Epstein, 1970); 2) the correlation of incidence of these types of skin cancer and latitude of residence of the patient (Urbach and Scotto, 1975); 3) the prevention of skin cancer in cancer-prone xeroderma pigmentosum (XP) patients by limitation of ultraviolet exposure (Lynch et al., 1980) (XP is a hereditary, recessive disease of sun-sensitivity, hyper- and hypo-pigmentation and development of cancerous lesions on sunlight-exposed areas; see Robbins et al., 1974). The correlation of melanoma and sunlight exposure is less clear, although recent data suggest that production of these cancers may correlate with occasional acute sunburning (see Committee on Impacts of Stratospheric Change, 1979).

DNA DAMAGE, REPAIR AND SOLAR ONCOGENESIS

Ultraviolet light induces a wide variety of photoproducts in DNA. Of these, the cyclobutyl pyrimidine dimer, formed between adjacent dimers on the same DNA strand, is the major lesion leading to death and mutation in eucaryotic and procaryotic cells (Setlow, 1966). Cells have developed two major classes of repair mechanisms for dealing with UV-induced damage to their DNA: a light-dependent, one-enzyme pathway mediated by the photoreactivating enzyme (Cook, 1970; Sutherland, 1981), and several light-independent pathways. Among the light-independent processes constitutive in the cell are pre-replication excision repair, in which oligonucleotides containing dimers are removed from the DNA and the opposing DNA strand is used as template for repair synthesis (Hanawalt et al., 1979), and post-replication repair in which (in some but not all species) gaps left opposite dimers during semi-conservative DNA replication are filled in by a by-pass mechanism (Bridges, 1978; Lehman, 1975).

These pathways were first delineated in the bacterium *Escherichia coli*. Although early studies indicated that mammalian cells might not be capable of excision (Klimek, 1966), later investigators found that mammalian cells could carry out this process. Fibroblasts from normal humans remove dimers efficiently from their DNA, although the rates of removal obtained by different investigators vary from 70% excision in 6 h (Konze-Thomas et al., 1978), to no excision after 3 (Carrier et al., 1978) or 12 h (Ehmann et al., 1978).

Several lines of evidence indicate that DNA damage and failure of repair, or inaccurate repair, are related to solar oncogenesis in man. Cleaver's (1968) demonstration of defective DNA repair in xeroderma cells suggested strongly that xeroderma resulted from this defect. Later investigators showed that the colony-forming ability of XP cells exposed to ultraviolet light is also defective compared to normal cells, with good correlation between depression of colony-forming ability and the degree of defectiveness of DNA repair (Konze-Thomas et al., 1978). Epstein et al. (1970) showed that the deficiency in DNA repair seen in fibroblasts was also present in the skin of XP patients: they exposed the skin of normal and XP individuals to UV radiation, injected ^{3}H-thymidine and obtained punch biopsies after 1 h. When the skin samples were analyzed for repair synthesis, the normal cells showed high levels of unscheduled DNA repair synthesis, while the XP cells had undergone almost no repair.

Light-dependent repair, photoreactivation, was the first DNA repair pathway described in procaryotic or eucaryotic cells (Kelner, 1949; Dulbecco, 1950). In photoreactivation, repair is mediated by one enzyme, the photoreactivating enzyme or photolyase (Rupert, 1960). This enzyme binds to its substrate, a cyclobutyl pyrimidine dimer in a DNA polynucleotide (Wulff and Rupert, 1962; Setlow et al., 1968), and in the presence of light, monomerizes the dimer to two pyrimidines (Setlow, 1964; Setlow et al., 1965). This kind of repair offers several advantages to the cell: 1) since there is no incision into the phosphodiester backbone, there is no opportunity for DNA degradation, 2) since there is no *de novo* synthesis, there is no chance for mis-repair due to infidelity of the synthetic apparatus, and 3) since the only energy requirement of the reaction is light, the reaction does not call upon the cell's energy stores.

This process was studied extensively in *E. coli* and the photoreactivating enzyme from yeast was the first to be characterized (Rupert, 1962a, 1962b; Muhammed, 1966). Although early reports indicated that the enzyme might be absent in mammalian cells (Cleaver, 1966; Cook, 1970), later investigators found photoreactivating enzyme

(Sutherland, 1974; Harm, 1976), cellular photoreactivation of dimers (Sutherland et al., 1975a), and photoreactivation of infecting UV-irradiated viruses (Sutherland et al., 1975b; Henderson, 1978).

The specificity of the photoreactivating enzyme for pyrimidine dimers offers a unique test for the involvement of dimers in the production of biological damage (see Sutherland, 1978). In the photoreactivation test, one determines the effect of photoreactivating light treatment on the induction of UV of biological damage. If the detrimental biological effect of UV can be reversed in a true photoenzymatic reaction, pyrimidine dimers were involved in the production of that damage. Hart et al. (1977) took advantage of this test to show that while injection of UV irradiated cells into the fish Poecilia formosa led to tumor formation, if those cells were UV-irradiated and then photoreactivated, tumor formation was greatly reduced. These experiments offer the first evidence linking a specific DNA alteration with UV oncogenesis.

PYRIMIDINE DIMER FORMATION AND REPAIR IN SKIN

Conventional methods for quantitating pyrimidine dimers in skin require high specific activity radioactive labeling of the DNA. This requirement precluded measurement of dimers in human skin, although several investigators followed dimer formation in the skin of other mammals. Pathak et al. (1972) applied [^{3}H]-thymidine to the epilated skin of guinea pigs, hydrolyzed the DNA, and separated the radioactive dimers and pyrimidine monomers by chromatography. Bowden et al. (1975), Cooke and Johnson (1978) and Strickland (1978) examined dimer formation in mouse or rat skin by chromatographic analysis of radioactive DNA. Cooke and Johnson also examined the wavelength dependence of dimer formation in rodent skin; the resulting action spectrum, when convoluted with an estimated absorption spectrum of skin, lent support to the idea of nucleic acid as the absorbing chromophore.

Repair in Rodent Skin

Bowden et al. (1975) and Cooke and Johnson (1978) reported disappearance of dimers from UV-irradiated rodent skin. Ley et al. (1978) analyzed dimer formation in mouse skin by extraction of the radioactive DNA, treatment with a UV-endonuclease preparation (which makes a single strand nick adjacent to every dimer) and sedimentation on alkaline sucrose gradients. Analysis of the molecular weight distribution of the DNA from samples taken at different times after UV failed to show any excision or photoreactivation. Ananthaswamy et al. (1981) also found no photoreactivation in adult mouse skin, but showed that in neonatal mice photoreactivation treatment resulted in efficient dimer disappearance.

Mouse cells in culture undergo slow dimer excision (Regan and Setlow, 1973) and contain very low levels of photoreactivating enzyme (Sutherland et al., 1974). It seems likely then, that dimer excision and photoreactivation may both exist in rodent skin, with the levels varying with mouse strain and age, and experimental result perhaps depending on the sensitivity of the method of analysis.

Pyrimidine Dimer Formation and Repair in Human Skin

Measurement of pyrimidine dimers in human skin awaited the development of methods for dimer quantitation in non-radioactive DNA. Achey et al. (1979) adapted the alkaline agarose gel system of McDonnell et al. (1977) to dimer measurement in unlabeled DNA: in Achey's method, DNA is extracted from irradiated cells and treated with the UV-endonuclease to make a nick adjacent to each dimer. The pH is then raised to 10 to stop the reaction and separate the DNA strands. The DNA is then electrophoresed on alkaline agarose gels, migration in which depends on the molecular weight of the DNA. DNA without dimers remains intact during endonuclease treatment, and the resulting high molecular weight DNA does not travel very far into into the gel. DNA containing dimers, however, is nicked by the endonuclease, yielding lower molecular weight species which have higher mobilities in the gel. The gel is neutralized, and stained with ethidium bromide, which fluoresces brightly when bound to DNA. The gel is photographed, the negative scanned with a densitometer, and the resulting molecular weight profiles analyzed to give dimer content.

Sutherland et al. (1980) developed a method for measuring pyrimidine dimer formation and repair in human skin. Sunlight unexposed skin of normal human volunteers was subjected to sunlamp irradiation, and punch biopsies obtained immediately and after 20 or 40 min incubation in the absence or presence of photoreactivating light. These studies showed that even suberythymal doses of sunlamp radiation produce measurable numbers of dimers: $^1/_2$ the minimal erythymal dose (med) produces about 5 dimers per 10^8 daltons, with 1 med yielding 10 dimers per 10^8 daltons. These studies also showed that dimers are rapidly excised from the skin DNA, with about 40% removal in 20 min, and 60% removal in 40 min. Similar results were obtained by D'Ambrosio et al. (1981), who measured excision of dimers in non-radioactive human skin DNA by extraction of the DNA, sedimentation in alkaline sucrose gradients, collection of gradient fractions and quantitation of DNA in each fraction by a fluorescence assay. They found that about half the dimers were removed at 60 min.

Sutherland et al. (1980) also looked for photoreactivation in skin exposed to a 60 W white incandescent bulb at 25 cm from the skin. After 20 min of photoreactivation treatment, 60% of the dimers had disappeared from the DNA. Since excision could account for removal of 40% of the dimers in this time, the photoreversal added only an additional 20%, too small an effect to be probed further. D'Ambrosio et al. (1981) obtained strikingly different results on photoreactivation in skin; they showed that in 1.3 min 50% of the dimers disappeared during photoreactivating treatment. What could be the source of differences in the results of Sutherland et al., and D'Ambrosio et al.? Comparison of the methods used by the two groups shows two major differences: first, the skin samples obtained by Sutherland et al., were 3 or 4-mm punch biopsies which included both the entire epidermis and the upper portion of the dermis, while the samples of D'Ambrosio et al., were thin (4-8 cell layers) epidermal "bubbles." Perhaps the epidermis or the upper layers of the epidermis have higher photoreactivation capacity. The second difference is the photoreactivating light source. D'Ambrosio et al., used a high intensity mercury arc filtered to exclude wavelengths shorter than 455 nm. [The action spectrum for PR by the human enzyme peaks at about 400 nm, but extends as far as 577 nm (Sutherland and Sutherland, 1975).] Perhaps the lesser photoreactivation observed by Sutherland et al. (1980) resulted from their use of only a 60 W incandescent bulb - the reaction may have been limiting in light!

These studies present three major new findings in the photobiology of skin. First, detectable numbers of dimers are formed even at sub-erythymal doses. Second, excision of dimers is much more rapid (∿50% removal in 1 h) than would be predicted from results obtained in cell culture. Third, comparison of the rates of excision and photoreactivation in skin indicates that in normal sunlight exposure, photoreactivation may well be the predominant repair pathway in skin.

Future Research Areas

These results on human skin point the way to several important lines of research. First, what is the action spectrum for dimer formation in human skin? Second, is the photoreactivation phenomenon a physical photoreversal or a true enzymatic photoreactivation process? Third, is this photoreversal phenomenon responsible for the photoreactivation of erythema seen by van der Leun and Stoop (1969), by Van Weelden (1979) and by Parrish (personal communication)? The near future may offer solutions to these and other basic problems in photodermatology.

REFERENCES

Achey, P. M. Woodhead, A. D., and Setlow, R. B., 1979, Photoreactivation of pyrimidine dimers in DNA from thyroid cells of the teleost, Poecilia formosa, Photochem. Photobiol., 29:305.

Ananthaswamy, H. N., and Fisher, M. S., 1981, Photoreactivation of ultraviolet radiation-induced pyrimidine dimers in neonatal BALB/c mouse skin, Cancer Res., 41:1829.

Bowden, G. T., Trosko, J. E., Shapas, B. G., and Boutwell, R. K., 1975, Excision of pyrimidine dimers from epidermal DNA and non-semiconservative epidermal DNA synthesis following UV irradiation of mouse skin, Cancer Res., 35:3599.

Bridges, B. A., 1978, Workshop Summary: Conditioned Repair Responses, in: "DNA Repair Mechanisms," C. F. Fox, E. C. Friedberg, and P. C. Hanawalt, eds., Academic Press, New York.

Carrier, W. L., Smith, D. P., and Regan, J. P., 1978, Pyrimidine dimer excision in human cells, J. Supramol. Structure Suppl., 2:77.

Cleaver, J. E., 1966, Photoreactivation: A radiation repair absent from mammalian cells, Biochem. Biophys. Res. Commun., 24:569.

Cleaver, J. E., 1968, Defective repair replication of DNA in xeroderma pigmentosum, Nature, 218:652.

Committee on impacts of stratospheric change, 1979, Protection against depletion of stratospheric ozone by chlorofluorocarbons, National Academy of Sciences Press, Washington, D.C.

Cook, J. S., 1970, Photoreactivation in animal cells, in: "Photophysiology," A. C. Giese, ed., Vol. 5, Academic Press, New York.

Cook, J. S., and McGrath, J. R., 1967, Photoreactivating enzyme activity in metazoa, Proc. Nat. Acad. Sci. USA, 58:1359.

Cooke, A., and Johnson, B. E., 1978, Dose response, wavelength dependence and rate of excision of ultraviolet radiation - induced pyrimidine dimers in mouse skin DNA, Biochem. Biophys. Acta, 517:24.

D'Ambrosio, S., 1981 (in press), Photorepair of pyrimidine dimers in human skin in vivo, Photochem. Photobiol.

Dulbecco, R., 1950, Experiments on photoreactivation of bacterophages inactivated with ultraviolet radiation, J. Bacteriol., 59:329.

Ehmann, U. K., Cook, K. H., and Friedberg, E. C., 1978, in: "DNA Repair Mechanisms," P. C. Hanawalt and E. C. Friedberg, eds., Academic Press, New York.

Epstein, J. H., 1970, Ultraviolet Carcinogenesis, in: "Photophysiology," A. C. Giese, ed., Vol. V, Academic Press, New York.

Epstein, J. H., Fukuyama, K., Reed, W. E., and Epstein, W. L., 1970, Defect in DNA synthesis in skin of patients with xeroderma pigmentosum demonstrated in vivo, Science, 168:1477.

Hanawalt, P. C., Copper, P. K., Ganesan, A. K., and Smith, C. A., 1979, DNA repair in bacteria and mammalian cells, Ann. Rev. Biochem., 48:783.

Harm, H., 1976, Damage and repair in mammalian cells after ultraviolet and/or visible light treatment, in: "Symposium on Biological effects and measurement of light sources, proceedings," DeWitt G. Hazzard, ed., HEW Publication (FDA), 77-8002, Rockville, Maryland.

Hart, R., Setlow, R. B., and Woodhead, A., 1977, Evidence that pyrimidine dimers in DNA can give rise to tumors, Proc. Nat. Acad. Sci. USA, 74:5574.

Henderson, E. E., 1978, Host cell reactivation of Epstein-Barr virus in normal and repair-defective leukocytes, Cancer Res., 38:3256.

Kelner, A., 1949, Effect of visible light on the recovery of Streptomyces griseus conidia from ultraviolet irradiation injury, Proc. Natl. Acad. Sci. USA, 35:73.

Klimek, M., 1966, Thymine dimerization in L-strain mammalian cells after irradiation with ultraviolet light and the search for repair mechanisms, Photochem. Photobiol., 5:603.

Konze-Thomas, B., Dorney, D. J., Maher, V. M. and McCormick, J. J., 1978, Comparing the percent survival and extent of excision repair of thymine dimers following UV irradiation of confluent cultures of human cells or of synchronized populations at various times during the cell cycle, J. Supramol. Structure, Suppl. 2:77.

Lehmann, A. R., 1975, Postreplication repair of DNA in mammalian cells, Life Sci., 15:2005.

Ley, R. D., Sedita, B. A., and Grube, D. D., 1978, Absence of photoreactivation of pyrimidine dimers in the epidermis of hairless mice following exposures to ultraviolet light, Photochem. Photobiol., 27:483.

Lynch, H. T., Lynch, P. M., and Guirgis, H. A., 1980, Host-Environmental Interaction and Carcinogenesis in Man in Genetic Differences in Chemical Carcinogenesis, R. E. Kouri, ed., CRC Press, Boca Raton, Florida.

McDonell, M., Simon, M. N., and Studier, F. W., 1977, Analysis of restriction fragments of T7 DNA and determination of molecular weight by electrophoresis of neutral and alkaline gels, J. Molec. Biol., 110:119.

Muhammed, A., 1966, Studies on the yeast photoreactivating enzyme, J. Biol. Chem., 241, 516.

Pathak, M. A., Kramer, D. M., and Gungerich, U., 1972, Formation of thymine dimers in mammalian skin by ultraviolet radiation in vivo, Photochem. Photobiol., 15, 177.

Regan, J. D., and Setlow, R. B., 1973, Repair of chemical damage to human DNA, in: "Chemical mutagens, principles and methods for their detection," Vol. 3, Plenum Press, New York.

Robbins, J. H., Kraemer, K. H., Lutzner, M. A., Festoff, B. W., and Coon, H. G., 1974, Xeroderma pigmentosum: An inherited disease with sun sensitivity, multiple cutaneous neoplasms, and abnormal DNA repair, Ann. Int. Med., 80:221.

Rupert, C. S., 1960, Photoreactivation of transforming DNA by an enzyme from Baker's yeast, J. Gen. Physiol., 43:573.

Rupert, C. S., 1962a, Photoenzymatic repair of ultraviolet damage in DNA: I. Kinetics of the reaction, J. Gen. Physiol., 45:703.

Rupert, C. S., 1962b, Photoenzymatic repair of ultraviolet damage in DNA: II. Formation of an enzyme-substrate complex, J. Gen. Physiol., 45:725.

Setlow, J. K., 1964, Effects of UV on DNA: Correlation among biological changes, physical changes and repair mechanisms, Photochem. Photobiol., 3:405.

Setlow, J. K., Boling, M. E., and Bollum, F. J., 1965, The chemical nature of photoreactivable lesions in DNA, Proc. Nat. Acad. Sci. USA, 53:1430.

Setlow, R. B., 1966, Cyclobutane-type pyrimidine dimers in polynucleotides, Science, 153:379.

Setlow, R. B., Carrier, W. L., and Bollum, F. J., 1965, Pyrimidine dimers in UV-irradiated poly dI:dC, Proc. Nat. Acad. Sci. USA, 53:1111.

Strickland, P. T., 1978, Pyrimidine dimer formation in epidermal DNA and oncogenesis in rat skin exposed to ultraviolet radiation, Ph.D. Thesis, New York University.

Sutherland, B. M., 1974, Photoreactivating enzyme from human leukocytes, Nature, 248:109.

Sutherland, B. M., 1978, Photoreactivation in mammalian cells, Int. Rev. Cytol., Suppl. 8, 301.

Sutherland, B. M., 1981, Photoreactivating enzymes, in: "The enzymes," Vol. 15, Part B (in press), P. Boyer, ed., Academic Press, New York.

Sutherland, B. M. Kochevar, I., and Harber, L., 1980, Pyrimidine dimer formation and repair in human skin, Cancer Res., 40:3181.

Sutherland, B. M., Rice, M., and Wagner, E. K., 1975, Xeroderma pigmentosum cells contain low levels of photoreactivating enzyme, Proc. Nat. Acad. Sci. USA, 72:103.

Sutherland, B. M., Runge, P., and Sutherland, J. C., 1974, DNA photoreactivating enzyme from placental mammals: origin and characteristics, Biochem., 13:4710.

Sutherland, J. C., and Sutherland, B. M., 1975, Human photoreactivating enzyme: action spectrum and safelight conditions, Biophys. J., 15:435-440.

Urbach, F., and Scotto, 1975, Incidence of nonmelanoma skin cancer, in: "Impacts of climatic change on the biosphere," DOT-TST-75-55.

Van der Leun, J. C., and Stoop, T., 1969, Photorecovery of ultraviolet Erythema, in: "The Biologic Effects of Ultraviolet Radiation," F. Urbach, ed., Pergamon Press, Oxford.

Van Weelden, H., 1979, Photoreactivation in Human Skin, in: "Conference Digest, Europhysics Conference, Lasers in Photomedicine and Phototheraphy," p. 25.

Wagner, E. K., Rice, M., and Sutherland, B. M., 1975, Photoreactivation of herpes simplex virus in human fibroblasts, Nature, 254:627.

Wulff, D. L., and Rupert, C. S., 1962, Disappearance of thymine photodimer in ultraviolet irradiated DNA upon treatment with a photoreactivating enzyme from Baker's yeast, Biochem. Biophys. Res., 7:237.

DOSIMETRY BY MEANS OF MEASUREMENT OF HEMOGLOBIN ALKYLATION AND RISK ESTIMATION BASED ON THE RAD-EQUIVALENT APPROACH

S. Osterman-Golkar

Radiology Department
Wallenberg Laboratory
University of Stockholm
Stockholm, Sweden

To assist the regulatory agencies in protecting the public health it is not sufficient to identify genetic risk factors. As a basis for measures, such as setting of TLV, data have to be provided that make possible a prediction of the relation between the level of exposure and extent of the damage to human health. Despite extensive biological experimentation there is very little data which can be directly used in quantitative risk assessment of genotoxic compounds. The possibilities of estimating risk to man from experimental data are limited, especially, by lack of knowledge of qualitative and quantitative differences between experimental organisms and man in metabolism of foreign compounds and in efficiencies of repair functions. A further drawback of tests for genotoxic activity of conventional scope is a low resolving power. If for some reason, such as a high toxicity or low solubility, a compound cannot be investigated at doses much higher than the one that occurs in human environments, an unacceptable risk may well be hidden in a negative result (Ehrenberg, 1974, 1977; Ehrenberg and Osterman-Golkar, 1980).

A dosimetry of ultimately reactive compounds/metabolites by a determination of stable reaction products with macromolecules gives data that are meaningful for quantitative risk estimations. Hemoglobin has been suggested as a suitable target molecule for such monitoring (Osterman-Golkar et al., 1976). The method utilizes the high resolving power of chemical analysis and is applicable to both animals and man. The relationship of covalent binding to hemoglobin and to DNA in specific tissues can be studied for individual compounds in animals. This relationship should provide a reasonable basis for estimating the alkylation of DNA from the alkylation of hemoglobin in man.

According to the approach suggested by Ehrenberg (Osterman-Golkar and Ehrenberg, 1977; Ehrenberg, 1980) the rad-equivalence of a chemical change in DNA may be established in experimental organisms and applied tentatively for quantitative assessments of risk to man posed by exposures to genotoxic compounds.

THEORETICAL AND EXPERIMENTAL BACKGROUND TO THE USE OF REACTION PRODUCTS OF HEMOGLOBIN FOR DOSE MONITORING

The degree of alkylation (arylation, etc.) of nucleophilic molecules in cells may be determined as a measure of the dose of an electrophilic compound/intermediate, provided that the target molecule and the alkylated product are sufficiently stable (Ehrenberg et al., 1974; Aaron, 1976; Lee, 1976). We define the dose, D, as the time integral of the concentration of the electrophilic compound, RX. The degree of alkylation (or other type of substitution), $[RY]/[Y^-]$, is directly proportional to the dose according to the equation

$$[RY]/[Y^-] = k_Y \cdot D \qquad (1)$$

where k_Y is the second order rate constant for reaction of the alkylating agent RX with the nucleophilic compound Y^-

$$(RY + Y^- \rightarrow RY + X^-).$$

Hemoglobin is a stable molecule. The life span equals that of the erythrocytes [126 days in man (- healthy persons), 40 days in the mouse]. Studies with methylating and hydroxyethylating agents, benzene and benzo[a]pyrene (Osterman-Golkar et al., 1976; Segerbäck et al., 1978; Segerbäck and Calleman, current work) have demonstrated that reaction products of these agents are persistent; the elimination of alkylated hemoglobin after acute exposure of mice corresponded to the life span of the erythrocyte. As a consequence, reaction products accumulate in a predictable way after repeated exposures. At chronic exposure the degree of alkylation of nucleophilic groups will reach a steady state value

$$[RY]_{acc}/[Y^-] = a \cdot t_{er.}/2 \qquad (2)$$

where a is the daily increment of the degree of alkylation and $t_{er.}$ is the life span of the erythrocytes (Osterman-Golkar et al., 1976).

About thirty radiolabelled compounds have been studied in rodents and found to bind to hemoglobin. These compounds (cf., Calleman, 1981) include both directly alkylating agents: alkyl methanesulfonates, methyl bromide, benzyl chloride, dichlorvos, and compounds that are activated chemically: *N*-alkyl-*N*-nitrosoureas, *N*-methyl-*N*-nitrosonitroguanidine, or metabolically: nitrosamines, polycylic aromatic hydrocarbons, aromatic amines, aflatoxin B_1, benzene, chloroform, carbon tetrachloride and vinyl chloride (Osterman-Golkar et al., 1976, 1977) Neumann et al., 1977; Segerbäck et al., 1978; Pereira and Chang, 1980; Farmer et al., 1980; Nguyen et al., 1981; Walles, 1981; and unpublished data). Also the simple unsaturated compounds ethylene (Ehrenberg et al., 1977; Segerbäck, 1981a) and propylene (unpublished data) produce metabolites that bind to hemoglobin.

The most important and nucleophilic groups of hemoglobin are cysteine-S, histidine-$\underline{N}^{\tau}$ and -$\underline{N}^{\pi}$, the amino group of the $\underline{N}$-terminal amino acid (valine in both chains), ε-NH_2 of lysine, and carboxylate groups. The reactivities of these specific groups in terms of the degree of alkylation obtained are determined by their nucleophilic strengths, abundance and degree of dissociation* and steric and solubility factors (cf. Ehrenberg and Osterman-Golkar, 1980). The combined effect of these factors results in a decreasing yield of products in the order: alkylated α-NH_2 (valine) - alkylated $\underline{N}^{\tau}$ and $\underline{N}^{\pi}$, respectively, of histidine - alkylated cysteine, after treatment of human red cells with, for example, ethylene oxide (s = 0.96 in the Swain-Scott scale; cf. Osterman-Golkar, 1975).

Analytical procedures have been worked out for a few alkylated products of cysteine and histidine (Calleman et al., 1978; Farmer et al., 1980). Briefly, these methods involve the isolation of globin from the erythrocytes, addition of internal standard (a trace amount of the alkylated product to be determined radiolabelled to a high specific activity) and hydrolysis of the protein in 6 M HCl. The hydrolysate is then chromatographed on ion exchange columns. Column fractions containing the radiolabelled tracer are analyzed directly on an amino acid analyzer or are derivatized for analysis by means of gas chromatography mass fragmentography. The large amount of hemoglobin that can be used in these procedures and the extremely high sensitivity of the chemical analysis makes the monitoring of human exposures to alkylating agents possible. Less time consuming techniques are currently under development.

DOSIMETRY BY DETERMINATION OF COVALENT BINDING TO HEMOGLOBIN AS A BASIS FOR RISK ESTIMATIONS

The fate of a mutagenic compound, from the appearance in the environment to the expression of a genotoxic effect is illustrated in Scheme 1. The model considers both compounds RX that are electrophilic <u>per se</u> and compounds A that are chemically or metabolically converted to such. In this model doses (D_i) and levels (L_i) have been defined at consecutive steps, 1-6, and their interrela-

---

*The fraction $[Y^-]$ of the total concentration of a nucleophile $([YH] + [Y^-])$ present as free base (Y^-) is, at low ionic strength given by $[Y^-]/([YH] + [Y^-]) = 1/(1 + 10pk_a\text{-}pH)$.

Scheme 1. System of steps from environmental level/dose of pollutants to biological response (simplified version in Table 1 in Ehrenberg et al., 1981; cf. also Ehrenberg and Osterman-Golkar, 1980).

Step*		Designation	Dimension (examples)
(D_0)	Emission		
	↓		
D_1	Exposure to premutagen A or ultimate mutagen RX	Exposure dose	ppm·h
	k_{12} ↓ uptake		
L_2	Absorbed amount of A or RX	Pharmacological dose	mg (kg b.w.)$^{-1}$
	k_{23} ↓ activation, deactivation transport		
D_3	RX in tissues	Tissue dose	mol (kg b.w.)$^{-1}$ h
	k_{34} ↓ transport diffusion		
D_4	RX in immediate environment of target molecules (often DNA)	Target dose ("DNA-dose")	-"-
	k_{45} ↓ alkylation, etc		
L_5	Chemically changed critical centers in target macromolecule	Molecular dose	mol RY (mol Y^-)$^{-1}$
	k_{56} ↓ repair, replication, promotion		
L_6	Expressed effect in the biological system studied		

*D denotes a dose in the strict sense with the dimension concentration x time; L is a level (concentration).

Scheme 2. Calibration scheme for quantitative risk esimations for humans from data obtained in experimental test systems. (Horizontal arrows indicate flow of information.)

Step in the model	Bacteria or mammalian cells in culture	Experimental animals	Exposed humans
D_1			Exposure dose
			↓ k_{12}
L_2	Concentration applied (known)	Amount administered (known)	Amount absorbed (estimated or known)
	↓ k_{23}	↓ k_{23}	↓ k_{23}
D_3	Dose in medium (determined)	Dose in blood (determined)	Dose in blood (determined
	↓ k_{34} →	↓ k_{34} →	↓ k_{34}
D_4	"DNA-dose" (determined)	"DNA-dose" (determined)	"DNA-dose" (estimated)
	↓ k_{46} →	↓ k_{46} →	↓ k_{46}
L_6	Biological effect Response (determined and expressed in suitable dose equivalents)	Biological effect Response determined and expressed in suitable dose equivalents)	Biological effect Response
	↓ →	↓ →	Risk (estimated and when possible checked with epidemiological data)

ships have been expressed in terms of transfer coefficients, $k_{i(i+1)}$. The relation between response (L_6) and dose determined at step i may be written

$$\text{Response} = D_i \prod_i^5 k_{i(i+1)} \tag{3}$$

An estimation of risk to man at a given dose D_i thus implies an estimation of the product (Π) of subsequent transfer coefficients. Scheme 2 shows the position of the hemoglobin dosimetry in this risk estimation and illustrates the type of information that may be obtained from laboratory test systems.

Relationship between Exposure Dose (D_1) or Pharmacological Dose (L_2) and Dose in Erythrocytes (D_3)

In laboratory experiments with mutagenic compounds (A or RX) the dose is usually expressed as the amount given per l or per kg body weight (L_2). This is also the common way to express the dose in treatments of patients or intake of food components, etc., L_2 thus has the dimension of a level (concentration). The dose in tissues of ultimately reactive compounds RX is determined by rates of transports and rates of chemical and enzyme-catalyzed reactions leading to the formation of RX from the premutagen A, elimination of A by other routes and elimination of RX. These processes may differ qualitatively as well as quantitatively between animals and man (and between individuals) and are not adequately represented in *in vitro* test systems.

From pharmacology it is known that the kinetics of processes such as diffusion, adsorption and metabolism are influenced by the level (concentration) (cf., e.g., Ehrenberg et al., 1981). Metabolic reactions leading to activation or deactivation of chemicals generally follow Michaelis-Menten kinetics:

$$-\frac{d[S]}{dt} = k\cdot[E]_{tot}\cdot\frac{[S]}{K_m + [S]} \tag{4}$$

where [S] = the substrate level ([A] or [RX] in the preceding text), $[E]_{tot}$ = total enzyme concentration, $k\cdot[E]tot$ (= V_{max}) = the rate of reaction at very high [S] and K_m = Michaelis constant (K_m = the concentration of the substrate where the rate of reaction is equal to $^1/_2\cdot V_{max}$). When [S] is small compared to K_m, Eq. (4) approaches first order kinetics and a *constant fraction* of [S] is converted per unit time. At high concentrations of S ([S] $\gg K_m$) zero-order kinetics is approached and a *constant amount* of S is converted per unit time.

It is important to recognize that, whereas exposures to humans of chemicals in the environment may be in the low dose region where processes can be assumed to follow first order kinetics, this is not always the case in laboratory experiments. Long-term assays for carcinogenicity are normally performed at extremely high levels (i.e., injected, ingested, or inhaled) in order to get a significant yield of tumors in a small number of animals. The results of such experiments may be very misleading because extrapolation to lower doses requires a knowledge of the relation between the level of chemical applied and the resulting dose of RX. A determination of the degree of binding of reactive metabolites to hemoglobin gives important information on this point.

The degree of binding to hemoglobin in rodents as a function of injected or inhaled amount of chemical has been determined for a few compounds of model character. For the compounds methyl methanesulfonate (Osterman-Golkar et al., 1976; Nguyen et al., 1981) and ethylene oxide (Ehrenberg et al., 1974) linear relationships between pharmacological dose (L_2) and the degree of alkylation of hemoglogin were obtained over the wide range of doses studied. The degree of alkylation of hemoglobin after i.p. administration of ethyl methanesulfonate (Murthy et al., 1981) increased proportionally to the injected amount in the range 0.25-50 μmol/kg b.w. Above this range a somewhat higher than proportional degree of alkylation was found, indicating that a saturation of some system for detoxification of the compound occurs, resulting in a decreased rate of elimination and consequently an increased dose in tissues of this directly akylating agent. (It is being investigated whether adsorption to lipophilic regions of plasma proteins is the cause of this phenomenon (cf. Borgå et al., 1970)).

The data on the degree of alkylation of hemoglobin after exposure of mice to ethylene are compatible with an enzymecatalyzed activation, following Michaelis-Menten kinetics; that is, the dose of the alkylating intermediate, ethylene oxide, as determined from the degree of alkylation of hemoglobin, is directly proportional to the level of ethylene in the atmosphere at low air concentrations. At high air concentrations the activating system is saturated and a constant amount of ethylene is transformed per unit time (Segerbäck, 1981, cf. also Ehrenberg et al., 1977; Andersen et al., 1980). Andersen and coworkers estimated the inhalational K_m of ethylene in rat to about 220 ppm and V_{max} to 8.6×10^{-6} mole ethylene per kg b.w. per hour. Assuming that ethylene oxide is the sole metabolite of ethylene - binding studies in mice indicated that it is the main metabolite (Segerbäck, 1981) - V_{max} corresponds to the exposure of rats at an air concentration of 6 ppm of ethylene oxide (Osterman-Golkar and Ehrenberg, 1981). From what is known at present about the results of the long-term study of the carcinogenicity of ethylene oxide in rats, carried out at the Carnegie-Mellon Institute of Research (Fishbein, 1980), it appears that 10 ppm is near the level where effects of chronic exposure could be detected with statistical significance. The expected dose-response curve of ethylene thus falls entirely below the detection limit of this test system. The implications to the interpretation of the negative results reported from long-term exposure of rats at levels up to 10,000 ppm of ethylene (CIIT, 1980) are obvious. For a comparison of the resolving power of test systems: a one-hour exposure of rats at 1 ppm of ethylene oxide or 33 ppm of ethylene), radiolabelled to the specific activity 100 mCi/mmole of ^{14}C, can easily be detected by determination of reaction products with hemoglobin.

Relationship between Dose in Erythrocytes (D_3) and "DNA-Dose" (D_4)

Model experiments with rodents have shown that for the alkylating agents methyl methanesulfonate (Segerbäck et al., 1978; Nguyen et al., 1981b), ethylene oxide (Ehrenberg et al., 1974; Segerbäck, 1981), ethyl methanesulfonate (Murthy et al., 1981) and benzyl chloride (Walles, 1981) - all of which are small uncharged molecules and soluble in both lipids and water - the dose determined by hemoglobin alkylation (application of Eq. (1) and rate constants determined in vitro) gives a good approximation of the dose to DNA. This is in general agreement with the demonstration by Frei et al. (1978) that the alkylating agents dimethyl sulfate, ethyl methanesulfonate, N-methyl-N-nitrosurea, and N-ethyl-N-nitrosourea give approximately the same degree of alkylation of DNA in different organs of the mouse. However, for many compounds effects of metabolism and compartmentalization are likely to affect the correspondence between the dose in red cells and the dose to DNA of different organs. These effects may be studied in animals. Extremely short-lived compounds, such as chloroethylene oxide (the main reactive metabolite of vinyl chloride) or the ultimately reactive intermediate from dimethylnitrosamine ($CH_3N_2^+$ or CH_3^+) give a high dose close to the site of formation. Nevertheless, it has been possible to determine hemoglobin alkylation as a measure of dose after exposure of mice to vinyl chloride (Osterman-Golkar et al., 1977) and dimethylnitrosamine (Osterman-Golkar et al., 1976).

Relationship between "DNA-Dose" (D_4) and Biological Effect (Response L_6)

But for the rare cases where clear-cut relationships between response and exposure dose of single mutagens/carcinogens can be established epidemiologically there is at present no direct method of quantitating the risk to man from exposure to genotoxic chemicals. Ionizing radiation is the environmental factor that has been most carefully subjected to quantitative risk estimates in terms of the number of cases of heritable damage and cancer expected to result from exposure of a population to a certain dose. Although the mechanisms of action of, and the primary lesions produced by, radiations and chemicals are not identical the similarities of the effects are large enough to suggest the value of radiological protection research as a model in efforts to evaluate genetic risks from chemicals. In order to be able to express the magnitude of a chemical risk and to compare the sensitivity of test systems γ-radiation has been suggested as a reference agent (Bridges, 1973; Committee 17, 1975; Heddle and Athanasiou, 1975; Latarjet, 1977; Ehrenberg and Osterman-Golkar, 1977; Ehrenberg, 1980). Although there seems to be an agreement that there is a need for a unit (units) to express a chemical risk, the "rad-equivalence" approach has been heavily criticized, partly because of the feeling that it might be unwise to tie a unit for chemical risks to effects of radiation, partly due to unawareness of the fact that the rad-equivalent has been defined in different ways. It may, therefore, be pertinent to define the two fundamentally different units in use with reference to Scheme 1. The "rec" unit used by Committee 17 (1975) expresses the biologically determined rad-equivalence of a chemical dose where dose is given as the amount of a mutagen or premutagen (e.g., in milligram) per kilogram body weight or per liter of a treatment solution (step $L_2 \rightarrow L_6$). Accordingly the rec unit does not consider concentrations and half lifes of ultimate mutagens and has to be established for each compound separately. The rad-equivalent as defined by Ehrenberg (step $L_5 \rightarrow L_6$) expresses the biologically determined rad-equivalence of a chemical dose where dose is given as the degree of alkylation of nucleophilic groups of DNA characterized by a low nucleophilic strength ($n = 2$ in the Swain Scott scale). The approach is based on the observation of a constant ratio between the mutagenic effectiveness of γ-radiation dose and molecular dose, L_5 (cf. Ehrenberg, 1979, 1980; Hussain, 1981). The relationship was established for simple monofunctional alkylating agents in a few forward mutation systems, and was found to be valid in organisms belonging to different phyla.

It is important that biological experiments are designed so that the biological background for the empirical relationship between degree of alkylation of groups of DNA with a low reactivity and mutagenic effectiveness of simple monofunctional alkylating agents can be clarified and similar relationships for other types of electrophilic agents developed.

Demonstration of the Procedure for Risk Estimation using Ethylene Oxide as a Model Compound

Possibilities of confirming the applicability of the suggested procedure to risk estimations for man are limited becuase of difficulties of finding populations with a predominanting exposure to one compound at sufficiently well-known exposure levels. Work environments where ethylene oxide is used for sterilization fulfill these requirements.

$D_1 \rightarrow D_3$) In a group of persons with a relatively well-known exposure situation the relationship between exposure dose and tissue dose (D_3 calculated according to Eq. (1) from degree of alkylation of histidine of hemoglobin and the corresponding rate constant) was estimated to be $0.1 \cdot 10^{-6}$ M·h (ppm·h)$^{-1}$ (= k_{13}) (Calleman et al., 1978).

$D_3 \rightarrow D_4$) The dose of ethylene oxide to DNA is assumed to be equal to the dose in erythrocytes as demonstrated in animal experiments (i.e., $k_{34} = 1$).

$D_4 \rightarrow L_5$) The degree of alkylation of sites of the nucleophilic strength n = 2 may be estimated using Eq. (1) and the rate constant for reaction of ethylene oxide with nucleophilic groups of this strength $k_{n=2} = 1.4 \cdot 10^{-2}$ M^{-1} h^{-1} (= k_{45}).

$L_5 \rightarrow L_6$) Data on the mutagenic effectiveness in submammalian systems of simple monofunctional alkylating agents including ethylene oxide show that the degree of alkylation $1 \cdot 10^{-7}$ of sites with the strength n = 2 is associated with a mutagenic response corresponding to that of 1 rad of γ-radiation, i.e., $k_{56} = 1 \cdot 10^7$ rad-equivalents per unit degree of alkylation at n = 2. The genetic effect in man from exposure to 1 ppm h of ethylene oxide would then, according to Eq. (3), correspond to that of 10^{-2} rad

$$(D_1\ k_{13}\ k_{34}\ k_{45}\ k_{56} = 1 \cdot 0.1 \cdot 10^{-6} \cdot 1 \cdot 1.4 \cdot 10^{-2} \cdot 1 \cdot 10^{7} = 10^{-2}).$$

Epidemiological Verification of the Risk Estimation for Ethylene Oxide

In a population with a relatively well-defined exposure to ethylene oxide the collective risk (in "man-rad equ.") has been estimated. Since this population had a recent exposure (from 1968) only leukemias would be expected to have appeared at the present time. Applying UNSCEAR's (1977) risk coefficient for induced leukemias, about 3 (1-10) leukemias were expected to have appeared up to 1978 (800 ppm h/wk × 40 wk/year × 8 years × 78 persons × 10^{-2} rad-equ./ppm h × $3 \cdot 10^{-5}$ cases/(man-rad) = 6 cases). The actual number found was 3, significantly above the expected value in the absence of exposure (about 0.1 cases in the investigated group) (Hogstedt et al., 1979a).

Although still uncertain, in view of the low number observed, this estimate has been further sustained by a follow-up of causes of death in a group of 89 workers exposed to ethylene oxide mainly in the 40's and 50's (Hogstedt et al., 1979b). In this group cancer had appeared also in other sites. The exposure levels could not be reconstructed with any certainty, but calculating back from the observed increase in cancer mortality, an average exposure concentration of 10 ppm was estimated to have prevailed. From independent measurements of exposure concentrations in chemical industry (cf. Joyner, 1964) it is hardly possible that, at that early period, the actual average concentration in air would have been below 3 or above 30 ppm. (In this study, exposure to some other chemicals has occurred, a fact that obscures the interpretation of the etiology of the cancers. However, ethylene oxide and to some extent 1,2-dichloroethane have to be considered the main causative agents.)

ACKNOWLEDGEMENT

The basic research was financially supported by grants from the Swedish Work Environment Fund, the Swedish Cancer Society and the Swedish Natural Science Research Council.

REFERENCES

Aaron, C. S., 1976, Molecular dosimetry of chemical mutagens. Selection of appropriate target molecules for determining molecular dose to the germ line, Mutat. Res., 38:303.

Andersen, M. E., Gargas, M. L., Jones, R. A., and Jenkins, L. J., 1980, Determination of the kinetic constants for metabolism of inhaled toxicants in vivo using gas uptake measurements, Toxicol. Appl. Pharmacol., 54:100.

Borgå, O., Hamberger, B. Malmfors, T., and Sjöqvist, F., 1970, The role of plasma protein binding in the inhibitory effect of nortriptyline on the neuronal uptake of norepinephrine, Clin. Pharmacol. Ther., 11:581.

Bridges, B. A., 1973, Some general principles of mutagenicity screening and a possible framework for testing procedures, Environ. Health Persp., 6:221.

Calleman, C. J., 1981, Monitoring and risk assessment by means of alkyl groups in hemoglobin in persons occupationally exposed to mutagens and carcinogens, Hemisphere, in press.

Calleman, C. J., Ehrenberg, L., Jansson, B., Osterman-Golkar, S., Segerbäck, D., Svensson, K., and Wachtmeister, C. A., 1978, Monitoring and risk assessment by means of alkyl groups in hemoglobin in persons occupationally exposed to ethylene oxide, J. Environ. Pathol. Toxicol., 2:427.

Chemical Industry Institute of Toxicology (CIIT), 1980, A twenty-four month inhalation toxicology study in Fisher-344 rats exposed to atmospheric ethylene gas - final report. Docket No. 12000, October 15 (1980).

Committee 17, appointed by the Council of Environmental Mutagen Society, 1975, Environmental mutagenic hazards, Science, 187: 503.

Ehrenberg, L., 1974, Genetic toxicity of environmental chemicals, Acta Biol. Yugoslav., Ser. B., Genetika, 6:367.

Ehrenberg, L., 1977, Aspects of statistical inference in testing for genetic toxicity, in: B. Kilbey, et al., eds., "Handbook of Mutagenicity Test Procedures," Elsevier/North Holland, Amsterdam.

Ehrenberg, L., 1979; Risk assessment of ethylene oxide and other compounds, in: V. K. McElheny and S. Abrahamson, eds., Banbury Report 1, "Assessing Chemical Mutagens: The Risk to Humans," Cold Spring Harbor Laboratory.
Ehrenberg, L., 1980, Purposes and methods of comparing effects of radiation and chemicals, in: "Radiobiological Equivalents of Chemical Pollutants," IAEA, Vienna.
Ehrenberg, L., Hiesche, K. D., Osterman-Golkar, S., and Wennberg, I., 1974, Evaluation of genetic risks of alkylating agents: Tissue doses in the mouse from air contaminated with ethylene oxide, Mutat. Res., 24:83.
Ehrenberg, L., Moustacchi, E., and Osterman-Golkar, S., 1981, Dosimetry of genotoxic agents and dose-response relationships of their effects, Working paper for ICPEMC.
Ehrenberg, L., and Osterman-Golkar, S., 1977, Reaction kinetics of chemical pollutants as a basis of risk estimates in terms of rad-equivalence, in: R. Chanet, ed., "Radiological Protection," First Eur. Symp. on Rad-Equivalence, Commission of the European Communities, Luxembourg.
Ehrenberg, L., and Osterman-Golkar, S., 1980, Alkylation of macromolecules for detecting mutagenic agents, Teratogenesis Carcinogenesis Mutagenesis, 1:105.
Ehrenberg, L., Osterman-Golkar, S., Segerbäck, D., Svensson, K., and Calleman, C. J., 1977, Evaluation of genetic risks of alkylating agents, III. Alkylation of hemoglobin after metabolic conversion of ethene to ethene oxide in vivo, Mutat. Res., 45:185.
Farmer, P. B., Bailey, E., Lamb, J. H., and Connors, T. A., 1980, Approach to the quantitation of alkylated amino acids in hemoglobin by gas chromatography mass spectrometry, Biomed. Mass. Spectrom., 7:41.
Fishbein, G. W., ed., Dec. 8, 1980, "Occupational Health & Safety Letter."
Frei, J. W., Swenson, D. H., Warren, W., and Lawley, P. D., 1978, Alkylation of deoxyribonucleic acid in vivo in various organs of C57Bl mice by the carcinogens N-methyl-N-nitrosourea, N-ethyl-N-nitrosourea and ethyl methanesulfonate in relation to induction of thymic lymphoma, Biochem. J., 174:1031.
Heddle, J. A., and Anthanasiou, K., 1975, Mutation rate, genome size and their relation to the rec concept, Nature, 258:359.
Hogstedt, C., Malmqvist, N., and Wadman, B., 1979a, Leukemia in ethylene oxide exposed personnel, JAMA, 241:1132.
Hogstedt, C., Rohlén, O., Berndtsson, B. S., Axelsson, O., and Ehrenberg, L., 1979b, A cohort study of mortality and cancer incidence in ethylene oxide production workers, Brit. J. Ind. Med., 36:276.
Hussain, S., 1981, Doctoral Thesis, Stockholm (in preparation).
Joyner, R. E., 1964, Chronic toxicity of ethylene oxide, Arch. Environ. Health, 8:700.

Latarjet, R., 1977, Quantitative mutagenesis by chemicals and by radiations: Prerequisites for the establishment of rad-equivalences, in: R. Chanet, ed., "Radiological Protection," First Eur. Symp. on Rad-Equivalence, Commission of the European Communities, Luxembourg.

Lee, W. R., 1976, Molecular dosimetry of chemical mutagens. Determination of molecular dose to the germ line, Mutat. Res., 38: 311.

Murthy et al., 1981 (Manuscipt in preparation).

Neumann, H. G., Metzler, M., and Töpner, W., 1977, Metabolic activation of diethylstilbestrol and amino-stilbene-derivates, Arch. Toxicol., 39:21.

Nguyen, L., Osterman-Golkar, S., Ward, J. B., Jr., and Legator, M. S., 1980, Detection of alkylating agents by the analysis of amino acid residues in hemoglobin and urine. II. Dosimetry in the rat of methyl methanesulfonate by amino acid analysis of N-methylhistidine in hemoglobin, manuscript.

Osterman-Golkar, S., 1975, Studies on the reaction kinetics of biologically active electrophilic reagents as a basis for risk estimates, Thesis, Stockholm University, Sweden.

Osterman-Golkar, S., and Ehrenberg, L., 1981, Covalent binding of reactive intermediates to hemoglobin as an approach for determining the metabolic activation of chemicals - Ethylene, Symposium on the "Metabolism and Pharmacokinetics of Environmental Chemicals in Man," Sarasota, Florida, June 7-12, 1981.

Osterman-Golkar, S., Ehrenberg, L., Segerbäck, D., and Hällström, I., 1976, Evaluation of genetic risks of alkylation agents. II. Hemoglobin as a dose monitor, Mutat. Res., 34:1.

Osterman-Golkar, S., Hultmark, D., Segerbäck, D., Calleman, C. J., Göthe, R., Ehrenberg, L., and Wachtmeister, C. A., 1977, Alkylation of DNA and proteins in mice exposed to vinyl chloride, Biochem. Biophys. Res. Commun., 76:259.

Pereira, M. A., and Chang, L., 1980, Binding of chemical carcinogens and mutagens to rat hemoglobin, Chem.-Biol. Interactions, 33: 301.

Segerbäck, D., Calleman, C. J., Ehrenberg, L. Löfroth, G., and Osterman-Golkar, S., 1978, Evaluation of genetic risks of alkylating agents. IV. Quantitative determination of alkylated amino acids in hemoglobin as a measure of the dose after treatment of mice with methyl methanesulfonate, Mutat. Res., 49:71.

Segerbäck, D., 1981a, Estimation of genetic risks of alkylating agents. V. Methylation of DNA in the mouse by DDVP (2,2-dichlorovinyl dimethyl phosphate), Hereditas, 94:73.

Segerbäck, D., 1981b, Alkylation of DNA and hemoglobin in hemoglobin in the mouse after exposure to ethylene, manuscripts.

UNSCEAR, 1977, "A report of the United Nations Scientific Committee on the Effects of Atomic Radiation, General Assembly with Annexes," Vol. II (A 8725), 27th Session, Suppl. No. 25, United Nations, New York.

Walles, S., 1981, Reaction of benzyl chloride with hemaglobin and DNA in various organs of mice, Toxicol. Letters (in press).

PUVA THERAPY: IMMUNOLOGIC AND GENOTOXIC APPROACHES TO RISK EVALUATION

G.H.S. Strauss

Centre for Medical Research and MRC Cell Mutation Unit
University of Sussex
Brighton, England

PUVA (psoralen and near ultraviolet light) is a DNA-damaging, clinically effective treatment. If we have patience, studies of PUVA therapy should give us a rare opportunity to learn much about not only the diseases it treats, but also about diseases it may cause. PUVA is a gamble, a calculated risk.

> "Leprosy is not exactly what I have, but what in the Bible is called leprosy (see Leviticus 13, Exodus 4:6, Luke 5:12-13) was probably this thing, which has a twisty Greek name it pains me to write. The form of the disease is as follows: spots, plaques, and avalanches of excess skin, manufactured by the dermis through some trifling but persistent error in its metabolic instructions, expand and slowly migrate across the body like lichen on a tombstone. I am silvery, scaly. Puddles of flakes form wherever I rest my flesh. Each morning, I vacuum my bed. My torture is skin deep: there is no pain, not even itching; we lepers live a long time, and are ironically healthy in other respects. Lusty, though we are loathsome to love. Keen-sighted, though we hate to look upon ourselves. The name of the disease, spiritually speaking, is Humiliation."

John Updike, "From the Journal of a Leper"

Psoriasis is a common chronic dermatologic disease which, when extensive, tests in the extreme the hypothesis that beauty is only skin deep. Its consequences in terms of morbidity are not severe, but, like leprosy, psoriasis can cause social debilitation and profound psychological anguish. It can occur in any part of the skin, but most commonly affects sites of trauma (elbows, knees, lower back, scalp). The primary lesion is a sharply demarcated, erythematous papule, which coalesces with others to form plaques covered with micaceous scale. About 6% of patients with psoriasis also have an associated arthritis.

Tissues affected by psoriasis display parakeratotic hyperkeratosis and acanthosis, and contain Monroe microabscesses, elongated dermal papillae, and engorged dermal capillaries. Accelerated epidermal turnover occurs such that cells multiply, mature, and exfoliate at 7-10 times the normal rate. The stratum granulosum is absent or diminished, and an inflammatory infiltrate invades the subpapillary dermis. The aetiology of common psoriasis is not known; the disease is not contagious, but it is probably a polygenic threshold disease most likely to occur in individuals carrying HL-A13 and HL-A17 (Svejgaard et al., 1974). There is no known cure for psoriasis.

Various treatment modalities have been used to achieve remission in widespread plaque psoriasis. As recently as ten years ago, arsenic trioxide and ionizing radiation were used to treat persistent lesions. Conventional approaches consist of topical applications of agents such as coal tar and dithranol, usually in combination with far ultraviolet light (UVB) irradiation during 2-4 week hospital admissions. Topical steroid preparations are popular, too, and are not unpleasant to the senses, as are the tars. However, steroids can produce unstable disease, and bear attendant risks of adrenocortical suppression after systemic absorption. Treatments using cytotoxic chemicals such as methotrexate are generally very effective but unsafe, at least with respect to their acute toxicity, especially evident in the liver.

In 1974 (Parrish et al., 1974), a new photochemotherapeutic approach to psoriasis employing psoralen and near ultraviolet light (UVA) was introduced. This treatment, known as PUVA, has come into widespread use for generalized psoriasis. It is also being used to treat several other conditions with dermatologic manifestations, including mycosis fungoides, urticaria pigmentosa, and vitiligo (hypopigmentation).

Psoralens are derived from the furocoumarins, which are naturally occurring compounds extractable from *Ammi majus*, a weed that grows in the Nile valley. The most commonly used derivative is 8-methoxy psoralen (8-MOP); its usual oral dose is 0.6 mg/kg body weight. The chemical is metabolized in the liver, and peak levels in skin are attained within 2-3 hours of ingestion. UVA exposure is timed to correspond with this peak period; the patient usually stands in a booth panelled with long, high-intensity fluorescent lamps. These lamps deliver radiations of 320-400 nm, with a peak at 365 nm. Between 40% and 50% of UVA penetrates the epidermis, dermis, and superficial blood vessels.

Alone, 8-MOP is virtually inactive in the skin; in the dark, it binds to DNA only loosely. On activation by UVA, 8-MOP passes through the reactive triplet state to transfer absorbed energy to DNA by forming monofunctional adducts with thymine bases. On further irradiation, interstrand cross-links form between opposite prymidine bases. The bifunctional adducts presumably inhibit DNA synthesis and cell division in the skin. Aside from a direct effect on skin cells, PUVA may act by causing damage to cells of the inflammatory infiltrate in the dermal papillae of psoriatic lesions.

The UVA exposures are initially low (about 1.0 J/cm^2) and are increased by 0.5 or 1.0 J/cm^2 with each treatment. Treatments are administered two or three times per week. The actual effective dose of PUVA depends on the interaction of several factors: intensity and duration of UVA exposure, level of active psoralen in the skin at the time of irradiation, and relative quality of protective pigmentation in the skin. The last parameter is described by an index of skin type (see Table 1). Individuals who have high skin-type indices become more deeply pigmented in response to PUVA, require greater UVA doses for therapeutic effect, and are not as likely to burn as those with low indices.

PUVA treatment protocols are designed to clear the lesions by producing regulated phototoxicity in the skin as frequently as

Table I. Index of Skin Type

Skin Type	Response to Sun Exposure
I	Always burn, never tan
II	Always burn, occasionally tan
III	Occasionally burn, always tan
IV	Never burn, always tan
V	Genetically hyperpigmented

possible without causing painful erythema and blistering. When clearance is accomplished, usually after three months and about twenty-five treatments, the last clearance dose may be used as the weekly maintenance dose. If remission persists, the frequency of the maintenance dose can be tapered to once in two, three, and four weeks (Parrish et al., 1980; Vella-Briffa et al., 1979).

The early results of PUVA therapy for psoriasis from the American Co-operative Clinical Trial are very promising indeed. Of 1308 patients with extensive disease, 88% were cleared completely and entered maintenance treatment, 3% failed to respond, 1% were withdrawn due to acute complications, and the remaining patients discontinued therapy for various reasons not associated with PUVA (Melski et al., 1977). The known acute side effects of PUVA include dryness and itching, nausea from 8-MOP, and erythema and blistering from over-exposure. These adverse reactions are generally easily managed or avoided on subsequent exposures and rarely force patients to abandon photochemotherapy. As PUVA gains worldwide popularity and restrictions are relaxed, understanding the chronic side effects will become increasingly important. In the following pages, I discuss the evidence that may enable us to predict adverse long-term consequences of PUVA.

In bacteria, 8-MOP can react with DNA in the dark to produce frame-shift mutations through non-covalent associations with DNA. Risks of similar interactions with DNA in human gonad cells are considered to be slight (Bridges, 1979). However, UVA-potentiated 8-MOP activity does result in covalent pyrimidine cross-linking, and these linkages have been found to be mutagenic in virtually every system tested (for reviews, see Bridges, 1978; Bridges et al., in press). Such alterations in the genetic apparatus lead to the induction of base-pair substitutions in bacteria (Igali et al., 1970), *in vitro* chromosome damage in Chinese hamster cells (Ashwood-Smith et al., 1977), *in vitro* gene mutations in mammalian cells (Arlett et al., 1977), and transformation to the malignant phenotype of mammalian cells in culture (Evans and Morrow, 1979). In light of this evidence, it is not surprising to learn that PUVA has been found to be carcinogenic to mammalian skin. In fact, the first studies suggesting that PUVA is carcinogenic to mammalian skin were completed more than two decades ago (Griffin, 1959). Since then, the evidence that PUVA is an initiator of carcinogenesis in animals has been well documented (see Bridges et al., in press, for references).

Proof that the viability and function of human lymphocytes are affected by PUVA comes from both *in vitro* (Morison et al., 1981) and *in vivo* (Kraemer and Weinstein, 1977) experiments. My first exposures to PUVA, both figuratively and literally, were during the development of the Strauss-Albertini test (described elsewhere in this volume). We endeavoured to use our system to evaluate PUVA effects on in vivo frequencies of thioguanine-resistant peripheral blood lymphocytes (TG^r PBLs) (Strauss et al., 1979).

We determined TG^r PBL frequencies in individuals from each of five groups. The first group consisted of eighteen psoriatics, each of whom had already received at least twenty-six PUVA treatments, were in the maintenance phase of therapy, and were appearing for treatments once a week. The normal control group included eleven healthy individuals. The third group consisted of sixteen psoriatics who were undergoing conventional therapies (topical steroids, UVB with and without topical coal tar, and methotrexate). The three groups were age- and sex-matched and were tested concurrently. Later, we tested two additional groups: seven vitiligo patients not on treatment of any kind and ten vitiligo patients receiving PUVA at doses similar to those of the PUVA-treated psoriatics. We tested vitiligo patients because we could not find untreated, severely diseased psoriatics; people who suffer from severe psoriasis apparently seek medical intervention or withdraw completely. Thus in testing psoriatics, we failed to separate the effects of PUVA, conventional therapies, and possible disease-state effects on PBLs. Vitiligo patients presented a useful alternative, because untreated patients are available, and the test cell (PBL) probably does not play a direct role in the pathogenesis of the disease. The results of tests with these five groups are depicted graphically in Figure 1.

Although the concurrent control group was small (11 individuals), variant frequency values from this group fit nicely into the distribution range reported from a standard reference group of sixty-three normal individuals (Strauss and Albertini, 1979). The PUVA-treated psoriasis patients presented a distribution of variant frequency values whose mean was significantly higher than that of the control group ($p < 0.001$; Wilcoxon's two-sample test). The median variant frequency of PUVA-treated psoriatics was 8.0×10^{-4} (the 10th and 90th percentiles were 5.9×10^{-5} and 3.5×10^{-3}, respectively). Similar results were seen in the conventionally-treated psoriasis patient group: the median variant frequency was 1.8×10^{-3} (the mean was 2.6×10^{-3}; the 10th and 90th percentiles were 1.2×10^{-4} and 7.5×10^{-3}, respectively). The psoriasis-patient groups were not different from each other in terms of variant-frequency distribution. However, the variant frequencies for the conventionally treated patients were significantly elevated ($p < 0.001$; Wilcoxon's two-sample test) over those of the cumulative control group.

The untreated vitiligo patients had a mean variant frequency of 1.4×10^{-4}, and all variant frequencies for this group fell between the 10th and 90th percentiles for the standard reference control group (Figure 1). In contrast, nine of ten variant frequencies determined from PUVA-treated vitiligo patients were above the 90th percentile value for the reference controls. The median variant frequency for the PUVA-treated vitiligo group was 5.1×10^{-4} (the mean was 1.1×10^{-3}, and the 10th and 90th percentiles were 9.6×10^{-5} and 4.2×10^{-3}, respectively). The variant frequencies in this group were significantly higher than those of the cumulative control group ($p < 0.001$; Wilcoxon's two-sample test). There were too few treated vitiligo patients to test for a statistically significant difference in variant frequencies between the two vitiligo groups (Strauss et al., 1979).

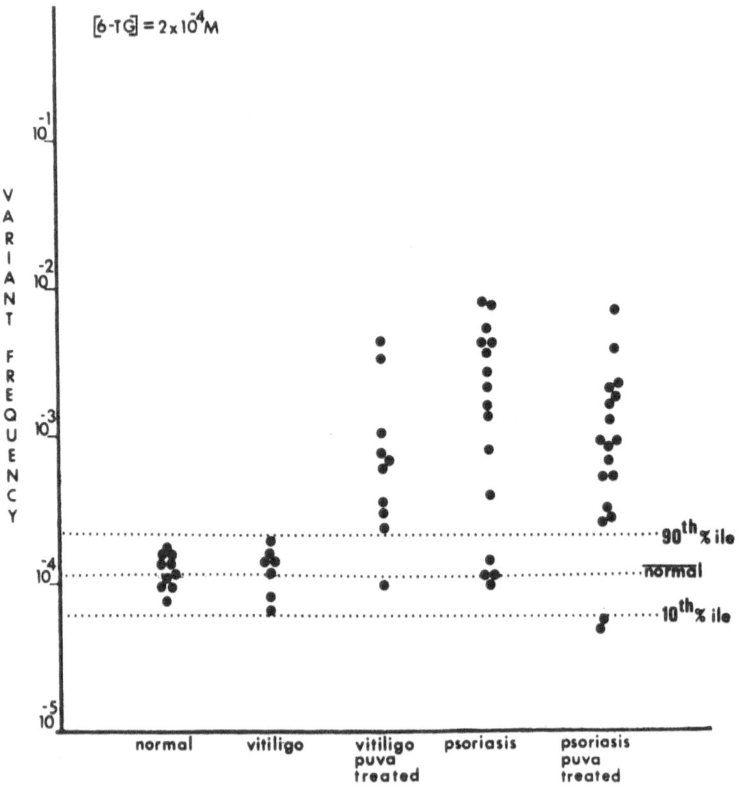

Figure 1. Frequency of TG^r PBLs as a function of treatment group; each point represents one test on one individual. The wavy line is the median variant frequency of 63 normal individuals.

A normal, healthy 28-year-old individual volunteered to receive intensive PUVA exposures and to be tested for TG^r PBL frequencies. He previously had been tested repeatedly over a two-year period and found to have variant frequencies consistently within the expected range for normal. Several tests were performed just before the first PUVA treatment; the variant frequencies were within the normal range. A second normal, healthy, untreated individual (21 years old) volunteered to be tested concurrently for TG^r PBLs. The variant frequencies for this normal, untreated control fell within normal limits during the entire period of the study (Figure 2). The PUVA-treated subject ingested the usual 8-MOP dose (0.6 mg/kg body weight) two hours before each UVA exposure. The subject received a high initial dose because, due to previous history of occupational sun

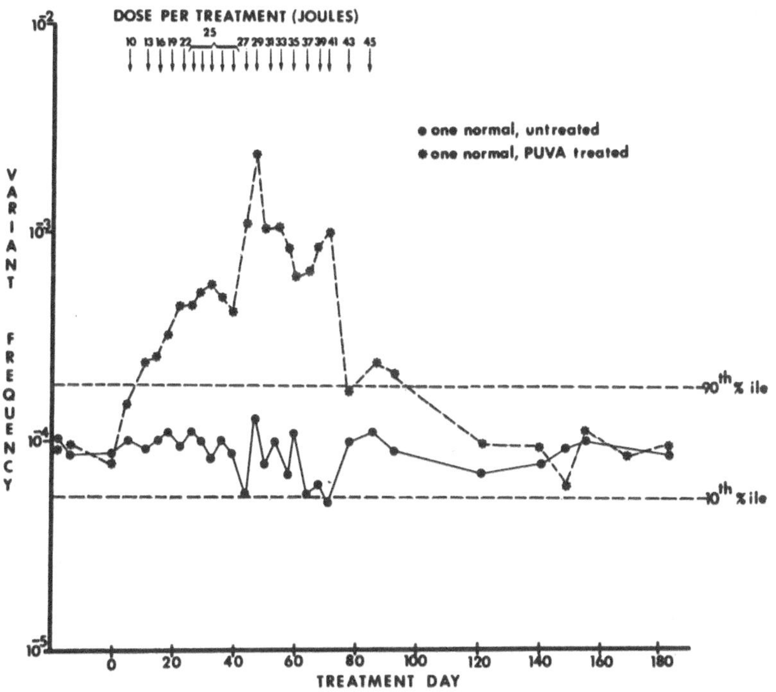

Figure 2. Frequency of TG^r PBLs in a normal, untreated individual and in a normal, PUVA-treated individual over a 180-day period. The broken horizontal lines indicate the 10th- and 90th-percentile values for variant frequencies from 63 normal individuals.

exposure (life-guard) and type IV colouring, it was felt that he could tolerate aggressive treatment. A response to the first dose was evident within about five or six days, when the variant frequencies climbed out of the normal range. They fell back to near normal when the rate of treatment was dropped from twice weekly to once weekly. The effective dose probably changed only slightly as the subject became progressively darker due to hyperpigmentation following each exposure. Soon after treatment was discontinued, the subject's variant frequencies returned to the normal range. If we assume that changes in variant frequencies are due to changes in the DNA, these results demonstrate that PUVA can cause mutations and, thus, presumptive initiation of carcinogenesis in man. The results also demonstrate that the effects of PUVA definitely extend to the capillary beds, with considerable peripheral blood exposure. It is reasonable to expect that the responses of skin cells in situ are similar to those of the PBLs (Strauss et al., 1979; Bridges et al., 1981).

In attempting to explain the results from psoriatics, we became fascinated with the possibility that the disease process itself could result in increases in variant frequency if immunological stimuli are mutagenic to mammalian cells (Malling, 1976; Kerkis and Skorova, 1973). We knew that the high mutability of normal lymphocyte DNA may be, in part, responsible for the diversity of responses of which normal lymphocyte populations are capable (Baltimore, 1974). Paradoxically, this high mutability may result in a constellation of benign and malignant disorders. It is possible, for instance, that psoriasis itself is a self-perpetuating, benign immunoregulatory disorder, in which lymphocytes respond to altered self-antigens in the basal cell layer of the skin (Cormane et al., 1979).

The question of lymphocyte involvement in the pathogenesis of psoriasis is a controversial one (Morhenn et al., 1980). Does the therapeutic efficacy of PUVA depend upon toxicity to keratinocytes directly, or to Langerhans cells and other immunocompetent cells in the skin that mediate cellular immune responses? PUVA undoubtedly does interfere with epidermal DNA synthesis and hyperproliferation, but these effects do not account for the positive responses observed when PUVA intervenes in vitiligo, alopecia areata, and mycosis fungoides. All of these disorders probably respond to cutaneous immunosuppression (Morhenn et al., 1980). In fact, virtually all the useful therapeutic approaches to psoriasis are, to a greater or lesser degree, immunosuppressive.

An incidental observation during the period of intensive PUVA exposure of the volunteer subject provides new insight into both the beneficial and adverse effects of PUVA therapy. The volunteer was coincidentally involved with immunological testing for clinical purposes not related to PUVA. Prior to PUVA exposures, he was repeatedly found to be a high-normal responder to the commonly used skin-test reagent, 2,4-dinitrochlorobenzene (DNCB). However, during the entire duration of PUVA treatment, he was unresponsive to DNCB. This was discovered by serendipity, and no careful analysis of the phenomenon was attempted at the time. When the treatment period ended, normal reactivity to DNCB returned. The DNCB test measures cell-mediated immunocompetency by evaluating delayed cellular hypersensitivity in the skin. A low response to DNCB indicates low cell-mediated immunocompetency. It occurred to us that indeed PUVA may cause measurable immunosuppression in man, at least in the skin (Strauss et al., 1980; Bridges et al., 1981).

We used the DNCB skin test (Catalona et al., 1972) to survey delayed cellular hypersensitivity in PUVA-treated psoriatics (Strauss et al., 1980). The volar surface of an arm was cleansed with acetone, and doses of 50 μg and 2000 μg of DNCB in 0.1 ml acetone were applied to 3-cm areas of forearm and upper arm, respectively. The sites were protected with plasters for 24-48 h. After this period, the 2000-μg site was examined for evidence of an irritative reaction (oedema and/or erythema). The presence of such a reaction indicates that the primary inflammation response is intact. Test sites were examined 7-14 days after attempted sensitization for evidence of a delayed cellular hypersensitivity (DCH) reaction. This reaction, a response to residual DNCB in the skin, is characterized by erythema and induration over the entire test site. A grade of 4 was assigned to subjects who responded to both the 50-μg and 2000-μg doses. A flare at the higher dose site only was recorded as a grade 3 response. Grades 3 and 4 are regarded as normal. If after fourteen days no reaction occurred, an additional challenge dose of 50 μg DNCB was applied to the other forearm and covered for 48 h. If a grossly apparent cutaneous delay hypersensitivity reaction occurred, it was assigned a grade of 2. If no such reaction was apparent, a 2-mm punch biopsy was examined for histological evidence of a DCH reaction. (Such a reaction is characterized by increased inflammatory cell infiltration around mid- and upper-dermal blood vessels, which may be dilated.) If microscopically positive, the reaction was graded 1; if negative, a grade of 0, indicating anergy (diminished reactivity), was assigned. Grades 2, 1, and 0 are regarded as sub-normal and indicative of impaired cutaneous DCH.

Twelve normal, untreated individuals all showed grades of 3 or 4, which is consistent with published reports for large groups of normals (Catalona et al., 1972). Nine untreated psoriatics also showed normal responses. On the other hand, 55 of the

102 PUVA-treated psoriatics had sub-normal responses to DNCB sensitization. PUVA-treated psoriatics differed significantly from disease-state controls ($p = 0.005$; chi-square test) and normal controls ($p = 0.001$; chi-square test) in their DCH reactions to DCNB. Figure 3 presents DCH grades as a function of dose rate and skin type. Dose rate is very important to interpretation of the results. Skin pigmentation, as might be expected, had a dramatic influence on effective dose (i.e., the amount of penetrant UVA available in the skin to promote psoralen-DNA interactions). Correlations between age, sex, duration of treatment, disease activity, total number of treatments received, and DCH grade were not significant.

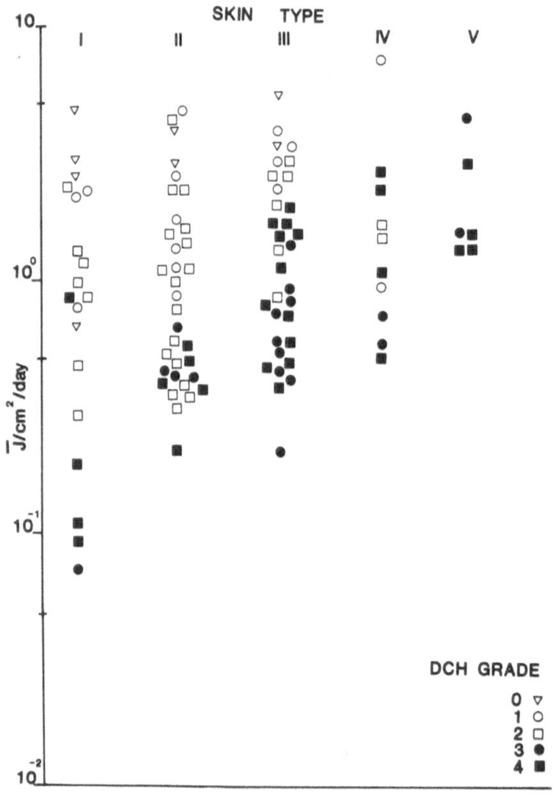

Figure 3. The interaction of a range of delayed cellular hypersensitivity (DCH) reactions (0-4), skin type (I-V), and dose rate ($\bar{J}/cm^2/day$).

In showing that PUVA impairs cutaneous DCH, these studies did not differentiate between failure to respond to sensitization and diminished challenge-response ability. To examine challenge-response ability, we tested patients who were in PUVA therapy and who had previously been DNCB-sensitized. The results from longitudinal studies on one individual are presented in Figure 4.

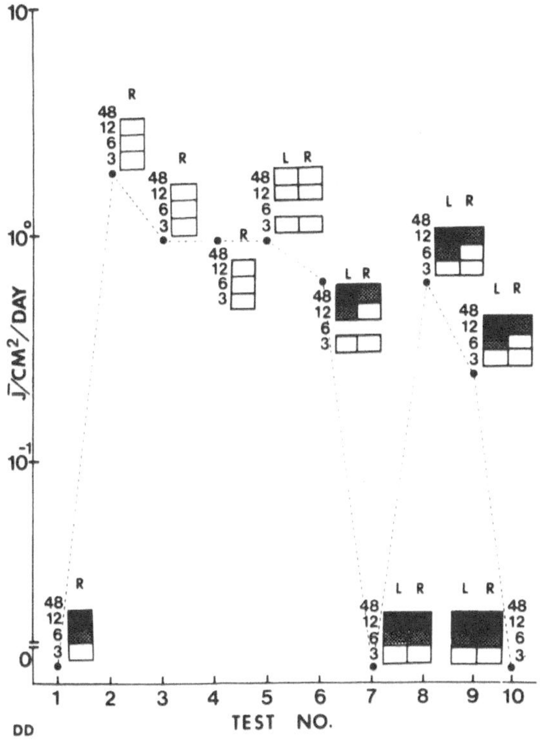

Figure 4. Results of DNCB challenge tests performed on one individual at 6-8 weeks intervals (no response, □; weak positive, ▩; strong positive, ■). The four numbers at each point refer to the DNCB challenge dose in μgs. R refers to challenge tests performed on the volar surface of the upper arm exposed to UVA; L refers to tests performed on a site masked from UVA.

These results are representative of those from eighteen other PUVA-treated individuals studied in this fashion. The individual was tested immediately before (test no. 1), during (test nos. 2-9), and at the end of an eighteen-month course of treatment (test no. 10). The intensity of treatment at the time of testing was determined by averaging UVA doses during the three weeks before testing.

There are at least four possible explanations of our findings: (i) PUVA blocks challenge response to DNCB in previously sensitized individuals; (ii) impairment, albeit to a lesser extent, is seen at sites masked from PUVA, indicating a systemic, as well as a local, effect; (iii) impairment is temporary, and normal responses return within three weeks of discontinuation or with dramatic decreases in intensity of treatment; and (iv) impairment is not simply linear with UVA dose, in that threshold doses of UVA are apparent below which little or no suppression of response can be seen (Bridges et al., 1981). We do not know yet whether PUVA blocks sensitization in man.

In studies similar to those we performed with human subjects, PUVA has been shown to impair DNCB responses in guinea pigs (Morison et al., 1979). Further animal studies by other investigators suggested that alterations in regulatory mechanisms within the immune system (e.g., suppressor T-cells) may be responsible for decreased responsiveness to antigenic stimuli (Roberts et al., 1979). These investigators also showed that when UV-induced skin tumours carrying strong tumour-associated antigens are transplanted to syngenic mice that have received PUVA treatment, the tumours are accepted. When the hosts are not treated, the transplants are rejected immediately. Langerhans cells of the skin are extremely sensitive to UV (Toews et al., 1980); in rodents, loss of these cells is directly related to impairment of DCH.

In man, skin cancer is certainly under immunological control mechanisms. This is evident in patients receiving immunosuppressive drugs, who develop a pronounced susceptibility to skin carcinoma (Kinlen et al., 1979). The earliest evidence of PUVA-induced carcinogenesis in humans came from an attempt to induce protective melanogenesis in patients afflicted with xeroderma pigmentosum (XP). XP is a hereditary disease; affected individuals are unable to repair DNA damage caused by various mutagens, including UV. XP is therefore characterized by extreme sensitivity to the carcinogenic effects of sun exposure. The PUVA-treated XP patients developed multiple cutaneous neoplasms, in one case within only one month of exposure, and one patient developed lymphatic leukemia as well (Reed, 1976). The rapidity with which these tumours developed was inconsistent with the usual long latency periods following initiation by agents normally associated with skin carcinogenesis. There may be a PUVA-associated promotional effect on pre-existing malignant foci. Regression of multiple cutaneous tumours in seven of eight XP patients was accomplished by using indomethacin to block suppressor cell interference in killer cell function (Al-Saleem et al., 1980). Prior to this, evidence for impaired cell-mediated immunity in XPs had been demonstrated (DNCB skin sensitization was attempted but failed), and it was suggested that this might contribute to factors resulting in cancer susceptibility in these patients. We subsequently proposed (Bridges and Strauss, 1980) that agents that damage DNA in the skin may well elicit neoplasms from pre-existing foci by a pseudopromoting effect on immunoregulatory processes rather than through new mutations. The excess tumours seen in immumosuppressed transplant recipients are mainly lymphoreticular or squamous cell cutaneous tumours. The excess skin tumours seen in PUVA-treated psoriasis patients are also mainly of squamous-cell origin. This is an important point, because the predominant skin tumour in the general population is of basal-cell origin.

There is already evidence of increased incidence of skin cancer within three years of starting PUVA treatments in subjects who might be expected to bear pre-malignant foci. Such foci would be due to DNA damage either from agents that had produced skin cancer prior to PUVA, from therapeutic exposures to X-rays, or from the combination of topical coal tar and far-UV. The magnitude of increase in cancer rate among these patients is not yet known, but the apparent relationship between early tumour expression and previous exposure to carcinogens is impressive (Stern et al., 1979). Among others, we reported case studies of apparent PUVA-induced skin cancers. We found (Strauss et al., 1980) that of 350 patients treated over the last four years, six developed multiple cutaneous tumours. In two of these patients, tumours were diagnosed after sub-normal responses to DNCB had been recorded. Moreoever, in both patients, the lesions, which included squamous cell carcinomas and keratoacanthomas, showed signs of regression soon after discontinuation of the PUVA therapy.

We continue to regard the role of immunosuppression in skin cancer as speculative. We should like to suggest, however, that it might be wise to attempt to control PUVA exposures so that DNCB responses remain within the normal range. Ideally, a more convenient approach, perhaps utilizing circulating lymphocytes, can be used to calibrate treatment intensity against therapeutic response and immunological impairment. Individuals at increased risk due to low skin-type index, previous skin cancer, or exposure to carcinogens should be excluded from PUVA therapy (Strauss, in press).

We believe a registry should be established to include all PUVA-treated patients, so that we can assess the long-term hazards through sound epidemiology. This is especially important in view of our prediction that, as well as apparently promoting carcinogenesis, PUVA might prove to be an initiator. PUVA might thereby produce a dramatic second wave of malignancies, possibly including those of lymphoid origin. However, if we use our information wisely, we may learn from the PUVA experience how to effect a cure for psoriasis and to develop a clearer picture of cancer.

It is my pleasure to thank my friend Dr. Patrick Hall-Smith, FRCP, for considerable moral support during my time in Great Britain. I am indebted to Dr. Bryn Bridges, F.I. Biol., for his great kindness and expert tutelage. I also wish to express my deep gratitude to my wife, Pamela Alix, for the graphs and so much more.

The author is presently supported by the British Cancer Research Campaign.

REFERENCES

Al-Saleem, R., Ali, Z.S., and Qassah, M., 1980, Skin cancers in xeroderma pigmentosum: response to indomethacin and steroids. Lancet, ii:264.

Arlett, C.F., Heddle, J.A., Broughton, B.C., and Rogers, A.M., 1980, Cell killing and mutagenesis by 8-methoxypsoralen in mammalian (rodent) cells. Clin. Exp. Dermatol., 5:147.

Ashwood-Smith, M.J., Grant, E.L., Heddle, J.A., and Friedman, G.B., 1977, Chromosome damage in Chinese hamster cells sensitized to near-ultraviolet light by psoralen and angelicin, Mutation Res., 43:377.

Baltimore, D., 1974, Is terminal deoxynucleotidyl transferase a somatic mutagen for lymphocytes?, Nature, 248:409.

Bridges, B.A., 1978, Possible long-term hazards of photochemotherapy with psoralens and near-ultraviolet light, Clin. Exp. Dermatol., 3:349.

Bridges, B.A., 1979, An estimate of genetic risk from 8-methoxypsoralen photochemotherapy, Hum. Genet., 49:91.

Bridges, B.A. and Strauss, G.H., 1980, Possible hazards of photochemotherapy for psoriasis, Nature, 218:523.

Bridges, B.A., Greaves, M., Polani, P.E., and Wald, N., in press, Do treatments available for psoriasis patients carry a genetic or carcinogenic risk? A report from an expert group of the International Commission for Protection against Environmental Mutagens and Carcinogens, Mutation Res. and Biol. Zentr.

Bridges, B.A., Strauss, G.H., Hall-Smith, P., and Price, M., 1981, Induction of somatic mutations and impairment of immune capacity by PUVA treatment and their relation to skin cancer in man, in: "Psoralens in Cosmetics and Dermatology", Pergamon Press, Paris.

Catalona, W.J., Taylor, P.T. and Chretieu, P.B., 1972, Quantitative dinitrochlorobenzene contact sensitization in a normal population, Clin. Exp. Immunol., 12:325.

Cormane, R.H., Hamerlinck, F. and Siddiqui, A.H., 1979, Immunologic implications of PUVA therapy in psoriasis vulgaris, Arch. Dermatol. Res., 265:275.

Evans, D.L., and Morrow, K.J., 1979, 8-methoxypsoralen induced alterations of mammalian cells, J. Invest. Dermatol., 72:35.

Griffin, A.C., 1959, Methoxsalen in ultraviolet carcinogenesis in the mouse. J. Invest. Dermatol. 31:367.

Igali, S., Bridges, B.A., Ashwood-Smith, M.J., and Scott, B.R., 1970, Mutagenesis in Escherichia coli IV, Photosensitization to near-ultraviolet light by 8-methoxypsoralen, Mutation Res., 9:21.

Kerkis, J.J., and Skorova, S.V., 1973, Humoral factors of "spontaneous" mutagenesis in mammals and man. Mutation Res., 18:179.

Kinlin, L., et al., 1979, Collaborative United Kingdom/Australian study of cancer patients treated with immunosuppressive drugs, Brit. Med. J., ii:1461.

Kraemer, K.H. and Weinstein, G.D., 1977, Decreased thymidine incorporation in circulating leukocytes after treatment of psoriasis with psoralen and long-wave ultraviolet light, J. Invest. Dermatol., 69:211.

Malling, H.V., 1976, Mutagenesis testing: mammalian systems. Mutation Res., 41:171.

Melski, J.W., Tanenbaum, L., Parrish, J.A., et al., 1977, Oral methoxsalen photochemotherapy for the treatment of psoriasis: a co-operative clinical trial, J. Invest. Dermatol., 68:328.

Morhenn, V.B., Benike, B.S., and Engleman, E.G., 1980, Inhibition of cell mediated immune response by 8-methoxypsoralen and long-wave ultraviolet light: a possible explanation for the clinical effects of photo-activated psoralens, J. Invest. Dermatol., 75:249.

Morison, W.L., Woehler, M.E., and Parrish, J.A., 1979, PUVA and systemic immunosuppression in guinea pigs. J. Invest. Dermatol., 72:273.
Morison, W.L., Parrish, J.A., McAuliffe, D.J. and Bloch, K.J., 1981, Sensitivity of mononuclear cells to PUVA: effect on subsequent stimulation with mitogens and on exclusion of trypan blue dye, Clin. Exp. Dermatol., 6:273.
Parrish, J.A., Fitzpartick, T.B., Tanenbaum, L., and Pathak, M.A., 1974, Photochemotherapy for psoriasis with oral methoxsalen and longwave ultraviolet light, New Engl. J. Med., 291:1207.
Parrish, J.A., LeVine, M.J., and Fitzpatrick, T.B., 1980, Oral methoxsalen photochemotherapy of psoriasis and mycosis fungoides, Int. J. Dermatol., 19:379.
Reed, W.D., 1976, Treatment of psoriasis with oral psoralens and longwave ultraviolet light, Acta Dermato-vener., 56:315.
Roberts, L.K., Schmitt, M., and Daynes, R.A., 1979, Tumour susceptibility generated in mice treated with subcarcinogenic doses of 9-methoxypsoralen and longwave ultraviolet light, J. Invest. Dermatol., 72:306.
Stern, R.S., Thibodeau, L.A., Kleinerman, R.A., Parrish, J.A., Fitzpatrick, et al., 1979, Risk of cutaneous carcinoma in patients treated with oral methoxsalen photochemotherapy for psoriasis, New. Engl. J. Med., 300-309.
Strauss, G.H., in press, PUVA - Gambling with a system? Int. J. Dermatol.
Strauss, G.H., and Albertini, R.J., 1979, Enumeration of 6-thioguanine peripheral blood lymphocytes as a potential test for somatic cell mutations arising in vivo, Mutation Res., 61:353.
Strauss, G.H., Albertini, R.J., Krusinki, P.A., and Baughman, R.D., 1979, 6-thioguanine-resistant peripheral blood lymphocytes in humans following psoralen longwave UV light therapy, J. Invest. Dermatol., 73:211.
Strauss, G.H., Bridges, B.A., Greaves, M., Hall-Smith, P., Price, M., and Vella-Briffa, D. 1980, Inhibition of delayed hypersensitivity reaction in skin (DNCB test) by 8-methoxypsoralen photochemotherapy: possible basis for pseudo-promoting action in skin carcinogenesis? Lancet, ii:556.
Svejgaard, A., Nielsen, L., Svejgaard, E., Kissmeyer-Nielsen, F., Hjortshφj, A., and Zachariae, H., 1974, HL-A in psoriasis vulgaris and in pustular psoriasis - population and family studies, Brit. J. Dermatol., 91:145.
Toews, G., Borgstresser, P.R., and Streilein, J.W., 1980, Epidermal Langerhans cell density determines whether contact hypersensitivity or unresponsiveness follows skin painting with DNFB, J. Immunol., 124:445.

Updike, J., 1979, From the journal of a leper, *in*: "Problems and Other Stories", Knopf, New York.
Vella-Briffa, D., and Warin, A.P., 1979, Photochemotherapy in psoriasis: A review, *J. R. Soc. Med.*, 72:440.

PARVOVIRAL PROBE OF DNA REPLICATION IN MAMMALIAN CELLS EXPOSED TO GENOTOXIC AGENTS

J. Rommelaere,[1,2,3] J.-M. Vos,[1] and D. C. Ward[2]

[1]Department of Molecular Biology
Université Libre de Bruxelles
B 1640 Rhode Saint Genèse, Belgium

[2]Yale University School of Medicine
New Haven, Connecticut 06510, USA

A. RATIONALE

Exposure of mammalian cells to a variety of chemical and physical agents depresses the overal rate of DNA synthesis [1]. Part of this inhibition can be ascribed to a disturbance of the initiation of cell DNA replication. The cellular genome comprises numerous units which contain each one replication origin and are replicated sequentially. Genotoxic agents, in particular direct or indirect inducers of DNA breaks, apparently delay the initiation of the replication of units normally programmed for a time subsequent to the treatment of the cells [2]. Single-strand breaks might lead to the loss of chromosomal segments if not sealed at the time of replication. The temporary inhibition of the initiation of DNA replication lowers this risk by providing cells with more time for DNA repair. The lack of a delay in DNA replication displayed by human cells derived from Ataxia telangiectasia patients is associated with an increased sensitivity to the lethal effect of the treatment [3].

The main replication block caused by UV-radiation and a variety of chemicals inducing gross alterations in DNA structure seems, however, to occur at the level of the elongation of growing nascent strands [1]. Some DNA lesions formed by these agents pose obstacles to the replication machinery. Pyrimidine dimers induced in a natural single-stranded DNA template by UV-radiation were found to

---

[3]To whom correspondence should be addressed in Brussels.

block the *in vitro* elongation of a complementary strand by DNA polymerase α, the enzyme thought to be involved in cell DNA replication [4]. *In vivo*, intrastrand pyrimidine dimers in parental DNA are responsible for the presence of discontinuities in newly synthesized DNA [5, 6, 7]. The structure of blocked replication intermediates in mammalian cells is controversed. It is disputed whether replication halts at blocking lesions [8, 9], or whether it resumes beyond them to leave gaps in the daughter strands synthesized from damaged templates [10-13]. Another intriguing phenomenon is the recovery of the ability of mammalian cells to synthesize DNA of normal size [6, 14] at a normal rate [8, 15] late after the genotoxic treatment despite the persistence of many lesions [16-18]. The mechanism of this delayed tolerance of DNA damage is not known. In this paper we investigated these questions, using a parvovirus as a probe of repair and/or replication activities displayed by mouse cells.

The analysis of the fate of damaged nulcear DNA in mammalian cells is obscured by the complexity of the genome and of its mode of replication. This problem can be alleviated by the use of a virus whose DNA metabolism relies on host functions and is therefore assumed to reflect the processing of cellular DNA. Thus, repair and/or replication activities encoded by the cell are identified through their action on the genome of an infecting virus serving as a probe. Viral DNA can be extracted selectively from infected cells, allowing the analysis of an homogeneous population of well-defined replication units. This strategy was used to investigate the ability of monkey kidney cells to replicate UV-irradiated Simian virus 40(SV40) [19-20]. The SV40 genome constitutes a small double-stranded DNA unit which is replicated bidirectionally from a single origin. Sarasin and Hanawalt [20] concluded that (i) UV-lesions, presumably pyrimidine dimers, interrupted the elongation of SV40 nascent DNA strands, and (ii) some of these blocks halted the replication fork (upper prong) whereas others did not (lower prong):

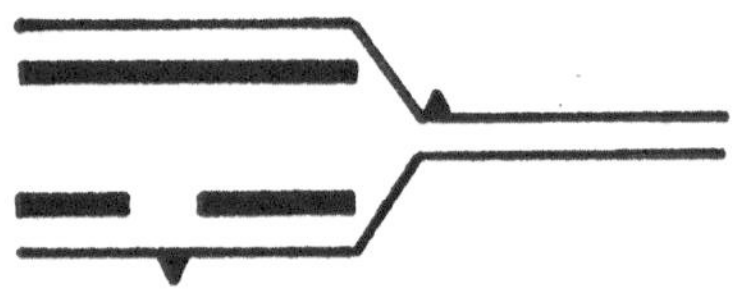

These data are consistent with a model [21, 22] proposing that damage, such as pyrimidine dimers, blocks the progression of the replication fork if present in the leading strand because synthesis is not reinitiated beyond the lesions (upper prong). In contrast, damage in the lagging strand would not impede the movement of the fork since the discontinuous mode of replication on that strand would reinitiate DNA synthesis downstream from the lesions (lower prong):

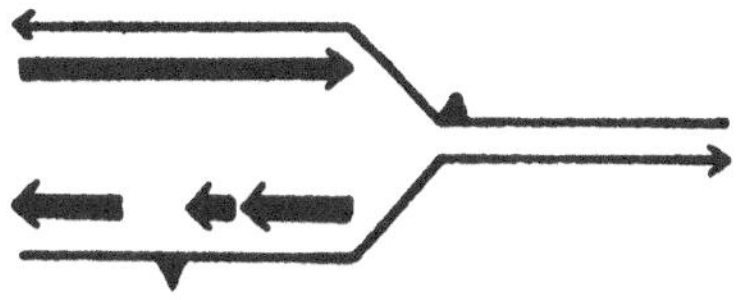

This general context prompted us to investigate the structure and persistence of blocked replication intermediates by using an even simpler animal virus, namely the Minute-Virus-of-Mice (MVM). MVM belongs to the group of autonomous parvoviruses and causes lytic infection of various mammalian cells [23]. As depicted in Fig. 1 the parvoviral genome is a linear single-stranded DNA molecule of about 5×10^3 nucleotides, which comprises short 3' and 5' terminal palindromes. The 3' end hairpin serves as a unique origin of replication by providing a natural primer for the conversion of viral DNA to a duplex replicative form [24, 25]. This conversion results from the continuous and unidirectional elongation of the 3' terminal palindrome and is likely to rely entirely on cellular functions [26].

It occurred to us that replicative form synthesis in parvoviruses might be representative of replication in the leading prong of a fork. In this respect, parvoviruses might be especially suitable to test the model of damaged DNA replication discussed above.

Exposure of bacteria to low doses of UV-radiation prior to infection with UV-damaged bacteriophage ϕX174, was found to increase the fraction of parental viral single-stranded DNA which was converted to duplex replicative forms [27]. Thus, preirradiation confers to bacteria the ability to tolerate UV-lesions which would otherwise inhibit viral DNA replication. A similar phenomenon might occur at apurinic sites [28]. Although the molecular events leading to the tolerance are not known, these data suggest that non- or sublethal doses of genotoxic agents such as UV-light might activate the expression of repair and/or replication processes which are not or less available in untreated bacteria. On the analogy of these observations, the induction of a tolerance mechanism might account for the recovery in mammalian cells, of normal DNA synthesis despite the persistence of many lesions [6, 8, 14-18]. However, alternative explanations for this recovery without the need of an induction step are possible [6, 17]. Whether some genotoxic agents trigger the expression of repair and/or replication activities in mammalian cells is a much debated question [29-32]. One difficulty is to dissociate the potential inducing effect of a treatment from its damaging action. The use of a viral probe allows one to alleviate this problem since the "inducer" can be administered to the cells and removed prior to virus infection. The virus may thus take advantage of the inducing effect of the treatment given to the cells without suffering its damaging action. In this context, we compared the replica-

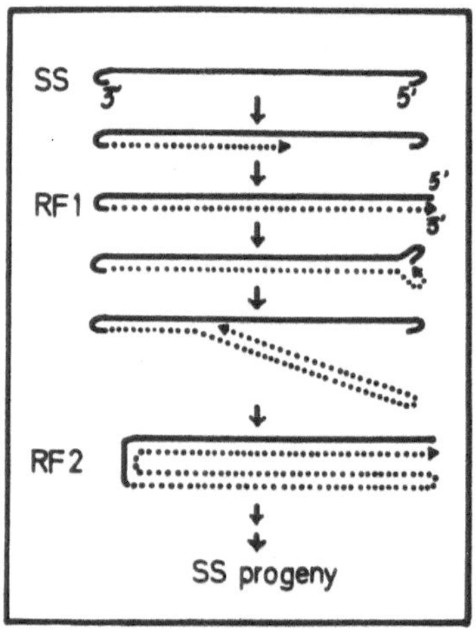

Fig. 1. Model for MVM DNA replication (after refs. 24, 25). The viral single-stranded (SS) DNA is converted into a monomer-length duplex replicative form (RF 1) by unidirectional and continuous elongation of a 3' terminus palindrome. RF 1 DNA is amplified by a process in which both monomeric (RF 1) and concatemeric (RF 2) DNA species are generated. RF 2 formation might involve the rearrangement of RF 1 in a "rabbit-eared" structure providing a new 3' end hairpin which can prime the copy of the complementary and viral strands. Subsequent steps leading to the synthesis of progeny SS DNA are not yet fully elucidated and are not depicted.

tion of UV-irradiated parvovirus MVM in normal cultures and in cells preexposed to mild UV-doses prior to infection. These experiments aimed at determining whether UV-radiation activated cellular repair and/or replication functions participating in the conversion of viral single-stranded DNA.

B. SUMMARY

UV-irradiation of parvovirus MVM prior to infection of A9 mouse cells decreases virus infectivity as well as viral capsid protein and DNA synthesis. As illustrated by Fig. 2, virus infectivity was measured by plaque formation in indicator A9 cells. Viral structural protein synthesis was revealed *in situ* by immunoenzymatic staining of infected cultures. Viral DNA replication intermediates were extracted from infected cells and analyzed by electrophoresis through agarose and polyacrylamide gels. Virus UV-irradiation was found to inhibit the *in vivo* conversion of ^{32}P-labeled parental single-stranded DNA to duplex replicative forms. UV-lesions, presumably pyrimidine dimers, appear to block irreversibly the elongation of the complementary strand.

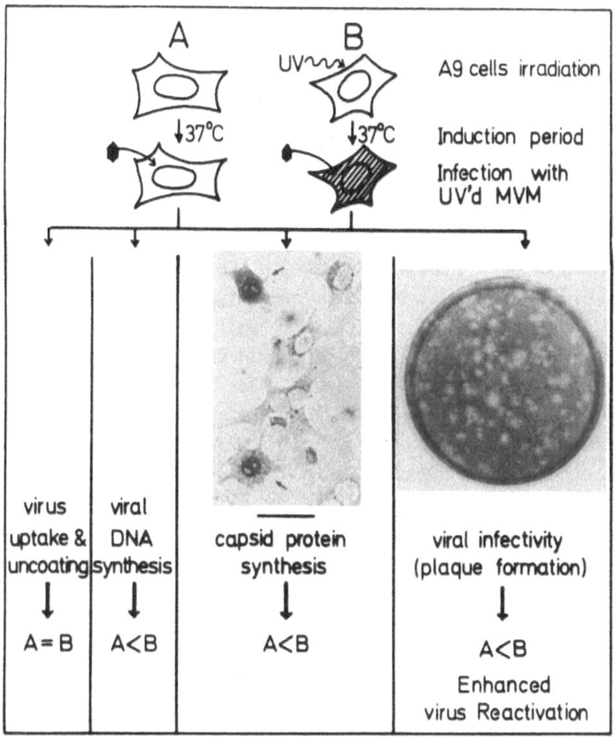

Fig. 2. Scheme of the experimental protocol and main conclusions. Untreated (A) and UV-irradiated (B) mouse A9 cells were infected with UV-damaged parvovirus MVM and compared for their ability to replicate the virus. Irradiated cultures were incubated prior to virus infection, in order to allow the expression of inducible cellular activities. Four end-points were measured. Cells supporting capsid protein synthesis were quantitated at 0-2.5 days post-infection (p.i.), using an *in situ* immunoenzymatic assay; arrows point to positive-staining cells showing the early accumulation of viral proteins in the nucleus; bar represent 50 μm. Virus infectivity was measured 5 days p.i., by plaque formation in growing monolayers of A9 cells. Cell UV-preirradiation had no detectable effect on the uptake of UV-damaged MVM nor on its uncoating (0-20 h p.i.). In contrast, the cell pretreatment was found to enhance the synthesis of viral DNA replicative forms (0-2 days p.i.) and to increase the fraction of the culture supporting either viral protein synthesis or the production of infectious particles. The higher survival of damaged virus in pretreated cells defines the enhanced virus reactivation phenomenon.

Exposure of the cells to sublethal UV-doses prior to infection was found to stimulate their capacity to replicate UV-damaged MVM. As depicted in Fig. 2, the survival of the virus ability to form plaques was higher in preirradiated cells (UV-enhanced virus reactivation phenomenon). Cells supporting the primary virus cycle and staining positively for protein synthesis were also more frequent in pretreated cultures. UV-irradiation is therefore likely to enhance virus survival by stimulating a step of the primary virus cycle rather than the subsequent rounds of infection required for plaque formation. Cell preirradiation had no detectable effect on virus uptake nor uncoating. In contrast, the fraction of input viral single-stranded DNA which was converted to replicative forms, was increased in cells which were treated prior to infection with UV-irradiated MVM. These parental replicative forms were amplified and gave rise to progeny single-stranded DNA. The expression of the enhanced call capacity to replicate UV-damaged virus was delayed and transient; moreover, it required active protein synthesis during the interval between cell treatment and virus infection.

Although the molecular mechanism giving rise to enhanced virus reactivation is not known, the data presented in this report suggest that the processing of viral single-stranded DNA is a likely candidate for (one of) the step(s) of the MVM cycle which is stimulated in irradiated cells. Cell exposure to sublethal doses of agents such as UV-light might activate the expression, availability or use of cellular repair and/or replication functions which are limiting for virus survival.

C. INTRODUCTION

The survival of UV-irradiated, nuclear-replicating DNA viruses is increased if the mammalian host cells are exposed to low doses of radiation or chemical carcinogens prior to infection (reviewed in refs. 33-36). A typical protocol for the measurement of this response, termed enhanced virus reactivation (ER), is illustrated by Fig. 1. ER is phenomenologically similar to Weigle reactivation of phages in pretreated bacteria [37-39].

Usually, virus survival is measured by plaque formation, an endpoint rather far removed from the initial treatment given to the cells. The target of ER in the sequence of events leading to plaque formation is not known. ER of herpes simplex virus [40] and parvovirus MVM [41] could be shown using an infectious center assay whereby UV-preirradiated cells were infected, transferred onto untreated indicator cells and tested for their ability to initiate plaque formation. Moreover, the survival of viral capsid protein synthesis in primary infected cells was also found to be increased when UV-irradiated adenovirus [42] or parvovirus [43] were propagated in γ-irradiated human fibroblasts and in UV-irradiated mouse cells, respectively. Altogether, these data suggest that ER results from an effect of the treatment on cells supporting the primary virus cycle rather than on indicator cells revealing the plaques. Thus, the stimulation of a step preceding virus release and secondary infection seems to be responsible for the enhancement of virus survival.

The pre-exposure of mammalian cells to UV-light or various chemicals has been shown to induce concomitantly an ER of UV-irradiated herpes simplex virus, simian virus 40 or parvovirus H-1 and an enhanced mutagenesis (EM) of intact and/or UV-damaged virus (see Cornelis et al., this volume). Because ER and EM display similar dose-responses and kinetics and share dependence on active protein synthesis following cell treatment, both phenomena may be performed by the same function. Alternatively, the effectors of ER and EM may be different but regulated coordinately as part of a set of functions whose expression is under a common control. The latter situation would be reminiscent of the SOS pleiotropic response which is triggered in bacteria exposed to various genotoxic agents and includes Weigle reactivation, a function involved in the survival of infecting phages [38, 39]. Actually, ER of virus survival in treated mammalian cells was found to be expressed concomitantly with an enhanced cell capacity to replicate untreated virus; yet, both responses could be dissociated in certain cell lines, suggesting that the underlying processes are at least partly independent [44]. Whether ER is similarly related to EM is not known. Therefore, the coordinate expression of ER and EM does not prove by itself that ER involves modification, repair, and/or replication of viral DNA. Moreover, as discussed in an accompanying paper (Cornelis et al., this volume), EM of irradiated virus is sometimes undetectable under conditions producing ER.

This general context prompted us to investigate directly whether ER conditions affected the metabolism of viral DNA. We showed previously that the survival of UV-irradiated parvovirus MVM was increased in mouse A9 cells exposed to subtoxic doses of UV-light prior to infection [41, 43, 44]. Owing to the unique structure and mode of replication of the parvoviral genome (see RATIONALE), this system was selected to analyze the effect of UV-preirradiation of the cells on their ability to process UV-damaged viral DNA. This work aims at testing whether certain treatments can induce an enhanced expression or availability of cellular functions involved in DNA repair and/or replication.

D. MATERIALS AND METHODS

Virus and Cell

The plaque-purified prototype strain of Minute-virus-of-mice [45] (MVM) was propagated in the A9 variant of mouse L cells [46]. Conditions for cell synchronization, virus infection, cell and virus

UV-irradiation (λ = 254 nm) and preparation of ^{32}P- or ^{3}H-labeled MVM virions have been described elsewhere [41, 47].

Experimental Protocol

Cells arrested in Go by isoleucine deprivation were UV-irradiated (0 or 4.5 J m^{-2}) further incubated in depleted medium for various times and infected with untreated or UV-irradiated MVM. Infected cultures were transferred to complete medium and processed for the assays described below. These cultures enter into S phase about 15 h following transfer, at which time viral DNA replication is initiated [41, 47].

Titration of Virus Infectivity

Virus titers were determined by plaque formation in growing monolayers of A9 cells, using either a direct plaque assay or an infectious center assay [41]. In the direct assay, treated cultures were used as indicators to reveal the plaques; the ranges of the multiplicity of infection (MOI, see Definitions) were 2×10^{-2}-2×10^{-4} and 2×10^{-2}-2.0 for intact and UV-irradiated (22-70 J m^{-2}; survival $\approx 10^{-3}$-10^{-4}) MVM, respectively. For the infectious center assay, irradiated cells were harvested after infection and seeded onto untreated A9 indicator cells; the MOIs were 2×10^{-3}-10^{-1} and 4.0-10 for intact and UV-irradiated (35-55 J m^{-2}; survival $\approx 10^{-2}$-10^{-3}) MVM, respectively. Plates were stained and plaques were counted 5 days post-infection.

Immunoenzymatic Assay

Monolayers of cells infected with intact (MOI = 10^{-1}) or UV-irradiated (35 J m^{-2}; survival $\approx 10^{-2}$; MOI = 10) MVM were fixed at intervals and incubated successively with goat anti-MVM serum and rabbit anti-goat serum-conjugated peroxidase. Cells which had accumulated viral capsid proteins were then revealed *in situ* using a peroxidase dependent staining with diaminobenzidine [43].

Virus Uptake

Cells were inoculated at 4°C with UV-irradiated (70 J m^{-2}) MVM labled with ^{3}H-thymidine (10^{-3} cpm/plaque-forming-unit; MOI = 25), they were incubated at 37°C and harvested at intervals. The medium and the nuclear and cytoplasmic cell fractions were isolated and acid-insoluble radioactivity was measured after TCA precipitation [41].

Infectivity of Cell-Associated Viral Particles

Monolayers of infected cells were incubated under conditions preventing secondary rounds of infection and were collected at intervals. Virus was extracted by freeze-thawing and titered by direct plaque assay [41].

Isolation of Intracellular Viral DNA

Cells were infected with approximately 15 plaque-forming-units/cell of MVM labeled with ^{32}P-orthophosphate or ^{3}H-thymidine. Viral DNA had an initial specific activity around 10^{6} cpm/μg. Infected cells were incubated in complete medium and harvested at intervals. Intracellular DNA was extracted and fractionated, using a modification of the Hirt procedure [48]. The viral DNA from the Hirt supernatant was treated with proteinase K, extracted with phenol and precipitated with ethanol [47].

Analysis of Viral DNA Extracted from Infected Cells

Parental Viral DNA. DNA radiolabeled with $^{32}P\text{-}PO_4$ in input parental strands was electrophoresed through 1 and 1.4% nondenaturing agarose vertical slab gels for 450 and 750 V·h, respectively [47]. Viral DNA was located in dry gels by autoradiography.

Total Viral DNA. DNA radiolabeled with ^{3}H-thymidine in input parental strands was electrophoresed through 1.4% nondenaturing agarose horizontal slab gels for 550 V·h. DNA was transferred onto cellulose nitrate filters essentially as described [49] and it was hybridized with ^{32}P-labeled DNA complementary to the viral strand. The probe was an Hinf I digest of monomeric replicative forms resulting from the *in vitro* conversion of purified virion single-stranded DNA by *E. coli* Klenow DNA polymerase in the presence of α-^{32}P-deoxyribononucleotides [50]. Blots were exposed to x-ray films for autoradiography.

Quantification. Autoradiographs were quantitated by scanning with a Joyce-Loebl densitometer. Bands of ^{32}P-labeled DNA were excised from dried gels and counted by liquid-scintillation spectrometry.

Definitions

Multiplicity of Infection (MOI). The MOI is the number of infectious (plaque forming) virus particles per cell for an equivalent inoculum of unirradiated virus titered by direct-plaque assay on untreated A9 cells.

Survival. The virus surviving fraction is defined as the ratio of the titer of UV-irradiated virus to that of intact virus. Since higher MOIs were used for irradiated virus, results were normalized for the same MOI as unirradiated virus, knowing that the titer of UV-damaged virus was found to be proportional to the MOI [41].

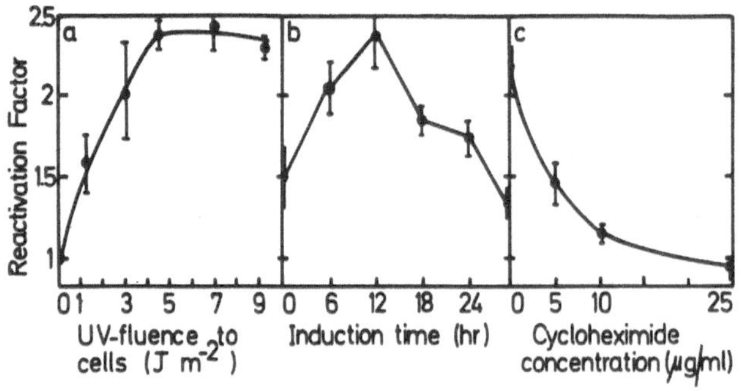

Fig. 3. Parameters of UV-enhanced virus reactivation. The survival of UV-irradiated MVM (70 J m^{-2}; survival $\simeq 10^{-4}$) was compared in untreated A9 cells and in cultures exposed to UV-radiation prior to virus infection. The reactivation factor is the ratio of the virus surviving fraction in irradiated cells to that in similarly treated but unirradiated cells. The magnitude of enhanced reactivation is shown in function of: a) the UV-dose administered to cells 6 h prior to virus infection; b) the time between cell UV-irradiation (4.5 J m^{-2}) and virus infection (induction period at 37°C); c) the concentration of cycloheximide given during a 12 h induction period at 37°C. Average values and standard deviations (bars) of 4 independent experiments (direct plaque assays).

Enhanced Virus Reactivation (ER). The ER factor is given by the ratio of the surviving fraction of UV-irradiated virus on UV-irradiated cells to that on similarly treated but unirradiated cells.

E. RESULTS

1. UV-Enhanced Virus Reactivation

Phenomenon. Parvovirus MVM forms lysis plaques in growing monolayers of A9 cells (Fig. 2). This property allows one to quantitate virus infectivity by titering its plaque-forming ability [45]. Exposure of MVM to UV-radiation decreases its titer. The ratio of the titer of damaged virus to that of untreated virus gives the surviving fraction. When UV-irradiated MVM was titered in cells which had been exposed themselves to mild UV-doses prior to virus infection, its survival was found to be increased [41, 43, 44]. A ratio of virus survival in treated cells to that in control cultures greater than 1.0 defines the UV-enhanced virus reactivation (ER) phenomenon. ER was demonstrated with several nuclear-replicating DNA viruses [33-36], including parvoviruses closely related to MVM [33, 51, 52]. Changes in the multiplicity of infection did not affect detectably the magnitude of ER [33, 41, 53]. A mechanism involving genetic interactions between input damaged genomes is therefore unlikely to account for this phenomenon. Five days elapse between MVM infection and plaque counting. The following sections describe our attempts to identify, within this time interval, the step of MVM propagation which is responsible for increased plaque formation by irradiated virus in pretreated cells.

Parameters of Enhanced Virus Reactivation. As shown in Fig. 3a, the magnitude of ER increases with the UV-dose administered to the cells and saturates around 4-5 J m^{-2}, a dose which is only slightly cytotoxic [41, 44]. ER is expressed after a delay following cell treatment and it decays at later times (Fig. 3b). ER was maximal when a 12 h interval was allowed between cell UV-irradiation and MVM infection [41]. The actual "induction period" might be longer since in our protocol, viral DNA replication is initiated parasynchronously around 15 h post-infection (see Materials and Methods). The inhibition of cellular protein synthesis by cycloheximide during the 12 h induction period prevents the expression of ER (Fig. 3c). The concentration of cycloheximide required to abolish ER had no or little effect on plaque formation in untreated cells [41, 44]. These data thus indicate that important metabolic events occur shortly after exposure of A9 cells to mild UV-doses. These events involve or induce protein effectors and generate transient condition which eventually promote plaque formation by irradiated MVM. In experiments with several other cell lines and viruses, a similar time [33, 51, 52, 54] and protein synthesis [52, 54, 55]-dependence of ER was observed.

Involvement of Primarily Infected Cells. In the direct-plaque assay, treated cultures are infected and used as indicators to reveal the plaques. ER could therefore result from an effect of UV-radiation on cells supporting either the primary infection or the secondary rounds of infection required for the formation of visible plaques. Data illustrated in Table 1 strongly suggest that the target cells are those producing the primary viral burst. Firstly, ER of herpes simplex virus [40] and MVM [41] was demonstrable using an infectious center assay whereby UV-irradiated infected cells were collected, transferred onto untreated indicator cells and tested for their ability to initiate plaque formation (Table 1A). Secondly, the magnitude of ER was not affected by a 4-fold increase in the average size of the plaques [41] (Table 1B) UV-radiation is therefore unlikely to act by delaying the growth of indicator cells, which causes enlargement of the plaques and might have accounted for the scoring of otherwise undetectably small plaques. Thirdly, pretreated cultures infected with UV-damaged adenovirus [42] or MVM [43] also contained a higher frequency of cells supporting the primary virus cycle and staining positively for viral capsid protein synthesis (Table 1C). Altogether these data narrow the ER-sensitive window of virus replication to a step of the primary virus

Table 1. Involvement of Primarily Infected Cells in Enhanced Virus Reactivation

	Experimental conditions	Reactivation factor
A	Direct-plaque assay	1.9 ± 0.4
	Infectious center assay	1.9 ± 0.5
B	Infectious center assay	
	Average plaque size = 2.2 mm	2.7
	Average plaque size = 8.2 mm	2.5
C	Infectious center assay	1.4 ± 0.1
	Immunoenzymatic assay	1.5 ± 0.2

A9 cell monolayers were UV-irradiated (0 or 4.5 J m^{-2}), incubated for 12 h at 37°C and infected with intact or UV-irraduated MVM. Dose to MVM was 55 J m^{-2} (A, B; survival $\approx 10^{-3}$) or 35 J m^{-2} (C; survival $\approx 10^{-2}$). The reactivation factor is the ratio of the survival of irradiated virus on irradiated cells to that on untreated cells. The survival of virus infectivity (A, B, C) was measured by plaque formation using a direct-plaque or an infectious center-assay as described in Materials and Methods. Plaques of different average sizes were obtained by transferring infectious centers onto monolayers of indicator cells seeded at different densities. The survival of viral capsid protein synthesis (C) was measured by *in situ* immunoenzymatic staining of primary infected cells at 2 days post-infection. Results from 1 (B) -3 (A, C) experiments.

cycle preceding release and secondary infection. We showed previously [41] that cell UV-irradiation did not alter significantly the kinetics of production of progeny particles from UV-damaged virus. Cell pretreatment is therefore most likely to affect the level of virus production in the primary burst, i.e., to increase the number of producer cells or the size of limiting bursts.

2. Effect of Cell Pre-Irradiation on Virus Uptake and Uncoating

Uptake. During the parvorvirus internalization process, viral DNA becomes progressively associated with the nucleus where DNA replication and progeny particle assembly occur [56]. As shown in Fig. 4a, no significant difference between UV-irradiated and control cells was detected with respect to the kinetics and the extent of MVM nuclear-association [41].

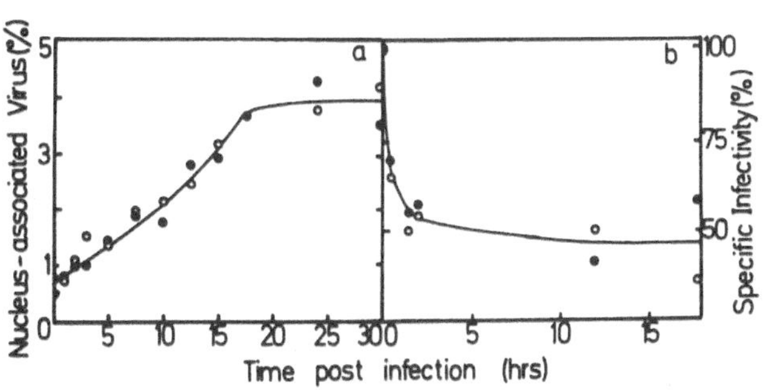

Fig. 4. Effect of cell UV-irradiation on the uptake and uncoating of UV-damaged MVM. A9 cell monolayers were UV-irradiated (0 or 4.5 J m^{-2}), incubated for 12 h at 37°C and infected at 4°C with UV-irradiated (70 J m^{-2}; survival $\approx 10^{-4}$) MVM labeled with ^{3}H-thymidine (MOI = 25 [a] or 10 [b]). Infected cells were incubated at 37°C, harvested at intervals and processed for the measurement of virus uptake (a) and cell-bound virus infectivity (b), as described in Materials and Methods. Panel (a) shows the percentage of ^{3}H-labeled input virus which is associated with the nuclear fraction of control (○) and UV-irradiated (●) cells. Panel (b) shows the infectivity of a given amount of virus taken up by control (○) and UV-irradiated (●) cells; the infectivity of virus bound to unirradiated cells at time 0 is considered as 100%.

Uncoating. Since replicating parvoviral DNA forms a complex with a capsid-like structure [57], uncoating could not be measured directly by the appearance of free DNA. It was therefore assumed that the loss of infectivity of internalized particles could be taken as an indirect test for uncoating. As shown in Fig. 4b, no significant quantitative nor kinetic difference in the eclipse of viral infectivity was observed between treated and control cultures [41]. Similar results were obtained using the vulnerability of intracellular MVM DNA to nuclease digestion as a second test for uncoating [41].

Early phases of the viral cycle, such as adsorption to cellular receptors, migration to the nucleus and uncoating, are therefore unlikely targets of the ER function(s).

3. Effect of Cell Pre-Irradiation on Viral DNA Replication

MVM UV-Irradiation Inhibits DNA Conversion. ^{32}P-labeled MVM irradiated with increasing UV-doses was inoculated onto A9 cells monolayers. Cells were harvested at intervals post-infection. In-

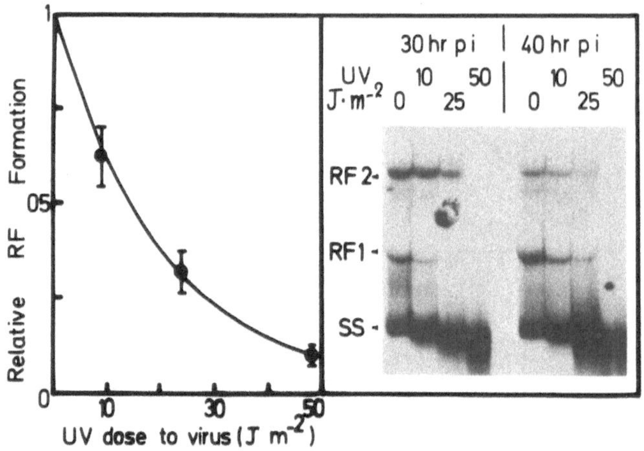

Fig. 5. Effect of MVM UV-irradiation on the conversion of parental viral DNA to duplex forms in untreated A9 cells. ^{32}P-labeled MVM was irradiated with increasing UV-doses (0-50 J m^{-2}) and inoculated onto untreated cell monolayers. Infected cultures were incubated at 37°C and harvested at 30 and 40 h post-infection (p.i.). Intracellular viral DNA was isolated and fractionated at 1.4% nondenaturating agarose gels. Right panel, autoradiograph of a dried gel. Samples applied to different lanes were count-matched. SS: Single-stranded DNA; RF 1: monomer-length DNA duplex; RF 2: oligomeric DNA duplex (see Fig. 1). Left panel, dose response of RF formation at 40 h p.i. The fraction of labeled viral DNA converted to duplex RF is shown relative to that given by unirradiated virus (●). The line drawn is the theoretical curve expected if every UV-induced pyrimidine dimer (as measured by Proctor et al. [58] for equivalent survivals of the closely related parvovirus KRV) constituted an absolute block to DNA-conversion. Average values and standard deviations (bars) from 2 independent experiments.

tracellular viral DNA was isolated and fractionated by agarose gel electrophoresis. As depicted in Fig. 1 and illustrated by Fig. 5 (right panel), native viral DNA migrates as a series of bands corresponding to unreplicated single-stranded DNA (SS) and duplex replicative forms of monomeric (RF1) and oligomeric (RF2) length. It is apparent from the autoradiograph shown in Fig. 5, that UV-irradiation of the virus inhibits the conversion of labeled parental single-strands to replicative forms. The total radioactivity recovered from infected cells was not affected by virus irradiation (not shown), suggesting that the lower fraction of RF molecules cannot be ascribed

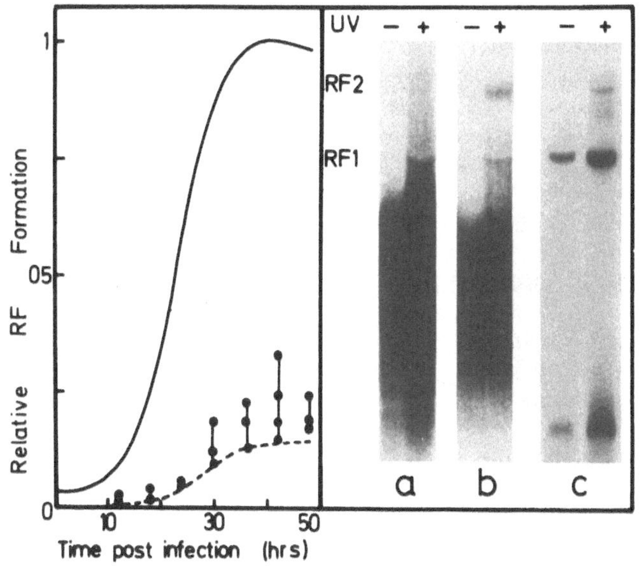

Fig. 6. Effect of cell UV-preirradiation on viral DNA replication after infection with UV-irradiated MVM. A9 cell monolayers were irradiated with UV-light (0 or 4.5 J m^{-2}), incubated for 12 h at 37°C and infected with UV-irradiated (50 J m^{-2}) MVM. Input virus was radiolabeled with ^{32}P-PO_4 or ^{3}H-thymidine. Infected cultures were incubated for 42 h (right panel) or various times (left panel) at 37°C and harvested. Viral DNA was isolated and run in nondenaturing agarose gels. Right panel (a, b) illustrates the processing of parental viral single-stranded DNA; input virus was ^{32}P-labeled; gels were dried. Right panel (c) illustrates the total synthesis of viral DNA strands; input virus was labeled with ^{3}H-thymidine; DNA was transferred from the gel onto a cellulose nitrate filter and hybridized with ^{32}P-labeled DNA complementary to the viral strand; input viral DNA was not detectable under those conditions. Autoradiographs of the dried gels (a, b) or blot (c) are shown. (-) and (+) on top of lanes denote untreated and UV-irradiated cells, respectively; for each pair of lanes, samples applied to the gel contained the same amount of radiolabeled input parental DNA. Symbols as in Fig. 5. Left panel shows the time courses of the conversion of ^{32}P-labeled parental single-strands to duplex replicative forms (RF) for intact MVM in untreated cells (——) and for UV-irradiated virus in untreated (---) or pretreated (●) cells. Data are from agarose gels as illustrated by Fig. 5 and Fig. 6a, b. RF formation is shown relative to that given by intact virus in untreated cells at 40 h post-infection. For each time, (●) values obtained in independent experiments are plotted.

to the degradation or loss of viral DNA species [47]. The quantitation of the inhibition of RF formation shown in Fig. 5 (left panel) is consistent with a linear UV-induction of replication blocks which occur at a frequency similar to that reported [58] for pyrimidine dimers. These DNA lesions might thus constitute the major obstacle to the conversion of parvoviral DNA. Restriction fragments analysis, to be described elsewhere [47], suggests that UV-radiation inhibits the conversion of viral parental strands mainly by blocking the elongation of growing complementary strands; there is no evidence for reinitiation of DNA synthesis downstream from the arrest sites.

As shown in Fig. 6 (left panel), MVM irradiation caused a permanent inhibition of RF formation but no significant delay in the residual DNA conversion.

Cell UV-Preexposure Enhances UV-Irradiated MVM DNA Conversion. Cell pretreatment conditions giving rise to maximal ER of UV-irradiated MVM were tested for their effect on viral DNA replication. Figure 6 (right panel, a, b) illustrates the processing of ^{32}P-labeled parental viral DNA in control and UV-preirradiated cells infected with UV-damaged MVM. It is apparent that the fraction of the activity which migrates as replicative forms is higher in pretreated cells. Cells irradiation did not affect detectably the total activity recovered from infected cultures (not shown) [47]. Differences in the gel profiles are therefore likely to be accounted for by a higher level of duplex DNA synthesis rather than the specific loss or degradation of single-stranded DNA in treated cells. Subtoxic UV-doses apparently stimulate the cell's ability to process parental viral DNA to replicative forms after infection with UV-irradiated MVM. Figure 6 (left panel) shows that the increase in the level of DNA conversion does not merely result from an earlier onset of viral DNA synthesis and varied in magnitude from one experiment to the other. Moreover, results not shown indicate that the enhancement of viral DNA conversion in preirradiated cultures (i) is hardly detectable for untreated virus and (ii) shares with ER its dependence on active protein synthesis during the interval between cell treatment and virus infection [47]. As illustrated by Fig. 6 (right panel, c) cell irradiation prior to infection with UV-damaged MVM also enhances the total amount of viral strands which are synthesized as part of the amplification of RF molecules and the displacement of progeny single-strands. The similar magnitude of the increase in parental DNA conversion and in the synthesis of viral strands suggests that (i) parental RF molecules formed in pretreated cells are metabolically active, and (ii) the conversion of input single-strands is the step of viral DNA replication which becomes less limiting under ER conditions.

F. DISCUSSION

1. Target of UV-Enhanced Reactivation in the Viral Life Cycle

Cell UV-irradiation prior to infection with UV-damaged MVM enhances the survival of the viral ability to form plaques (enhanced virus reactivation phenomenon). A first goal was to identify the viral function(s) which become(s) less limiting for virus survival in pretreated cells. Evidence was presented showing that the target of enhanced virus reactivation is a step which follows virus uptake and uncoating but precedes the release of the primary burst and secondary infection. In particular, the earliest viral function whose survival was found to be enhanced by cell pretreatment was the conversion of parental single-stranded DNA to duplex replicative forms. The data suggest that cell irradiation generates conditions promoting the processing of input viral single-strands to duplex forms. This increased processing is likely to account for a higher level of progeny viral DNA synthesis in pretreated cultures. Moreover, a treatment known to inhibit the expression of ER was also found to prevent the increase in viral DNA conversion [47]. Altogether, these results point to single-stranded DNA repair and/or conversion as a likely candidate function whose greater availability in pretreated cells eventually enhances the survival of UV-damaged parvovirus MVM.

2. Induction Process

Phenomenologically, the exposure of A9 cells to UV-light induces an enhancement of their ability to replicate viral DNA and to produce virus after infection with UV-irradiated MVM. At least three different processes might account for this induction. Firstly, an altered kinetics of the ongoing viral cycle in irradiated cells might change the time available for viral DNA repair and/or replication. This possibility is unlikely since the cell pretreatment had no or little effect on the time course of viral DNA synthesis and of infectious particles production [41].

Secondly, preirradiation of the cells might affect their ability to compete with infecting viruses for cellular functions operating on both cell and viral genomes. Direct damaging of the cells is, however, not a prerequisite since intact cells were found to display ER of UV-irradiated parvovirus H-1, provided that they were preinfected with another UV-inactivated virus (Cornelis et al., unpublished).

Thirdly, UV-radiation might alter the level, properties or availability of cellular functions participating in or antagonizing repair and/or replication. The delayed expression of ER and its dependence on *de novo* protein synthesis following cell treatment might

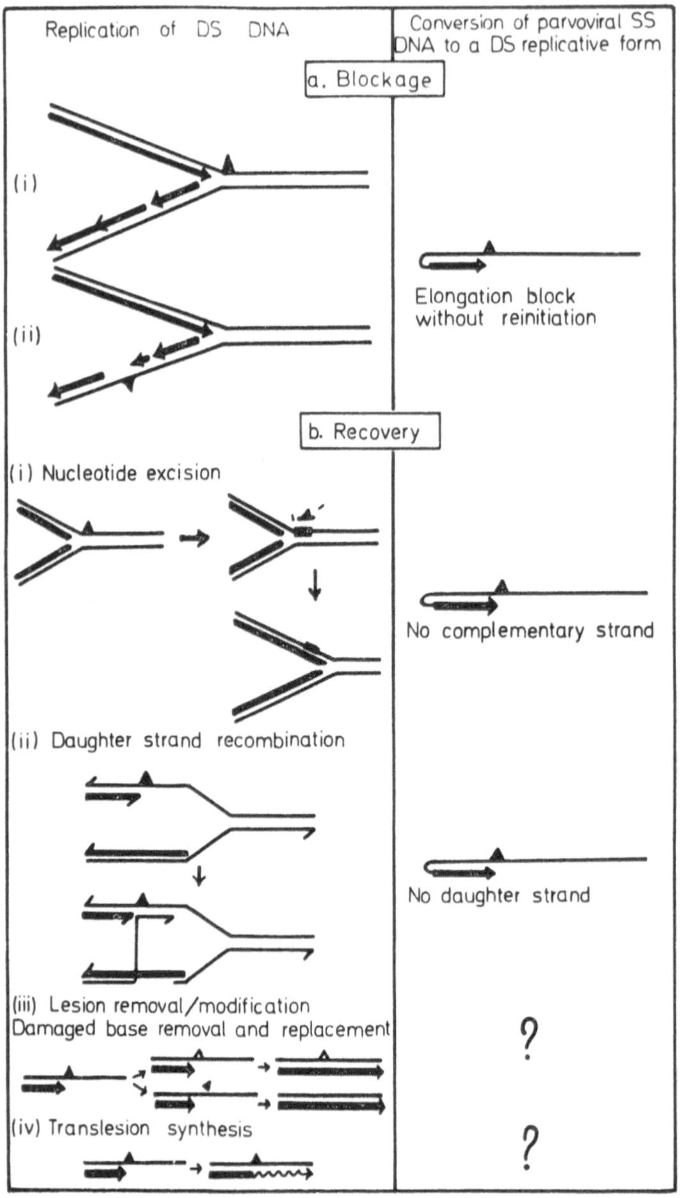

Fig. 7. Model for replication of damaged DNA induction of, and recovery from, elongation blocks. Left column: a) Proposed model [21, 22] for the blockage of DNA replication on a leading (i) or lagging (ii) strand. b) Possible mechanisms for the recovery from elongation blocks [1]: (i) excision and replacement of a patch of DNA comprising damaged nucleotides(s); (ii) insertion of a preformed DNA segment by recombination with the homologous daughter molecule; (iii)

reflect the involvement of non-constitutive protein effectors whose synthesis is triggered by UV-radiation. However, short-lived or cell-cycle-dependent proteins normally produced by cells, might as well account for these properties.

3. Molecular Mechanism of Enhanced Virus Reactivation

The conversion of parvoviral single-stranded DNA to duplex replicative forms is thought to rely entirely on cellular enzymes [26]. Moreover, it is very unlikely that the virus encodes for a repair function which might facilitate the conversion of damaged DNA. Therefore, enhanced parental RF formation in pretreated cultures is presumably performed by host cell functions.

Most UV-induced blocks to the conversion of MVM DNA could be ascribed to the irreversible arrest of the elongation of the growing complementary strand (Fig. 7a, right column). Owing to its continuous mode of synthesis, parvoviral DNA conversion might be considered as a simplified model for replication in the leading prong of the fork. In this respect, our results support the scheme proposing that DNA synthesis does not get reinitiated downstream from blocking lesions in a leading strand [20-22] (Fig. 7a, left column). The overcome of such elongation blocks in pretreated cells might account for the enhanced conversion of input single-strands to duplex forms after infection with UV-irradiated MVM. Figure 7b (left column) depicts candidate recovery mechanisms. The single-strandedness of parvoviral DNA tends to limit these possibilities to either the bypass of the lesions or the removal or modification of the damage leaving the DNA backbone intact. Either of these mechanisms could be a single- or multi-step process. Moreover, irradiated cells might also display activities antagonizing the misprocessing of input strands which is responsible for the generation of many defective genomes after infection with untreated MVM [59].

Although most replication intermediates generated from UV-damaged templates appear to be partially converted molecules, it cannot be ruled out that a fraction of the blocks occurs at the level of initiation, as the result, e.g., of lesions within the 3' terminus

---

removal or modification of the lesion or replacement of the damaged base(s); (iv) bypass of the lesion by a modified replicase. Right column: Parvoviral DNA conversion provides a simplified system for continuous and unidirectional replication on a leading strand (a). Moreover, the absence of a complementary strand precludes the involvement of excision repair or daughter strand recombination in the recovery from elongation blocks. Symbols: ——) parental DNA; ■) newly synthesized DNA (normal replicase); ∿∿) newly synthesized DNA (modified replicase); ▲) lesion; △) modified lesion.

palindrome which primes DNA conversion. Moreover, a significant proportion of input viral single-strands does not initiate replication even if the virus has not been treated [25, 47]. Therefore, another potential effect of cell preirradiation could be the removal of UV-induced or spontaneous barriers to the initiation of MVM DNA conversion. We are presently attempting to discriminate between these various possible mechanisms.

4. Relevance of Enhanced Virus Reactivation to Cell Survival

As discussed previously, ER might result from an enhanced level, availability or use of cellular effectors involved in viral DNA metabolism. These same effectors may also operate upon the genome of the host cell. This raises the intriguing possibility that cell exposure to inducers of ER generates conditions allowing the cell itself to better tolerate the damaging effect of the treatment. No conclusive evidence in favor of this possibility has been found so far. No straightforward correlation was observed between the magnitude of ER displayed by related cell lines and their resistance to UV-killing [44]. However, differences in other parameters involved in overall survival might obscure this comparison. The higher cell survival observed when the total dose of genotoxic agent is fractionated in time indicates that a first exposure may allow cells to better resist subsequent ones [60]. It is unclear, however, whether such a split-dose protocol results in any enhancement of the cell capacity to tolerate lesions [29-32].

During incubation following treatment with a DNA damaging agent, mammalian cells are eventually able to seal daughter strand discontinuities [1] and to perform normal DNA synthesis despite the persistence of many lesions [6, 8, 14, 15]. This recovery contrasts with our failure to detect any release of the blockage of UV-irradiated MVM DNA conversion in untreated cells. This finding might indicate that the recovery mechanism(s) are not expressed constitutively by mammalian cells. However, the persistence of the blockage of MVM DNA replication might as well be ascribed to the peculiar structure of the parvoviral genome. As depicted in Fig. 7b (right panel), the single-strandedness of MVM DNA prevents it from being a substrate for nucleotide excision repair and daughter strand recombination. Excision repair is very unlikely to account for the recovery of DNA replication in mammalian cells [16-18]. Although large single-strand exchanges do not appear to be involved either [21, 61, 62], recombinational insertion of short segments might still participate in the tolerance of the lesions in cellular DNA.

The role, if any, played by the ER process in the physiology of the cell, is therefore a matter of speculation. Some of the possible mechanisms mentioned above for the induction and operation of ER would likely affect the host cell whereas others would be specific to infecting viruses. It is also conceivable that the triggering of the ER process is superfluous with respect to cell survival but is associated with the induction of cell mutations (see Cornelis et al., this volume). Further characterization of the molecular mechanism of ER together with the analysis of related cells differing in their ER ability should help elucidating the relevance of ER to cell survival.

ACKNOWLEDGMENTS

We are indebted to Drs. D. Baltimore and M. Errera for stimulating discussions. This work was supported by CEC (156-76-1 BIOB; ENV/355/B), FRSM (3.4514.80), IHE(0392-1980) and US PHS (GM-20124; CA-16038). J. R. and J. M. V. are Chercheur Qualifié and Aspirant du Fonds National Belge de la Recherche Scientifique.

REFERENCES

1. J. D. Hall and D. W. Mount, Mechanism of DNA replication and mutagenesis in ultraviolet-irradiated bacteria and mammalian cells, Prog. Nucl. Acid Res. and Mol. Biol., 25:53 (1981).
2. R. B. Painter, Effect of caffeine on DNA synthesis in irradiated and unirradiated mammalian cells, J. Mol. Biol., 143: 289 (1980).
3. M. D. Ford and M. F. Lavin, Ataxia telangiectasia: an anomaly in DNA replication after irradiation, Nucleic Acids Res., 9: 1395 (1981).
4. P. D. Moore, K. K. Bose, S. D. Rabdkin, and B. S. Strauss, Sites of termination of *in vitro* DNA synthesis on ultraviolet- and N-acetylaminofluorene-treated ϕX174 templates by prokaryotic and eukaryotic DNA polymerases, Proc. Natl. Acad. Sci. USA, 78:110 (1981).
5. A. R. Lehmann, The relationship between pyrimidine dimers and replicating DNA in UV-irradiated human fibroblasts, Nucleic Acids Res., 7:1901 (1979).
6. J. E. Cleaver, G. H. Thomas, and S. D. Park, Xeroderma pigmentosum variants have a slow recovery of DNA synthesis after irradiation with ultraviolet light, Biochim. Biophys. Acta, 564:122 (1979).
7. B. S. Rosenstein and R. B. Setlow, DNA repair after ultraviolet irradiation of ICR 2A frog cells, Biophys. J., 31:195 (1980).
8. H. J. Edenberg, Inhibition of DNA replication by ultraviolet light, Biophys. J., 16:849 (1976).
9. D. Dahle, T. D. Griffiths, and J. G. Carpenter, Inhibition and recovery of DNA synthesis in UV-irradiated Chinese hamster V-79 cells, Photochem. Photobiol., 32:157 (1980).
10. A. R. Lehmann, Postreplication repair of DNA in ultraviolet-irradiated mammalian cells, J. Mol. Biol., 66:319 (1972).
11. S. N. Buhl, R. B. Setlow, and J. D. Regan, Steps in DNA chain elongation and joining after ultraviolet-irradiation of human cells, Int. J. Radiat. Biol., 22:417 (1972).

12. J. Doniger, DNA replication in ultraviolet light irradiated Chinese hamster cells: nature of replicon inhibition and post-replication repair, J. Mol. Biol., 120:433 (1978).
13. R. Meneghini, M. Cordeiro-Stone, and R. I. Schumacher, Size and frequency of gaps in newly synthesized DNA of Xeroderma pigmentosum human cells irradiated with ultraviolet light, Biophys. J., 33:81 (1981).
14. S. N. Buhl, R. B. Setlow, and J. D. Regan, Recovery of the ability to synthesize DNA in segments of normal size at long times after ultraviolet irradiation of human cells, Biophys. J., 13: 1265 (1973).
15. J. E. Cleaver, Investigations into the effects of UV-light on the rate of deoxyribonucleic acid synthesis in mammalian cells, Biochim. Biophys. Acta, 108:42 (1965).
16. R. E. Meyn, M. R. Kasschan, and R. R. Hewitt, The recovery of normal DNA replication kinetics in UV-irradiated Chinese hamster cells, Mutation Res., 44:129 (1977).
17. S. D. Park and J. E. Cleaver, Recovery of DNA synthesis after ultraviolet irradiation of Xeroderma pigmentosum cells depends on excision repair and is blocked by caffeine, Nucleic Acids Res., 6:1151 (1979).
18. J. Doniger and J. A. DiPaolo, The early and late modes of DNA replication in ultraviolet irradiated Syrian hamster embryo cells, Biophys. J., 31:247 (1980).
19. J. I. Williams and J. E. Cleaver, Perturbations in Simian virus 40 DNA synthesis by ultraviolet light, Mutation Res., 52:301 (1978).
20. A. R. Sarasin and P. C. Hanawalt, Replication of ultraviolet-irradiated Simian virus 40 in monkey kidney cells, J. Mol. Biol., 138:299 (1980).
21. R. Meneghini and P. C. Hanawalt, T4-endonuclease V-sensitive sites in DNA from ultraviolet-irradiated human cells, Biochim. Biophys. Acta, 425:428 (1976).
22. M. Cordeiro-Stone, R. I. Schumacher, and R. Meneghini, Structure of the replication fork in ultraviolet light-irradiated human cells, Biophys. J., 27:287 (1979).
23. P. Tattersall and D. C. Ward, the parvoviruses: an introduction, in: "Replication of Mammalian Parvoviruses," D. C. Ward and P. Tattersall, eds., p. 3, Cold Spring Harbor Laboratory, New York (1978).
24. P. Tattersall and D. C. Ward, Rolling hairpin model for replication of parvovirus and linear chromosomal DNA, Nature, 263:106 (1976).
25. D. C. Ward and D. K. Dadachanji, Replication of minute-virus-of-mice DNA, in: "Replication of Mammalian Parvoviruses," D. C. Ward and P. Tattersall, eds., p. 297, Cold Spring Harbor Laboratory, New York (1978).
26. S. L. Rhode, H-1 DNA synthesis, in: "Replication of Mammalian Parvoviruses," D. C. Ward and P. Tattersall, eds., p. 279, Cold Spring Harbor Laboratory, New York (1978).

27. P. Caillet-Fauquet, M. Defais, and M. Radman, Molecular mechanism of induced mutagenesis: replication *in vivo* of bacteriophage ϕ174 single-stranded ultraviolet light-irradiated DNA in intact and irradiated host cells, J. Mol. Biol., 117:95 (1977).
28. R. M. Schaaper and L. A. Loeb, Depurination causes mutations in SOS-induced cells, Proc. Natl. Acad. Sci. USA, 78:1773 (1981).
29. S. M. D'Ambrosio, P. M. Aebersold, and R. B. Setlow, Enhancement of postreplication repair in ultraviolet light-irradiated Chinese hamster cells by irradiation in G2 or S-phase, Cancer Res., 38:1147 (1978).
30. R. B. Painter, Response of Chinese hamster ovary cells to DNA damages after a conditioning exposure to ultraviolet light, Biochim. Biophys. Acta., 609:257 (1980).
31. E. Moustacchi, U. K. Ehmann, and E. C. Friedberg, Defective recovery of semi-conservative DNA synthesis in Xeroderma pigmentosum cells following split-dose ultraviolet irradiation, Mutation Res., 62:159 (1979).
32. R. Waters, The repair of human DNA following fractionated doses of ultraviolet irradiation, Carcinogenesis, 1:9 (1980).
33. C. D. Lytle, Radiation-enhanced virus reactivation in mammalian cells, J. Natl. Cancer Inst. Monogr., 50:145 (1978).
34. M. Radman, Is there SOS induction in mammalian cells?, Photochem. Photobiol., 32:823 (1980).
35. L. E. Bockstahler, Induction of enhanced reactivation of mammalian viruses by light, Prog. Nucl. Acid Res. and Mol. Biol., 26:303 (1981).
36. M. J. Defais, P. C. Hanawalt, and A. R. Sarasin, Viral probes for DNA repair, Adv. in Radiat. Biol., 10:in press (1981).
37. J. J. Weigle, Induction of mutations in a bacterial virus, Proc. Natl. Acad. Sci. USA, 39:628 (1953).
38. M. Radman, SOS repair hypothesis: phenomenology of an inducible DNA repair which is accompanied by mutagenesis, in: "Molecular Mechanisms for Repair of DNA," P. C. Hanawalt and R. B. Setlow, eds., p. 355, Plenum Press, New York (1975).
39. E. M. Witkin, Ultraviolet mutagenesis and inducible DNA repair in *Escherichia coli*, Bacteriol. Rev., 40:869 (1976).
40. C. D. Lytle, J. G. Goddard, and Chen-ho Lin, Repair and mutagenesis of herpes simplex virus in UV-irradiated monkey cells, Mutation Res., 70:139 (1980).
41. J. Rommelaere, J.-M. Vos, J. J. Cornelis, and D. C. Ward, UV-enhanced reactivation of minute-virus-of-mice: stimulation of a late step in the viral life cycle, Photochem. Photobiol., 33:845 (1981).
42. W. P. Jeeves and A. J. Rainbow, Gamma-Ray-enhanced reactivation of UV-irradiated adenovirus in normal human fibroblasts, Mutation Res., 60:33 (1979).
43. Luo Zu Yu, J. J. Cornelis, J.-M. Vos, and J. Rommelaere, UV-enhanced reactivation of capsid protein synthesis and infectious center formation in mouse cells infected with UV-irradiated minute-virus-of-mice, Int. J. Radiat. Biol., in press (1981).

44. J.-M. Vos, J. J. Cornelis, S. Limbosch, F. Zampetti-Bosseler, and J. Rommelaere, UV-iradiation of related mouse hybrid cells: similar increase in capacity to replicate minute-virus-of-mice but differential enhancement of survival of UV-irradiated virus, Mutation Res., in press (1981).
45. P. Tattersall, Replication of the parvovirus MVM, J. Virol., 10:586 (1972).
46. J. W. Littlefield, Three degrees of guanylic acid-inosinic acid pyrophosphorylase deficiency in mouse fibroblasts, Nature, 203: 1142 (1964).
47. J. Rommelaere and D. C. Ward, Effect of virus and cell UV-irradiation on parvovirus minute-virus-of-mice DNA replication in mouse fibroblasts, in preparation (1981).
48. P. Tattersall, L. V. Crawford, and A. J. Shatkin, Replication of the parvovirus MVM, J. Virol., 12:1446 (1973).
49. E. M. Southern, Detection of specific sequences among DNA fragments separated by gel electrophoresis, J. Mol. Biol., 98:503 (1975).
50. G. J. Bourguignon, P. J. Tattersall, and D. C. Ward, DNA of minute-virus-of-mice: self-priming, non permuted, single-stranded genome with a 5'-terminal hairpin duplex, J. Virol., 20:290 (1976).
51. M. Gunther, R. Wicker, S. Tiravy, and J. Coppey, Enhanced survival of ultraviolet-damaged parvovirus Lu III and herpes virus in carcinogen pretreated transformed human cells, in: "Chromosome Damage and Repair," E. Seeberg, ed., Plenum Press, New York (1980).
52. Zao Zhong Su, J. J. Cornelis, and J. Rommelaere, Mutagenesis of intact parvovirus H-1 is expressed co-ordinately with enhanced reactivation of ultraviolet irradiated virus in human and rat cells treated with 2-nitronaphthofurans, Carcinogenesis, 10:in press (1981).
53. A. R. Sarasin and P. C. Hanawalt, Carcinogens enhance survival of UV-irradiated Simian virus 40 in treated monkey kidney cells: induction of a recovery pathway? Proc. Natl. Acad. Sci. USA, 75:346 (1978).
54. U. Das Gupta and W. C. Summers, Ultraviolet reactivation of herpes simplex virus is mutagenic and inducible in mammalian cells, Proc. Natl. Acad. Sci. USA, 75:2378 (1978).
55. C. D. Lytle and J. G. Goddard, UV-enhanced virus reactivation in mammalian cells: effects of metabolic inhibitors, Photochem. Photobiol., 29:959 (1979).
56. P. Linser, H. Bruning, and R. W. Armentrout, Uptake of minute-virus-of-mice into cultured rodent cells, J. Virol., 31:537 (1979).
57. D. Revie, B. Y. Tseng, R. H. Grafstrom, and M. Goulian, Covalent association of protein with replicative form DNA of parvovirus H-1, Proc. Natl. Acad. Sci. USA, 76:5539 (1979).

58. W. R. Proctor, J. S. Cook, and R. W. Tennant, Ultraviolet photobiology of Kilham rat virus and the absolute ultraviolet photosensitivities of other animal viruses: influence of DNA strandedness, molecular weight and host-cell repair, Virology, 49:368 (1972).
59. E. A. Faust and D. C. Ward, Incomplete genomes of the parvovirus minute-virus-of-mice (MVM): selective conservation of the genome termini, including the origin for DNA replication, J. Virol., 32:276 (1979).
60. P. Todd, H. Dalen, and C. B. Schroy, Survival of synchronized cultured human liver cells following single and fractionated exposures to ultraviolet light, Radiat. Res., 69:573 (1977).
61. J. Rommelaere and A. Miller-Faurès, Detection by density equilibrium centrifugation of recombinant-like DNA molecules in somatic mammalian cells, J. Mol. Biol., 98:195 (1975).
62. A. R. Lehmann and S. Kirk-Bell, Pyrimidine dimer sites associated with the daughter DNA strands in UV-irradiated human fibroblasts, Photochem. Photobiol., 27:297 (1978).

ULTRAVIOLET-LIGHT-INDUCED TRANSFORMATION

OF HUMAN PRIMARY CELLS

Betsy M. Sutherland

Biology Department
Brookhaven National Laboratory
Upton, New York

INTRODUCTION

Understanding solar induction of skin cancer in man at the molecular level demands the development of experimental systems for probing this, the most frequent of all human cancers. A good model system should fulfill at least three criteria: first, the response should be light-dependent, with a low background (light-independent) response. Second, the system should be based on human cells, preferably primary skin cells from normal individuals. Third, after the oncogenic treatment, the responding cells should have properties similar to those cancers produced in man. Such systems should provide an excellent complement to the experimental UV-oncogenesis systems in rodents, which allow experimental manipulation of the intact animal but are subject to differences between rodents and humans in response to UV damage. They will also be useful in conjunction with the human epidemiological studies, which provide both prospective and predictive information on human populations, but are not amenable to experimental manipulation.

Two major problems impeded the development of such systems. First, human cells were recalcitrant to transformation by agents other than oncogenic viruses. Second, ultraviolet light had failed to produce transformation in any mammalian cultured cell, whether human or rodent.

In the mid-1970s, several systems were developed which met at least two of these criteria, Chan and Little (1976) reported a system for UV transformation of mouse C3H/10T$^{1}/_{2}$ cells. [Although note that Mondal and Heidelberger (1978) were unable to obtain transformation of the same cells by UV light unless a promoter was present.] DiPaolo and Donovan (1978) developed a system for UV transformation of Syrian hamster cells. Kakunaga (1978) obtained transformants of human cells using chemical carcinogens. Sutherland (1978) reported transformation of human diploid fibroblasts by ultraviolet light; I shall discuss the latter system below, since because it involves both human cells and ultraviolet light, and because I am most familiar with it.

The system for UV transformaton of human cells was developed from three major premises. First, most sunlight-induced human skin cancers (squamous cell and basal cell carcinomas) arise in sunlight-exposed areas in individuals with histories of chronic sunlight exposure. The experimental protocol thus subjects cultured human skin fibroblasts to multiple exposures of UV radiation. Second, in many bacterial mutagenesis experiments, it is necessary to allow growth to allow gene expression before requiring the mutagenized cells to use the new (acquired through mutation) gene product. The treated cells will therefore be allowed to grow before selection. (This requirement for growth before expression has also been found in other systems of oncogenesis.)

Third, one must choose a selection system for distinguishing transformed from nontransformed cells. Although many systems have been developed to distinguish transformed from nontransformed cells - ability to grow in low serum concentrations, loss of density-dependent growth control, etc. - the characteristic best correlated with tumorigenicity in rodent cells is the ability to grow without anchorage (Shin et al., 1975). The UV-treated cells will therefore be plated in soft agar; non-transformed cells will not grow, while cells transformed to anchorage-independent growth will develop into clones or colonies ranging from about one hundred to several thousand cells. In developing any system, one must consider the type of cell to use as a basis for the assay. This system was originally developed with human embryonic skin and muscle fibroblasts (HESMs), which grew rapidly (generation time about 24 h), were available commercially, and were supplied as primary cells. Recently, the transformation system has been extended for use on other mammalian cells; differences and similarities among the various cells types will be discussed below.

THE UV TRANSFORMATION SYSTEM

I shall first describe the experimental protocol for induction of transformation of human cells to anchorage-independent growth. I shall then discuss factors affecting transformation frequencies, and shall describe properties of the transformants. Finally I shall briefly note results obtained with other mammalian cells, and shall describe a use of the system in probing human health hazards.

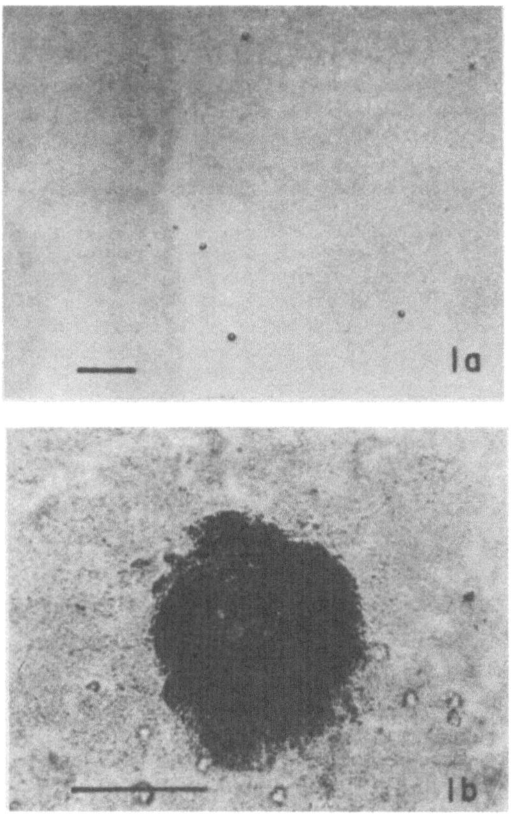

Fig. 1. a) Unirradiated HESM cells 14 days after plating in soft agar b) anchorage-independent clone arising from UV-irradiated HESM cells, 14 days after plating in soft agar. Bar, 0.2 mm. Photograph taken from Sutherland et al. (1980) Cancer Res., 40:1934, with permission of the authors and publisher.

Protocol for UV Transformation

This procedure is described in detail in Sutherland et al. (1980). Early passage, rapidly growing cells are maintained in a Dulbecco's modified Eagle's medium containing 20% fetal bovine serum (Sutherland and Oliver, 1976) and tested before each experiment for mycoplasma. Cells are seeded into 60 mm dishes at densities ranging from (1-3) $\times 10^5$ cells/dish. (All cell handling is performed under yellow fluorescent room lights, with no additional lighting in the sterile hood.) From the first irradiation till the end of the experiment, all cell handling (including opening of the incubator) is done only in red fluorescent light ($\lambda > 600$ nm). After

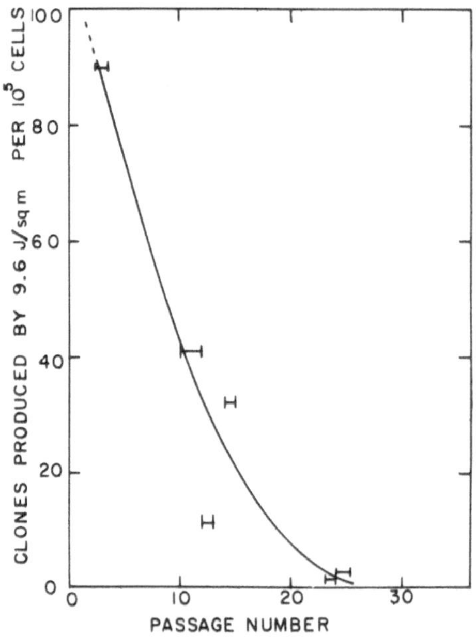

Fig. 2. Production of anchorage-independent clones by 9.6 J/m^2 of 254 nm radiation as a function of cell passage number. The length of the horizontal bars represents the span of passages for cells used in an individual experiment. Data taken from Sutherland et al. (1980), Cancer Res., 40:1934, with permission of the authors and publisher.

overnight growth of the cells, the medium is removed from the cells, they are washed twice with 1-ml portions of phosphate buffered saline (PBS), and 1 ml PBS is layered over the cells. They are exposed to ultraviolet radiation, the PBS is removed and fresh medium placed over the cells. After 24 and 48 h growth, the cells are washed, irradiated and fed. (Thus, each radiation treatment contains one-third of the total UV exposure.) After the last treatment, cells are allowed to grow for five days. The cells are detached from the dishes by trypsin treatment, counted, and 10^5 cells are placed in a 3-ml layer of 0.33% agar over a 10 ml base of 0.5% (MacPherson, 1973). After the upper agar layer has solidified, the dishes are scored for cell clumps (which might grow into aggregates resembling transformed clones). The cells are fed once every 3.4 days with 0.5 ml medium to prevent drying of the agar layers. After 14 days' growth, the dishes are counted for clones not previously marked as the sites of clumps. Figure 1a shows the appearance of unirradiated HESM cells 14 days after plating in soft agar and Fig. 1b shows an anchorage-independent clone from UV-irradiated cells (also photographed 14 days after plating).

Factors Affecting the Transformation Frequency

We have explored four major factors which affect the frequency of transformation to anchorage-independent growth of the HESM cells. The first factor is UV dose. Sutherland et al. (1980) showed that in dose-ranges where there was >95% viability, the number of transformants increased with increasing UV dose. They found, however, that although the shapes of the dose-response curves were similar from experiment to experiment, the absolute number varied from 2 to 80 transformants per 10^5 cells produced by 10 J/m^2 of 254 nm radiation. They showed that this variation reflected the passage number of the cells: low passage (in the sense of population doubling) cells gave high transformation rates, while the rate of transformation decreased sharply with increasing passage number. Figure 2 shows that HESM cells of greater than passage 15 gave many fewer transformants; it is therefore of great advantage with these cells to obtain cells at the earliest passage possible.

The frequency of transformation also depends on the wavelength of the UV. This provides a powerful tool for determining the cellular target for absorption of the transforming photon: if wavelengths absorbed by nucleic acids are most efficient in producing transformation, one has evidence for the role of DNA in UV light absorption in the cell. If, on the other hand, the most efficient wavelengths are in the 280 nm region (where most proteins absorb strongly because of their tryptophan content) it would be likely that absorption by aromatic amino acids in proteins was important in the transformation process. Jagger (1967) has outlined several criteria which must be met for the establishment of valid action spectra from dose-response data at different wavelengths. First, reciprocity of time and dose must hold. Second, the dose-response curves at the different wavelengths must be similar, indicating the existence of a common molecular process underlying the observed biological effect. Sutherland et al. (1981) found that the reciprocity of time and dose held in the HESM system, and that the dose-response curves at the various wavelengths (248, 265, 270, 280, 289, and 297 nm) were similar. These data allowed them to compute an action spectrum (shown as the solid symbols in Fig. 3; the filled triangles show the reciprocals of photon fluences required to produce 150 transformants per 10^6 cells, and the filled circles those for the production of 75 transformants/10^6 cells). These action spectra are compared with data of Kantor et al. (1980) for killing of human fibroblasts, shown as open circles, and of Rothman and Setlow (1978), shown as the open triangles, for formation of pyrimidine dimers in isolated V-79 hamster DNA. All these spectra have maxima at 265 nm, and do not provide evidence for absorbing moieties other than nucleic acids. Recently action spectra for transformation and pyrimidine dimer formation in the Syrian hamster embryo system were reported to have a rather sharp maximum at 270 nm (Doniger et al., 1981). The sharpness of this peak is rather sur-

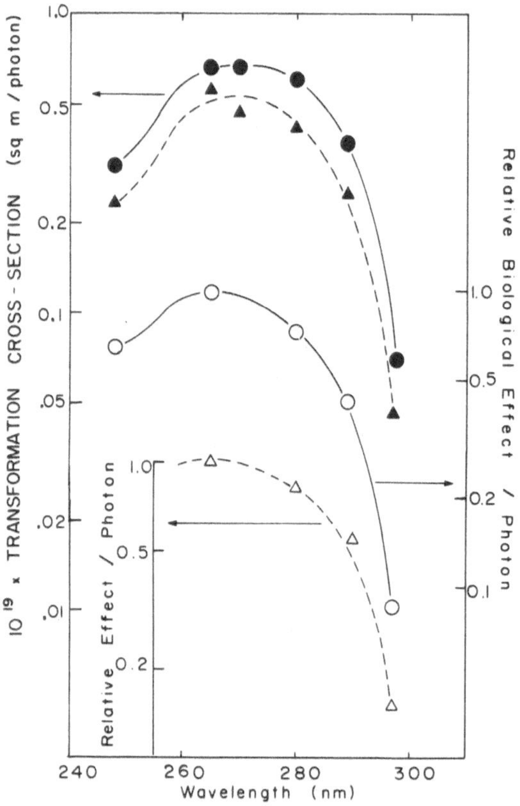

Fig. 3. Action spectra of transformation to anchorage-independent growth (solid symbols), killing of human fibroblasts (open circles; Kantor et al., 1980; and pyrimidine dimer formation in V79 cells (open triangles; Rothman and Setlow, 1978). The upper curve (filled circles) represents the reciprocals of photon fluences required to produce 75 transformants per 10^6 viable cells, and the solid triangles those for the production of 150 transformants per 10^6 cells. Data taken from Sutherland et al. (1981), Cancer Res., 41:2211, with permission of the authors and publisher.

prising, since the absorption spectra of biological molecules are broad in this wavelength range. The possibility of an instrumental artifact should be excluded [since a similar sharp peak at 270 nm was obtained in an action spectrum for cell killing and mutagenesis in mouse cells by Jacobson et al. (1981) using the same monochromator and dosimetry apparatus] before the molecular cause of this peak be sought.

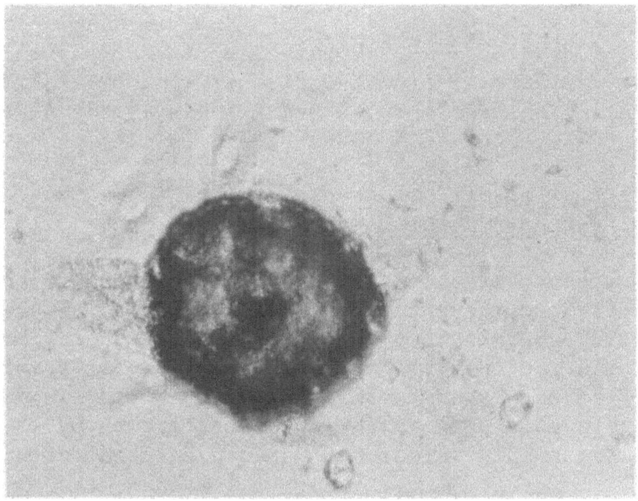

Fig. 4. Anchorage-independent clone removed from soft agar, shown with cells growing from the clone attached to a plastic surface. Bar is 0.2 mm.

A further modification of the transformation rate results from repair processes. One repair process, photoreactivation, results in the light-dependent, enzyme-mediated reversal of cyclobutyl pyrimidine dimers in DNA. Sutherland et al. (1980) found that exposure of UV-irradiated HESM cells to photoreactivating light immediately after each UV treatment resulted in the reduction of the yield of transformants. As a light-mediated process, photoreactivation has a strong wavelength dependence; the action spectrum for photoreactivation of dimers in human cells, and for dimer photoreactivation by isolated human enzyme in vitro shows a broad maximum at 400 nm, and extends to shorter wavelengths of about 310 nm, and to wavelengths as long as 577 nm (Sutherland and Sutherland, 1975). If the photoreversal observed by Sutherland et al. (1980) results from true photoenzymatic repair, its action spectrum should resemble that for action by the enzyme. This identification will allow direct assessment of the role of pyrimidine dimers, the only known substrate for the photoreactivating enzyme, in UV transformation.

Repair processes may also be responsible for the differences in the UV dose-response curves seen in the various rodent transformation systems and in human system. At low doses, DiPaolo and Donovan (1978) and Doniger et al. (1981) found a linear UV dose-transformation relation in the Syrian hamster system, and Chan and Little (1976) also reported a linear dose-response relationship in the mouse embryo C3H/10T$^1/_2$ system. However, the data of Sutherland et al.

(1980, 1981) can not be adequately represented by a straight line, showing a paucity of transformants at very low doses. Since rodent cells in culture undergo much slower excision repair than do human cells (Regan and Setlow, 1973), the paucity of human transformants at low UV doses may result from repair by excision of lesions in the normal human, but not in the rodent cells.

Characterization of the Transformants to Anchorage-Independent Growth

Before one can characterize the transformed cells, one must be able to grow sufficient quantities of each clone for study. On the human cell system, development of suitable conditions (choice of serum lot, quantity of medium, isolation conditions) required some year's work. Figure 4 shows cells growing on a plastic surface from a clone transformed to anchorage-independent growth by UV-treatment. These cells grow rapidly in culture and can be used for characterizations.

The first characteristics which must be determined for each strains are those which mark its integrity of origin and freedom from contamination. The HESM transformants cultures are first checked for mycoplasa contamination [MacPherson (1973) notes that mycoplasma contamination can lead to increased frequency of growth in soft agar] and maintained in antibiotic-free medium to allow immediate detection of bacterial or fungal contamination. The species of origin is checked by analysis of isozymes of lactate dehydrogenase (Shannon and Macy, 1973), which are distinct and quite different among the human and rodent cells in our laboratory (Sutherland et al., 1980). The karyotype is determined to insure against contamination with other human cell lines, for example, HeLa (HeLa cells are not permitted to be grown in our laboratory).

After ascertaining the integrity of the cultures of transformants, one can begin to characterize the cells. In the case of the human UV-induced transformants to anchorage-independent growth, transformation, the variation from one clone to another precludes characterization of "the" transformant, but instead requires description of a full range of cell types. The transformant clones differ in ability to attach to plastic surface (even under apparently optimal conditions), growth rate of the cultures as anchored cells growing on a plastic surface, and in ability to grow in soft agar (Sutherland et al., 1980). One clone was found to be non-tumorigenic when injected into immune deficient mice (the mice dies 3-4 months after cell injection, presumably of other causes). Other clones from this system must be evaluated before a valid assessment of their tumorigenic potential can be made.

The UV Transformation System Using Other Mammalian Cells

The recent unavailability of HESMs from their commerical supplier has led us to test other mammalian cells in our UV-transformation system. We examined the UV-transformability of several strains of mouse 3T3 cells; like Withrow et al. (1980) who used single dose irradiation schedules - we obtained transformation to anchorage independent growth. However, we, like Withrow, found high background (anchorage independent clones appearing in unirradiated samples); for example, a maximum number of 30 clones/10^5 viable cells might be produced with 254 nm exposure over a background of 10 per 10^6. This contrasts strongly with the HESM system, in which the irradiated samples might contain 80/10^5 viable cells, while the unirradiated cell contained <1/10^6-10^7 cells. We have now developed a system using neonatal foreskin fibroblasts cells; this system has only a slightly higher backgroun ($\sim$ 1 per 10^6 cells) and a good transformation rate ($\sim$ 30 per 10^6 cells). The first results using this system are described in the following section.

Transformation by Sunlamp Exposure in the Presence of Para-amino Benzoic Acid

Para-amino benzoic acid (paba) is the parent compound upon which many sunscreen preparations are based. This compound is similar in structure and energy levels to many compounds which sensitize pyrimidine dimer formation in DNA by wavelengths not absorbed by the DNA itself (Lamola, 1966; Sutherland and Griffin, 1981). Hodges et al. (1977) showed that paba-and-UV light induced damage in *E. coli* was photoreactivable, implying the formation of pyrimidine dimers. We thus examined the effects of sunlamp exposure on neonatal foreskin fibroblasts with any and without 0.2% in the overlying PBS. The sunlamp alone was inefficient in producing transformation; 19 sec. of FS40 sunlamp exposure produced only 0.7 ± 0.3 transformant per cells. We showed that even this low rate of transformation resulted from the shorter wavelengths (less than about 310 nm) present in the sunlamp by interposing a thin mylar film between the cells and the sunlamp to exclude the shorter wavelength. At the range of doses we used, the filtered sunlamp produced no transformants to anchorage-independent growth. In the presence of paba, the number of transformants increased by a factor of $\sim$10. These results are compatible with those of K. Griffin and J. C. Sutherland (1981), who found that paba + 313 nm light produced dimers in DNA, and was mutagenic to Salmonella tested in the Ames system. They are also compatible with the data of R. Daynes (personal communication) who showed that although paba reduced skin thickening and abnormal pigmentation induced by UV in mice, it did not affect the rate of UV-induced tumor formation in the mice.

These *in vitro* systems offer great promise for probing and understanding damage to human cells at the molecular level. They should complement both the systems for experimental oncogenesis in rodents and the human epidemiological studies. Development of these systems to provide a fuller understanding of their potential and limitations, strengths, and blind spots, will allow a more accurate assessment of their adaptability to detection of potential carcinogens.

REFERENCES

Chan, G. L., and Little, J. B., Induction of oncogenic transformation in vitro by ultraviolet light, Nature, 264:442 (1976).

DiPaolo, J. A., and Donovan, P. J., Transformation frequency of Syrian golden hamster cells and its modulation by ultraviolet irradiation, in: "International Conference on Ultraviolet Carcinogenesis," M. L. Kripke, E. R. Sass, eds., National Cancer Institute Monograph 50, U.S. Government Printing Office, Washington, D.C. (1978).

Doniger, J., Jacobson, E. D., Krell, K., and DiPaolo, J. A., Ultraviolet light action spectra for neoplastic transformaton and lethality of Syrian hamster embryo cells correlate with spectrum for pyrimidine dimer formation in cellular DNA, Proc. Natl. Acad. Sci. USA, 78:2378 (1981).

Griffin, K. P., and Sutherland, J. C., Sensitized formation of cyclobutyl pyrimidine dimers in DNA in vitro, Abstracts, Am. Soc. for Photobiol., 9th Ann. Meeting, Williamsburg, Virginia (1981).

Hodges, N. D. M., Moss, S. H., and Davies, D. J. G., The sensitizing effect of a sunscreening agent, p-amino benzoic acid, and near UV induced damage in repair deficient strain of Escherichia coli, Photochem. Photobiol., 26:493 (1977).

Jacobson, E. D., Krell, K., and Dempsey, M. J., The wavelength dependence of ultraviolet light-induced cell killing and mutagenesis in L5178Y mouse lymphoma cells, Photochem. Photobiol., 33:257 (1981).

Jagger, J., Introduction to research in ultraviolet photobiology, Prentice-Hall, Englewood Cliffs, New Jersey (1967).

Kakunaga, T., Neoplastic transformation of human diploid fibroblasts cells by chemical carcinogens, Proc. Natl. Acad. Sci. USA, 75: 1334 (1978).

Kantor, G. J., Sutherland, J. C., and Setlow, R. B., Action spectra for killing nondividing normal human and xeroderma pigmentosum cells, Photochem. Photobiol., 31:459 (1980).

Lamola, A. A., Specific formation of thymine dimers in DNA, Photochem. Photobiol., 9:291 (1966).

MacPherson, I., Soft Agar Techniques, in: "Tissue Culture," P. F. Kruse and M. K. Patterson, eds., Academic Press, New York (1973).

Mondal, S., and Heidelberger, C., Ultraviolet light in the oncogenic transformation of cultured C3H/10T$^1/_2$ mouse embryo cells, in: "International conference on ultraviolet carcinogenesis, M. L. Kripke and E. R. Sass, eds., National Cancer Institute Monograph 50, U.S. Government Printing Office, Washington, D.C. (1978).

Regan, J. D., and Setlow, R. B., Repair of chemical damage to human DNA, in: "Chemical mutagens, principles, and methods for their detection," A. Hollaender, ed., Vol. 3, Plenum Press, New York (1973).

Rothman, R. H., and Setlow, R. B., An action spectrum for cell killing and pyrimidine dimer formation in Chinese hamster V-79 cells, Photochem. Photobiol., 29:57 (1978).

Shannon, J. E., and Macy, M. L., Enzymatic Fingerprinting, in: "Tissue culture, methods, and application," P. F. Kruse and M. K. Patterson, Jr. (1973).

Shin, S. I., Freedman, V. H., Risser, R., and Pollack, R., Tumorigenicity of virus-transformed cells in nude mice is correlated specifically with anchorage independent growth in vitro, Proc. Natl. Acad. Sci. USA, 72:4435 (1975).

Sutherland, B. M., Photoreactivation: Evaluating the role of pyrimidine dimers in UV-induced cell transformation, in: "International Conference on Ultraviolet Carcinogenesis," M. L. Kripke, E. R. Sass, eds., National Cancer Institute Monograph 50, DHEW, Publication No. (NIH) 78-1532 (1978).

Sutherland, B. M., Cimino, J. S., Delihas, N., Shih, A., and Oliver, R. P., Ultraviolet light-induced transformation of human cells to anchorage-independent growth, Cancer Res., 40:1934 (1980).

Sutherland, B. M., Delihas, N. C., Oliver, R. P., Sutherland, J. C., Action spectra for ultraviolet light-induced transformation of human cells to anchorage-independent growth, Cancer Res., 41: 2211 (1981).

Sutherland, B. M., and Oliver R., Culture conditions affect photoreactivating enzyme levels in human fibroblasts, Biochem. Biophys. Acta, 442:358 (1976).

Sutherland, J. C., and Sutherland, B. M., Human photoreactivating enzyme: action spectrum and safelight conditions, Biophys. J., 15:435 (1975).

Withrow, T. J., Lugo, M. H., and Dempsey, M. J., Transformation of BALB 3T3 cells exposed to a germicidal UV lamp and a sunlamp, Photochem. Photobiol., 31:135 (1980).

USE OF HUMAN LYMPHOBLASTOID CELL LINES TO DETERMINE CELLULAR HYPERSENSITIVITY TO PHYSICAL AND CHEMICAL AGENTS

Kenneth H. Kraemer

Laboratory of Molecular Carcinogenesis
National Cancer Institute
Bethesda, Maryland 20205

INTRODUCTION

During the past decade, human lymphoblastoid cell lines have become recognized as providing a convenient source of material for studies of human genetic diseases [1-7]. Lymphocytes may be transformed with Epstein-Barr (EB) virus to produce immortal cell lines [8-10]. They are termed lymphoblastoid because of their morphological similarities to the immature lymphocytes called lymphoblasts.

USE OF LYMPHOBLASTOID CELL LINES

Table 1 lists some of the advantages and disadvantages of lymphoblastoid cell lines for use in laboratory studies. Using EB virus for transformation only a small volume of blood, usually less than 10 ml is commonly sufficient to establish a line, making the procedure usable for children as well as adults [8, 9].

The lymphoblastoid cell lines appear to be immortal in that they can be passed (subcultured) indefinitely. They thus avoid the problems of senescence found in fibroblast cultures. Further, passing the lymphoblastoid cell lines does not involve trypsinization which is time consuming and may alter cell properties.

Lymphoblastoid cell lines may be grown rapidly in suspension culture in RPMI 1640 medium supplemented with 10-20% fetal calf serum. They grow exponentially to a plateau concentration of 1-3 × 10^6 cells/ml with a doubling time of 15-30 h. Refeeding may be easily accomplished by removing a portion of the culture and adding fresh medium.

Table 1. Advantages and Disadvantages of Human Lymphoblastoid Cell Lines for Laboratory Investigations

A. Advantages
- Small volume of blood to initiate line
- Immortal
- Suspension culture
- Rapid doubling time
- High concentration
- Suitable for cellular and biochemical studies
- Retain characteristic sensitivities

B. Disadvantages
- Theoretical EB virus risk to workers
- Cells from some patients difficult to transform
- Possible alteration of cellular properties due to transformation or to presence of viral antigens

Large numbers of lymphoblastoid cells are much easier to obtain for biochemical studies than are adherent fibroblasts. Most established lines are B lymphocytes and may produce antibodies. Lymphoblastoid lines retain many of the characteristic genetic hypersensitivities found in fibroblasts or lymphocytes [1-7].

The disadvantages of the lymphoblastoid cell lines mainly relate to the presence of EB virus. This virus has been associated with infectious mononucleosis, African Burkett's lymphoma and nasopharyngeal carcinoma [11]. The transformed cells express certain viral antigens but typically do not produce infectious virus. Low levels of infectious virus have been induced by treatment of lymphoblastoid cells with agents such as bromodeoxyuridine [12, 13] or TPA [14]. Thus these cells should be handled carefully using conditions appropriate for low risk oncogenic viruses including vertical laminar flow hoods, gloves, mechanical pipettes and decontamination of all waste material. We routinely inactivate liquid waste with povodine iodine (Wescodyne), autoclave all disposable waste and decontminate reusable materials such as hemocytometers with dilute sodium hypochlorite, soap and 95% ethanol.

A proportion of adults have serum antibodies to EB virus indicating that they probably had clinical infectious mononucleosis or sub-clinical exposure to EB virus [11]. These people are presumably immune to re-infection with EB virus. Those laboratory workers without EB virus serum antibodies are followed with periodic antibody testing. However, I am not aware of any EB virus infection of laboratory workers which has been shown to be caused by exposure to lymphoblastoid cell lines.

Table 2. Tests of Cellular Sensitivity to Physical or Chemical Agents Using Human Lymphoblastoid Cell Lines

A.	Intact cell function
	Growth rate
	Colony forming ability
	DNA synthesis
	Viral host cell reactivation
	Mutagenesis
B.	Chromosomal integrity
	Chromosome breakage
	Sister chromatid exchanges
C.	DNA repair

Cellular properties may be altered by the viral transformation. SV_{40} viral transformation has been shown to alter the ability of some fibroblast strains to remove alkylation damage to DNA [15]. Similar alterations may be induced by EB virus transformation of lymphocytes [7].

Many measurements of cellular sensitivity to physical or chemical agents can be assayed with lymphoblastoid cell lines (Table 2).

The remainder of the paper will describe two of the assays used to test intact cell function: growth rate and colony forming ability using examples from human diseases. Descriptions of other assays may be found in the following references: DNA synthesis, and DNA repair in reference 16; viral host cell reactivation in reference 2; mutagenesis in reference 17; and chromosomal integrity in the sections by P. Perry and by M. Taylor in this book.

TESTS OF INTACT CELL FUNCTION

Tests of intact cell function generally are used to determine if any cellular defect is present without pinpointing the site of the defect. One of the simplest and most useful tests is the determination of the growth rate in mass culture following treatment with the damaging agent [1, 6, 18-21]. The change in total cell concentration may be assessed by use of a Coulter counter. A somewhat more sensitive assessment may be made by hemocytometer counts of the concentration of cells that exclude the vital dye, trypan blue. This viable cell count changes more rapidly than the total cell count after agents such as ultraviolet radiation that generally do not lyse the cells.

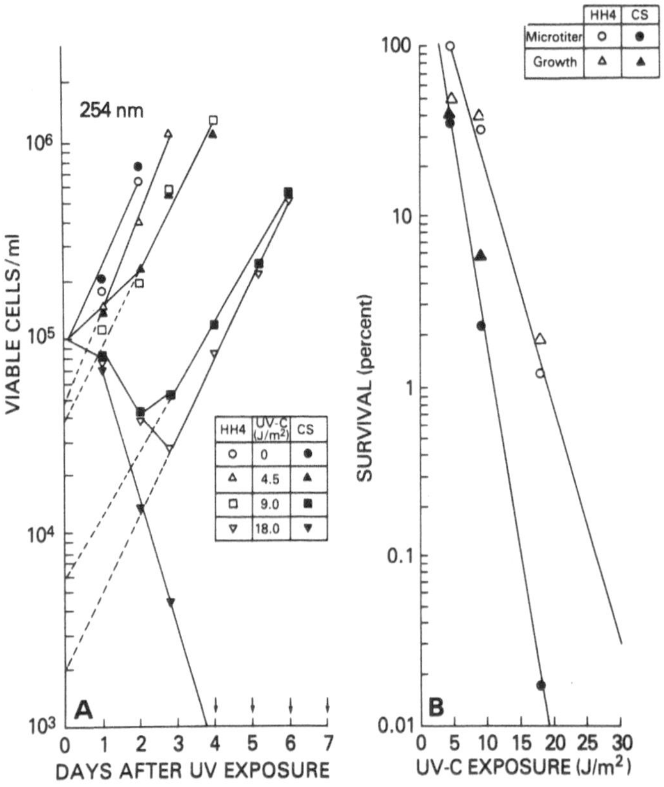

Fig. 1. Survival of normal and Cockayne syndrome lymphoblastoid cell lines after treatment with 254 nm ultraviolet radiation (UV-C). A) Growth curve assay. B) Microtiter well assay and extrapolation results from growth curve assay.

An example demonstrating ultraviolet hypersensitivity of a Cockayne syndrome (CS) lymphoblastoid cell line (GM 2964) [22] is shown in Fig. 1A. Daily hemocytometer counts of the viable cell concentration of the untreated CS cells showed a similar growth rate to that of the normal lymphoblastoid cell line (HH4). Exposure to 254 nm ultraviolet radiation (UV-C) diminished the rate of growth in both cell lines but the effect was more marked in the CS line. These growth curves generally have one of 3 shapes [19]: 1) exponential increase from day zero (untreated cells); 2) lag or fall for several days followed by exponential increase (cells treated with 4.5 or 9.0 J/m^2); or 3) inexorable fall without increase until no viable cells are found (treatment of CS cells with 18 J/m^2). Inspection of Fig. 1A reveals that there was much more growth inhibition in the CS line than in the normal line after UV treatment.

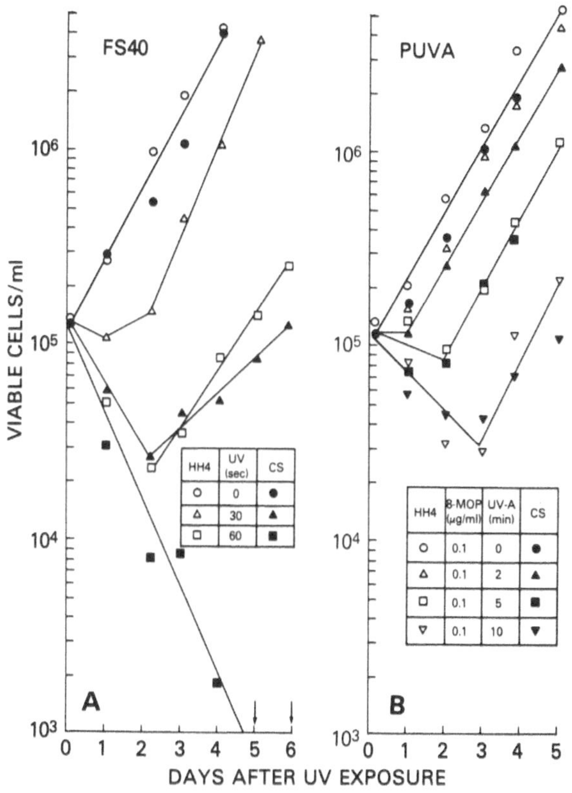

Fig. 2. Survival of normal and Cockayne syndrome lymphoblastoid cell lines after treatment with fluorescent sunlamp or 8-methoxypsoralen plus ultraviolet radiation (PUVA). A) Growth curves after treatment with sunlamp (UV-B). B) Growth curves after treatment with 8-MOP plus long wavelength ultraviolet radiation (UV-A).

Data from growth curves may be quantified by comparing the ratio of cell concentrations of treated and untreated test cells at a uniform time after treatment [5, 6]. An alternative method of analysis involves back-extrapolation of the exponential portion of the growth curve to day zero (as shown in Fig. 1A) [18]. The ratio of the intercept of the treated cells to the intercept of the untreated cells is the surviving fraction. These values for the experiment shown in Fig. 1A are plotted in Fig. 1B as triangles so they form survival curves as a function of UV-C exposure for the normal and the CS line. It is apparent that lymphoblastoid cell survival decreases exponentially with increasing UV exposure. Further, the CS cells are more sensitive to UV-C than the normal cells.

Figure 2A shows the results of a similar experiment comparing survival of the CS line after treatment with a fluorescent sunlamp (predominantly 313 nm ultraviolet radiation, UV-B). There is a greater inhibition of cell growth in the CS cells than with the normal line (HH4).

In contrast, Fig. 2B shows the effect of treatment of these same cell lines with 8-methoxypsoralen (8-MOP) followed by exposure to long wavelength (predominantly 360 nm ultraviolet radiation, UV-A). This treatment results in photo-dependent covalent binding of 8-MOP to DNA forming monoadducts and interstrand crosslinks [19, 20, 21]. Figure 2B shows that the CS line had a similar response to the normal line after 8-MOP plus UV-A. Taken together, Figs. 1 and 2 show that the CS line is hypersensitive UV-C and UV-B but has normal sensitivity to inhibition of growth by 8-MOP plus UV-A.

Another method of assessing lymphoblastoid cell line survival involves analysis of the efficiency of cells to initiate microcultures in microtiter wells [18]. Sterile plastic trays with 96 wells in a rectangular grid array are commercially available. In the microtiter well survival assay 0.2 ml of culture medium containing different dilutions of cells is innoculated into a series of wells (for example: 20 wells each with 20 cells per well, 6.6 cells per well, and 2 cells per well). After 1-3 weeks incubation the wells are scored under the microscope for evidence of cell proliferation. Microculture initiative efficiency, S, is calculated from the Poisson formula:

$$S = (-\ln P_0)/n$$

where P_0 is the experimentally determined fraction of negative wells and n is the mean number of cells innoculated per well. The surviving fraction is obtained by dividing the S of the treated cells by the S of the untreated control cells in an experiment.

Survival of cells treated with 254 nm ultraviolet radiation from the experiment shown in Fig. 1A was also measured with the microtiter well assay. The results are plotted as circles in Fig. 1B. By this assay also the CS line is hypersensitive to ultraviolet killing. Figure 1B also shows that similar results are obtained by survival measurements with the microtiter well assay and with the growth curve extrapolation assay.

Table 3 lists several human genetic diseases where abnormalities have been manifested in lymphoblastoid cell lines. Establishment of lymphoblastoid cell lines from patients suspected as having these disorders and performing the appropriate test may be of assistance in clinical diagnosis. On the other hand, human lymphoblastoid cell lines with defined hypersensitivity may serve as indicator cells,

Table 3. Human Genetic Diseases with Abnormalities Manifested in Lymphoblastoid Cell Lines*

Disease	Cellular abnormality	Reference
Xeroderma pigmentosum	Ultraviolet hypersensitivity	1-3, 6
Ataxia telangiectasia	X-Ray hypersensitivity	3, 4
Cockayne's syndrome	Ultraviolet hypersensitivity	3
Fanconi's anemia	DNA crosslink hypersensitivity (some lines)	3
Bloom's syndrome	Increased spontaneous sister chromatid exchanges (some lines)	3
Huntington's disease	X-Ray hypersensitivity	5

*Lymphoblastoid cell lines frm patients with many genetic disorders are available to qualified laboratories from the Human Genetic Mutant Cell Repository at the Institute for Medical Research, Copewood and Davis Streets, Camden, New Jersey 08103, U.S.A.

analogous to the Ames bacterial tester strains, for the assessment of risk from physical or chemical agents. In this regard, the end point analysis of the microtiter well assay can be automated for processing of large numbers of samples [18].

SUMMARY

Human lymphoblastoid cell lines, obtained by EB virus transformation of peripheral blood lymphocytes, are a convenient source of cells from patients with genetic diseases. These immortal lines grow to high density in suspension culture, rapidly producing large numbers of cells for biological or biochemical studies. Cell survival may be assessed by growth in mass culture or in microtiter wells. Lymphoblastoid cell lines retain many of the characteristic cellular hypersensitivities seen in fibroblasts from patients with gnetic diseases such as xeroderma pigmentosum, Cockayne's syndrome, and ataxia telangiectasia. Lymphoblastoid cell lines may be useful to clinical diagnosis or as indicator cells in risk assessment.

ACKNOWLEDGMENT

The author wishes to acknowledge the excellent technical assistance of Mr. H. Waters, Mr. D. Whyte, and Ms. M. Jones in the performance of the survival assays.

REFERENCES

1. A. D. Andrews, J. H. Robbins, K. H. Kraemer, and D. N. Buell, Xeroderma pigmentosum long-term lymphoid lines with increased ultraviolet sensitivity, J. Natl. Cancer Inst., 53:691-693 (1974).
2. E. E. Henderson, Host cell reactivation of Epstein-Barr virus in normal and repair-defective leukocytes, Cancer Res., 38: 3256-3263 (1978).
3. E. E. Henderson and R. Ribecky, DNA repair in lymphoblastoid cell lines established from human genetic disorders, Chem. Biol. Interactions, 33:63-81 (1980).
4. P. H. Kohn, K. H. Kraemer, and J. K. Buchanan, Influence of ataxia telangiectasia gene dosage on bleomycin-induced chromosome breakage and replication inhibition in human lymphoblastoid cell lines, Exp. Cell Res. (in press).
5. A. N. Moshell, R. E. Tarone, S. F. Barrett, and J. H. Robbins, Radiosensitivity in Huntington's disease: Implications for pathogenesis and presymptomatic diagnosis, Lancet, i:9-11 (1980).
6. A. N. Moshell, R. E. Tarone, S. A. Newfield, A. D. Andrews, and J. H. Robbins, A simple and rapid method for evaluating the survival of xeroderma pigmentosum lymphoid lines after irradiation with ultraviolet light, In vitro, 17:299-307 (1981).
7. M. Altamirano-Dimas, R. Sklar, and B. Strauss, Selectivity of the excision of alkylation products in a xeroderma pigmentosum-derived lymphoblastoid line, Mutat. Res., 60:197-206 (1979).
8. E. Henderson, G. Miller, J. Robinson, and L. Heston, Efficiency of transformation of lymphocytes by Epstein-Barr virus, Virology, 76:152-163 (1977).
9. H. Tohda, A. Oikawa, T. Kudo, and T. Tachibana, A greatly simplified method of estabishing B-lymphoblastoid cell lines, Cancer Res., 38:3560-3562 (1978).
10. E. E. Henderson and R. Ribecky, Transformation of human leukocytes with Epstein-Barr virus after cellular exposure to chemical or physical mutagens, J. Natl. Cancer Inst., 64:33-39 (1980).
11. J. L. Ziegler, I. T. Magrath, P. Gerber, and P. H. Levine, Epstein-Barr virus and human malignancy, Ann. Internal Med., 86:323-336 (1977).
12. B. Hampar, J. G. Derge, L. M. Martos, and J. L. Walker, Synthesis of Epstein-Barr virus after activation if the viral genome in a "virus-negative" human lymphoblastoid cell (Raji) made resistant to 5-bromodeoxyuridine, Proc. Natl. Acad. Sci., 69:78-82 (1972).

13. P. Gerber, Activation of Epstein-Barr virus by 5-bromodeoxyuridine in "virus-free" human cells, Proc. Natl. Acad. Sci., 69:83-85 (1972).
14. N. Yamamoto and H. zurHausen, Tumor promoter TPA enhances transformation of human leukocytes by Epstein-Barr virus, Nature, 280:244-245 (1979).
15. R. S. Day, C. H. J. Zoilkowski, D. A. Scudiero, S. A. Meyer, A. S. Lubiniecki, A. J. Girardi, S. M. Galloway, and G. D. Bynum, Defective repair of alkylated DNA by human tumor and SV40-transformed human cell strains, Nature, 288:724-727 (1980).
16. E. C. Friedberg and P. C. Hanawalt, eds., "DNA Repair: A Laboratory Manual of Research Procedures, Vol. 1," Marcel Dekker, New York (1981).
17. W. G. Thilly, J. G. DeLuca, E. E. Furth, H. H. Hoppe, IV, D. A. Kaden, J. J. Krolewski, H. L. Liber, T. R. Skopek, S. A. Slapikoff, R. J. Tizard, and B. W. Penman, Gene-locus mutation assays in diploid human lymphoblast lines, in: "Chemical Mutagens, Vol. 6," F. J. de Serres and A. Hollaender, eds., Plenum Press, New York (1980), pp. 331-364.
18. K. H. Kraemer, H. L. Waters, and J. K. Buchanan, Survival of human lymphoblastoid cells after DNA damage measured by growth in microtiter wells, Mutat. Res., 72:285-294 (1980).
19. K. H. Kraemer, H. L. Waters, O. L. Ellingson, and R. E. Tarone, Psoralen plus ultraviolet radiation-induced inhibition of DNA synthesis and viability in human lymphoid cells in vitro, Photochem. Photobiol., 30:263-270 (1979).
20. L. F. Cohen, K. H. Kraemer, H. L. Waters, K. W. Kohn, and D. L. Glaubiger, DNA crosslinking and cell survival in human lymphoid cells treated with 8-methoxypsoralen and long wavelength ultraviolet radiation, Mutat. Res., 80:347-356 (1981).
21. K. H. Kraemer, H. W. Waters, L. F. Cohen, N. C. Popescu, S. C. Amsbaugh, J. A. DiPaolo, D. L. Glaubiger, O. A. Ellingson, and R. E. Tarone, Effects of 8-methoxypsoralen and ultraviolet radiation on human lymphoid cells in vitro, J. Invest. Dermatol., 76:80-87 (1981).
22. R. M. Kennedy, V. D. Rowe, J. J. Kepes, Cockayne syndrome: An atypical case, Neurology, 30:1268-1272 (1980).

CELLULAR STUDIES ON PATIENTS WITH AN UNUSUAL CLINICAL SENSITIVITY TO IONIZING RADIATION

A. M. R. Taylor

Department of Cancer Studies
The Medical School
Birmingham, B15 2TJ
England

There are people in the population who show an unusual sensitivity to ionizing radiation compared with normal individuals. This effect has been demonstrated in the course of bona fide radiotherapy for malignant conditions in these patients with the result proving either lethal to the patient or subsequently giving rise to tumors in the irradiated field. These individuals are members of a small group with inherited disorders showing a predisposition to malignant disease. Although some attempts have been made to study the variation in radiosensitivity in normal members of the population (Weichselbaum et al., 1976) most work has been done on the inherited disorders. The underlying causes of the different responses to radiation are at present not understood, but it seems likely that more than a single factor is important. In ataxia telangiectasia, for example, particular tumor types are associated with radiation sensitivity in these patients. This suggests that particular cell types or differentiation states are more susceptible to the consequences of the possible repair deficiency in these patients.

There is some controversy over the numbers of inherited disorders which demonstrate a truly increased radiosensitivity compared with normal.

The usefulness of cells derived from these patients in the assessment of risk from physical and chemical agents to the general population is probably quite limited although of course the patients may themselves benefit from such an assessment of risk to their own cells. One only has to consider the wide range of cytotoxic drugs plus radiation used in the treatment of malignant disease or for example in the preparation of bone marrow transplantation.

Differential Radiosensitivity between Different Groups of Individuals with an Increased Susceptibility to Cancer

Cancer susceptibility is associated in different syndromes with a wide range of defects including immune deficiency, chromosomal defects, DNA repair deficiency and loss of host growth control. Some syndromes have no other associated feature other than the tumor susceptibility. In one such disorder, retinoblastoma, there have been suggestions of an unusual radiosensitivity.

i. Retinoblastoma

Retinoblastoma is a tumor seen only in children and is a malignant tumor of the immature retinocyte. Susceptibility to the tumor is inherited as an autosomal dominant gene, and almost half the cases are familial, although half are also sporadic.

There is some evidence for an unusual radiosensitivity. Strong (1977) suggests that the number of radiation induced sarcomas of the orbit is greater in these patients than would be expected for a comparative radiation dose in patients not having retinoblastoma. An additional group of patients have been described with a deletion in chromosome 13. This is associated with congenital abnormalities and retinoblastoma.

Cells from retinoblastoma patients have been examined for radiosensitivity by cell survival. Although there is some controversy over the radiosensitivity of these cells, we have been unable to show an unusual radiosensitivity in familial cases of retinobalstoma, and single strain of cells from a patient with D-deletion retinoblastoma (Harnden et al., 1980).

We have recently undertaken a comparative radiosensitivity study of chromosomes in lymphocytes from patients with familial retinoblastoma, Down's syndrome and normal individuals. For each retinoblastoma blood sample received a sample from a Down's patient and a normal individual were also taken. All blood samples were irradiated simultaneously and the induced chromosome aberrations scored on coded slides. The results showed that the level of chromosome damage in lymphocytes from 10/11 retinoblatomas patients irradiated with 400r at G_0 was intermediate between normal and the level of damage in Down's patients (Morten et al., 1981). Following exposure to 200r the ranking pattern was less clear and no significant difference between retinoblastoma patients' cells and normals was observed. It is clear therefore that any increased radiosensitivity compared to normal as measured by colony assays, or the level of induced chromosome aberrations is at best small and the biological significance of any statistical significant difference is unknown. By these criteria increased radiosensitivity as measured by cell killing compared with normals is not a major consequence of the retinoblastoma gene. How the clinical observation of a possibly increased susceptibility to radiation induced malignancy is related to these experimental findings is not known.

ii. Basal Cell Naevus Syndrome

In this dominantly inherited disorder there is again clinical evidence that patients are unusually sensitive to the carcinogenic effects of ionizing radiation. This has been shown following irradiation of these patients for medulloblastoma. Basal cell carcinomas arose in the irradiated field at a much greater frequency and with a much shortened latent period, compared with other individuals receiving similar doses of radiation (Strong, 1977). The latent period for basal cell carcinomas arising in the irradiated field is normally greater than ten years (Strong, 1977).

Multiple naevoid basal cell carcinomas occur spontaneously in these patients. Histologically these tumors are undistinguishable from those found in non BCNS patients. Another tumor type associated with this gene is medulloblastoma. Various benign growths including ovarian fibroma have been reported (Strong, 1977). Patients who show other features such as skeletal abnormalities, jaw cysts and pitting of the palms (Gorlin et al., 1972) also have been reported.

From the clinical evidence, Strong has suggested that BCNS patients represent a special subgroup with a hereditary predisposition to basal cell carcinoma in whom radiation may supply the subsequent mutation for tumor development and so lead to the rapid onset of multiple radiogenic basal cell carcinomas.

We have investigated possible causes for the basis of this apparent clinical radiosensitivity. The lethal effects of ionizing radiation are however, no greater in BCNS cells compared with normal cells (Taylor et al., 1975; Harnden et al., 1980; Featherstone, 1981). It should be made clear, however, that the cells treated are fibroblasts and the target cells for malignant change in the patients are epithelial. Whether or not the gene would act differently in these cells with respect to cell killing is not known.

Potential lethal damage repair in these basal cell naevus syndrome fibroblasts is no different from normal, suggesting that there is no repair deficiency expressed at least in the fibroblasts (Featherstone, 1981).

Lymphocytes from BCNS patients have been found to have a significantly higher number of dicentric and ring chromosomes and chromosome deletions following either 200 or 400r γ-rays compared with irradiated lymphocytes from normal individuals (Featherstone, 1981). The increase in aberration frequency in BCNS patients is small and similar to that seen in retinoblastoma lymphocytes (Morten et al., 1981). Although there is no direct evidence BCNS lymphocytes are likely to be less radiosensitive than lymphocytes from Down's patients. Overall, therefore again cells from BCNS patients are not markedly more radiosensitive compared with normals using lethality as the measure of sensitivity. Whether or not the increased frequency of radiation induced tumors is due to an increased mutability of these cells, is not at present known (Featherstone, 1981).

iii. Ataxia Telangiectasia

An unusual radiosensitivity was first recognized clinically following radiotherapy (Gotoff et al., 1967; Morgan et al., 1968; Cunliffe et al., 1975). This observation has been confirmed at the cellular level (Taylor et al., 1975). There is an approximately 2-3 fold differential in radiosensitivity between normal and A-T fibroblasts. This clear increased cell lethality is also seen in the increased level of chromosome aberrations in A-T cells following radiation exposure. There are increases in distinct types of chromosome aberrations following both G_0 and G_2 irradiation (Taylor et al., 1976; Taylor, 1978; Taylor, 1982). Unlike retinoblastoma and basal cell naevus syndrome there is a large unambiguous increase in radiosensitivity in A-T cells. A-T cells are also unusually sensitive to bleomycin (Taylor et al., 1979; Lehmann et al., 1979), neocarcinostatin (Shiloh -personal communication) and streptonigrin (unpublished results), all of which are DNA strand breaking anti-tumor agents. The evidence for a DNA repair deficiency has come from various sources (Taylor 1978; Paterson et al., 1979; Inoue et al., 1977), but perhaps the most compelling evidence is the absence of potential lethal damage repair (Cox et al., 1982; Weichselbaum 1978).

Following γ-irradiation A-T cells do not show the same degree of inhibition of DNA synthesis as normals (Edwards and Taylor, 1980; Painter and Young, 1980; Houldsworth and Lavin, 1980; de Wit et al., 1980). This differential effect is also seen following treatment of cells with drugs which cause a differential lethal effect (Cramer and Painter, 1981; Edwards et al., 1981; Jaspers et al., 1982; Shiloh - personal communication). Despite these findings the nature of the fundamental defect in A-T cells remain unknown. It seems unlikely that it is the abnormal response to DNA synthesis as an unusual response to ionizing radiation can be shown following irradiation at G_0 and post mitosis at G_2 (Taylor, 1978; Natarajan and Meyers, 1979). A more feasible explanation is that a repair defect, as shown particularly by the potential lethal damage repair experiments and the chromosomal results is the fundamental defect. The anomalous DNA synthesis may result from a failure to recognize the radiation induced damage which would in turn trigger a shut-down of DNA synthesis. The precise nature of the non-repairable lesion in A-T remains unknown, but some form of DNA strand break remains a strong possibility. The types of chromosome damage observed and the sensitivity of A-T cells to DNA strand breaking agents support this notion.

Although the frequency of ataxia telangiectasia in the population is low, the frequency of heterozygotes may be of the order of 1%. If such people had an intermediate sensitivity to ionizing radiation by virtue of being carriers of the gene this might also be important in relation to the reported increased levels of some malignancies in these patients (Swift et al., 1979; Swift, 1982). Some evidence has been put forward to suggest that such an intermediate radiosensitivity is seen in these patients (Chen et al., 1978; Kidson et al., 1982), but there is no consensus on this point. Our own work on cell survival and induced chromosome damage following exposure of A-T heterozygote cells suggests that their radiosensitivity is no different from normal (unpublished work).

iv. Other Syndromes

Reports of increased radiosensitivity have been made for Fanconi's anaemia cells (Remsen and Cerutti, 1976; Bigelow et al., 1979). Fanconi's anaemia is clearly a heterogeneous disorder and it seems quite possible that a proportion of these patients may in addition to showing an increased sensitivity to DNA crosslinking agents also show increased radiation sensitivity.

Down's syndrome lymphocytes have long been known to be more radiosensitive than normals as shown chromosomally (Kucerova, 1967; Countryman et al., 1977). Our own work suggests that this radiosensitivity cannot be shown by normal colony survival techniques.

Several other disorders, have also been associated with increased radiosensitivity. The most important of these perhaps is Hungtington's chorea. Patients with this disorder do not apparently show an increased susceptibility to malignant disease. There is no consensus over whether these patients are truly unusually radiosensitive and much controversy exists over this (Moshell et al., 1980; Kidson et al., 1981; Arlett et al., 1980). Our own limited data on cell survival and induced chromosome aberrations following exposure to x-rays have failed to show any difference between these patients and normals (unpublished results).

The Role of Cells Derived from These Patients in Assessment of Risk

As outlined in the introduction it is clear that cells from *bona fide* radiosensitive cells from individuals with the various disorders mentioned have a limited application in risk assessment. In risk assessment what is required presumably is an estimate of the effect of a particular level of an agent on a representative sample of the population. This end will not be achieved by using cells from rare groups of patients with poorly defined gene defects.

If, ultimately, these defects are defined then the cells may be useful in some circumstances; for example, in screening agents whose mode of action is unknown and cannot be discovered by other means. If the cells from a known disorder are sensitive to a particular agent by virtue of a very specific effect of the agent on the cells then other drugs can be tested for a similar effect. Clearly this approach has limitations as there will be very few agents with the same specific effects. In many cases, e.g., ionizing radiation, the problem will be the reverse; being able to sort out from a variety of induced effects the one(s) to which the cells are unusually sensitive.

For a general assessment of risk therefore there are severe limitations on the usefulness of these cells for this purpose. The great advantage of these disorders, particularly ataxia telangiectasia with respect to ionizing radiation, is that they serve as model systems for studying development of malignant disease.

Assessment of risk from various sources to the patients own cells is a different matter and it would certainly be an advantage to them to known to which agents they were unusually sensitive especially when the probability of their having treatment for malignant disease is known to be high.

The use of the techniques described here to measure sensitivity to ionizing radiation highlights their differential sensitivity. The evidence is that there is no increased lethal effect of radiation on cells derived from retinoblastoma patients, basal cell naevus patients and Down's patients compared with normals as measured by colony assays. Cytogenetic analysis however following exposure to x-rays would suggest that differences can be seen between some of these disorders and normals. Although the biological significance of this may be small in retinoblastoma patients and basal cell naevus syndrome patients the effect is larger for Down's patients, but its significance is unknown at present.

A further important point when considering possible small differences between individuals or individual cell strains is the use of a sufficient number of strains from normal individuals to obtain a measure of the true range of sensitivity. Also the simultaneous measurement of normal control strains and the strain under investigation will help to avoid finding spurious differences.

Conclusions

Patients with ataxia telangiectasia show a very clear unequivocal increased radiosensitivity as measured clinically and in the laboratory. The clinical radiosensitivity reported for retinoblastoma and basal cell naevus syndrome is not associated with cell killing, but appears to result in an unusually increased level of malignant disease in the irradiated field, perhaps as a result of a further mutation necessary for this process. For Fanconi's anaemia there is compelling evidence that perhaps some patients may be unusually sensitive to ionizing radiation. Down's syndrome patients do appear again to be slightly more radiosensitive than normals as measured by induced chromosome changes. There is therefore a range of both type and degree of radiosensitivity in man linked to various gene defects.

The usefulness in general terms of chromosome aberration production, cell survival, etc., for measurement of risk assessment has been discussed by others. These particular disorders may not be of any additional usefulness to currently used systems, but with the exceptions of ataxia telangiectasia they do highlight the problems generally encountered in measuring small increases in radiosensitivity.

References

Arlett, C. F., Presymptomatic diagnosis of Huntington's disease, Lancet (i), 540 (1980).

Bigelow, S. B., Rary, J. M., and Bender, M. A., G_2 chromosomal radiosensitivity in Fanconi's anaemia, Mutation Res., 63, 189-199 (1979).

Chen, P., Lavin, M. F., Kidson, C., and Moss, D., Identification of ataxia telangiectasia heterozygotes, a cancer prone population, Nature, 274, 484-486 (1978).

Chen, P., Kidson, C., and Imray, F. P., Huntington's chorea: implications of associated cellular radiosensitivity, Clin. Genet., 20, 331-336 (1981).

Countryman, P. I., Heddle, J. A., and Crawford, E., The repair of x-ray induced chromosomal damage in trisomy 21 and normal diploid lymphocytes, Cancer Res., 37, 52-58 (1977).

Cox, R., A cellular description of the repair defect in ataxia telangiectasia, in: B. A. Bridges, D. G. Harnden, eds., Ataxia telangiectasia - A cellular and molecular link between cancer, neuropathology and immune deficiency, pp. 141-153, John Wiley and Sons, Ltd. (1982).

Cramer, P., and Painter, R. B., Bleomycin resistant DNA synthesis in ataxia telangiectasia cells, Nature, 291, 671-672 (1981).

Cunliffe, P. N., Mann, J. R., Cameron, A. H., Roberts, K. O., and Ward, H. W. C., Radiosensitivity in ataxia telangiectasia, Brit. J. Radiol., 48, 374-376 (1975).

Edwards, M. J., and Taylor, A. M. R., Unusual levels of (ADP-ribose)$_n$ and DNA synthesis in ataxia telangiectasia cells following γ-irradiation, Nature, 287, 745-747 (1980).

Edwards, M. J., Taylor, A. M. R., and Flude, E. J., Bleomycin induced inhibition of DNA synthesis in ataxia telangiectasia cell lines, Biochem. Biophys. Res. Commun., 102, 610-616 (1981).

Featherstone, T., A study of cultured cells from basal cell naevus syndrome patients, Ph.D. Thesis, University of Birmingham, England (1981).

Gorlin, R. J., and Sedano, H. O., The multiple naevoid basal cell carcinoma syndrome revisited, Birth Defects, 7(8), 140-148 (1972).

Gotoff, S. P., Amirmokri, E., and Liebner, E. J., Ataxia telangiectasia: Neoplasia, untoward response to x-irradiation and tuberous sclerosis, Am. J. Dis. Child., 114, 617-625 (1967).

Harnden, D. G., Edwards, M. J., Featherstone, T., Morten, J., Morgan, G. R., and Taylor, A. M. R., Studies on cells from patients who are cancer prone and may be radiosensitive, in: H. V. Gelboin, B. MacMahon, T. Mutsushima, T. Sugimura, S. Takayama, and H. Takebe, eds., Genetic and Environmental Factors in Experimental and Human Cancer, pp. 231-246, Tokyo: Japan Scientific Societies Press (1980).

Houldsworth, J., and Lavin, M. F., Effect of ionizing radiation on DNA synthesis in ataxia telangiectasia cells, Nucleic Acids Res., 8, 3709-3720 (1980).

Inoue, T., Hirano, K., Yokoiyama, A., Kada, T., and Kato, H., DNA repair enzymes in ataxia telangiectasia and Bloom's syndrome fibroblasts, Biochim. Biophys. Acta, 479, 497-500 (1977).

Jaspers, N. G. J., de Wit, J., Regulski, M. R., and Bootsma, D., Abnormal regulation of DNA replication and increased lethality in ataxia telangiectasia cells exposed to carcinogenic agents, Cancer Res., 42, 335-341 (1982).

Kidson, C., Chen, P., and Imray, P., Ataxia telangiectasia heterozygotes: dominant expression of ionizing radiation sensitive mutants, in: B. A. Bridges and D. G. Harnden, eds., Ataxia telangiectasia - A cellular and molecular link between cancer, neuropathology and immune deficiency, pp. 363-372, John Wiley and Sons (1982).

Kucerova, M., Comparison of radiation effects in vitro upon chromosomes of human subjects, Acta Radiol., 6, 441-448 (1967).

Lehmann, A. R., and Stevens, S., The response of ataxia telangiectasia cells to bleomycin, Nucleic Acids Res., 6, 1953-1960 (1979).

Morten, J. E. N., Harnden, D. G., and Taylor, A. M. R., Chromosome damage in G_0 x-irradiated lymphocytes from patients with hereditary retinoblastoma, Cancer Res., 41, 3635-3638 (1981).

Morgan, J. L., Holcomb, T. M., and Morrissey, R. W., Radiation reaction in ataxia telangiectasia, Am. J. Dis. Child., 116, 557-558 (1968).

Moshell, A. N., Tarone, R. E., Barratt, S. F., and Robbins, J. H., Radiosensitivity in Huntingston's disease: implications for pathogenesis and presymptomatic diagnosis, Lancet (i), 9-11 (1980).

Natarajan, A. T., and Meyers, M., Chromosomal radiosensitivity of ataxia telangiectasia cells at different cell cycle stages, Hum. Genet., 52, 127-132 (1979).

Painter, R. B., and Young, B. R., Radiosensitivity in ataxia telangiectasia: a new explanation, Proc. Natl. Acad. Sci. USA, 77, 7315-7317 (1980).

Paterson, M. C., Smith, B. P., Lohmann, P. H. M., Anderson, A. K., and Fishman, L., Defective excision repair of gamma ray damaged DNA in human (ataxia telangiectasia) fibroblasts, Nature, 260, 444-447 (1976).

Remsen, J. F., and Cerutti, P. A., Deficiency of gamma-ray excision repair in skin fibroblasts from patients with Fanconi's anaemia, Proc. Natl. Acad. Sci. USA, 73, 2419-2423 (1976).

Strong, L. C., Theories of pathogenesis: mutation and cancer, in: J. J. Mulvihill, R. W. Miller, and J. F. Fraumeni, eds., Genetics of human cancer, pp. 401-415, Raven Press (1977).

Swift, M., Sholman, L., Perry, M., and Chase, C., Malignant neoplasms in the families of patients with ataxia telangiectasia, Cancer Res., 36, 209-215 (1976).

Swift, M., Disease predisposition of ataxia telangiectasia heterozygotes, in: B. A. Bridges and D. G. Harnden, eds., Ataxia telangiectasia - A cellular and molecular link between cancer, neuropathology and immune deficiency, pp. 355-361, John Wiley and Sons (1982).

Taylor, A. M. R., Unrepaired DNA strand breaks in irradiated ataxia telangiectasia lymphocytes suggested from cytogenetic observations, Mutation Res., 50, 407-418 (1978).

Taylor, A. M. R., Cytogenetics of ataxia telangiectasia, in: B. A. Bridges and D. G. Harnden, eds., Ataxia telangiectasia - A cellular and molecular link between cancer, neuropathology, and immune deficiency, pp. 53-81, John Wiley and Sons (1982).

Taylor, A. M. R., Harnden, D. G., Arlett, C. F., Harcourt, S. A., Lehmann, A. R., Stevens, S., and Bridges, B. A., Ataxia telangiectasia: a human mutation with abnormal radiation sensitivity, Nature, 258, 427-429 (1975).

Taylor, A. M. R., Metcalfe, J. A., Oxford, J. M., and Harnden, D. G., Is chromatid type damage in ataxia telangiectasia after irradiation at G_0 a consequence of defective repair? Nature, 260, 441-443 (1976).

Taylor, A. M. R., Rosney, C. M., and Campbell, J. B., Unusual sensitivity of ataxia telangiectasia cells to bleomycin, Cancer Res., 39, 1046-1050 (1979).

Weichselbaum, R. R., Epstein, J., and Little, J. B., In vitro radiosensitivity of human diploid fibroblasts derived from patients with unusual clinical responses to radiation, Radiology, 121, 479-482 (1976).

Weichselbaum, R. R., Nove, J., and Little, J. B., Deficient recovery from potentially lethal radiation damage in ataxia telangiectasia and xeroderma pigmentosum, Nature, 271, 261-262 (1978).

de Wit, J., Jaspers, N. G. J., and Bootsma, D., The rate of DNA synthesis in normal human and ataxia telangiectasia cells after exposure to ionizing radiation, Mutation Res., 80, 221-226 (1981).

ELECTROPHILIC REACTIVITY AS A MEASURE OF GENOTOXIC POTENCY

Lars Ehrenberg and Siv Osterman-Golkar

Department of Radiobiology, Wallenberg Laboratory
University of Stockholm, S-106 91 Stockholm
Sweden

The mutagenic effectiveness in forward mutation systems of a number of monofunctional alkylating agents with large differences in absolute reactivity and with different s-values (Swain and Scott, 1953) have been compared in the low-dose region of the dose-response curves. It was shown that the mutation frequency, R, at equal dose, D* (D is the time integral of the concentration of the alkylating agent, RX), was proportional to the second order rate constant, $k_{n=2}$, for reaction with some nucleophilic center with a low nucleophilic strength (n=2 in the Swain-Scott scale, see Fig. 1) (Hussain and Ehrenberg, 1975; Osterman-Golkar, 1975; Ehrenberg, 1980; Hussain, 1981)

$$R = \text{const.} \cdot k_{n=2} \cdot D \quad (1)$$

The degree of alkylation, $[RY]/[Y^-]$, of a nucleophilic center, Y^-, is proportional to the dose of the alkylating agent according to the equation

$$[RY]/[Y^-] = k_Y \cdot D \quad (2)$$

---

*Abbreviations and symbols used: L_i, level (concentration); D_i, dose ($D = \int L(t)dt$); Indices i in L_i, D_i refer to system of steps from environmental level/dose (i=1) to biological response (i=6); i=2 absorbed amount of a chemical given e.g. in mg/kg b.w. (pharmacological dose); i=3 dose of an electrophilic compound in tissues; i=4 dose of an electrophilic compound in immediate environment of target molecules (DNA-dose); i=5 level of potentially mutagenic lesions in DNA (molecular dose); $k_{i(i+1)}$, transfer coefficient between consectutive steps in this system (Cf. Osterman-Golkar this journal and Ehrenberg et al., 1981).

This means that the mutation frequency is proportional to the degree of alkylation of nucleophilic centers of the nucleophilic strength n=2 independent of the chemical used (see Fig. 2).

Nucleophilic sites of DNA, critical or non-critical, are alkylated at random - with rates > 0, determined by the nucleophilic strengths of these groups, by the reactivity and the s-value of the alkylating agent, in several cases also by steric factors, etc. (cf. Ehrenberg and Osterman-Golkar, 1980). Therefore reactions at sites of the reactivity n=2 occur along with reactions at all other reactive sites, and *vice versa*.

It follows, that the *demonstration* of alkylating activity of RX in DNA or its immediate environment (or outside the cell nucleus if it can be assumed that $k_{34} > 0$), is a sufficient criterion on risk of genetic damage.

It is probably valid for all other types of electrophilic agents as well (cf. Table II of Ehrenberg and Osterman-Golkar, 1980), that, if they can at all penetrate membranes, they will give rise to critical as well as non-critical chemical changes in the DNA.

Miller and Miller (1971) have claimed that all carcinogens (i.e. cancer initiators), which according to the same authors are (in general) also mutagenic, are electrophilically reactive ($\longrightarrow$ in the expression):

$$\left.\begin{array}{l}\text{cancer initiators}\\ \\ \text{mutagens}\end{array}\right| \;\rightleftarrows\; \left|\begin{array}{l}\text{electrophilic}\\ \\ \text{reagents}\end{array}\right. \qquad (3)$$

It follows from the random distribution of reactions with different nucleophilic sites in the DNA that the conversion of expression (3) is also valid. The implication is that a demonstration of electrophilic reactivity *in vivo* is a sufficient criterion on genetic risk, including cancer risk.

The conversion of (3) concerns the qualitative risk identification. If somebody would like to show that this conversion is not valid in a specific case a knowledge of quantitative parameters determining the rate of reaction with critical sites of DNA is required. The absence of a biological effect (i.e. response = 0) in a test for mutagenicity or carcinogenicity can, for statistical reasons, never prove the absence of genotoxic activity. Therefore, the proof for non-validity of the conversion (3) has to be based on the demonstration that the mutation frequency (etc) is significantly lower than the expected frequency ($R_{expect.}$) or a certain fraction, a, thereof. On the analogy of corresponding calculations for

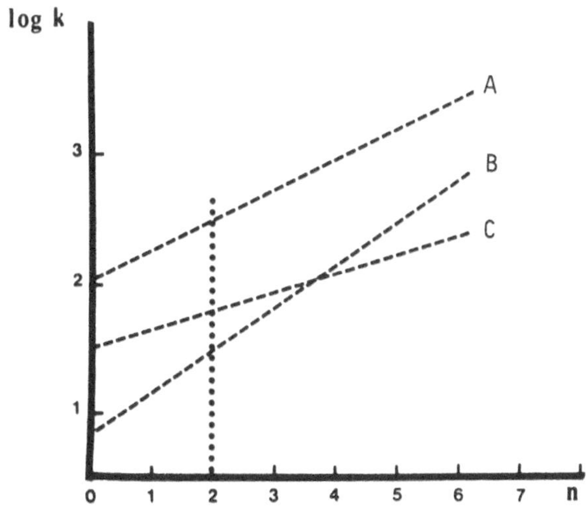

Fig. 1. Swain-Scott relationships for the alkylating agents A, B and C. (Logarithms of second order rate constants for the reactions $RX + Y^- \longrightarrow RY + X^-$ as a function of the nucleophilic strength (n) of Y^-.) The approximate n-value at which rate constants are proportional to the mutagenic effectiveness in the linear low-dose region of dose-response curves is indicated.

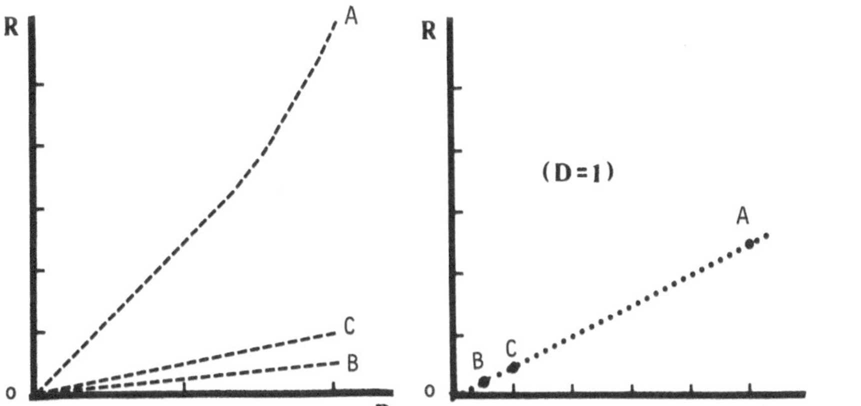

Fig. 2. a) The mutagenic effectiveness of the alkylating agents A, B and C, respectively, as a function of dose.
b) The mutagenic effectiveness of the alkylating agents A, B and C, respectively as a function of the degree of alkylation of groups with the nucleophilic strength n=2.

simple alkylating agents, $R_{expect.}$ is estimated from the equation

$$R_{expect.} = D_4 \cdot k_{45} \cdot k_{56} \tag{4}$$

From the value of the expected response the scope of a test can be determined, which has, for example, the statistical power $(1 - \beta) = 95\%$ to detect $R_{expect.}$ (or a fraction thereof) at e.g. 99% significance level. A negative result in this test, i.e. the Null Hypothesis being accepted, means that the substance with a high probability is non-mutagenic, or strictly, less effective than expected. If the true activity of the substance is equal to the expected activity a negative result would be obtained in only 5% of repeated experiments. The significance level should, in a case like this, be as high as 99% in order to avoid false positive results (α-error = 1%) (Fig. 3).

It should be stressed that at present no compound is known for which the conversion (3) is not valid. For the relevance of protein (hemoglobin) alkylation, etc., as a monitor of risk it is further important to note that no electrophilic compound is known to react with DNA or proteins exclusively. In our view, claimants of the non-validity of (3) should carry the burden to sustain their claim experimentally.

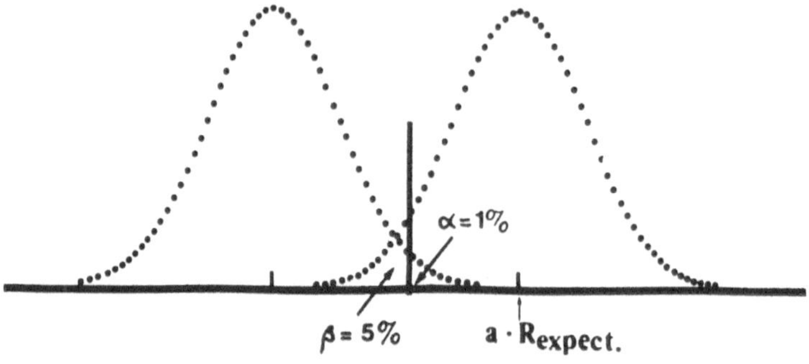

Fig. 3. Illustration of sampling distributions for the Null Hypothesis (difference d=0) and for the hypothesis that $d=R_{expect.}$ (or $a \cdot R_{expect.}$, $a < 1$) is true, at a size of the experiment giving $\alpha=0.01$, $\beta=0.05$ in single-sided statistical test. (For details see Ehrenberg, 1977.)

The sole condition for the validity of (3) is the existence of a linear component in the dose - response relationship, predominating at low doses/levels. This condition means that $k_{56} > 0$ at all doses/levels > 0, or, that there is no dose/level below which repair is fully effective. Certain agents (e.g. UV light, methylating agents) may give rise to lesions which, at low L_5, are subjected to a highly effective repair in certain organs and in certain individuals. Strong arguments may however be presented in favour of the general validity of the linear hypothesis (Segerbäck and Ehrenberg, 1981; Ehrenberg et al., 1981). Although, in experiments with cultivated cells, painstaking work is able to show that a linear component is at hand at the lowest doses we may think of, viz., corresponding to $L_5 <$ one potentially mutagenic "hit" per cell, data are still lacking, which could give convincing information on the true shape of the dose-response curve in gonads and other tissues of human beings.

In this situation a practice has developed to make a "conservative" risk estimate by assuming the dose-response curve to be linear down to dose zero; "conservative" is given here with quotation signs because in some cases mutagens may be more effective at very low doses than is expected from linear extrapolation through the response at intermediate - high doses (cf. Ehrenberg et al., 1981).

Following this practice, we may state that the demonstration of electrophilic reactivity means the identification of a risk, which might be, but can not be proved to be, infinitesimally or negligibly small.

ACKNOWLEDGEMENT

This article is based on research supported by grants from the Swedish Work Environment Fund and the Swedish Natural Science Research Council.

REFERENCES

Ehrenberg, L., 1977, Aspects of statistical inference in testing for genetic toxicity, in: "Handbook of Mutagenicity Test Procedures," B. Kilbey, et al., eds., Elsevier/North Holland, Amsterdam.

Ehrenberg, L., 1980, Purposes and methods of comparing effects of radiation and chemicals, in: "Radiobiological Equivalents of Chemical Pollutants," IAEA, Vienna.

Ehrenberg, L., Moustacchi, E., and Osterman-Golkar, S., 1981, Dosimetry of genotoxic agents and dose-response relationships of their effects, Working paper for ICPEMC.

Ehrenberg, L., and Osterman-Golkar, S., 1980, Alkylation of macromolecules for detecting mutagenic agents, Teratogenesis Carcinogenesis Mutagenesis, 1:105.

Hussain, S., 1981, Doctoral Thesis, Stockholm (in preparation).

Hussain, S., and Ehrenberg, L., 1975, Prophage inductive efficiency of alkylating agents and radiations, Int. J. Radiat. Biol., 27:355.

Miller, E. C., and Miller, J. A., 1971, The mutagenicity of chemical carcinogens: Correlations, problems and interpretations, in: "Chemical Mutagens," vol. 1, A. Hollaender, ed., Plenum Press, New York.

Osterman-Golkar, S., 1975, Studies on the reaction kinetics of biologically active electrophilic reagents as a basis for risk estimates, Doctoral Thesis, Stockholm.

Segerbäck, D., and Ehrenberg, L., 1981, Alkylating properties of dichlorvos (DDVP), Acta Pharmacol. Toxicol., in press.

Swain, C. G., and Scott, C. A., 1953, Quantitative correlation of relative rates. Comparison of hydroxide ion with other nucleophilic reagents towards alkyl halides, esters, epoxides and acyl halides, J. Am. Chem. Soc., 75:141.

SOS FUNCTIONS INDUCED IN CARCINOGEN-TREATED MAMMALIAN CELLS

Alain Sarasin and Mauro Mezzina

Institut de Recherches Scientifiques sur le Cancer
B.P. 8-94802 Villejuif
Cedex, France

INTRODUCTION

It is now well established that treatment, which blocks semiconservative DNA synthesis, induces in bacteria a series of pleiotropic effects called SOS functions [1-3]. The bacterial RecA protein, in the presence of single-strand DNA, displays a protease activity, which will specifically cleave its own repressor - the LexA protein - and the repressor of λ phage leading to prophage induction in a lysogenic bacteria. The cleavage of the LexA protein turns on several other genes which belong to the SOS response such as recA, umuC, sfiA, uvrA, uvrB genes (see Fig. 1). Among these responses, the umuC gene product seems to be partly responsible for the error-prone repair pathway expressed in treated-bacteria. Since SOS functions in bacteria are strongly mutagenic and can lead to virus induction, it is of great interest to determine if such functions could also be induced in mammalian cells treated with carcinogens. The expression of some specific mutations and/or the induction of some integrated viral genomes could very well represent one of the first steps in the initiation of carcinogenesis. In order to approach this problem, we have studied the properties of the DNA replication process in SOS conditions (i.e., in cells treated with chemical or physical carcinogens) trying to answer two specific questions: 1) Does an error-prone replication pathway exist in mammalian cells? 2) Are any specific replication enzymes induced in carcinogen-treated mammalian cells?

ERROR-PRONE REPLICATION IN CARCINOGEN-TREATED MONKEY CELLS

The induction of an error-prone DNA replication process in bacteria treated by carcinogens has been essentially demonstrated by

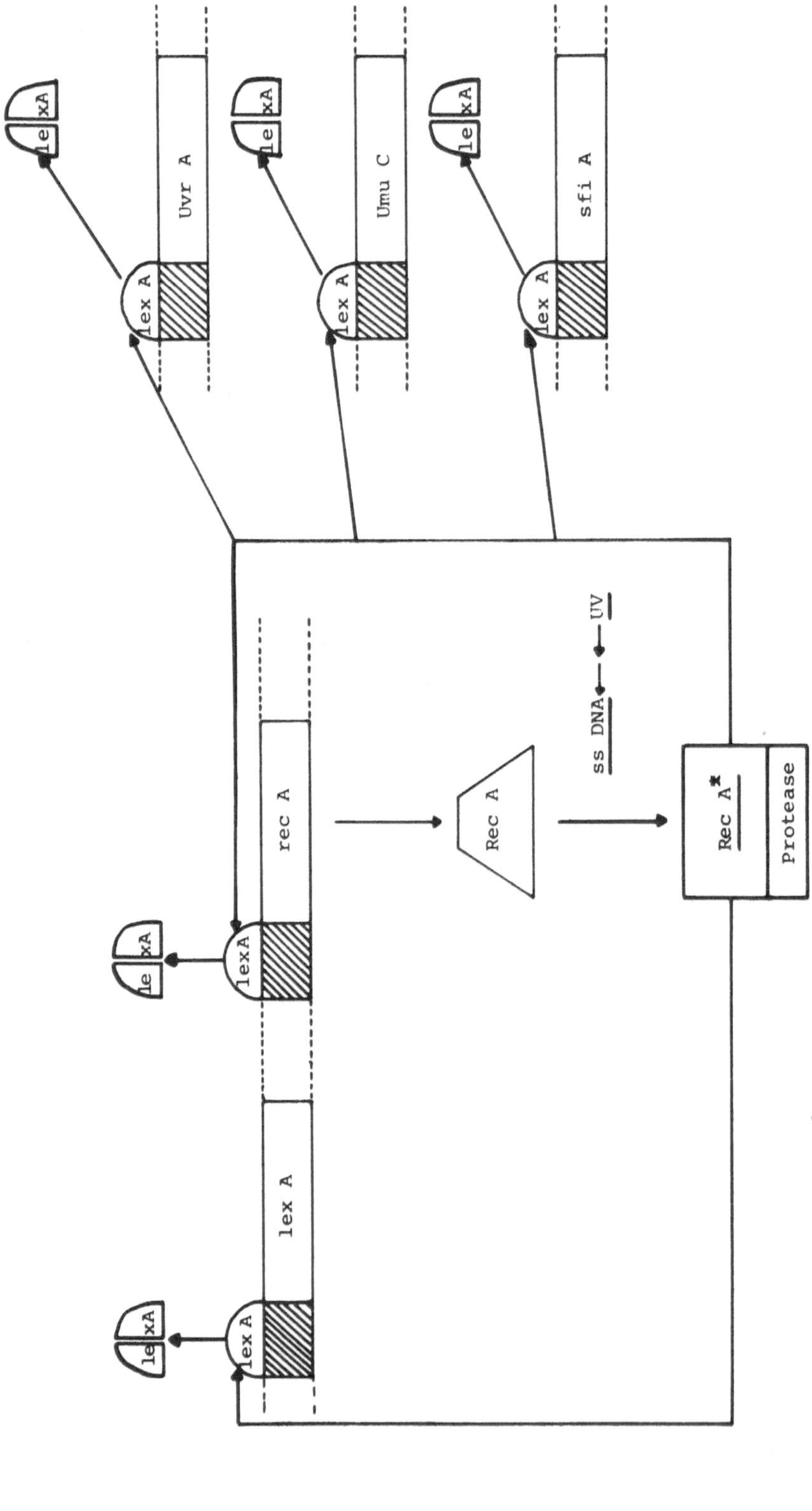

Fig. 1. Current view of the SOS pathway regulation. Single-stranded DNA due to DNA damages activates the protease activity of RecA protein which will cleave its LexA repressor. Then several SOS genes are turned on such as <u>recA</u>, <u>uvrA</u>, <u>uvrB</u>, <u>umuC</u>, <u>sfiA</u>, ...

using various UV-damaged bacteriophages as a molecular DNA probe [4]. Results have shown that UV-irradiated λ phage has a better survival in UV-irradiated or carcinogen-treated host cell than in unirradiated one. Moreover, this UV-reactivation process is associated with a high level of mutations in the repaired phage genome. The most likely explanation for this error-prone replication is the induction in the treated bacteria of some type of DNA synthesis past pyrimidine dimers (or other lesions) which will produce mutations on newly synthesized strand opposite to the lesions [5].

As in bacteria, treatment of mammalian cells with various physical or chemical agents which damage DNA, prior infection with UV-irradiated virus, enhances virus survival. This phenomenon which has been called induced virus reactivation or enhanced virus reactivation, by analogy with bacteriophage, has been obtained with various animal viruses such as Herpes virus [6], simian adenovirus [7], simian virus 40 [8, 9] and parvoviruses [10-12]. Chemical carcinogen treatment of monkey kidney cells has also been shown to be very efficient in enhancing the survival of UV-irradiated SV40 [8]. This effect was obtained both with compounds producing "UV-like" damages (such as metabolized aflatoxin B_1 or N-acetoxyacetyl-aminofluorene) or those producing "X-ray" like damages (such as methyl-methane-sulfonate or ethyl-methane-sulfonate). These results have been confirmed using UV-irradiated herpes virus [13] and Lu III parvovirus [11]. SV40 reactivation was also promoted in monkey cells which were treated by drugs inhibiting DNA replication such as hydroxyurea or cycloheximide [8]. We have hypothesized that the inhibition of scheduled DNA synthesis is a direct or indirect signal inducing a new repair process able to replicate UV-irradiated DNA [8]. This induced pathway might be related to the phenomenon in which enhanced post-replication repair is observed in carcinogen-treated Chinese hamster or human fibroblast cells with a split-dose protocol [14].

If this virus reactivation phenomenon resembles bacteriophage reactivation, it should be accompanied by an increased mutagenesis of the repaired virus. In order to approach this problem, we used simian virus 40 as a molecular probe. The lytic infection of SV40 in monkey kidney cells is well characterized and consists of early functions (virus absorption, uncoating, early mRNA transcription and early protein synthesis producing the small t and large T antigens), followed by initiation of viral DNA replication and then expression of late functions (late mRNA transcription and late protein synthesis producing the VP-1, VP-2, and VP-3 coat proteins) [15]. Due to its limited genetic content, SV40 is extremely host dependent and therefore SV40 is an excellent tool to investigate the induction of cellular enzymes particularly those involved in DNA metabolism. A number of SV40 mutants have been isolated and well characterized. We used thermosensitive SV40 mutants either at the level of the early genes (tsA58) or of the late genes (tsB201). tsA58 SV40

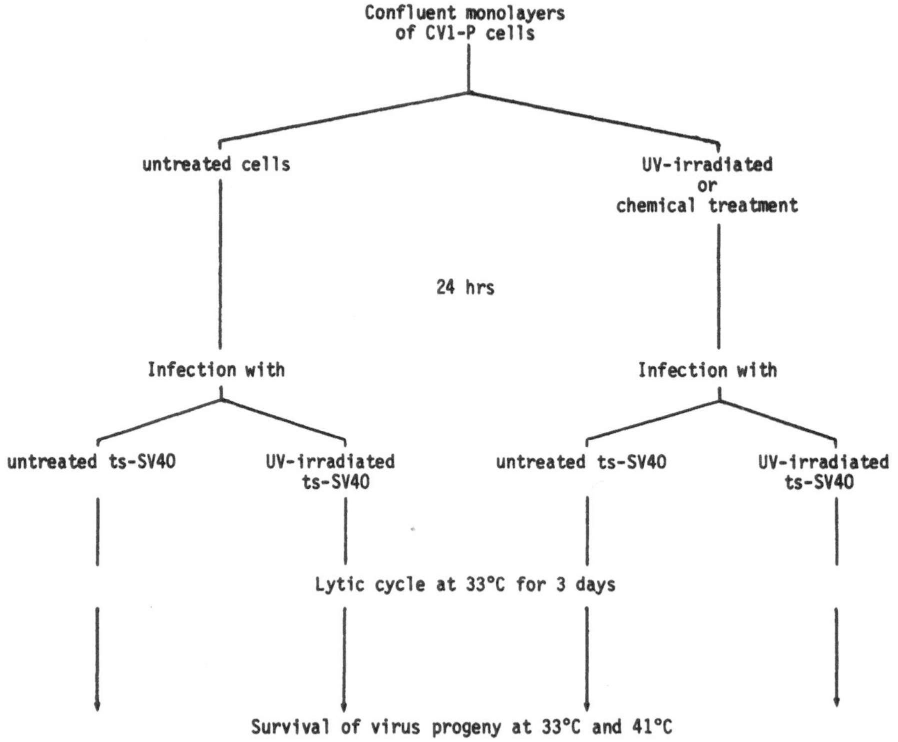

Fig. 2. Experiment protocol used to study the inducible mutagenesis of SV40 in pretreated monkey cells.

mutant is defective in the initiation of viral DNA replication at 41°C due to a single base-pair substitution in the large T antigen gene [16-18]. tsB201 SV40 mutant is defective in virus production at 41°C due to a mutation in the VP-1 protein gene. Moreover, SV40 DNA which is a small supercoiled molecule (3.5×10^6 daltons) is easy to isolate and its DNA sequence is completely known. Finally, the idea that SV40 DNA should be repaired in the same way as cellular DNA is strengthened by the fact that SV40 minichromosome shares structural similarities with mammalian chromosome [19].

The experimental protocol, we have used to study the induced mutagenesis of SV40 in carcinogen-treated cells, is schematized in Fig. 2: virus infection, with unirradiated or UV-irradiated thermosensitive SV40, occurs 24 h after cell treatment and one lytic cycle is carried out at the permissive temperature (72 h at 33°C), and then viral progeny survival is measured at 33°C and 41°C in untreated CV1-P cells. The mutation frequency is equal to the ratio of virus survival at 41°C to virus survival at 33°C.

Table 1. Mutation Frequencies Towards Wild-Type Phenotype of tsB201 SV40 Mutant Grown in AAAF-Treated Cells

AAAF-treatment of cells (μM)	Reversion frequency after infection with	
	unirradiated SV40*	1500 J/m^2-UV'd SV40**
0	8.8×10^{-8}	1.25×10^{-5}
0.5	-	6×10^{-5}
1	5.9×10^{-8}	30×10^{-5}
2	7.7×10^{-8}	55×10^{-5}
3	3.1×10^{-8}	14×10^{-5}
4	-	20×10^{-5}
5	$<9.2 \times 10^{-8}$	33×10^{-5}
6	-	32×10^{-5}
7	$<8.7 \times 10^{-8}$	27×10^{-5}

*Multiplicity of infection: 5 PFU/cell.
**Multiplicity of infection: 7×10^{-3} PFU/cell.
Control or UV-irradiated tsB201 SV40 mutants were used to infect control or acetoxy-acetyl-aminofluorene-treated CV1-P monkey cells during one lytic cycle at 33°C (72 h). Survival of progeny was measured at 33°C and 41°C to evaluate the reversion frequency by the plaque assay technique already described.

Table 1 shows that the reversion frequency towards wild-type phenotype of tsB201 SV40 mutants is strongly increased when host cells have been pretreated with the carcinogen N-acetoxy-acetyl-aminofluorene (AAAF), before the infection with the UV-irradiated virus. An amount of carcinogen as small as 1 μM is enough to induce the mutagenic process. This phenomenon is essentially detectable with UV-irradiated SV40 (1500 J/m^2) and no significant increased mutagenesis is observed with unirradiated SV40 mutant (Table 1). Since we are using a tsB SV40 mutant which has a wild-type behavior for DNA replication, the lytic cycle could be carried out at the non-permissive temperature of 41°C. Table 2 shows that enhanced mutagenesis could be observed whatever the temperature of the lytic cycle of UV-irradiated tsB mutant in AAAF-treated cells. Similar results have been obtained after cell treatment with mitomycin C (MMC) which is a very potent inhibitor of DNA synthesis due to its DNA cross-link activity (Table 3).

To ensure that the SV40 revertants were genetically stable, some viral plaques appearing at 41°C were picked up and viruses were assayed for survival at 33°C and 41°C. The results show that the viruses present in these plaques grow as well at 41°C as at 33°C

Table 2. Mutation Frequencies Towards Wild-Type Phenotype of Temperature-Sensitive tsB201 Mutant during the AAAF-Induced Virus Reactivation Process at Different Temperatures

AAAF-treatment of cells (μM)	Reversion frequencies when the lytic cycle has been carried out at	
	33°C	41°C
0	1×10^{-5}	5×10^{-3}
0.5	6×10^{-5}	140×10^{-3}
1	30×10^{-5}	300×10^{-3}
2	55×10^{-5}	60×10^{-3}
4	20×10^{-5}	220×10^{-3}
6	32×10^{-5}	40×10^{-3}

We used the same protocol as the one described under Table 1. The lytic cycle was carried out at 33°C for 72 h or at 41°C for 52 h.

Table 3. Mutation Frequencies Towards Wild-Type Phenotype of Temperature-Sensitive tsB201 Mutant during the Mitomycin C-Induced Virus Reactivation Process

Mitomycin C-treatment of cells (μg/ml)*	Virus survival in PFU/ml at		Reversion frequencies
	33°C	41°C	
0	6×10^{4}	<1	$<2 \times 10^{-5}$
0.5	1.2×10^{6}	72	6×10^{-5}
1	3×10^{6}	660	22×10^{-5}
2	3×10^{6}	390	13×10^{-5}
3	1.5×10^{6}	540	36×10^{-5}
5	8×10^{6}	1440	18×10^{-5}
10	0.4×10^{6}	480	120×10^{-5}

*CV1-P cells have been treated with mitomycin C for 3 h at 37°C in the dark.

or even better (data not shown). This result indicates that the mutation assay we have developed is really measuring a true genetic reversion from thermosensitive to wild-type phenotype. The molecular mechanisms of the SV40 induced mutagenesis in chemical carcinogen-treated cells is not known yet. However, we have studied the mutagenesis induced in UV-irradiated monkey kidney cells before infection with UV-irradiated tsA58 SV40 mutant [17, 20]. Results indicate that UV-irradiated tsA58 SV40 mutant [17, 20]. Results indicate that revertants were composed of two mutation sites compared to wild-type SV40: the tsA58 mutation site is still present (this mutation is due to a base-pair substitution from C-G to T-A) and another base-pair substitution which occurs opposite a possible pyrimidine dimer. These two mutations are close from each other and restitute a normal wild-type behavior to the viral large T antigen [21].

In conclusion, our results support the hypothesis that treatment of monkey cells with carcinogens induces some type of error-prone replication pathway, which will allow a better replication efficiency on UV-damaged templates. Consequently, a higher survival and a higher mutagenesis of UV-irradiated virus are observed in carcinogen-treated cells. These results could be partly explained by a bypass of DNA lesions via a somewhat modified DNA polymerase activity, which has already been observed in treated *E. coli* [22]. However, no evidence has been obtained that this error-prone pathway is active on cellular DNA. Since we do not think that mammalian cells would have conserved such an erroneous pathway only for viruses, this discrepancy could be due to experimental protocols. In fact, viral mutants are much more well characterized and easier to manipulate than cellular mutants. However, the recent generation of various "mutator" mutants of mammalian cells can provide in the near future a good tool for the analysis of this induced mutagenesis.

DNA LIGASE INDUCTION IN CARCINOGEN-TREATED CELLS

Many evidences have been provided showing the role of DNA ligase in the semi-conservative DNA replication mode by joining Okazaki's fragments to produce mature daughter DNA strand both in bacteria and in eucaryotic cells [23]. It has been generally postulated that a DNA ligase must play a crucial role also in DNA excision-repair process by sealing the newly-repaired DNA to the parental strand [24]; genetic evidences have shown in fact that temperature-sensitive mutants of *E. coli* [25] and yeast [26] defective in ligating activity are highly sensitive to UV-irradiation. Such a genetic approach is not yet possible in mammalian cells because of the lack of this type of mutants. However, by biochemical analysis, the direct role of ligase in DNA replication has been proven in different mammalian cell systems [27-30] and two different forms of ligating activity have been purified from mammalian cells [31]. Söderäll has suggested that these two enzymes could be differently regulated during DNA replication and DNA repair processes [27].

In previous experiments, we have shown that ligase activity increases considerably after UV-irradiation of monkey kidney cells [32] and human fibroblasts [33]. In an attempt to study the enzymes involved in DNA repair mechanisms induced by carcinogen treatment in mammalian cells, we have carried out several experiments, with confluent monkey cells and human fibroblasts treated with chemical car-

Table 4. Specific Activity of DNA Ligase in Different Cell Strains after Various Carcinogen Treatments

Cell strains	Controls	UV-irradiated	MMC-treated	AAAF-treated	SV40 infected	MMC-pre-treated and SV40 infected
Monkey kidney cells (CV1)	5.1	10	10.8	9.8	10.5	15.7
Normal human fibroblasts	3.1	6	6.5	7.2	-	-
XP-fibroblasts (complementation group A, 12BE-CRL 1223)	2.7	6	-	-	-	-

UV-irradiation fluences at 254 nm were 17.5 J/m^2 for control cells and 2 J/m^2 for XP cells. Mitomycin C treatment was done for 3 h at 5 μg/ml and acetoxy-acetyl-aminofluorene treatment was done for 1 h at 1 μg/ml. The determination of specific activity of ligase (units/μg of proteins) in crude extracts were performed as already described [32-33].

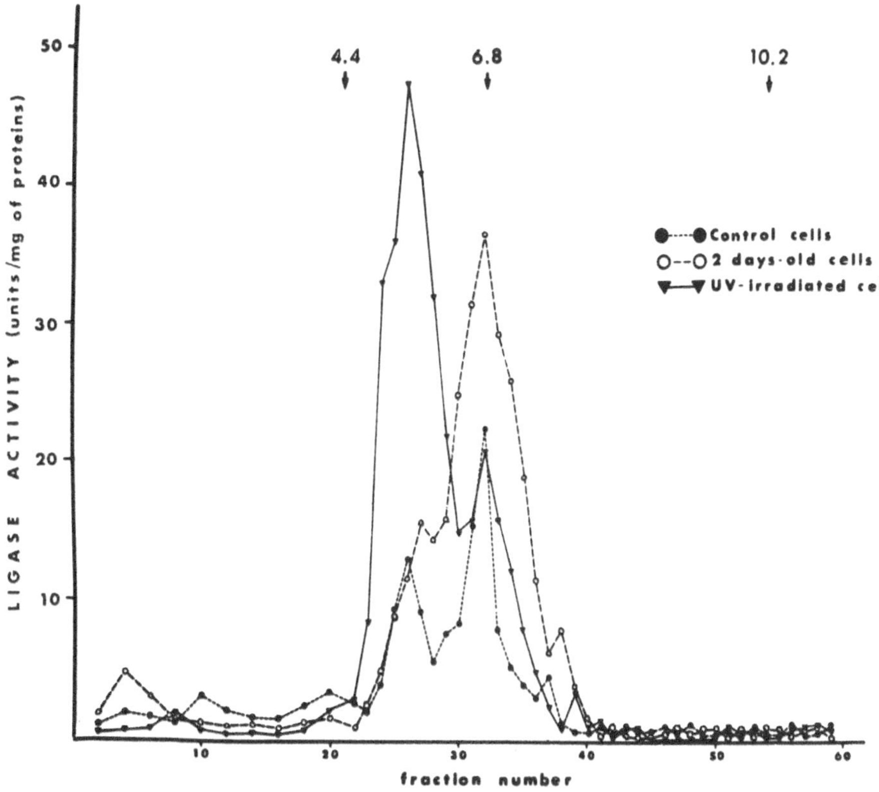

Fig. 3. Partial purification of DNA ligases in 5-20% sucrose gradients. Cellular crude extracts were loaded onto 12 ml-5-20% linear sucrose gradients in 0.5 M KCl, 20 mM Tris-HCl pH 7.5, 2 mM DTE, 2 mM β-mercaptoethanol and the gradients were run at 40,000 rpm for 40 h at 4°C in Beckman SW41 rotor. Bovine serum albumin (4.4S), bacterial alkaline phosphatase (6.8S) and catalase (10.2S) were used as external markers in a parallel gradient. Ligase activity was determined in each fraction as described [32]. Confluent control monkey kidney cells (--●--); exponentially growing monkey kidney cells (---o--); UV-irradiated monkey kidney cells (—▼—).

cinogens such as mitomycin C and N-acetoxy-acetyl-aminofluorene. Results show that such cell treatment induces an increase of DNA ligase activity of about 2-3 times over that measured in untreated cells.

As shown in Table 4, the increase of DNA ligase activity after carcinogen treatment is observed both in excision-proficient cells (fibroblasts from Xeroderma pigmentosum group A patient) indicating that this disease is not due to the lack of DNA ligase inducibility. The characteristics of this enzyme increase is: a) of the same order of magnitude of that measured in UV-irradiated cells; b) it seems to be dependent on *de novo* protein synthesis; c) it is independent on a semiconservative DNA synthesis, since these drugs block also the scheduled DNA synthesis.

In parallel experiments we have measured the enzyme activity in exponentially-growing and SV40 infected confluent monkey cells. The ligase activity level in these extracts is two times higher than in confluent control cells, according with other results already published [32]. Table 4 shows also that SV40 infection with MMC-pretreated cells induces an increase of enzyme activity which is identical to the sum of the ligase activity induced by each treatment alone. In order to test if several enzymes are induced during these processes, a partial purification of the ligase activities was carried out by sedimentation through 5-20% sucrose gradients of crude extracts obtained from confluent exponentially growing and UV-irradiated monkey kidney cells. Figure 3 shows the profile activity of ligase in each gradient fraction. Two distinct peaks of enzyme activity of different S values (about 4S and 6S) were detected. In exponentially growing cells, the 6S peak of ligase activity is two times higher, whereas in UV-irradiated cells, the 4S peak is about three times higher compared to the ligase profile of confluent control cells. The same S values of the enzyme profiles are detected after sucrose gradient sedimentation of MMC-treated and SV40 infected monkey kidney cells: MMC-treatment seems to increase the 4S-peak of enzyme activity profile, whereas SV40-infection increases the 6S peak of enzyme activity (submitted to publication). The possibility exists that, in these experiments, two different ligases could be detected. A tempting hypothesis might be that the heavy form of ligase would be preferentially induced during semiconservative DNA replication, according to the results previously reported by Söderäll [27] and the light form of the enzyme would be induced preferentially during the DNA repair process.

CONCLUSIONS

The analysis of the SOS functions in bacteria has been very fruitful both in terms of fundamental genetic regulation and in terms of research applied to carcinogen detection, since almost all bacterial screening methods are based upon SOS responses in treated-bacteria [34]. At least for these two reasons, the study of inducible functions in mammalian cells opens a new era in terms of fundamental cancer research.

Treatment of mammalian cells with physical or chemical carcinogens gives rise to specific DNA lesions. These lesions are normally repaired by the constitutive repair pathways without important con-

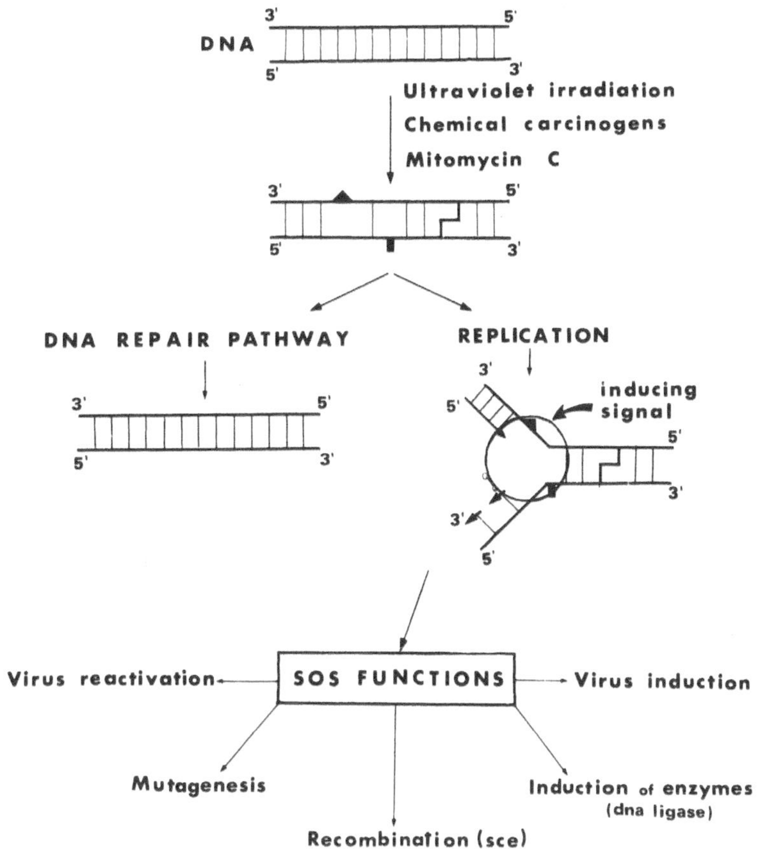

Fig. 4. Hypothetical scheme of SOS function induction in mammalian cells treated with carcinogens.

sequence for the cells (Fig. 4). However, the absence of constitutive excision repair, as it is observed in cells isolated from Xeroderma pigmentosum patient, leads to the accumulation of DNA lesions and subsequently to the appearance of tumors. During the replication of cellular DNA, the presence of residual DNA lesions (especially those induced by the UV-like compounds) constitutes a block to the progression of replication forks. We have hypothesized that such a block could constitute a direct or indirect signal for the activation of some specific cellular functions (Fig. 4). Among these functions, we have shown in this paper evidences for the induction of an error-prone mode of DNA replication and some specific enzymes such as DNA ligases. Other functions seem to be expressed at the same time. For example, induction of mammalian viruses from some transformed cells treated with physical or chemical carcinogens presents a dose-response and a time-course very similar to the error-prone repair pathway induction [35, 36]. The induction of mammalian viruses resembles the bacteriophage induction although the molecular mechanism might be completely different.

Recombination processes have not been clearly studied in somatic mammalian cells yet. Although the use of cytological indicators such as sister chromatid exchanges or chromosomal rearrangements, indicates that physical or chemical carcinogens may activate some kind of recombination event in the treated cell [37], it is clear that blockage of replication forks by DNA lesions constitute a substrate for recombinational processes. Is this mechanism part of the SOS functions?

ACKNOWLEDGMENTS

We thank very much Mrs. A. Benoit and A. Margot for their excellent technical assistance and Dr. S. Nocentini and Dr. H. G. Suarez for providing us the cells from which DNA ligase activity was measured. This work was supported by grants from ATP-DGRST No. A650-7886 (Paris, France), from INSERM No. 77-79-109 (Paris, France) and from the Commission of the European Communities No. B10-E-427-81-F (Brussels, Belgium).

REFERENCES

1. E. M. Witkin, Ultraviolet mutagenesis and inducible DNA repair in *Escherichia coli*, Bacteriol. Rev., 40:869 (1976).
2. M. Radman, SOS repair hypothesis: phenomenology of an inducible DNA repair which is accompanied by mutagenesis, in: "Molecular Mechanism for Repair of DNA," P. C. Hanawalt and R. B. Setlow, eds., Plenum Press, New York (1975).
3. R. Devoret, A. Goze, Y. Moulé, and A. Sarasin, Lysogenic induction and induced phage reactivation by aflatoxin B_1 metabolites, in: "Mécanismes d'altération et de réparation du DNA: relation avec la mutagénèse et la cancérogénèse chimique," R. Daudel, Y. Moulé, and F. Zajdela, eds., C.N.R.S., Paris (1977).
4. M. Defais, P. C. Hanawalt, and A. Sarasin, Viral probes for DNA repair, Adv. in Radiat. Biol., 10 (1982).
5. P. Caillet-Fauquet, M. Defais, and M. Radman, Molecular mechanism of induced mutagenesis, replication *in vivo* of bacteriophage ϕX174 single-stranded, ultraviolet light-irradiated DNA in intact and irradiated host cells, J. Mol. Biol., 117:95 (1977).
6. L. E. Bockstahler, and C. D. Lytle, Ultraviolet light enhanced reactivation of a mammalian virus, Biochem. Biophys. Res. Commun., 41:184 (1970).
7. L. E. Bockstahler and C. D. Lytle, Radiation enhanced reactivation of nuclear replicating mammalian viruses, Photochem. Photobiol., 25:477 (1977).

8. A. Sarasin and P. C. Hanawalt, Carcinogens enhance survival of UV-irradiated Simian Virus 40 in treated monkey kidney cells: Induction of a recovery pathway? Proc. Natl. Acad. Sci. USA, 75:346 (1978).
9. A. Sarasin, Induced DNA repair processes in eucaryotic cells, Biochimie, 60:1141 (1978).
10. C. D. Lytle, Radiation-enhanced virus reactivation in mammalian cells, J. Natl. Cancer Instit. Monograph., 50:145 (1978).
11. M. Günther, R. Wicker, S. Tiravy, and J. Coppey, Enhanced survival of ultraviolet-damaged parvovirus Lu III and Herpes virus in carcinogen pretreated transformed human cells, in: "Chromosome Damage and Repair," E. Seeberg, ed., Plenum Press, New York (1981).
12. J. Rommelaere, J. M. Vos, J. J. Cornelis, and D. C. Ward, UV-enhanced reactivation of Minute-Virus-of-Mice: stimulation of a late step in the viral cycle, Photochem. Photobiol., 33:845 (1981).
13. C. D. Lytle, J. Coppey, and W. D. Taylor, Enhanced survival of ultraviolet-irradiated Herpes simplex virus in carcinogen-pretreated cells, Nature, 272:60 (1978).
14. S. M. D'Ambrosio and R. B. Setlow, Defective and enhanced postreplication repair in classical and variant Xeroderma pigmentosum cells treated with N-acetoxy-2-acetyl-aminofluorene, Cancer Res., 38:1147 (1978).
15. J. Tooze, "DNA tumor viruses," Cold Spring Harbor Laboratory, Cold Spring Harbor (1980).
16. P. Tegtmeyer and H. L. Ozer, Temperature-sensitive mutants of Simian virus 40: infection of permissive cells, J. Virol., 8:516 (1971).
17. A. Sarasin, C. Gaillard, and A. Benoit, Molecular mechanism of error-prone DNA replication induced in UV-irradiated or acetoxy-acetyl-aminofluorene treated monkey cells, J. Supramol. Struct. Cell. Biochem., 5:203 (1981).
18. C. J. Lai and D. Nathans, A map of temperature-sensitive mutants of simian virus 40, Virology, 66:70 (1975).
19. P. Chambon, The molecular biology of the eukaryotic genome is coming of age, Cold Spring Harbor Quant. Biol., 42:1209 (1977).
20. A. Sarasin and A. Benoit, Induction of an error-prone mode of DNA repair of UV-irradiated monkey kidney cells, Mutation Res., 70:71 (1980).
21. A. Sarasin, C. Gaillard, and J. Feunteun, Induced mutagenesis of simian virus 40 in carcinogen-treated monkey cells, in: "Induced Mutagenesis: Molecular Mechanisms and their Implications for Environmental Protection," C. W. Lawrence, L. Prakash, and F. Sherman, eds., Plenum Press, New York, in press.
22. D. Lackey, S. W. Krauss, and S. Linn, Isolation of an altered form of DNA polymerase I from *Escherichia coli* cells induced for recA/lexA functions, Proc. Natl. Acad. Sci. USA, 79:330 (1982).
23. S. Söderhäll and T. Lindhal, DNA ligases of eukaryotes, FEBS Lett., 67:1 (1976).

24. J. E. Cleaver, "Advances in Radiation Biology," J. T. Lett, H. Adler, and M. Zeller, eds., Academic Press, New York (1974).
25. C. Pauling and L. Himm, DNA ligase mutants of *E. coli*, Proc. Natl. Acad. Sci. USA, 60:1595 (1967).
26. K. A. Nasmyth, Temperature-sensitive lethal mutants in the structural gene for DNA ligase in the yeast Schizosaccharomyces pombe, Cell, 12:1109 (1977).
27. S. Söderhäll, DNA ligases during rat liver regeneration, Nature, 260:640 (1976).
28. K. Tsukada, Changes in polynucleotide ligase during rat liver regeneration, Biochem. Biophys. Res. Commun., 57:758 (1974).
29. P. Beard, Polynucleotide ligase in mouse cells infected by polyoma virus, Biochim. Biophys. Acta, 269:385 (1972).
30. S. Spadari, Purification and properties of polynucleotide ligase in HeLa cells infected with Herpes simplex virus, Nucl. Acids Res., 3:2155 (1976).
31. S. Söderhäll and T. Lindhal, Mammalian DNA ligases: serological evidence for two separate enzymes, J. Biol. Chem., 250:8438 (1975).
32. M. Mezzina and S. Nocentini, DNA ligase activity in UV-irradiated monkey kidney cells, Nucl. Acids Res., 5:4317 (1978).
33. S. Nocentini and M. Mezzina, Effectsof ultraviolet irradiation of DNA ligase activity of human fibroblasts from normal and Xeroderma pigmentosum donors, in: "Chromosome Damage and Repair," E. Seeberg, ed., Plenum Press, New York (1981).
34. R. Devoret, Bacterial tests for potential carcinogens, Scientific American, 241:40 (1979).
35. G. B. Zamansky, L. F. Kleinman, P. H. Black, and J. C. Kaplan, Reactivation of Herpes simplex virus in a cell line inducible for simian virus 40 synthesis, Mutation Res., 71:1 (1980).
36. L. E. Bockstahler, Induction and enhanced reactivation of mammalian viruses by light, Prog. Nucl. Acid Res. Mol. Biol., 26: 303 (1981).
37. A. Gentil, Effects of tumor promoters on sister chromatid exchange, in: "Sister chromatid exchanges," Alan R. Liss, New York, in press (1982).

RADIATION-INDUCED TRANSFORMATION IN RODENT AND HUMAN CELLS: ASSAY SYSTEMS AND USES IN RISK ESTIMATES

Carmia Borek

Radiation Research Laboratory and
Department of Pathology
Columbia University, College of Physicians and Surgeons
New York, NY 10032

INTRODUCTION

In recent years public concern has focussed on the hazards of low dose radiation, at the levels of 0.1 to 1.0 rad. This is a dose level involved in public exposure from nuclear installation as well as from medical diagnostic x-rays. While radiation is a weak carcinogen and mutagen compared to some chemicals it is the most ubiquituous and measurable at low doses.

Chemicals which pervade the environment are also a source of great concern. Epidemiological studies as well as data from experimental animals clearly indicate that cancer incidence is greatly influenced by environmental factors including diet (Doll and Peto 1981). Thus, we aim to detect the various factors which present potential biological hazards, to identify them and prevent their influence. We also endeavor to find means to inhibit their action, at early stages when possible, to eliminate the irreversible process of initiation as well as at later stages where expression and promotional events take place in the classic multistage carcinogenesis process (Berenblum 1978).

While much of our knowledge on cancer causing agents and cancer risk estimates comes from epidemiology and animal data (Doll and Peto 1981), these sources have their limitations in studies at low dose levels. Human data cannot supply the information and inordinately large numbers of the animals are required to evaluate the effects of low doses. In addition, efforts to elucidate the cellular and molecular mechanisms underlying the process of carcinogenesis are limited by the complex homeostatic conditions which prevail *in vivo*.

The development of cell culture systems has made it possible to study the effects of chemicals and radiation under defined conditions. Using in vitro systems free of host mediated influences one is afforded the opportunity to assess qualitatively and quantitatively dose related and time dependent interactions of radiation and chemicals with single cells. One can study the modifying influences of agents present in the cellular milieu at genetic level as well as on gene expression, and one can also evaluate the role of cell-cell interaction in the process of neoplastic development.

CELL TRANSFORMATION IN VITRO

Cell transformation in vitro was first suggested by Alexis Carel in 1925, however, the direct oncogenic effects of chemicals was demonstrated in 1962 in the hamster cell system by Berwald and Sachs, and in 1966 Borek and Sachs first reported the direct oncogenic effect of x-rays by exposing diploid hamster embryo cells to 300 rad of x-rays and transforming a fraction of them (Fig. 1). The transformed cells gave rise to tumors upon injection into hamsters while untreated cells showed no spontaneous transformation (Borek and Sachs 1966, 1967, 1968). The work indicated that in order to fix radiation transformation as a hereditary property, cell divisions must take place soon after exposure and that subsequent additional replications are required for expression of the neoplastic state. The studies also indicated that there exists among cells a differential physiologic and genetic competence to be transformed and that surface mediated cell recognition was modified in culture upon transformation.

Transformation of mammalian cells in vitro by radiation was later approached in mouse cell systems (Terzaghi and Little 1976a, 1976b, Han and Elkind 1979, Miller and Hall 1978) and in human cells (Borek 1980) making it possible to evaluate the effects of radiation on cells across the lines of various species.

Cell systems currently used in radiation transformation studies are similar to those used with chemicals (Borek 1979, 1982) and are comprised of fibroblast-like cells, where morphological criteria serve well in quantitative assays of transformation. Since in man the preponderance of carcinomas over sarcomas is unequivocal there is a constant and urgent need to develop epithelial cultures to study transformation. A number of epithelial cell systems have been developed and used in studies on chemically induced transformation (reviewed in Borek 1979, 1981, 1982) but so far not applied to studies in radiation carcinogenesis. There is a particular uniformity in fibroblast-like cells which does not exist in epithelial cells whose nature and susceptibility to radiation transformation may depend on the particular differentiated qualities and the source and age of tissue from which they are

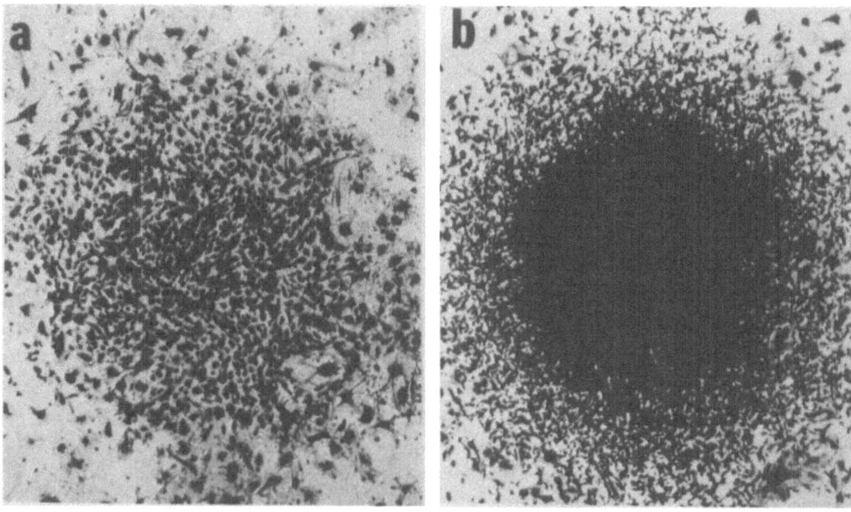

Fig. 1. 1a. An 8 day colony of normal hamster embryo cells. 1b. An 8 day colony of x-ray transformed hamster embryo cells. (Giemsa X 125).

derived. Human as well as animal data have clearly indicated that in radiation carcinogeneses latency, age dependence and specific organ susceptibility determine the frequency of cancer. A further difficulty with epithelial cells arises from the fact that criteria for early stages in the neoplastic state of epithelial cells are expressed phenotypically in a less consistent manner than in fibroblasts (Borek 1979, 1982).

Among the fibroblast lines there are two main cell systems in radiogenic transformation studies.

(a) Primary Cultures and Cell Strains

Primary cells are fresehly derived from animal or the human tissue. They are direct descendents of the cells *in situ* and consist of diploid cells. These cultures have a finite life span which differs from one cell type to another and is related to the longevity of the species from which they originate.

The primary cultures which are used most commonly in radiation transformation studies are those of mixed cell populations derived from hamster embryo cells (Borek and Sachs 1966, Borek and Hall 1973). The advantage of these cultures lies in the fact that they are comprised of normal diploid cells. They senesce upon continuous subculture allowing "immortal" transformants to emerge against a background of dying cells thus confirming *in vitro* their distinct transformed state. Cell survival and cell transformation can be scored simultaneously in the same dishes and the rate of spontaneous transformation in these cells is less than 10^{-6}.

Expression time for transformation is 8-10 days, a relatively short period of time. Transformed colonies are identifiable by dense multilayered cells, random cellular arrangement and haphazard cell-cell orientiation accentuated at the colony edge (Fig. 1). Normal counterparts are usually flat, with an organized cell to cell orientation. Because of the mixed population of cells there exist untransformed cells which may possess a higher cell density than the usual flat colonies. These however do not exhibit the randomness at the colony edge described above.

Human primary cultures used in radiation transformation studies are fibroblasts derived from adult human skin (Kakunaga 1978, Borek 1980), human embryos (Sutherland 1980) or foreskin (Milo and DiPaolo 1978, Silinkas et al. 1981). The assay is growth in agar or a focus assay where the loss of cell density inhibition among the transformed fibroblasts renders them capable of proliferating over the untrans - formed sheets of cells thus forming distinct recognizable foci (Fig. 2).

(b) Established Cell Lines

Established cell lines possess an unlimited life span. They represent cell population which originated as primary cultures. Following a continuous and meticulously timed regime of subculturing a selected population emerged which had undergone a "crisis" enabling the cells to grow indefinitely at a constant rate. The karyotype of these cells is usually characterized by various chromosomal rearrangements and heteroploidity. Often, these cell lines are cloned and the cloned cells are further propagated into large populations. An example of cell lines which have been used extensively in transformation studies are the Balb 3T3 cell line (Todaro and Green 1963) and the C3H 10T½ clone 8 cell line (Reznikoff et al. 1973). Both cell lines originated from mouse embryos. They are transformable by a variety of oncogenic agents and used extensively in radiation transformation studies. The advantage of these systems lies in the fact that they are "immortal" and one can continuously utilize particular cell passage by maintaining "banks" of frozen cells. The disadvantages are that the cells are not diploid, and if not treated meticulously as originally described they can give rise at high passage to spontaneous transformants. Transformation assay is a focus assay thus survival must be scored in separate sets of dishes. In the C3H 10T½ system three types of transformed foci are identifiable (Reznifoff et al. 1973b), types I, II and III. Their morphology can be related to their oncogenic potential, type III being the most malignant.

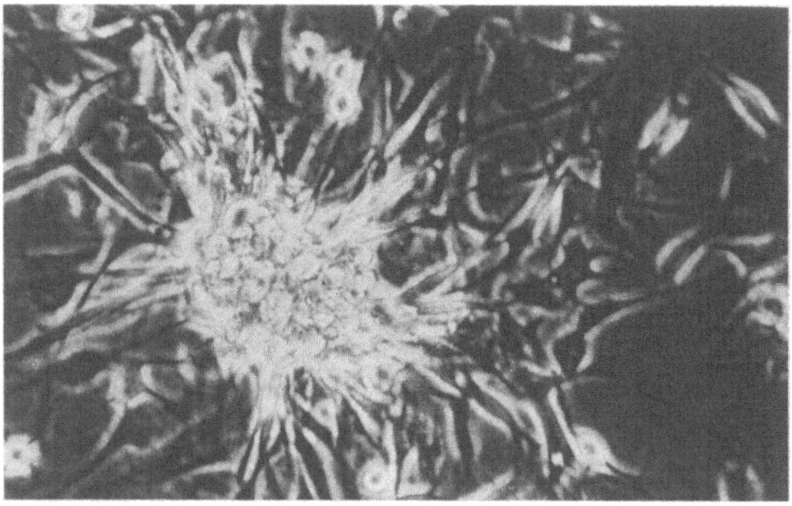

Fig. 2. A focus of x-ray transformed human fibroblasts.

(c) IN UTERO - IN VITRO Systems

Here exposure to radiation is carried out in utero and the tissues are cultured and assayed for transfromation in vitro (Borek et al. 1977).

INITIATION AND PHENOTYPIC EXPRESSION OF TRANSFORMATION

One of the basic conundrums in cancer research evolves from our inability at the present time to unequivocally distinguish primary events associated with initiation of neoplastic transformation from those which function as secondary events. While we aim to identify the process of initiation and consequently hope to modulate it, we are faced with the fact that at present we determine the occurance of initiation by its phenotypic expression. Thus, although radiation carcinogenesis was recognized some 85 years ago we are still relatively ignorant of the mechanisms involved and must judge the events determining neoplastic transformation by a variety of phenomena associated with the neoplastic phenotype. These phenomena appear to be similar irrespective of the initiation oncogenic agent; whether it is a virus whose contribution is the introduction of new genetic material, a chemical carcinogen forming aducts with cellular DNA or radiation, whose initiating action on the cell is established and over within a fraction of a second.

We therefore strive at defining various steps within the processes of transformation and try to associate cellular and molecular events with each step.

A. Sequence of Events in Transformation IN VITRO

a) Initiation i.e. exposure of cultured cells to the carcinogen.

b) Fixation of the transformed state requiring cell replication within hours after initiation (Borek and Sachs 1966, 1967, 1968. Reznikoff et al. 1973b, Terzaghi and Little 1976a, Kakunaga 1974, 1975, Little 1979).

c) Expression of the transformed state of a single cell requiring several cell replications depending on the cell type. The results are the growth of a focus or a colony (depending on the assay), which in fibroblasts and some epithelial cells are morphologically distinct from control (Berwald and Sachs 1963, Borek and Sachs 1966, 1967, 1968, Reznikoff et al. 1973b, Kakunaga 1974, 1975, Little 1979). It should be added that there is little information on the neoplastic characteristic of exposed fibroblasts which do not differ morphologically from the normal. So far, the assessment of the transformed state in fibroblasts has consistently adhered to the premise that the earliest observable phenotypic change in the process of transformation is morphological.

B. Methods Used for Transformation Studies

a) Exposure of mass cultures to radiation or other oncogenic agents and continuous subculturing for several weeks or months until transformed cells are selected out and form foci. Periodic clonings are made to assess the frequency of transformation (Borek and Sachs, 1966, 1967).

b) Treatment of mass cultures and cloning out at various periods of time after exposure. Transformation can then be scored in a colony or focus assay (Borek 1980).

c) Treatment of single cells seeded at a low density clonal level. Each cell is then allowed to proliferate into a distinct clone. Cultures are fixed and stained. Transformed clones are distinguished morphologically from normal by high cell density and random cell orientation. This method is used routinely in quantitative studies and has been applied in the hamster system (Borek and Hall 1973) where incubation time is 8-10 days.

d) Treatment of single cells seeded at low density. Cells are allowed to proliferate to high density. Transformed cells form foci clearly distinct against a background of flat density-inhibited cells. The characteristics of the foci are high cell density as well as randomness of cell organization especially in the peripheral area of the focus invading into the surrounding area. Incubation time for the appearance of these foci ranges from 4 to 8 weeks depending on the cells employed. The method is widely used, for the 3T3 and 10T½ transformation assays (4-6 weeks incubation time, respectively) (Reznikoff et al. 1973b, Terzaghi and Little 1976a, Miller and Hall 1978, Little 1979) and can be applied in human transformation studies where incubation is approximately 8 weeks (Borek 1980).

C. Criteria For Transformation

The establishment of criteria for transformation is based on the characterization of transformed cells as compared to their untransformed parental cells. These studies utilize mass cultures of mixed cell populations as well as cultures propagated from single isolated clones. Most of the characteristics associated with the transformed state of fibroblasts hold true for epithelial cells though in the latter case less consistency is observed (Borek 1979, 1982).

DNA and Chromosomes

Since in the case of ionizing radiation no specific DNA repair enzymes have been identified, in mammalian cells exploration of the effects of radiation on transformation at the level of DNA damage and repair and at a chromosomal level is a study of associated phenomena. This is especially true since the frequency of transformation is low, so that the relationship of chromosomal changes or DNA damage and repair, carried out on parallel cultures, can be inferred but not conclusively stated.

Once one has observed a morphologically changed colony or focus one can then explore with more certainty the relationship between the karyotypic alteration and the phenotypic expression of the cells, though admittedly one can evaluate the neoplastic nature of these cells only later when progressive culture has taken place and most probably karyotypic changes. Another critical factor in studying chromosomal changes associated with transformation is the starting material. The utilization of diploid cultures in the study may differ from the study of heteroploid cell lines where chromosomal imbalance has already taken its course.

While subtle chromosomal alterations following exposure to radiation may denote genetic rearrangements and instability (Kinsella and Radman 1978) which may be associated with transformation, no changes in chromosomal number or in banking patterns have been observed in diploid hamster or human cells studied within several passages after initiation and expression of transformation, i.e. at early stages after having expressed other criteria associated with their transformed state (Borek et al. 1977, 1978, DiPaolo and Donovan 1973, Borek 1980).

Loss of "Contact Inhibition" and Changes in Cell Topography

The most obvious phenotypic changes observed in transformed fibroblasts are mediated via the cell surface. A loss of contact inhibition of movement and replication reduced density dependent inhibition, irregular growth patterns and ability to grow in multilayers represent features which characterize the transformed nature of fibroblasts derived from solid tissue and differentiate them from normal counterparts grown under the same conditions.

These morphological differences so distinct in dense populations of cells are not apparent at low density when cells are not in contact with one another. Changes at a single-cell level can be found when cell topography is evaluated using scanning electronmicroscopy (Borek and Fenoglio 1976). At early stages, following initiation, within 8 days after exposure to radiation and expression of transformation the relatively smooth and simple surface of normal hamster fibroblasts acquires a variety of excrescences and a marked cellular pleomorphism (Fig. 3). These topographic changes comprising of ruffles and blebs are present on the transformed cell surfaces throughout the cell cycle and remain as an integral part of the transformed cell after many years of culture. The normal parental cells exhibited these complex features only during mitosis (Borek and Fenoglio 1976) thus affirming other observations indicating that a variety of membrane associated properties characteristic of the neoplastic state are found in normal cells in mitosis (see Borek 1979).

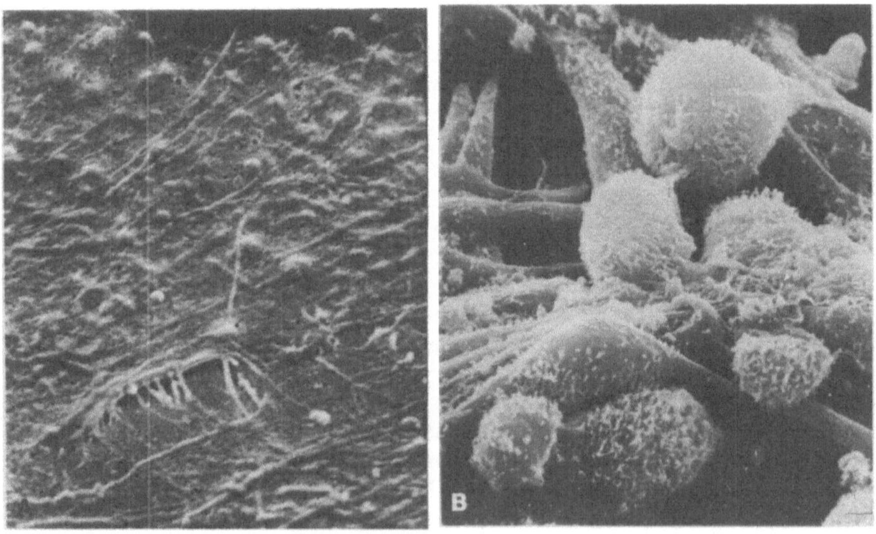

Fig. 3. Scanning electron microscopy of normal (3a) and x-ray transformed (3b) hamster embryo cells. Note the flat adherent normal cells in contrast to the polymorphism and abundant surface features of the neoplastic cells.

C. Decreased Serum and Calcium Dependence

Once rodent fibroblasts are initiated by radiation as well as other oncogenic agents and undergo several replications to express their transformed state their dependence on nutrients decreases and they are capable of proliferating well in medium containing low serum concentrations, as low as 1% serum, while their untransformed counterparts remain essentially in the non-proliferating state (Borek et al. 1977). This feature which serves well in selecting out low frequency transformants from a background of normal cells holds true for rodent cells but not necessarily for human fibroblasts where some normal as well as the transformants grow at low serum concentrations (Borek 1980). Low calcium dependence namely the ability to proliferate in medium containing less than 0.5% calcium seems to be a feature common to transformed fibroblasts and epithelial cells of rodent origin (Swierenga et al. 1978) as well as transformed human fibroblasts (Borek 1980). In all cases it has served as a selective feature for transformants since normal cells die within days after exposure to maintenance medium containing low calcium while the transformed cells thrive and can form distinct foci (Borek 1980).

D. Membrane Structural Changes

The cell membrane is a complex dynamic organelle which is thought to exert control over a variety of cellular patterns of behavior (Puck 1977, Nielson and Puck 1980). This control system may function by the coordination of interacting molecules of both surface receptors and submembranous fibrilar elements. This control appears to be transmembraneous in nature in extricably related to the structure of the cell membrane and to the molecular features of its surface receptors. These are glycolipids and glycoproteins which traverse the matrix of the membrane as integral membrane proteins. Their glycosylated portions project into the cytoplasm where a number of interactions with cytoplasmic components such as cytoskeletal elements take place and can be affected by antimitotic drugs, horomes and cyclic AMP (Puck 1977).

Upon neoplastic transformation the cell membrane undergoes a variety of structural and functional changes (for review see Borek 1982). Neoantigens are observed, glycoproteins decrease, disappear or are no longer completely glycosylated similarly sialoglycolipids (gangliosides), a major group of membrane glycolipids are incompletely glycosylated showing a reduction in higher gangliosides Na/K ATPase, a Na transport membrane associated enzyme is altered. Intercellular communication is modified (Borek et al. 1969). Some fibroblasts and epithelial cells acquire an enhanced sensitivity to undergo agglutination following exposure to low levels of plant lectins (Borek et al. 1973) in contrast to the normal counterparts which exhibit this property in mitosis or following trypsinization.

E. Proteolytic Enzymes Produced by Transformed Cells

The amount of proteases produced by transformed fibroblasts depends on the origin of the cells studied and must be related to the production of these proteases by the untransformed counterparts. Such proteases include the plasminogen activator (Unkeless et al. 1973) which can be identified at a clonal level using an overlay agar method (Jones et al. 1975) as well as other proteases including a series of acid hydrolases (Borek 1977). Thus, while radiation transformed hamster embryo cells exhibit an increased level of plasminogen activator (Borek et al. 1977) and a serine protease MIF factor (Borek 1979) an examination of 15 different acid hydrolazes indicated that only acid phosphatases were elevated in the radiation transformed cells (Borek et al. 1977).

F. Growth in Agar

Agar suspension assays as a selective assay for transformed cells was first applied to virally transformed cells (MacPherson and Montagnier 1964). The underlying premise is the observation that normal cells derived from solid tissues cannot proliferate in suspension or in semi-solid medium such as agar or methylcellulose. Thus, the acquisition of the ability to grow in semi-solid medium following exposure to oncogenic agents including radiation has been associated with the neoplastic state of the transformed cells for both rodent fibroblasts and epithelial cells (Borek 1979) as well as for human cells transformed in vitro (Borek 1980, Kakunaga 1978, Sutherland et al 1980, Silinkas et al. 1981, Milo and DiPaolo 1978).

While the growth in agar is an accepted criterion for transformation and considered to be closely associated with the malignant potential of the cells, one can find instances whereby transformed cells did not grow in agar yet gave rise to tumors (Borek and Sachs 1966) and others of both rodent and human origin which grew in agar yet did not give rise to tumors (Borek 1980).

Thus, growth in agar or on agar (Borek 1980) can be used as a selective criterion for transformation when the employed conditions are minimal, namely they do not favor the growth of normal counterparts. To evaluate the neoplastic nature of the cells in an unequivocal way the innoculation of transformed cells into appropriate hosts should be carried out in conjunction with growth in agar.

G. Tumorogenicity

The Ultimate and unequivocal demonstration of malignancy is the induction of tumors in syngeneic inbred hosts or in immunosuppressed animals. In the case of human cell transformation the animal of choice is the immunologically crippled nude mouse nu/nu (Kakunaga 1978, Milo and DiPaolo 1978, Borek 1980, Sutherland et al. 1980, Silinkas et al. 1981). Since radiation transformation studies utilize fibroblasts the injection of transformed cells gives rise to sarcomas with different degrees of differentiation. It is of interest to note that when hamsters were irradiated in Utero and the embryos cultured in vitro the transformed lines which arose were capable of inducing both sarcomas and carcinomas (Borek et al. 1977) indicating that while the neoplastic epithelial cells were not visible in culture they developed in the host as epithelial tumors.

RADIATION ONCOGENESIS IN VITRO

Though the various criteria for transformation have been dealt with in the above section, the following will summarize these criteria as they have been utilized by various investigators in radiation oncogenesis studies.

1. THE ONCOGENIC EFFECTS OF SPARSELY IONIZING RADIATION

a) Single Dose Effects

1) Neoplastic Transformation of Diploid Cell Studies

The successful induction of neoplastic cell transformation in vitro by x-rays was first reported by Borek and Sachs (1966). Short term primary cultures derived from midterm golden hamster embryos were used as the source of normal cells. Mass cultures were irradiated with 300 rad and subcultured at low density three days later onto rat feeder layers. Further progressive subculturing without feeders of both irradiated and controls resulted in senescence in control cultures, and a gradual enhancement of mitotic rate in the x-irradiated cells. Within three to four weeks after exposure foci of fusiform cells began to pile up and over - took the culture. Quantitative evaluation of this transformation event was carried out by irradiating mass cultures and cloning them out immediately. Results showed an 0.7-0.8% transformation in the treated cultures and no observable transformants in the controls ($<10^{-6}$). It is of interest to note that transformability of the embryonic cells by x-rays declined with cell passage in vitro and at passage 3 to 4 no transformation was observed following irradiation with 300 rad (Borek and Sachs 1967). The ability of the transformed cells to grow in agar was tested as well as their ability to form tumors in six week old hamsters.

Subsequent studies to ascertain conditions and requirements for x-ray induced transformation indicated that one to two cell replications were required for the fixation of the transformed state (Borek 1967). Replication had to take place within 24 hrs. after exposure of log phase cultures to x-rays. Irradiation of mass cultures and trypsinization soon after gave similar results. Inability to divide resulted in a loss of fixation of the transformed state (Borek and Sachs 1967, 1968). This was indicated by maintaining cultures at plateau phase in liquid holding for 24 to 72 hrs. post irradiation. Transformation rate following trypinization of these cultures declined progressively. The frequency of transformation was inversely proportional to the length of time of maintenance in plateau phase. Loss of fixation was inhibited by maintaining the plateau phase cells at 25°C for 24 to 72 hrs. When cells were cloned after liquid holding at low temperature transformation frequency was fully restored (Borek and Sachs 1967). This suggested that repair mechanisms were involved in the loss of fixation and that maintenance at low temperatures where repair was slowed prevented this loss. Further experiments indicated that expression of transformation could occur within two days after treatment. Irradiation of cloned cells at different stages of growth resulted in partial clonal transformation whose expression was related to the number of days in culture (Borek and Sachs 1967). Once cells were transformed by x-rays they acquired specific surface properties which were characteristic to every transformed line individually derived. Thus, cells transformed at different times by x-rays were incapable of proliferating over other x-ray transformed cell lines as well as upon various chemically and virally transformed cell lines (Borek and Sachs 1966).

Surface mediated changes following radiogenic transformation were also indicated by the loss of intercellular communication in some x-ray transfomed hamster embryo lines, as measured by ionic movement via permeable membrane junctions (Borek et al. 1969) and in modification of cellular gangliosides (Brady et al.1969, Borek et al. 1977).

The first dose response for radiation induced <u>in vitro</u> transformation was shown by Borek and Hall (1973) using the hamster clonal cell system. Single cells seeded onto syngeneic feeder cells were exposed 24 hrs. later to x-ray doses ranging from 1 rad to 600 rad. The results shown in Fig. 6 indicated that a transformation incidence per survivor was evident at doses as low as 1 rad and that the frequency rose exponentially with dose from 1 rad up to a plateau of 150 to 300 rad. At higher doses radiation toxicity appeared to be a competing factor in these asynchronmous mixed cell populations and transformation rate declined. Current ongoing experiments using the same system indicate that cell transformation can be detected at doses as low as 0.3 rad of x-ryas (fig. 4) and that at low doses the effectiveness of x-rays per rad in producing transformation is about twice as high as that induced by ^{60} Cobalt γ rays (Borek et al., in preparation), a fact predicted on

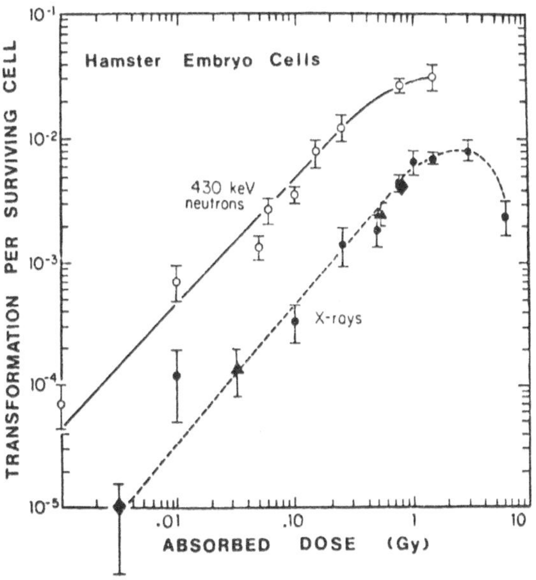

Fig. 4. Dose response curve for cell transformation by x-rays and neutrons.

microdosimetric grounds and of important implications in radiation protection. When transformed clones were isolated and propagated they were tested for their agglutinability by 20 μg/ml of concanavalin A, for their ability to grow in 0.33% agar and for their malignant potential in animals. Positive results served as an affirmation of the neoplastic potential of the isolated cells (Borek and Hall 1973).

2) Transformation of Established Cell Lines

Utilizing the C3H/10T½ mouse embryo cell line (Reznikoff et al. 1973a) and following the transformation assay described for chemically induced transformation (Reznikoff et al. 1973b), Terzaghi and Little (1976) and Miller and Hall (1978) Han and Elkind (1979) established dose response relationships for these cells.

b) Split Dose Effects

As seen above the ability to directly transform cells *in vitro* by x-rays has enabled detailed quantitiative assessment of radiation effects over a wide range of doses. A logical extention of these studies has been to investigate the influence of the temporal distribution of radiation on transformation, to evaluate the oncogenic potential of radiation delivered as protracted doses or at low dose rates, the types of exposure which are of a continuous concern to man. Some unexpected information was obtained. Borek and Hall in 1974 first reported with the hamster embryo cell system that fractionation of an x-ray dose results in an elevated transformation incidence (Fig.5) In these experiments it was shown that two doses of 25 rad separated by five hours produced more transformation than a single dose of 50 rad. and that two doses of 37.5 rad were much more effective than a single exposure of 75 rad.

Splitting the dose resulted in a 70% enhancement in transformation rate as compared to the same dose delivered as a single exposure but fractionation also produced a sparing effect on cell survival, indicating that cellular mechanisms involved in repair for survival differ from those associated with cell transformation. At higher doses above 200 rad splitting the dose results in enhanced survival and decreased transformation (Borek 1979). Similar results were obtained by Miller and Hall (1978) and Little (1979).

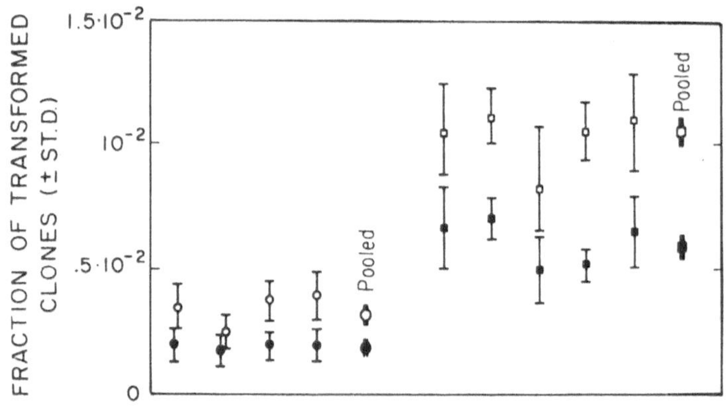

Fig. 5. Incidence of cell transformation following irradiation of hamster embryo cells with single and split doses of x-rays. The consequences of a single dose of 50 rad (●) is compared with 2 doses of 25 rad (O) and the results of 75 rad (■) with 2 doses of 37.5 rad (□).

These results indicate that the use of linear interpolation from high to low dose levels may lead to cancer risk estimates that are neither conservative nor prudent depending on the distribution of the dose in time.

2. HAMSTER CELLS INITIATION IN UTERO AND ASSAY IN VITRO

The available data on the subject of in utero carcinogenesis are sparse (Storer 1975). Experiments conducted by Borek et al. (1977) set out to compare transformation incidence in hamster embryo cells exposed in utero to 300 rad and then cultured in vitro immediately with those of embryos cultured in vitro and later exposed to the same dose radiation. The results indicated that transformation incidence induced in utero was tenfold lower than that induced in vitro, thus closer to the frequency of oncogenesis in vivo. One cannot discount modifying effects of various cell populations, and some differences in plating efficiency. However, these striking differences in incidence support some other factors which may be involved, such as host mediation, repair and loss of fixation at high density, inhibition of expression by cell-cell interaction or other influences created by the tissue specific organization on present in vivo. When cells are transformed in vitro they are devoid of tissue specific arrangements, and are able to replicate under conditions where normally they may remain in a non-replicating state. Thus, the in vitro situation may yield an exaggerated rate of transformation since fixation of transformation can be carried out with ease in log phase cultures.

A number of transformed cell lines were developed from these in utero experiments and studied for a variety of properties. The most striking finding was that injection of the mixed populations of transformed cells into hamsters yielded carcinomas as well as sarcomas.While these epithelial transformed embryonic cells went undetected in culture, because of their unaltered morphology they proliferated in the animal to form carcinomas.

THE ONCOGENIC EFFECTS OF NEUTRONS

As an oncogenic agent neutrons are more effective than x-rays . They are also more toxic. The effectiveness in cell transformation is matched by the enhanced killing effect. The importance of neutrons lies in the fact that neutrons are a type of radiation used in therapy as well as being a product of nuclear energy. Using the hamster embryo clonal system Borek 1975 and Borek et al. 1978 reported the induction of cell transformation in vitro following exposure to 430 keV neutrons in the dose range of 0.1 to 150 rad. A 430 keV Van Graaff accelerator was used where protons accelerated onto a tritium source produced the spectrum of neutrons. The angle of the cells with respect to the source determined the neutron energy they received (Borek et al. 1978). The results indicated that while neutrons were much more efficient than x-rays in producing cell transformation they were also more effective in cell killing. Transformation was observed with neutron doses as low as 0.1 rad. It increased exponentially as a function of the dose to 150 rad indicating a much higher frequency than that observed for x-rays. When transformation frequency is expressed as the number of transformants per exposed cell (Fig. 5), and evaluation more closely related to the in vivo situation, both neutrons and x-ray curves rise to the same peak value. Thus, while the RBE for survival varies and is inversely proportional to the square root of the neutron dose, RBE for transformation per exposed cell does not reflect this wide variation. Qualitatively, the hamster cells transformed by neutron did not differ from those transformed by x-rays.

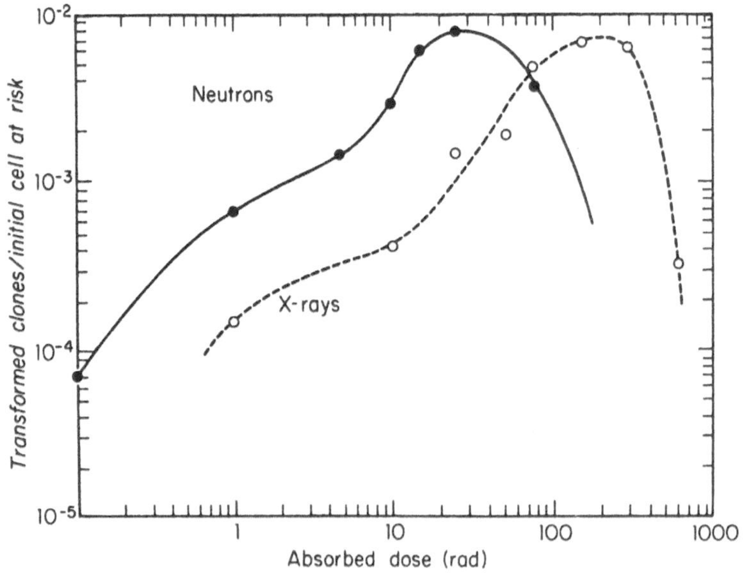

Fig. 6. Dose response relationship for transformation by neutrons or x-rays wherein the number of transformed clones per initial cell at risk is plotted as a function of dose.

HUMAN CELL TRANSFORMATION BY X-RAYS

In 1980 Borek demonstrated the transformation of human skin fibroblasts by 400 rad x-rays into cells which progressed in vitro to malignancy and were able to grow in agar and give rise to tumors when injected into nude mice (Borek 1980). The cells used were a strain of diploid skin fibroblasts, the KD strain, previously used for studies in chemical transformation (Kakunaga 1978). Early passage cells were used and their diploid nature was ascertained by chromosome G banking analysis. Their doubling time is 30-32 hours. Survival curves indicated that survival fraction following a a dose of 400 rad was close to 12% of the total population. No shoulder was observed indicating the different response of the human cells compared to that of the hamster (Borek and Hall 1973). The protocol used for transformation was synthesis between two methods employed for chemically induced human cell transformation, that of Kakunaga (1978), the focus assay, and that of Milo and DiPaolo (1978) where cells were synchronized prior to exposure to the oncogenic agent (Borek 1980).

The protocol took advantage of the following: The cells were quiescent by serum deprivation thus entered a synchronous wave of DNA Synthesis when released from quiescence by medium change. Treatment of the cells at this point enabled the capturing of cells entering S phase. Within 60 to 80 days after treatment foci appeared in treated cultures which were clearly distinguishable from the untreated controls. (Fig. 7) They grew progressively when medium changed to a low calcium medium, the transformed morphology of the foci was enhanced while the normal died within 24 hrs. These clearly distinguishable foci were isolated and propagated in vitro. Chromosome G banding indicated a near diploid range of chromosomes (46-49), saturation density was twofold compared to the normal and the transformed but not the normal were agglutinable by 25 μg/ml of conconavalin A, when seeded into 0.33% agar or grown on agar (0.5% concentration) the KD transformed cells formed colonies. None of the unirradiated or the irradiated but untransformed cells formed colonies in this semisolid medium.

The ultimate proof of the neoplastic nature of the cells transformed in vitro is their ability to form tumors in an appropriate host. Whereas the five transformed lines tested formed colonies in agar, three gave rise within 6 weeks both in irradiated (450 rad) unirradiated nude mice to tumors which have been characterized as a human karyotype.

Cultures which were treated, irradiated but not allowed to replicate more than 4 or 5 times before reaching confluency did not exhibit transformation. This indicated that as in the rodent cells replication is required following radiation for the fixation and expression of the transformed state.

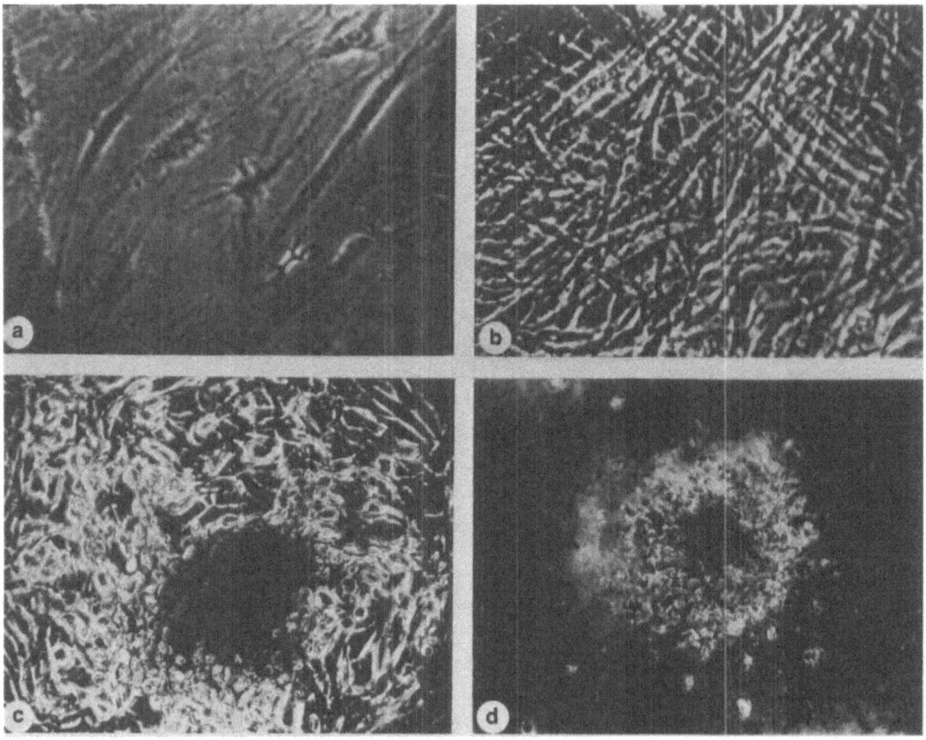

Fig.7. 7a. Normal human KD diploid cells. 7b. The same cells transformed in vitro by 400 rad x-rays. 7c. Cellular morphology of 7b in calcium depleted medium.
7d. Transformed KD cells growing in agar.
Note the flatness of the normal cells (a) in contrast to the criss-cross morphology of the transformed human cell (b) Also note that under conditions of low calcium transformed cells appear as defined foci.

At the present time quantitative assays for human cells transformation are not firmly established, though a number of labs have utilized growth in agar as an assay (Sutherland et al., 1980, Silinkas et al., 1981, Milo and Dipaolo 1978). The correlation between the malignant nature of the cells and their ability to grow in agar is clearly not established. Growth in agar is suggestive of malignancy but not indicative. Another problem with using agar as the sole endpoint for analysis of dose response relationships in transformation studies is the inability to evaluate plating efficiency in agar. For example, do the number of clones growing in agar reflect the total cells which have undergone transformation or does it reflect only a fraction of transformants, those with a higher plating efficiency in this semi-solid medium and an ability to proliferate under those conditions, other transformants having had a better chance to grow into high density cultures and in the animal?

Though the quantitative aspects of x-ray induced human transformation are currently not precise, a number of observations can be stressed. The incidence of transformation in the human cells appears to be much lower than that observed in the rodent cells given the same dose of radiation. While in the human cells the frequency per treated cells is approximately 10^{-6} at 400 rad, a frequency associated with mutational events, rodent cells have significantly higher incidence of 10^{-4} at that dose level. The number of doublings required for the expression of the transformed state of the human cells was approximately 13-15. The longer doubling period of the human cells (30-32 hrs.) compared to that of rodent cells (16 hrs.) may account in part for the increased length of time required to detect morphological transformation in the human diploid cultures as compared to that in diploid rodent cells. Other observations on the transformed human cells can be stressed. a) Initial loss of contact inhibition is not as striking as that seen in rodent cells . b) In contrast to rodent cells the ability to proliferate in medium with low serum (1%) is not confined to the transformed cells; our normal KD cells as well as the transformed proliferated in medium containing low serum . c) The transformed state is associated with membrane changes and as in rodent cells, agglutinability by plant lectins can be used as a distinguishing probe. d) Surface topography in the x-ray transformed human cells is altered but not as dramatically as in the rodent cells. Microvilli found in abudnance on rodent cells were (Borek and Fenoglio 1976) not as abundant in transformed human cells (C. Borek, unpublished).

Currently we cannot yet assess the roles played by growth inhibition and release from this arrest in the process of x-ray induced transformation. Recent experiments indicate that while these steps are not essential for observing transformation, without growth arrest transformation is decreased and latency in appearance of transformed foci is lengthened (as long as four months). A tempting thought is provoked by reports of Woodcock and Cooper (1979). The work indicates that following the inhibition of DNA by certain drugs replication initiates at the same origins. Quiescence by serum deprivation and refeeding (Borek 1980) could lead to similar results. Resulting events may include disproportional DNA replication and gene amplification (Schimke et al. 1981) which may play a role in potentiating the induction of radiogenic transformation and enhancing its frequency.

More recently adult skin fibroblasts from patients with Xeroderma Pigmentosum (Setlow et al. 1969, Cleaver 1969) have been transformed in vitro by UV into anchorage independent cells UVB, a sun lamp type of irradiation, of relevance to human skin carcinogenesis. Single cells were exposed to wavelengths of 280 and 320 nm. Both morphological foci as well as ability to grow in agar were assessed. It appears as mentioned earlier that here too in human cells transformed by UV, ability to grow in agar was exhibited concommitantly with the appearance of foci comprising piled up, randomly oriented cells which were clearly distinguishable morphologically from the flat oriented control cells.

COCARGINOGENS AND MODULATORS OF RADIOGENIC TRANSFORMATION

In Recent years it has become increasingly clear that environmental factors including diet play a crucial role in determining cancer incidence in man (Peto and Doll 1981). While radiation is a weak oncogenic agent compared to some chemicals it is the most universal. Thus, in assessing the effects of radiation from the point of view of cancer risk to man (Beir 1972, Storer 1975, Upton 1975, UNSCEAR 1977, Sinclair 1981) one cannot exclude the possibility that a multitude of genetic, physiological and environmental factors influence cancer incidence initiated by radiation. The difficulty lies in indentifying the carcinogens which act in an additive or synergistic manner. Once recognized measures may be sought to alter exposure to these agents and to find ways to modify their effects and interactions.

In vitro, under defined conditions we can evaluate some of these interactions at a cellular level though admittedly the absence of host mediated effects or intact tissue organization give us a somewhat slanted view. Within the context of the accepted concept of cancer development (Berenblum 1975) one thinks of neoplastic transformation as being comprised of the early phases of initiation and a later stage of expression by which we recognize initiation. Agents that modify expression can interact at early or at later stages serving as promotors. While initiation by radiation is irreversible it can sometimes be prevented (Guernsey, Ong and Borek 1980, Guernsey, Borek and Edelman 1981, Borek 1982). Expression or promotion can be reversed (Borek et al. 1979, Miller et al. 1981, Borek et al. 1981, Kennedy and Little 1978, Borek 1982, 1982a).

1. Enhancement of Transformation

Chemicals

Pre-exposure of hamster embryo cells to x-ray doses of 150 to 250 rad rendered them more responsive to transformation by Benzo (a) pyrene (DiPaolo and Donovan 1976). A synergistic interaction was reported (Borek and Ong 1981) between x-rays and the food pyrolysate product 3 amino-1 methyl-5H-pyriode (4,3-b) indol (Trp-P-2). Isolated in Japan from broiled meat and fish, foods widely consumed there, this compound has been shown to be a mutagen and a carcinogen in vivo and in vitro (Nago and Sugimura 1978). Pre-exposure of hamster embryo cells to 50 or 150 rad of x-rays followed by treatment with Trp-P-2 resulted in an enhanced transformation which was dose dependent indicating a synergistic interaction at 150 rad. The study of the mechanisms of action between these two agents is complex since both x-rays and Trp-P-2 damage DNA and the exposure of the irradiated cells to Trp-P-2 took place within the period of fixation of radiation transformation. The interaction however is of interest. Though we are clearly aware that these are studies in vitro, that the compound is in concentrated form, and that we are not exposed daily to doses of 50 or 150 rad, the fact that these two agents interact is of importance; it further compounds the interpretation of some of the data from Hiroshima and Nagasaki, the largest source of evidence on radiation carcinogenesis.

Enhancing agents can also be of the family of tumor promotors. The most widely studied in conjunction with radiation transformation has been the phorbol ester derivative 12-0-Tetradecanoyl-Phorbol-13 acetate (TPA) (Hecker 1971). Promotors in themselves are considered non-carcinogens and TPA has been considered a classic promotor. In studies on radiation transformation TPA shows an interaction with both chromosomes as well as having an effect on membrane associated enzymes within the same cell system (Borek et al. 1982, Borek 1982a). The enhancement of x-ray induced transformation by TPA has been studied in detail (Kennedy et al. 1978, Miller et al. 1981, Borek et al. 1981).

Antipain (AP) (umazawa et al. 1979) is a protease inhibitor which has been shown to have anticarcinogenic activity (Troll 1976). It's action in vitro on influencing radiation induced transformation has been of dual nature (Borek et al 1979, Geard et al., in press). Antipain potentiated x-ray induced transformation in human (Borek 1980), hamster, and 10T½ mouse cells. When added to the cells prior to radiation it has a protective effect or reduces x-ray induced transformation when added after irradiation (Kennedy and Little 1978, Borek et al. 1979, Geard et al., in press). These dual actions are exerted without any effect on cell survival. The enhancing effects of AP are more pronounced if AP is removed after irradiation as compared to the situation where it is added before and kept on for the duration of the experiment, whereby its protective effect reduces the enhancing actions. The dual activity of AP was not reflected in chromosomal alterations as measured by sister chromatid analysis (Geard et al., in press). AP has been shown by Kinsella and Radman (1980) to modify chromosomal aberration but not SCE. AP had no effect on DNA damage or replication (Borek and Cleaver, 1981).

Clearly, the mechanisms of the protease inhibitors AP call for more inquiry. One can only speculate that the two diametrically opposed actions of AP on transformation are mediated via different mechanisms; some associated with the direct cellular interactions with radiation at which time cascading events could occur as compared to later events when its inhibitory activity acting in a temporal fashion (Borek et al. 1979) may be mediated via an effect on specific cellular proteases.

2. Inhibition of Radiogenic Transformation

While we try to identify agents which act as cocarginogens or promotors we aim at finding compounds or conditions which may inhibit the progression of transformation and even better prevent initiation.

Retnoids

Within the last decade analogs of Vitamin A (retinoids) have been shown to modulate malignancy both in laboratory animals as well as in the clinic (Sporn 1976, Lotan 1980, Peto et al. 1981). Their effectiveness on inhibiting x-ray induced transformation in vitro was first shown using the 10T½ cells (Harisiadis et al. 1978) indicating that these compounds could act in vitro and that their action was not limited to an effect on neoplastic epithelial cells, as previously observed in vivo. The ability of retinoids to inhibit not only x-ray induced transformation but also the enhancement of this transformation by TPA in both 10T½ and hamster embryo cells was reported more recently (Miller et al. 1981), Borek et al. 1981). The effect was striking. Two analogs, β all trans retinoic acid (RA) and trimethyl methoxy phenyl analog of N-ethyl retinamide (TMMP-ERA), were used. Retinoids were present in the medium at the time of irradiation and TPA was added after irradiation to part of the experimental plates. The retinoids were kept in contact with the cells for four days only and thereafter removed with an exchange of medium. TPA was maintained for two weeks (hamster) or six weeks (10½) for the total length of the experiment. Thus, inhibitory action of the retinoids had to be exercised within four days to override the enhancing effect of TPA. The retinoids did indeed inhibit both x-ray transformation and TPA enhancement of this transformation thus indicating that their action on radiogenic transformation takes place within a short time and is irreversible

Studies to evaluate the mechanisms of action indicated that the inhibitory action of retinoids on transformation and on TPA action was not reflected in an inhibition of sister chromatid exchanges (SCE) (Miller et al. 1981, Borek 1981). Radiation enhanced SCE about twofold, TPA caused a slight enhancement of SCE but so did the retinoids. The retinoids inhibited the small enhancement of SCE by TPA. When added after irradiation TPA slightly enhanced the x-ray induced SCE but so did the retinoids to the same degree. When retinoids were present along with x-ray and TPA, a combination which resulted in inhibition of transformation, one observed the highest degrees of SCE enhancement. Thus, the retinoids were not exercising inhibition at the chromosomal levels. Their action was reflected at the membrane level on the membrane associated Na^+ transport enzyme Na^+/K^+ ATPase, but not on Mg^+ ATPase or on 5' nucleotidase (Borek 1982, 1982a). TPA enhanced the level of the enzyme. Retinoids decreased it. When cells were exposed to both agents concommitantly the Na^+/K^+ level returned to control level. Thus the retinoids appear to exercise their effect at the level of gene expression.

Once cells are transformed and exhibit a neoplastic phenotype their membrane Na^+/K^+ ATPase alters (Borek 1982a). It's activity is no longer modulated by either retinoids or TPA.

While the mechanisms of action of the retinoids are not clear the data lend support to the notion that these compounds are effective suppressors of carcinogen induced neoplastic progression. They increase cell adhesion to the plates as well as alter the cellular morpology into fusiform elongated cells. While we considered their action on TPA as an effect on a promotor, we cannot rule out their action on x-ray and TPA as an inhibition of cocarinogensis.

A clear effect to inhibit the synergistic interaction between two oncogenic agents has been reported (Borek 1982). Retinyl acetate was found to inhibit in hamster embryo cells the oncogenic effect of tryptophan pyrolsate 3 amino-1methyl-5 H-pyrido (4, 3-b) indol (Trp-P-2), to suppress radiation transformation and also to markedly inhibit the synergistic interaction between Trp-P-2 and radiation. The inhibitory action by retinoids was exercised within four days in an irreversible manner. The retinoid action to inhibit synergism between x-rays and these pyrolysates is of significance. The potential role in carcinogenesis of food products presents a complex dilemma in terms of assessing the risk to the general public and any agent which may decrease the effectiveness of the carcinogenic action and inhibit synergism and cocarcinogenesis offers hope in prevention especially since retinoids are derivatives of a natural product, vitamin A.

Selenium, a micronutrient and a ubiquitous element in nature, has long been considered a chemopreventive agent though it does possess some carcinogenic action under certain conditions (Griffin 1979). One of its major functions may be related to its role as a co-factor in glutathione peroxidase (Griffin 1979). A recent report (Borek 1982 indicates that selenium inhibits in 10T½ cells both x-ray induced transformation as well as that induced by pyrolysate products and Benzo (a) pyrene. Its effectiveness on radiogenic transformation indicates that its inhibitory action follows a path other than the one thought previously, in relation to chemical carcinogenesis, namely its action to inactivation of the carcinogen. A possibility which seems more plausible is the suggestion that its inhibitory action on radiation transformation is via an interference with the availability of free oxygen radicals which are closely associated with the action of radiation and may be mediating, in part, the oncogenic action of x-rays (Borek and Troll, in press).

The generation of reactive oxygen species in living systems exposed to radiation has long been recognized as well as the protective action by *radical scavengers* (Bacq and Alexander 1955). More recently tumor promotors have been shown to produce free radicals. These include TPA and Teleocydine. Utilizing hamster embryo cells the effects of superoxide dismutase (SOD) and catalase on x-ray induced transformation (300 rad) and its SOD and catalase were added to the cells at seeding, or combined during irradiation and were removed immediately after exposure or at the end of experiment. TPA was used and was added after irradiation and SOD and catalase were kept on (alone or in combination) for the full course of the experiment. The results indicate that SOD, and to a lesser extent catalase, inhibited both x-ray induced transformation (inhibition of 50% by SOD) as well as the TPA enhancing effect, while having a less marked effect in enhancing cell survival. Their effectiveness on lowering x-ray transformation was similar to that exhibited by β all trans retinoic acid and Antipain.

The results suggest that x-ray induced transformation and TPA action may be in part mediated via the action of free radicals. SOD, (which was not detected in the serum used in these experiments) will convert $\bar{O}_2$ to H_2O_2 thus preventing it from forming toxic compounds such as $\bar{O}H_2$, Ocl and singlet oxygen (McCord and Fridovich 1969). The prevailing H_2O_2 which is a substrate for many toxic peroxidases is then converted by catalase into oxygen. The modest action of catalase in reducing transformation rate may be due to the finding that the hamster embryo cells contain a high level of this enzyme, this may be sufficient to convert the toxic H_2O_2.

Though we are relatively ignorant of the mechanisms by which free radicals may influence neoplastic transformation one could speculate that their effect may be mediated via an action involving membrane lipid peroxidation which may result in a cascade of events with cell death and transformation being some of the consequences.

The Role of Thyroid Hormone in Radiation Transformation

Little is known about the cellular and molecular mechanisms involved in the process of initiation and the physiological requirements for the induction of transformation. Recent reports indicate that thyroid hormones play a crucial role in the process of initiation of x-ray induced transformation (Guernsey et al. 1980, 1981, Borek 1981). Experiments conducted using hamster embryo cells as well as the 10T½ cells indicate that while removal of thyroid hormone from serum used in the medium does not modify cell growth rate nor cell survival, the hypothyroid conditions completely inhibit the initiation of transformation by radiation (Guernsey et al. 1980, 1981) as well as chemicals (Borek et al. 1981). In the experiments cells grown in medium containing resin treated serum, which selectively removes triiodothyronin (T_3) and thyroxin (T_4) (Samuels et al. 1979), were considered hypothyroid ($-T_3$)/ Others grown in medium with untreated serum were fortified with 10^{-7}M T_3 were hyperthyroid ($-T_4$). When both types of cells were irradiated (300 or 400 rad) under these three conditions no transformation was observed in the (T_3-) cells while euthyroid and hyperthyroid showed neoplastic transformation (Fig.8). When T_3 was added to the hypothyroid medium prior to irradiation transformation was observed.

A dose related role of T_3 in the transformation process was illustrated by the fact that when T_3 was added to the hypothyroid milieu, prior to irradiation at doses of 10^{-12}M to 10^{-7}M, transformation incidence was T_3 dose dependent (Fig. 9). The action of T_3 was specific to the active hormone and was not mimicked by reverse T_3, an inactive isomer. The involvement of thyroid hormone in initiation of transformation was further indicated by the fact that maximum transformation was achieved when T_3 was added at least 12 hours prior to irradiation (Fig. 10). If added at the time of radiation, transformation was dramatically decreased and if added after radiation no transformation was observed. The activity of T_3 when added prior to irradiation was exercised within 24 hours and its removal after radiation had no effect in reducing transformation.

The action of T_3 in transformation was inhibited by cyclohexamide, no transformation was observed when 100 ng/ml of cyclohexamide were added along with T_3 at 12 hours prior to

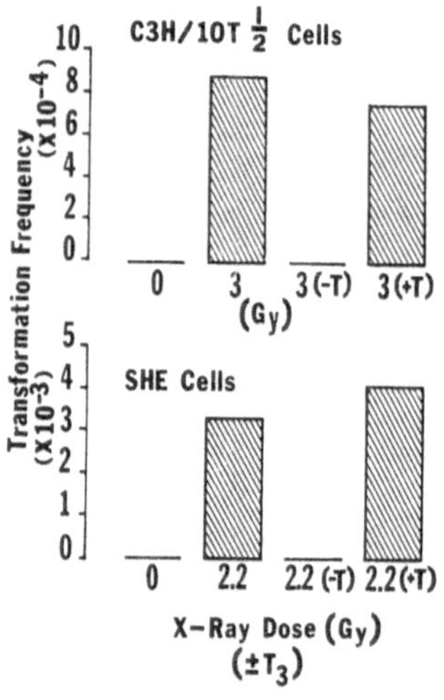

Fig. 8. Histogram relating inhibition of radiation induced transformation by maintaining cells under hypothyroid conditions ($-T_3$). Prior and during irradiation. In cells maintained under euthyroid conditions and hyperthyroid ($+T_3$) radiation induced transformation.

irradiation and removed 24 hours after exposure. This suggested that active protein synthesis is required for the T_3 effect in x-ray induced initiation. A further indication of protein synthesis involvement in the process of T_3 effect is seen by the fact that the induction of Na^+/K^+ ATPase, an enzyme inducible by T_3, is related to T_3 dose in a similar manner as the T_3 dose dependent x-ray induced transformation. These and the fact that a 12 hour preincubation with T_3 results in the highest transformation

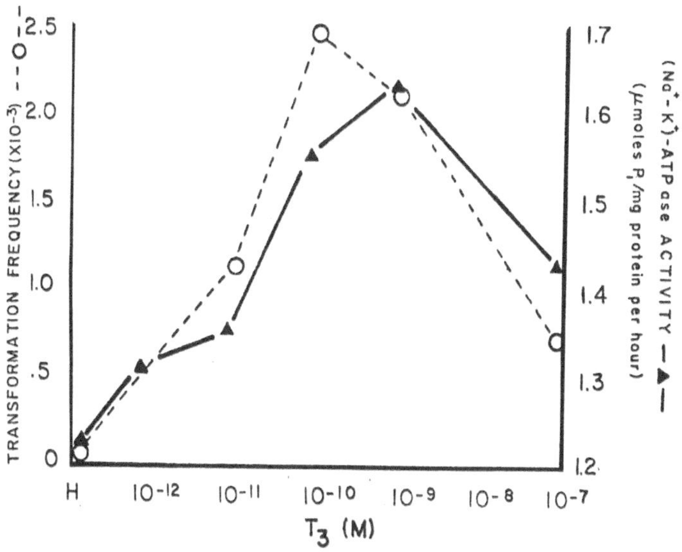

Fig. 9. The effect of various triiodothyronine (T_3) on transformation rate (-0-) Na/K ATPase.

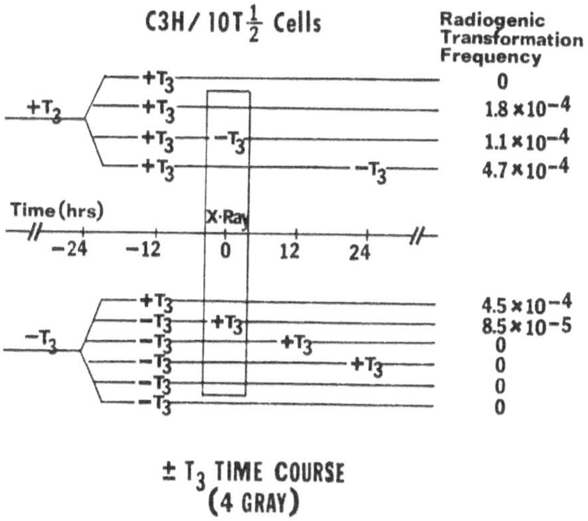

Fig. 10. Time course relating exposure of cells at different time prior to and after irradiation to media devoid of triiodethyroine ($-T_3$) as well as supplemented with T_3 ($+T_3$) maxiumum transformation is observed when T_3 is added 12 hrs. prior to irradiation and no transformation if added after irradiation.

rate suggest the possibility that T3 is inducing the synthesis of a specific "transforming protein" involved in initiation and this is currently being pursued.

These results are the first demonstration at a cellular level that a specific hormone plays a crucial role in the initiation of transformation. They indicate the importance of the cellular milieu in influencing cellular competence to transformation and invite a wide range of investigations to assess the role of other physiological agents in the processes of oncogenesis. Current research indicated that thyroid hormone plays a crucial role in chemically induced transformation (Borek et al., in preparation) and that under hypothyroid condition, no transformation by Benzo (a) pyrene is observed (Borek 1882a) (Fig. 11).

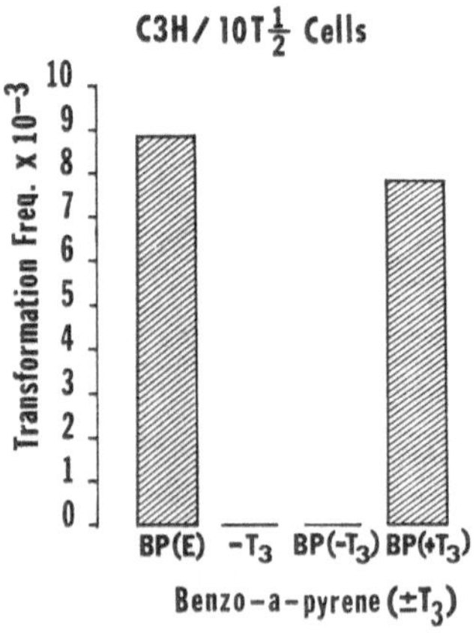

Fig. 11. Histogram representatian of the inhibition Benzo (a) Pyrene induced transformation in the absence of thyroid hormone ($-T_3$) in contrast to control serum (E) or hyperthyroid serum ($+T_3$).

DISCUSSION

In recent years public concern has focussed on the potential biological hazards of low dose radiation within the range of 0.1 to 1 rad. This is the dose level involved in public exposure from nuclear installations as well as from medical diagnostic x-rays. We cannot discount the effect of low doses in the initation of an event. It may later be amplified. For any carcinogens given at the right dose to a competent and specific target cell may serve as effective initiators and promotors. The need to develop suitable systems to directly assess the oncogenic potential of low dose radiation is clearly urgent. Epidemiological studies do not lead themselves to evaluate the carcinogenic effect of low doses of radiation. The contributions from epidemiology have been through extrapolation from incidences where limited numbers of individuals have received high doses of radiation delivered in most cases as single acute exposure (Rossi) and Kellerer 1974). In practice public exposure is comprised of multiple small doses. Animal systems where the induction of tumor by radiation serves to assess the oncogenic action of the x-rays are limited for studies in the low dose range.

Cell cultures offer the best systems to evaluate the varied biological effects of radiation at a cellular level and to investigate the mechanisms involved.

The use of cell culture to study radiation oncogenesis (Borek and Sachs 1966) and the opportunity to study cellular and molecular mechanisms associated with radiation oncogenesis have advanced our knowledge on quantitative cancer risk estimates related to radiation quality, dose rates, cocarcinogenesis and the modification of the initiation and promotion (Fig. 12).

While cell cultures offer defined systems which afford the opportunity to evaluate various aspects of transformation they must be recognized as such and their response to a variety of agents and conditions suggests rather than definitely establishes a situation comparable to that *in vivo*. "Suggestion" may vary among cell strains and lines including cells from human origin where the genetic makeup of the donor cannot be excluded. We use *in vitro* cultures as simplified systems yet these cells are derived of proliferating and non-proliferating tissue and "forced" to grow freely *in vitro*. While cell strains from freshly explanted cultures such as the hamster systems or human origin age *in vitro*, cell lines such as the 10T½ are populations of selected cells which are no longer subject to the control of time clocks and finite life spans. In risk assessment these systems are useful.

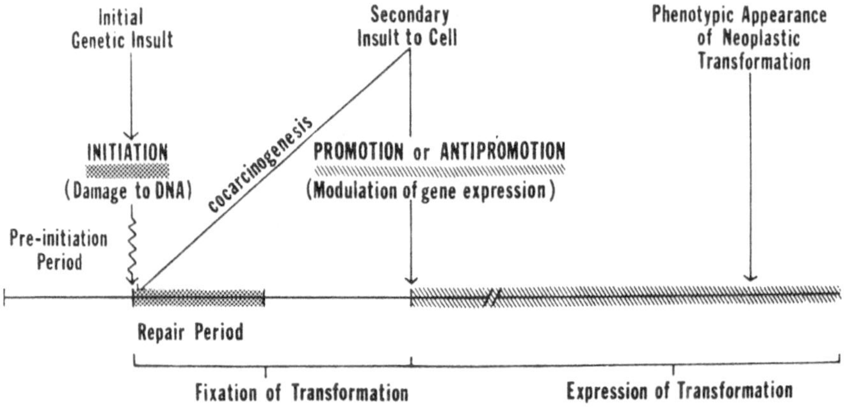

Fig. 12. Representation of initiation expression and progression of neoplastic transformation in vitro.

We can assess the success of cell cultures in studies related to radiation oncogenesis by the current acquiring of information which would be unobtainable via other biological systems. Some of the following findings illustrate that, indeed, the in vitro systems have been useful and hold promise for the future.

1) The number of assay systems based on rodent fibroblasts offer excellent tools to estimate quantitatively the incidence of radiation induced oncogenic transformation under conditions where high and low toxicity prevail (Borek and Hall 1973, Borek et al.1978, Terzaghi and Little 1976, Little 1979, Han and Elkind 1979, Lloyd et al. 1979).

2) Using these systems it is possible to obtain dose response relationships over a wide range of doses and with a level of precision that cannot be rivalled by epidemiological studies of carcinogenesis in man. a) High LET radiation is more oncogenic than x-rays (Borek et al. 1978). b) Transformation can be detected at doses as low as 0.3 rad of x-rays. c) The RBE for γ rays as compared to x-rays at low dose level is 0.5 which has important implications in medical radiation. (Borek and Hall, in preparation). d) The incidence of neutron induced transformation peaks higher than x-ray transfromation when assayed per cell survivor; but when evaluated on this basis of cells at risk which is more relevant to the in vivo situation. X-rays and neutrons rise to the same peak value (Borek et al. 1978, Han and Elkind 1979).

3) Assessment of transformation frequency can be made with in vitro assay systems at doses that are relevant to public

health concern for exposure to medical radiation. No extrapolation is necessary.

4) Dose response relationships established in vitro indicate that the data are poorly fitted by a simple linear relationship between dose and incidence. A linear extrapolation from data derived at high doses does not accurately predict transformation at low dose (Miller et al. 1978).

5) Data from several in vitro transformation systems indicate that fractionation of an x-ray dose leads to an enhanced transformation for total doses less than about 150 rad. A linear interpolation from single acute large doses therefore does not lead to cancer risk estimates that are either conservative or prudent for low doses as delivered as a series of fractions (Borek and Hall 1974, Miller and Hall 1978, Little 1979).

6) Human fibroblasts can be transformed in vitro by x-rays and UV (Borek 1980, Sutherland et al. 1980). The temporal process of transformation is different (Andrews and Borek unpublished, McCloskey and Milo 1977, Milo et al. 1981) from that seen in rodent cells as well as some aspects of the phenotypic expression of the cells. Potential to grow in agar appears concomitantly with morphological changes, and the frequency of human cell transformation by x-rays is lower than that of rodent cells given the same dose of radiation (Borek 1980).

7) Agents which interact with radiation to enhance radiation transformation have been identified. These include tumor promotors, chemicals, pyrolysate products, Antipain added before radiation, and estradiol.

8) We can successfully identify agents which suppress radiation induced carcinogenesis and its cocarcinogenic interactions with other agents. These include the protease inhibitors Antipain (added after radiation) (Borek et al. 1979, Kennedy and Little 1978).

9) Other agents which inhibit radiation induced transformation and its enhancement by TPA are SOD and catalase, agents which scavenge free radicals, suggesting that x-ray induced oncogenesis may be mediated in part via the effect of free radical. The cellular content of catalase and SOD may determine to some extent cellular response to radiation (Borek and Troll, in press).

10) It has been possible to evaluate underlying cellular and molecular mechanisms which regulate the effect of modulating compounds on radiation transformation. Thus, the action of retinoids is not mediated by the type of damage inflicted on DNA which can be monitored by sister chromatid (SCE) analysis (Borek et al. 1981, Miller et al. 1981). It is mediated at the level of gene expression at the membrane level, expressed by altered adhesion and morphology and by changed levels of the Na transport enzyme Na/K ATPase (Borek et al. 1982, Borek 1982a). The molecular effects of Antipain which has diametrically opposed action on transformation depending on its temporal interaction with the cells being irradiated, does not alter DNA damage and

replication. (Borek and Cleaver 1981). AP does not alter SCE in a direction parallel to its effect on transformation (Geard et al., in press).

11) The surface expression of a variety of cellular features associated with the neoplastic state of x-ray induced transformation can be identified within a week after exposure to radiation allowing the identification of early transformants (Borek and Fenoglio 1976). Such surface changes and other cytoskeletal modifications which may be associated could conceivably be intricately related to a cascade of events affecting the genetic apparatus (Puck 1979). In chemically transformed cells a cytoskeletal element has been identified as a mutational product associated with transformation (Hamada et al., in press).

12) The role of chromosomal fine structure changes and instability as associated with radiation induced transformation can only be inferred though it is compelling. Diploid stranis of hamster and human origin remain near diploid or diploid even after transformation has taken place and other phenotypic changes have been expressed (Borek et al. 1977, 1980). But "near diploid" is perhaps sufficient instability.

13) In the course of evaluating the role of repair in transformation it is worth stressing that the variety of studies described above clearly indicate that mechanisms associated with repair of cell survival probably differ from those responsible for cell transformation. The increased survival associated with splitting the x-ray doses is paralleled by higher transformation at low doses and lower when the higher doses are split. (Borek and Hall 1974, et al 1978).

Some important goals for the future in studies on _in vitro_ transformation in radiation must be:

A. To develop quantitative systems using differential epithelial cells derived from various organs.

B. To refine the human cell transformation assay in fibroblasts for quantitative assessment of radiation incidence in human cells, a task which is difficult because of the lower frequency of human cell transformation by radiation compared to rodent cells.

It is of prime importance to assess how frequency, latency, expression, and mechanisms of transformation in human cells are related to those observed in the rodent systems. Most of our current data are from rodent cells and we are at a loss as to which of these cell systems matches most closely the human situation.

In terms of studying the mechanisms underlying radiation induced transformation we are limited by techniques and knowledge of cellular and biochemical products which may be modified following radiation. New techniques to study gene transfection

(Shilo and Weinberg 1981) could help us evaluate genetic mechanisms associated with transformation, as well as establish the cellular physiological milieu required to provide a competent state for neoplastic conversion.

References

Andrews, A., and Borek, C., (unpublished)

Bacq, A.M., and Alexander, P. (1955) In "Fundametnals of Radiobiology". Academic Press, N.Y.

Beir, (1972) The Effects on Populations of Exposure to Low Levels of Ionizing Radiation. Natl. Res. Coun. Acad. Sci., Washington, D.C.

Berenblum, I (1975) Sequential Aspects of Chemical Carcinogenesis: Skin, In "Cancer, A Comprehensive Treatise". Vol. 1. 323-344 F.F. Becker, ed., Plenum Press, N.Y.

Berenblum, I, (1978) Historical Perspective, In: "Carcinogenesis", Vol. 2. T.J. Slaga, A. Siraic and R. K. Boutwell, eds., Acad. Press, N.Y.

Berwald, Y., and Sachs, L. (1963) In Vitro Cell Transformation with Carcinogens, Nature 200: 1182-1184.

Borek, C., (1979). Malignant Transformation In Vitro: Criteria, Bioliogical Markers, and Application in Environmental Screening of Carcinogens. Radiat Res. 79, 209-232.

Borek, C., (1980) X-Ray-Induced In Vitro Neoplastic Transformation of Human Diploid Cells. Nature, 283: 776-778.

Borek, C., (1981) In "Advances in Environmental Toxicology". Vol. 1. 297-318. N. Mishra, V. Dunkle, and M. Mehlman, eds. Senate Press, Inc. Princeton, N.J.

Borek, C. (1982) Advances in Cancer Research (in press).

Borek, C., (1982a) In "Molecular Interactions of Nutrition and Cancer", 337-349. M. S. Arnott, and J. vanEys, eds. Raven Press, N.Y.

Borek, C., and Cleaver, J. E., (1981), Protease Inhibitors neither damage DNA nor Interfere with DNA Repair or Replication in Human Cells. Mutation Res. 82, 373-380.

Borek, C., and Fenoglio, C.M., (1976). Scanning Electron Microscopy of Surface Features of Hamsters Embryo Cells Transformed In Vitro by X-Irradiation. Cancer Res. 36: 1325-1334

Borek, C., Grob, M., and Burger, M.M., (1973). Surface Alterations in Epithelial and Fibroblastic Cells in Culture: A Disturbance of Membrane Degradation Versus Biosynthesis. Exp. Cell Res. 77, 207-215.

Borek, C., and Hall, E.J., (1973). Transformation of Mammalian Cells In Vitro by Low Doses of X-Rays. Nature 243: 450-453.

Borek, C., and Hall, E.J., (1974) Effect of Split Doses of X-Rays on Neoplastic Transformation of Single Cells. Nature 252: 499-501.

Borek, C., Hall, E.J., and Rossi, H.H. (1978) Malignant Transformation in Cultured Hamster Embryo Cells Produced by X-Rays,

430-keV Monenergetic Neutrons, and Heavy Ions. Cancer Res. 38: 2997-3005.

Borek, C., Higashino, S., and Loewenstein, L.R., (1969) Intercellular Communication and Tissue Growth. J. Memb. Biol. 1: 274-293.

Borek, C., Miller. R.C., Pain, C., and Troll, W., (1979). Conditions for Inhibitors and Enhancing Effects of the Protease Inhibitors Antipain on X-Ray-Induced Neoplastic Transformation in Hamster and Mouse Cells Proc. Natl. Acad. Sci., (U.S.A.) 76: 1800-1803.

Borek, C., Miller, R.C., Geard.,C.R., Guernsey, D.L., Osmak, R.S., Rutledge-Freeman, M., Ong, A., and Mason H., (1981) In "Modulation of Cellular Interaction by Vitamin A and its Analogs". L.M. DeLuca and S.S. Shapiro, eds. Annals of New York Acad. of Sci. 359: 237-250.

Borek, C., Pain, C., and Mason, H., (1979). Neoplastic Transformation of Hamster Embryo Cells Irradiated In Vitro and Assayed In Vitro. Nature, 266: 452-454.

Borek, C., and Sachs, L., (1966) In Vitro Transformation by X-Irradiation, Nature, 210: 276-278.

Borek, C., and Sachs, L., (1967) Cells Susceptibility to Transformation by X-Irradiation and Fixation of the Transformed State. Proc. Natl. Acad. Sci. U.S.A. 57: 1522-1527.

Borek, C., and Sachs, L., (1968) The Number of Cell Generations Required to Fix the Transformed State by X-Ray Induced Transformation Proc. Natl. Acad. Sci. (U.S.A.) 59: 83-85.

Borek, C., and Troll.W., (1981) in press.

Brady, R.O., Borek, C., Bradley, R.M., (1969). Composition and Synthesis of Ganglioside in Rat Hepatocyte and Hepatoma Cell Lines. J. Biol. Chem. 244: 6552-6554.

Di Paolo, J.A., Nelson, R.L., Donovan, P.J., and Evans, C.H., (1973) Host-Mediated In Vivo-In Vitro Assay for Chemical Carcinogenesis. Arch. Pathol. 95: 380-385.

Doll, R., and Peto, R., (1981) The Causes of Cancer: Quantitative Estimates of avoidable Risks of Cancer in the U.S.A. Today. J. Natl. Cancer. Inst: 66: No. 6, 1191-1308.

Geard, C.R., Freeman, M.L., Miller, R.C., and Borek,C., Carcinogenesis (in press)

Griffin, A.C., (1979) Role of Selenium in the Chemoprevention of Cancer. Adv. In Cancer Res. 29: 419-441.

Guernsey, D.L., Borek, C., and Edelman, I.S. (1981) Proc. Natl. Acad. Sci. U.S.A. (in press)

Guernsey, D.L., Ong, A., and Borek, C., (1980) Thyroid Hormone Modulation of X-Ray-Induced In Vitro Neoplastic Transformation. Nature, 288: 591-592.

Hamada, H., Leavitt, J., and Kakunaga, T., (1981) Proc. Natl. Acad. Sci. U.S.A. (in press).

Han, A., and Elkind, M.M., (1979) Transformation of mouse

$C_3H/10T\frac{1}{2}$ cells by Single and Fractioned Doses of X-Rays an Fission Spectrum Neutrons. Cancer Res: 39, 123-130.

Harisiadis, L., Miller, R.C., Hall, E.J., and Borek, C., (1978) A Vitamin A Analogue Inhibits Radiation-Induction Oncogenic Transformation. Nature, 274: 486-487.

Hecker, E., (1971) In "Methods of Cancer Research." Vol. 6: 439-484. H.H. Busch, eds., Acad. Press, N.Y.

Jones, P.A., Benedict, W.F., Strickland, S., and Reich, E. (1975) Fibrin Overlay Methods for the Detection of Single Transformed Cells and Colonies of Transformed Cells. Cell, 5: 323-329.

Kakunaga, T., (1974), Requirement for Cell Replication in the Fixation and Expression of the Transformed State in Mouse Cells treated with 4-Nitroquinoline - 1 - Oxide. Int. J. Cancer. 14: 736-742.

Kakunaga, T., (1975) The Role of Cell Division in the Malignant Transformation of Mouse Cells Treated with 3 - Methycholanthrene. Cancer Res., 35: 1637-1642.

Kakunaga, T., (1978), Neoplastic Transformation of Human Diploid Cells by Chemical Carcinogens. Proc. Natl. Acad. Sci. U.S.A. 75: 1334-1338.

Kennedy, A.R., and Little, J.R. (1978) Protease Inhibitors Suppress Radiation Induced Malignant Transformation In Vitro. Nature, 276: 825-826.

Kinsella, A.R., and Radman, M., (1978) Tumor Promoter Induces Sister Chromatid Exchanges: Relevance to Mechanisms of Carcinogenesis. Proc. Natl. Acad. Sci. U.S.A. 75: 6149-6153.

Kinsella, A.R. and Radilian, M., (1980) Inhibition of Carcinogen-Induced Chromosal Aberrations by Anti-Carcinogenic Protease. Proc. Natl. Acad. Sci. U.S.A. 77: 3544-3547.

Little, J.B., (1979) Quantitative Studies of Radiation Transformation with A3I-11 Mouse Balb/3T3 Cell Line. Cancer Res. 39: 1474-1480.

Lloyd, E.L., Gemmell, M.A., Henning, D.S., Gemmell, D.S. and Zabransicy, B.J., (1979) Cell Survival Following Multiple-Track Alpha Particle Radiation. Int. J. Radiat. Biol. 35: 23-31.

Lotan, R. (1980) Effects of Vitamin A and its Analogs (Retinoids) on Normal and Neoplastic Cells. Biochem. Bio Ph. Acta. Rev. on Cancer, 26: 33-91.

McCloskey, J., and Milo, R., (1977) In Vitro transformation of normal diploid human cells by UV and X-rays.Proc. Am.Soc. 110.

McCord, J.M., and Fridovich, I. (1969) Superoxide Dismutase: An Enzymatic Function for Erythrocuprein (Hemocuprein) J. Biol. Chem. 244: 6049-6055.

McPherson, I., and Montagnier, L., (1964) Agag Suspension for the Selective Assay of Cells Transformed by Polyonia Virus. Virology, 23: 291-294.

Miller, R.C., and Hall, E.J., (1978) Effect of X-Ray Dose

fractionation on the Induction of Ocogenic Transformation of Single Cells. Nature 272: 58-60.

Miller, R.C., Geard, C.R., Osmak, R.S., Rutledge-Freeman, M., Ong,A., Mason,H., Napholz, A. , Perez, N., Harisiadis, L., and Borek, C., (1981). Retinoids and A Promotor Modify Radiation Induced Transformation but not Sister Chromatid Exchanges in Rodent Cells. Cancer Res. 41: 655-659.

Milo, G.E., DiPaolo, J.A. (1978) Neoplastic Transformation of Human Diploid Cells In Vitro after Chemical Carcinogen Treatment. Nature, 275: 130-132.

Milo, G.E., Noyes, I., Donahue, T., and Weisbrode, S., (1981) Induction of Neoplasia After In Vitro of Human Epithelial Cells to Carcinogens Proc. Am. Assoc. Cancer Res. 22: 117.

Nagao, M., Sigimira, T., and Matsushima, T., (1978) Environmental Mutagens and Carcinogens. Ann. Rev. Gengt. 12: 117-159.

Nielson, S.E., and Puck, T.T., (1980) Deposition of Fibronectin in the Course of Reverse Transformation of Chinese Hamster Ovary Cells by Cyclicamp. Proc. Natl. Acad. Sci. U.S.A. 77: 985-989.

Peto, R., Doll, R., Buckley, J.D., and Sporn, M.B., (1981) Can Dietary Beta-Carotene Materially Reduce Human Cancer Rates. Nature, 290: 201-207.

Puck, T.T., (1977) Cyclic Amp, The Microtubule-Microfilament system, and cancer Proc. Natl. Acad. Sci. U.S.A. 74: 4491-4495.

Puck, T.T., (1979) Studies on Cell Transformation, Somatic Cell Genetics, 5: 973-990.

Reznikoff, C.A., Brankow, D.W., and Heidelberger, C., (1973a) Establishment and Characterization of a Cloned Line of C_3H Mouse Embryo Cells Sensitive to Postconfluence Inhibition of Division. Cancer Res., 33: 3231-3238.

Reznikoff, C.A., Bertram, J.S., Brankow, D.W., Heidelberger, C., (1973b) Quantitative and Qualitative Studies of Chemical Transformation of Cloned C_3H Mouse Embryo Cells Sensitive to Postconfluence Inhibition of Cell Division. Cancer Res. 33: 3239-3249.

Rossi, H.H., and Kellerer, A.M., (1974) The Validity of Risk Estimates of Luekemia Incidence Based on Japanese Data. Radiat. Res. 58: 131-140.

Samuels, H.H., Stanley F., Casanov,J., (1979) Depletion of L-3,5, 3' - Triodothyronine and L-Thyroxine in Euthyroid Calf Serum for use in Cell Culture Studies of the action of Thyroid Hormone. Endocrinology; 105: 80-85

Schiwike, K.C., Kately, S.A., Tower, J.E., Maher, V.M., and McCormick, J.J. (1981). Induction of Anchorage - Independent growth in Human Fibroblasts by Propane Sultone. Cancer Res. 41: 1620-1627.

Sinclair, W.K. (1981) Effects of Low-Level Radiation of Comparative Risk. Radiology, 138: 1-9.

Sporn, M.B., Dunlop, N.M., Newton, D.L., and Henderson, W.R.,

1976. Relationships between Structure and Activity of Retinoids. Nature, 263:110-113.

Storer, J.B. (1975) In "Cancer A Comprehensive Treatise." Vol. 1: 453-479. F.F. Becker, ed., Plenum Publishing Co., N.Y.

Sutherland, B.M., Gimino, J.S., Delihas, N., Shih, A.C., and Oliver, R.P., (1980). Ultraviolet Light Induced Transformation of Human Cells to Anchorage. Dependent Growth. Cancer Res. 40, 1934-1939.

Swierenga, S.S.H., Whitfield, J.F., and Karasaki, S., (1978) Loss of Proliferative Calcium Dependre: Simple In Vitro Indicator of Tumorigenicity. Proc. Natl. Acad. Sci. U.S.A., 75: 6069-6072.

Terzaghi, M., and Little, J.B., (1976a) X-Irradiation Induced Transformation in a C_3H Mouse Embryo-Derived Cell Line. Cancer Res. 36: 1367-1374.

Terzaghi, M., and Little, J.B., (1976b) Oncogenic Transformation In Vitro following Split-Dose X-Irradiation, Int. J. Radiat. Biol. 29: 583-587.

Todaro, G.J., and Green,H., (1963) Quantitative Studies of the Growth of Mouse in Culture and their Development. J. Cell Biol. 29: 299-313, 583-587.

Umezawa, K., Sawamura, M., Matsushima, T., and Sugimura, T., (1979) Chem. Biol. Interactions, 24: 107-110.

Uniceless, J.C., Tobin, A., Ossowski, L., Quigley, J.P., Rifkin, D.B., and Reich, E., (1973), Menzymatic Function Associated with Transformation of Fibroblasts by Oncogenic Viruses. J. Exp. Med. 137: 85-111.

Unscear (1977) Report of the General Assembly on Sources and Effects of Ionizing Radiation (United Nations, N.Y.)

Upton, A.C., (1955) In "Cancer A Comprehensive Treatise." Vol. 1. 387-401. F.F. Becker, ed., Plenum Publishing Co. N.Y.

Woodcock, D.M., and Cooper, I.A., (1979) Aberrant Double Replication of Segments of Chromosomal Following DNA Synthesis Inhibition by Cytosine and Arabinoside. Exp. Cell Res. 123: 157-166.

CORRELATION OF NCI AND IARC CARCINOGENS WITH THEIR MUTAGENICITY IN SALMONELLA

B.L. Harper, S.J. Rinkus, M. Scott, M. Ammenhauser, K.M. Bang, M. Lowery and M.S. Legator

Department of Preventive Medicine and Community Health
University of Texas Medical Branch
Galveston, Texas 77550

SUMMARY

Carcinogens identified by the NCI Bioassay Program and by recent IARC monographs were reviewed for mutagenicity in the Salmonella/microsome assay. Out of 124 NCI carcinogens, 33 were mutagenic in Salmonella, 24 were non-mutagenic, 19 were incompletely tested in Salmonella, and 48 were not tested. Out of 60 IARC carcinogens, 30 were mutagenic, 15 were non-mutagenic and 15 incompletely or not tested. Of the 102 adequately-tested carcinogens, 63 were mutagenic, giving an overall "success rate" of 62% (i.e. 62% of carcinogens were also mutagenic). If incompletely-tested carcinogens are eventually proven to be non-mutagenic, the success rate would be far lower. The large number of carcinogens which have either been incompletely tested in the Salmonella/microsome assay or not tested at all clearly deserve priority for in vitro testing.

Many of the non-mutagenic carcinogens fall into predictable chemical classes, especially chlorinated aliphatics and mono-substituted or complex aromatic amines. Other instances of non-mutagenic carcinogens can be explained by the inability of in vitro bioactivation to mimic host metabolism, especially with reference to complex metabolic activation and to short- lived electrophiles.

The usefulness of mutagen-carcinogen correlations also depends on the quality of carcinogenicity data, and the statistical power to eliminate both false positives and false negatives. The quality of the Bioassay data was quite variable, often due to inconsistencies between experimental protocol and the established NCI guidlines. In several instances the maximum tolerated dose was not adequately determined, or was not used in lifetime studies. In other instances length of exposure was half-lifetime or three-quarter lifetime. Some reports utilized only one rodent species, and others used fewer than 50 animals per group. Finally, many chemicals contained varying amounts of impurities; although this may more accurately mimic human exposure and may provide some indication that an impurity has a biological effect, these impurities might also contribute to toxicity, or other effects (tumor promotion, induction of metabolizing enzymes and so on). In at least two instances, impurities were responsible for mutagenicity.

The statistical design of the Bioassays reflects a desire to detect only the most potent carcinogens, namely those which cause a 5-fold or greater increase in incidence over a very narrow range of spontaneous incidence. Only a few sites have the statistical sensitivity to detect significant increases in incidence, the most prominent of which is the liver. Historical controls are of little use for any purpose other than suggesting a causal appearance of rare tumors, primarily because of the extremely wide range of reported incidences at several sites. Even with these drawbacks, a comparison of relative carcinogenic potency can be made on the basis of the degree of response per dose of chemical.

INTRODUCTION

The final purpose of doing any biological test for mutagenicity or carcinogenicity is to provide data that can be used to calculate risks to humans. Extrapolation from animal cancer to human cancer based on some indication of carcinogenic potency in animals should be fairly straight-forward, although attempts to do so have been beset by arguments over details which are more important for regulation than for theories of chemical carcinogenesis. Since it is impractical to perform lifetime bioassays for any but the most highly suspect or widely used chemicals, we naturally rely on short-term tests to provide additional information. These short-term tests are designed to detect different parts of the carcinogenic process such as point mutation, transformation, structural chromosome damage, DNA synthesis and repair, and so on.

Many papers have discussed how well carcinogens are detected in the Salmonella/microsome assay, which is by far our widest used test for mutagenicity. Many of these arguments center in effect on which bacterial mutagens are also carcinogens, and therefore more attention is given to some chemical classes over others. This report examines chemicals defined as carcinogens by NCI bioassays and in recent monographs. This set of chemicals is also non-random, because the more potent carcinogens are not evenly distributed among chemical classes. However, it may be more realistic to start with potent animal and human carcinogens and examine how many are detected as Salmonella mutagens then to do the reverse. When this is done, certain classes of chemicals are seen to be non-mutagenic in Salmonella, for a variety of reasons discussed below and in other chapters. It is improtant to realize how much of the total human exposure can come from these classes of chemicals, which include particulates, inorganics and some widely used chlorinated pesticides and aromatic amines.

NATIONAL CANCER INSTITUTE BIOASSAY PROGRAM-BACKGROUND

The National Cancer Institute "Carcinogenesis Program" was responsible for planning, implementing and managing the coordinated research program of the NCI on carcinogenesis by chemical and physical factors, and on cancer prevention. It was established in 1961, and reorganized in 1973-1975, resulting in the current "Carcinogenesis Bioassay Program". Activities include resource development, standardization of guidelines, selection of chemicals, data analysis and retrieval, and publication of the NCI Carcinogenesis Technical Report Series (Page, 1977).

The average 40-month Bioassay includes 10 months of pre-chronic testing, 24 months of chronic exposure, 3 months for necropsy and histopathological analysis, and 3 months to prepare the technical report. Guidelines have been published: "Guidelines for Carcinogen Bioassay in Small Rodents" (NTIS-PB-264-061, Feb, 1976; or NCI-CG-TR-I). The main aspects of the guidelines are as follows:

1. Both sexes of two species (rat and mouse) are used. Animals should be started on the test as weanlings.

2. At least 2 dose levels should be used, the highest being the maximum tolerated dose that does not cause life shortening or toxicity unrelated to tumor induction. Determination of maximum tolerated dose should be measured over a period of 90 days (13 weeks).

3. Each group consists of 50 of each sex and at each dose level, including control groups.

4. The period of exposure is 24 months with an additional period without treatment as optional.

5. The exposure route should mimic that of human exposure.

6. 30 tissues are routinely examined in detail.

7. Chemical purity and stability should be determined.

The major strain of mouse used in the program is an F1 hybrid between a C57Bl/6 female and C3H male, designated B6C3F1. Strains of rats include Fisher 344, Osborne-Mendel, Sprague-Dawley and Charles River CD. Spontaneous tumor incidences at various sites for these strains have been compiled from historical control values reported in the Technical Reports.

Difficulty is still being encountered in estimating chronic tolerance in mice, even with a 90 day subchronic test. MTD estimation in rats has considerably improved with extension of subchronic tests to 90 days (Page, 1977).

Microscopic examination of 30 tissues plus blood smears, tissue masses and gross lesions are performed for each animal. This requirement is among the most stringent protocols, but is needed for completeness. All endpoints are noted, including hyperplasia, nodules and adenomas as well as carcinomas, but preneoplastic lesions (nodules) are not used in the statistical analysis.

IARC Background

In 1971, the International Agency for Research on Cancer (IARC) initiated a program on the evaluation of the carcinogenic risk of chemicals to humans. Reviews of data on carcinogenicity for groups of chemicals have been published in a series of monographs. Reports included in monographs 14 through 23 were evaluated for qualitative aspects (experimental parameters, background information available for the chemical, spectrum of neoplastic response) and quantitative aspects (dose-response affects, statistical analysis).

NCI Criteria for Determining Degree of Animal Evidence

We have evaluated reports from the NCI Bioassay Program (NTIS Technical Reports: NCI-CG-TR-1 through NCI-CG-TR-198) for methodology, results, problems with reporting and so on. Each chemical was ranked according to the degree of evidence for carcinogenicity. Several reports were eliminated from further consideration because of poor survival, chemical instability or deficient experimental design. After thorough critical evaluation, each report was ranked as to degree of animal evidence. This procedure was independently followed by Griesemer and Cueto (1980) and our evaluations are in almost complete agreement with theirs. For this reason, we have followed their categorization as published. We will henceforth refer to the following tables as NCI-Tables 1-9 (Griesemer and Cueto, 1980).

NCI-Table 1. Chemicals with very strong evidence (to an unusual degree and/or in multiple experiments) for carcinogenicity in two animal species (both sexes of both species).

- 3-amino-9-ethyl carbazole hydrochloride
- o-anisidine hydrochloride
- chlordecone
- chloroform
- 4-chloro-o-phenylenediamine
- p-cresidine
- cupferron
- 2,4-diaminoanisole sulfate
- 2,4-diaminotoluene
- dibromochloropropane
- 1,2-dibromoethane
- 1,2-dichloroethane
- 1,4-dioxane
- hydrazobenzene
- 4,4-methylene-bis(N,N-dimethyl) benzenamine
- Michler's ketone
- 1,5-naphthalenediamine
- 5-nitroacenaphthene
- nitrilotriacetic acid, trisodium salt
- nitrilotriacetic acid
- phenazopyridine HCl
- phenoxybenzamine HCl
- procarbazine
- reserpine
- selenium sulfide
- sulfallate
- 4,4'-thiodianiline
- thio-TEPA
- o-toluidine HCl
- tris(2,3-dibromopropyl) phosphate

NCI-Table 2. Chemicals with very strong evidence for carcinogenicity in one species and sufficient evidence in a second species.

- 2-aminoanthraquinone
- 1-amino-2-methyl-anthraquinone
- 5-nitro-o-anisidine
- nitrofen (2 reports)
- p-nitrosodiphenylamine
- phenestrin
- 2,4,6-trichlorophenol
- trimethylphosphate

NCI-Table 3. Chemicals with very strong evidence for carcinogenicity in one species and no evidence in a second species.

- acronycine
- 4-amino-2-nitrophenol
- aniline HCl
- azobenzene
- direct dye black 38
- direct dye brown 95
- heptachlor
- hexachloroethane

chlordane	lasiocarpine
chlorobenzilate	2-methyl-1-nitroanthraquinone
3-(chloromethyl pyridine HCl	6-nitrobenzimidazole
5-chloro-o-toluidine	n-nitrosodiphenylamine
4-chloro-o-toluidine HCl	5-nitro-o-toluidine
chlorothalonil	oestradiol mustard
cinnamylanthranilate	pivaloactone
m-cresidine	p-quinone dioxime
dapsone	1,1,2,2-tetrachloroethane
p,p'-DDE	tetrachloroethylene
n,n'-diethylthiourea	toxaphene
3,3'-dimethoxybenzidine-4,4-diisocyante	1,1,2-trichloroethane
direct dye blue 6	trichloroethylene
	trifluralin

NCI-Table 4. Chemicals with sufficient evidence for carcinogenicity in two species (one sex in each species).

4-chloro-m-phenylenediamine	isophosphamide
ICRF-159	nithiazide

NCI-Table 5. Chemicals with sufficient evidence for carcinogenicity in one species and no evidence in a second species.

aldrin	ethyl tellurac
3-amino-4-ethoxy-acetanilide	3,3'-iminobis-1-propanol dimethane-sulfonate (ester) HCl
2-amino-5-nitrothiazole	3-nitro-p-acetophenetide
5-azacytidine	2-nitro-p-phenylenediamine
captan	3-nitropropionic acid
chloramben	piperonyl sulfoxide
C.I. vat yellow 4	tetrachlorvinphos
daminozide	ß-TGdR
dicofol	trimethyl thiourea
2,4-dinitrotoluene	

NCI-Table 6. Chemicals with equivocal evidence for carcinogenicity in one or two species.

acetohexamide	dibutylindiacetate
allyl chloride	2,7-dichlorodibenzo-p-dioxin
p-anisidine HCl	1,1-dichloroethane
aroclor 1254	dichlorvos
aspirin, phenacetin and caffeine mixture	N,N'-dicyclohexylthiourea
	2,5-dithiobiurea

azinphosmethyl
1H-benzotriazole
butylated hydroxytoluene
4'-chloroaetyl-acetanilide
p-chloroaniline
2-chloro-p-phenylene-diamine sulfate
chloropicrin
clonitralid
p,p'-ethyl-DDD
fenthion
β-nitrostyrene and styrene
parathion
phosphamidon
picloram
proflavine
styrene
TDE

NCI-Table 7. Chemicals with no evidence for carcinogenicity in limited animal experiments. The evidence was considered too limited to draw conclusions about noncarcinogenicity without further tests.

aldicarb
anilazine
calcium cyanamide
carbromal
(2-chloroethyl)trimethyl-ammonium chloride
2-(chloromethyl)pyridine HCl
chlorpropamide
3-chloro-p-toluidine
coumaphos
diazinon
dieldrin
dimethoate
2,4-dimethoxyaniline HCl
dimethyl terephthalate
dioxathion
endosulfan
endrin
ethionamide
ethylene diaminetetra-acetate trihydrate
fluometuron
hexachlorophene
iodoform
lead dimethyldithiocarbamate
lindane
lithocholic acid
malathion
methoxychlor
methyl parathion
mexacarbate
4-nitro-o-phenylenediamine
pentachloronitrobenzene
phenformin
1-phenyl-3-methyl-5-pyrazolone
p-phenylenediamine dihydro-chloride
n-phenyl-p-phenylenediamine
1-phenyl-z-thiourea
photodieldrin
phthalamide
phthalic anhydride
piperonyl butoxide
pyrazinamide
pyrimethamine
sodium diethyldithiocarbamate
sulfisoxazole
3-sulfolene
tetraethylthiuram disulfide
tolazamide
tolbutamide
trichlorofluoromethane
triphenyltin hydroxide
L-tryptophan

NCI-Table 8. Chemicals with no evidence for carcinogenicity in both sexes of one species with limited information on a second species.

anthranilic acid
bis(2-chloro-1-methylethyl)ether
N-(1-naphthyl)ethylenediamine dihydroxhloride

diarylanilide yellow
dibenzo-p-dioxin
formulated fenaminosulf
malaoxon
4-nitroanthranilic acid
2,3,5,6-tetrachloro-6-nitroanisole
2,5-toluenediamine sulfate

NCI-Table 9. Chemicals with no evidence for carcinogenicity in both sexes of two species.

dl-menthol
titanium dioxide
1-nitronaphthalene

Discussion of Placement into NCI tables as NCI-Tables 109

We are in almost complete agreement with Griesemer and Cueto's judgement of degree of evidence. For example, NCI Table 5 contains 3 chemicals which were reported by the contract laboratories as having "no conclusive evidence for carcinogenicity" but for which there was, by our evaluation and by that of Griesemer and Cueto, clearly sufficient evidence in one species. These chemicals are ethyl tellurac, 3-nitropropionic acid and 2,4-dinitrotoluene. Such placement is of course partially subjective since it is ultimately dependent on the pathologists' judgement, particularly concerning "preneoplastic lesions". Furthermore, there is no accepted way to rank low incidence at multiple sites versus high incidence at one site only (Griesemer and Cueto, 1980).

We have included chemicals placed into NCI Table 6 ("equivocal") in the present analysis of proven and suspect carcinogens for the following reasons. Table 6 contains 20 chemicals for which the evidence is definitely suggestive. These 20 chemicals were judged by the reporting contract labs to give "no evidence" or "no conclusive evidence" of carcinogenicity. However, in our opinion and in the opinion of Griesemer and Cueto, and usually of the NCI critique group for each particular report, these chemicals definitely belong in a "suggestive" category. The reasons for this (discussed in more detail below) include the appearance of a rare tumor, borderline statistics (Fisher exact test $.05<p< .1$, or the Fisher exact test $p<.05$, but $>.025$ and therefore "not significant" when the Bonferoni inequality is invoked), only one of the two statistical tests is positive (for example when the Cochran-Armitage dose-response analysis is positive but no single treatement group is statistically different from the control group), the pathologist's judgement of a positive carcinogenic effect, or when the overall opinion of the NCI critique suggests some carcinogenic effect. Table 6 also contains 8 chemicals judged "positive" by the contract lab but only to be "suggestive" by other review groups. It is thus clear that independent and consistent evaluation of each report is necessary for accurate comparisons.

Chemicals from NCI Tables 1 through 6 are presented in Table 1 . For ease of information retrieval, chemicals are listed alphabetically. The chemical class or classes for each chemical are also indicated. Chemical classification is the same as that used by Rinkus and Legator (1980). This particular classification, although adopted by the GENE-TOX Committee, has been criticised by Ames et al (Cancer Res., in press) as being overstratified. As further discussed by Rinkus and Legator (Cancer Res., in Press), several categories could be even further stratified based on known routes of metabolisms. For example, hydrazines could be divided into symmetrical and non-symmetrical, while nitroso compounds could be divided into ultimate or proximate reactive forms. These factors are discussed in the section on metabolism, as appropriate.

We have also assigned many chemicals to secondary classes, as was done by the GENE-TOX Committee. This is based on the multiple potential routes of metabolism which exist for many chemicals. Such multiple classification can never be completely comprehensive since so many ultimate reactive species and their pathways of metabolism have not been determined. For example, metabolism of nitroaromatic compounds is predominantly at the nitro group, so such compounds are listed primarily under group 7 (nitroaromatic) and secondarily listed under phenyl or polyaromatic as appropriate, because of the possibility of ring epoxidation.

It should also be noted that this classification scheme does not attempt to measure carcinogenic potency per se. A chemical falling into NCI Table 2, for example may not be more carcinogenic (per weight of chemical) than chemicals in NCI Tables 4 or 5, because the doses used may vary considerably due to toxicity. Lastly, NCI Table 7 is not a list of non-carcinogens, although a glance at the summary page of each individual report might give that impression. Evidence for carcinogenicity of NCI Table 7 chemicals is inconclusive without further testing. It is unfortunate that 51 (26%) chemicals had to be placed in this table.

IARC Criteria for Determining Degree of Animal Evidence

We have also evaluated IARC monographs (volumes 14-23). Each chemical was ranked according to degree of evidence consistent with the criteria adopted by the IARC Working Group. This presented some difficulties since the monographs are literature reviews, and experimental parameters were quite varied, usually no statistical analysis was reported, and often there were conflicting reports in the literature. While each individual experiment could be roughly ranked similarly to the NCI ranking, each overall estimate of carcinogenicity is an average of all reports for each particular chemical, and more precise ranking is not possible. Therefore, we have followed the broad IARC categories of "sufficient", "limited" or "inadequate" evidence for carcinogenicity (IARC vol 20). "Sufficient evidence" is provided by experimental studies that show an increased incidence of malignancy: (i) in multiple species or strains, and/or (ii) in multiple experiments (routes and/or doses), and/or (iii) to an unusual degree with regard to incidence, site, type and/or latency of onset. A dose-response effect was considered as additional evidence. "Sufficient evidence" thus approximates NCI Tables 1-5, and does not provide further ranking of degrees of evidence within this overall positive category. It was furthermore felt by the IARC Working Group that further ranking is unwarranted since the objective of the reviews is to provide an approximate quantitative evaluation of human risk, and at present there is no defined predictable relationship between the dose required to produce cancer in test animals and the dose which would produce a similar incidence in humans.

Evidence for the carcinogenicity of some chemicals in experimental animals may be "limited" for two reasons. Experimental data may reflect qualitative or quantitative limitations but still be adequate for evaluation and suggestive of carcinogenicity. Such limitations may include testing in only one species, strain or sex, or inadequate dosage, duration of exposure, survival or reporting, or difficulty in determining the degree of malignancy. Secondly, certain neoplasms, including lung and liver tumors in mice, have been considered by the IARC group to be of lesser significance because of higher spontaneous incidence, although this is not a valid statement. "Limited" evidence is thus equivalent to NCI Table 6 ("equivocal").

We have evaluated monographs 14 - 23 and determined the degree of evidence for carcinogenicity of each chemical. Chemicals with "sufficient" or "limited" evidence are listed in Table 2. Some of these are not new carcinogens (for example DMN, DEN), but have been comprehensively reviewed in recent monographs.

(Text continues on Page 377)

Table 1. NCI Carcinogens

Chemical (Report No.)	Class[a]	Degree of Evidence (NCI Table)[b]	References	Salmonella Mutagenicity[c]
Acetohexamide (50)	8,31,12	6	--	NT
Acronycine (49)	24	3	--	NT
Aldrin (21)	18,29	5	13	Neg
Allyl Chloride (73)	25	6	10,62	pos 1535 - S9
2-Aminoanthraquinone (144)	10,16	2	16,63	Neg
3-Amino-4-ethoxyacetanilide (112)	10,12	5	--	NT
3-Amino-9-ethylcarbazole hydrochloride (93)	10,16,24	1	--	NT
1-Amino-2-methyl-anthraquinone (111)	10,16	2	16	0
4-Amino-2-nitrophenol (94)	11,10,12	3	29,30	pos 1538 + S9;pos 98 - S9
2-Amino-5-nitrothiazole (53)	11,10	5	29	pos 100 - S9
Aniline hydrochloride (130)	10,12	3		Neg
o-Anisidine hydrochloride (89)	10,12	1	29,31	weakly pos 1538 + S9
p-Anisidine hydrochloride (116)	10,12	6	3	Neg
Aroclor 1254 (38)	12	6	78,103	Neg
APC (Aspirin, phenacetin, caffeine) (67)	-	6	--	NT
5-Azacytidine (42)	34	5	58	pos 100 - S9
Azinphosmethyl (69)	2,32,24	6	21,85	0
Azobenzene (154)	4,12	3	61	pos 100 + S9
1H-Benzotriazole (88)	2	6	29	weakly pos 1535 + S9
Butylated hydroxytoluene (150)	12	6	--	NT
Captan (15)	25	5	27,84	pos 100, 1535, 98 - S9
Chloramben (25)	10	5	2	0
Chlordane (8)	29	3	82	pos 100 - S9 (desiccator)
Chlordecone (Kepone, no report)	29	1	38,60,78	Neg
4'-(Chloroacetyl)-acetanilide (177)	10	6	--	NT

Table 1. (continued)

Chemical (Report No.)	Class	Degree of Evidence (NCI Table)	References	Salmonella Mutagenicity
para-Chloroaniline (189)	10	6	29,81,108	pos 98 + S9
Chlorobenzilate (75)	14	3	77,97	Neg
Chloroform (no report)	25	1		0
3-(Chloromethyl) pyridine hydrochloride (95)	34	3	29	pos 100 - S9
4-Chloro-meta-phenylenediamine (85)	10	4	--	NT
4-Chloro-ortho-phenylenediamine (63)	10	1	--	NT
2-Chloro-para-phenylenediamine sulfate (113)	10,30	6	--	NT
Chloropicrin (65)	25	6	--	NT
Chlorothalonil (41)	12	3	--	NT
4-Chloro-ortho-toluidine hydrochloride (165)	10	3	--	NT
5-Chloro-ortho-toluidine (187)	10	3	--	NT
Cinnamylanthranilate (196)	16,12	3	29	Neg
C.I. Vat Yellow 4 (134)	16	5	--	NT
Clonitralid (91)	11	6	54	0
meta-Cresidine (105)	10	3	--	NT
para-Cresidine (142)	10	1	--	NT
Cupferron (100)	7,10	1	--	NT
Daminozide (83)	6	5	94	0
Dapsone (20)	10,30	3	51,72	Neg
para,para'-DDE (131)	28,14	3	8,90	Neg
2,4-diaminoanisole sulfate (84)	10,30	1	30	pos 1538 + S9
2,4-diaminotoluene (162)	10	1	79	pos 1538, 98 + S9
Dibromochloropropane (28)	25	1	11	0
1,2-Dibromoethane (86)	25	1	74,75,87	pos 100, 1535 ± S9
Dibutylin diacetate (183)	38	6	--	NT
2,7-Dichlorodibenzo-para-dioxin (123)	19	6	--	NT

Table 1. (continued)

Chemical (Report No.)	Class	Degree of Evidence (NCI Table)	References	Salmonella Mutagenicity
1,1-Dichloroethane (66)	25	6	83	0
1,2-Dichloroethane (55)	25	1	74	pos 100, 1535 ± S9
Dichlorvos (10)	28,32	6	15,55	pos 100, 1535 ± S9
Dicofol (90)	14	5	80	0
N,N'-Dicyclohexylthiourea (56)	8	6	--	NT
3,3'-Diethylthiourea (149)	8	3	--	NT
3,3'-Dimethoxybenzidine-4,4'-diisocyanate (128)	12	3	--	NT
2,4-Dinitrotoluene (54)	11	5	34	pos 98 + S9
1,4-Dioxane (80)	19	1	57	Neg
Direct dye Black 38 (108)	3	3	53	0
Direct dye Blue 6 (108)	3	3	--	NT
Direct dye Brown 95 (108)	3	3	--	NT
2,5-Dithiobiurea (132)	8	6	--	NT
Estradiol Mustard (59)	26,33	3	--	NT
para,para'-ethyl-DDD (156)	25,14	6	--	NT
Ethyl tellurac (152)	8	5	40	Neg
Fenthion (103)	32,12	6	37,84,85 102	Neg
Heptachlor (9)	29	3	59,80	0
Hexachloroethane (68)	25	3	--	NT
Hydrazobenzene (92)	6,12	1	25	Neg
ICRF-159 (78)	38	4	88,101	Neg
3,3'-Iminobis-1-propanol dimethanesulfonate (ester) hydrochloride (IPD) (18)	30	5	--	NT
Isophosphamide (32)	26	4	9	pos 1535 + S9
Lasiocarpine (39)	23	3	49,106	pos 100 + S9

Table 1. (continued)

Chemical (Report No.)	Class	Degree of Evidence (NCI Table)	References	Salmonella Mutagenicity
4,4'-methylene-bis(N,N-dimethyl) benzenamine (186)	10	1	29,81	weakly pos 100 + S9
2-methyl-1-nitroanthraquinone (29)	11,16	3	16	weak pos 100 98, 1537, 1538 ± S9
Michler's Ketone (181)	12	1	--	NT
1,5-Naphthalene diamine (143)	10,16	1	29	weakly pos 100 ± S9
Nithiazide (146)	11,8	4	--	NT
Nitrilotriacetic acid and trisodium salt (6)	38	1	29	Neg
5-Nitroacenaphthene (118)	11,16	1	104	pos 100, 98 ± S9
3-Nitro-para-acetophenetide (133)	11	5	--	NT
5-Nitro-ortho-anisidine (127)	11	2	23	pos 98 + S9
6-Nitrobenzimidazole (117)	11,24	3	64	Neg
Nitrofen (26, 184)	11	2	45	Neg
2-Nitro-para-phenylenediamine (169)	11,10	5	30	pos 1538, 98 ± S9
3-Nitropropionic acid (52)	38	5	--	NT
para-Nitrosodiphenylamine (190)	7,10	2	--	NT
N-Nitrosodiphenylamine (164)	7	3	--	Neg
B-Nitrostyrene and styrene (170)	11,12	6	--	NT
5-Nitro-ortho-toluidine (107)	11,10	3	--	NT
Parathion (70)	11,32	6	84	0
Phenazopyridine hydrochloride (99)	34,10,4	1	66	0
Phenesterin (60)	10,33	2	--	NT
Phenoxybenzamine hydrochloride (72)	26,12	1	--	NT
Phosphamidon (16)	8,28,32	6	--	NT
Picloram (23)	10,24	6	20,93	0
Piperonyl sulfoxide (124)	13	5	--	NT

Table 1. (continued)

Chemical (Report No.)	Class	Degree of Evidence (NCI Table)	References	Salmonella Mutagenicity
Pivalolactone (140)	20	3	--	NT
Procarbazine (19)	6	1	86	Neg
Proflavine (5)	10,24	6	29	pos 100 + S9
para-Quinone dioxime (179)	12	3	--	NT
Reserpine (193)	24	1	29	Neg
Selenium sulfide (194)	39	1	--	NT
Styrene (185)	12	6	19,65	Neg
(styrene oxide)	(18)		19	(pos 100, 1535 ± S9)
Sulfallate (115)	8,28	1	21,56	pos 100, 1535 ± S9
para,para'-TDE(1,1'-(2,2-dichloroethylidene) bis (4-chloro)-benzene (DDD) (131)	14,25	6	--	NT
1,1,2,2-Tetrachloroethane (27)	25	3	18	0
Tetrachloroethylene (13)	28	3	6	0
Tetrachlorvinphos (33)	28,12,32	5	48	0
B-TGdR(B-2'-deoxy-6-thioguanosine) (57)	34	5	--	NT
4,4'thiodianiline (47)	10	1	51	pos 100, 98 + S9
Thio-TEPA (Trus(1-aziridinyl) phosphine sulfide) (58)	17	1	61	pos 1535, 100 - S9
ortho-Toluidine hydrochloride (153)	10	1	39,81	Neg
Toxaphene (37)	29	3	44	pos 100, 98 ± S9
1,1,2-Trichloroethane (74)	25	3	75	0
Trichloroethylene (2)	28	3	5,6,36, 41,82,98	weak pos 100 + S9 closed system preincubation
2,4,6-Trichlorophenol (155)	12	2	52	0
Trifluralin (34)	11	3	--	NT
2,4,5-Trimethylaniline (160)	10	1	108	pos 100, 98 + S9

Table 1. (continued)

Chemical (Report No.)	Class	Degree of Evidence (NCI Table)	References	Salmonella Mutagenicity
Trimethylphosphate (81)	32	2	3	pos 100, 1535 + S9
Trimethylthiourea (129)	8	5	--	NT
Tris (2,3-dibromopropyl) phosphate (76)	32	1	73	pos 100, 1535 ± S9

Footnotes to Table I

[a]Chemical Class:

1. Cyanamide
2. Triazene
3. Diazo
4. Azo
5. Azoxy
6. Hydrazine
7. Nitroso
8. Carbamy, thiocarbamyl
9. Diaryl alkynyl carbamate
10. Aromatic amine
11. Nitroaromatic
12. Phenyl
13. Benzodioxole
14. Substituted diphenylethane
15. Stilbenediol
16. Polyaromatic
17. Aziridine
18. Oxiran, thiirane
19. Dioxane
20. Lactone
21. Anhydride
22. Pyrazolinone
23. Pyrrolizidine
24. Heteroaromatic
25. Halomethane, haloethane
26. N-,S- or O-mustard
27. Haloalkyl ether
28. Chloroethylene
29. Polychlorinated nonaromatic
30. Sulfate, sulfonate, sultone
31. Sulfanilamide
32. Phosphate
33. Steroid
34. Antimetabolite
35. Polysaccharide
36. Polymer
37. Metal complex
38. Miscellaneous
39. Inorganic

[b]NCI Tables: Carcinogenic potency

- Very strong evidence in two species
- Very strong evidence in one specie, sufficient evidence in second
- Very strong evidence in one specie only
- Sufficient evidence in two species
- Sufficient evidence in one species only
- Equivocal

[c]neg = at least 100, 98 ± S9, to toxicity; or 2 abstracts stating all strains ± S9 were used.
0 = incomplete; unavailable in-house reports or foreign journals; inconclusive overall results; not tested to toxicity; reported in abstract but no data given
pos: some "+S9" may also be pos "-S9" and vice versa
NT = not tested or no available reports in literature

REFERENCES FOR TABLE 1

1. D. E. Amacher and S. C. Paillet, Induction of trifluorothymidine-resistant mutants by metal ions in L5178Y/TK+ cells. Mutation Res., 78:279-288 (1980).
2. K. J. Anderson, E. G. Heighty, and M. T. Takahashi, Evaluation of herbicies for possible mutagenic properties, J. Ag. Food Chem., 20:649-656 (1972).
3. D. Anderson and J. A. Styles, An evaluation of 6 short-term tests for detecting organic chemical carcinogens. Appendix 2. The bacterial mutation test, Br. J. Cancer, 37:924-930 (1978).
4. A. E. Auletta, J. M. Kuzawa, and A. S. Parmar, Lack of mutagenicity of a series of food dyes for Salmonella typhimurium, Mutat. Res., 56:203-206 (1977).
5. J. M. Baden, M. Kelley, R. I. Mazze, and V. F. Simmon, Mutagenicity of inhalation anaesthetics: trichloroethylene, divinyl ether, nitrous oxide and cyclopropane, Br. J. Anaesth., 51:417-421 (1979).
6. H. Bartsch, C. Malaveille, A. Barbin, and G. Planche, Mutagenic and alkylating metabolities of halo-ethylenes, chlorobutadienes and dichlorobutenes produced by rodent or human liver tissues, Arch. Toxicol., 41:249-277 (1979).
7. A. Bartsch, et al., Validation and comparative studies on 180 chemicals with S. typhimurium strains and V79 Chinese hamster cells in the presence of various metabolizing systems, Mutat. Res., 76:1-50 (1980).
8. C. T. Bedford, Agricultural and industrial chemicals: miscellaneous organics, in: "Foreign Compound Metabolism in Mammals, Vol. 4," D. E. Hathaway, ed., The Chemical Society, London, p. 193-258 (1977).
9. W. F. Benedict, et al., Mutagenicity of cancer chemotherapeutic agents in the Salmonella/microsome test, Cancer Res., 37:2209-2213 (1977).
10. M. Bignami, G. Conti, L. Conti, et al., Mutagenicity of halogenated aliphatic hydrocarbons in Salmonella typhimurium, Streptomyces coelicolor and Aspergillus nidulans, Chem. Biol. Interact., 30:9-23 (1980).
11. R. W. Biles, T. H. Conner, N. M. Trieff, and M. S. Legator, The influence of contaminants on the mutagenic activity of dibromochloropropane (DBCP), J. Env. Path. Tox., 2:301-312 (1978).
12. L. F. Bjeldanes and H. Chew, Mutagenicity of 1,2-dicarbonyl compounds: maltol, Kojic acid, diacetyl and related substances, Mutat. Res., 67:367-371 (1979).
13. W. E. Blumberg, Enzymic modification of environmental intoxicants: the role of cytochrome P450, Quart. Rev. Biophys., 11:452-481 (1978).
14. A. M. Bonin, J. B. Farquharson, and R. S. Baker, Mutagenicity of aryl methane dyes in Salmonella, Mutat. Res., 89:21-34 (1981).
15. B. A. Bridges, On the detection of volatile liquid mutagens with bacteria: experiments with dichlorvos and epichlorohydrin, Mutat. Res., 54:367-371 (1978).
16. J. P. Brown and R. J. Brown, Mutagenesis by 9,10-anthraquinone derivatives and related compounds in Salmonella typhimurium, Mutat. Res., 40:203-224 (1976).
17. J. P. Brown, G. W. Roehm, and R. J. Brown, Mutagenicity testing of certified food colors and related azo, xanthene, and triphenylmethane dyes with the Salmonella/microsome system, Mutat. Res., 56:249-271 (1978).
18. H. Brown, A. B. Stein, and H. S. Rosenkranz, The mutagenicity and DNA-modifying effects of haloalkanes, Cancer Res., 34:2576-2579 (1974).
19. L. Busk, Mutagenic effects of styrene and styrene oxide, Mutat. Res., 67:201-208 (1979).
20. A. Carrere, G. Cardamone, V. A. Ortali, M. Bruzzone, and D. Di Giuseppi, Mutational studies with some pesticides in Streptomyces coelicolor and Salmonella typhimurium, Mutat. Res., 38:136 (1976) Abstract.
21. A. Carrere, V. A. Ortali, G. Cardamone, and G. Morpurgo, Mutagenicity of dichlorvos and other structurally related pesticides in Salmonella and Streptomyces, Chem. Biol. Interact., 22:297-308 (1978).
22. A. Carrere, V. A. Ortali, G. Cardamone, A. M. Torracca, and R. Raschetti, Microbiological mutagenicity studies of pesticides in vitro, Mutat. Res., 57:277-286 (1978).
23. C. W. Chiu, L. H. Lanfong, C. Y. Wang, and G. T. Bryan, Mutagenicity of some commercially available nitro compounds for Salmonella typhimurium, Mutat. Res., 58:11-22 (1978).
24. R. V. Cooney and A. A. Benson, Arsenic metabolism in Homarus americanus, Chemosphere, 9:335-341 (1980).

25. J. A. Cotruvo, V. F. Simmon, and R. J. Spanggard, Investigation of mutagenic effects of products of ozonation reactions in water, ANYAS, 298:124-140 (1977).
26. D. B. Couch and M. A. Friedman, Suppression of dimethylnitrososarcosine and other nitrosamines, Mutat. Res., 38:89-96 (1976).
27. S. DeFlora and V. Boido, Effect of human gastric juice on the mutagenicity of chemicals, Mutat. Res., 77:307-315 (1980).
28. C. DeMeester, M. D. Van Bogaert, M. L. Vandepaer, M. Roberfroid, F. Poncelet, and M. Mercier, Liver extract mediated mutagenicity of acrylonitrile, Toxicol., 13:7-15 (1979).
29. V. C. Dunkel and V. F. Simmon, Mutagenic activity of chemicals previously tested for carcinogenicity in the National Cancer Institute Bioassay Program, in: "Molecular and Cellular Aspects of Carcinogen Screening Tests," R. Montesano, ed., IARC, Lyon, pp. 283-302 (1980).
30. E. Dybing and S. S. Thorgeirsson, Metabolic activation of 2,4-diaminoanisole, a hair-dye component, Bioch. Pharm., 26:729-734 (1977).
31. F. J. Ferretti, W. Lu, and M. B. Liu, Mutagenicity of benzidine and related compounds employed in the detection of hemoglobin, Am. J. Clin. Path., 67:526-527 (1977).
32. R. C. Garner and C. A. Nutman, Testing of some azo dyes and their reduction products for mutagenicity using Salmonella typhimurium TA1538, Mutat. Res., 44:9-19 (1977).
33. H. R. Glatt, M. Metzler, and F. Oesch, Diethylstilbestrol and 11 derivatives, A mutagenicity study with Salmonella typhimurium, Mutat. Res., 67:113-121 (1979).
34. E. J. Green, M. A. Friedman, and J. A. Sherrod, In vitro mutagenicity and cell transformation screening of caprolactam, Env. Mut., 1:399-407 (1979).
35. M. R. Green and J. V. Pastewka, Mutagenicity of some lipsticks and their dyes, JNCI, 64:665-669 (1980).
36. H. Griem, et al., Mutagenicity and chromosomal aberrations as an analytical tool for in vitro detection of mammalian enzyme-mediated formation of reactive metabolites, Arch. Tox., 39:159-169 (1977).
37. N. P. Hajjar and E. Hodgson, Flavin adenine dinucleotide-dependent monooxygenase: its role in the sulfoxidation of pesticides in mammals, Science, 209:1134-1136 (1980).
38. D. Hallett, K. Khera, D. Stoltz, I. Chiu, D. Villeneuve, and G. Trivett, Photomirex: synthesis and assessment of acute toxicity, tissue distribution, and mutagenicity, J. Ag. Food Chem., 26:388-391 (1978).
39. S. S. Hecht, K. El-Bayoumy, and E. LaVoie, Structure-mutagenicity relationships of N-oxidized derivatives of aniline, o-toluidine, 2'-methyl-4-aminobiphenyl and 3,2'-dimethyl-4-aminobiphenyl, J. Med. Chem., 22:981-987 (1979).
40. A. Hedenstedt, U. Rannug, C. Ramel, and C. A. Wachmeister, Mutagenicity and metabolism studies on 12 thiouram and dithiocarbamate compounds used as accelerators in the Swedish rubber industry, Mutat. Res., 68:313-325 (1979).
41. D. Henschler and G. Bonse, Metabolic activation of chlorinated ethylenes: dependence of mutagenic effect in electrophilic reactivity of the metabolically formed epoxides, Arch. Tox., 39:7-12 (1977).
42. A. Hesbert, M. Lemonnier, and C. Cavelier, Mutagenicity of nitrosodiethanolamine on Salmonella typhimurium, Mutat. Res., 68:207-210 (1979).
43. J. A. Heddle and W. R. Bruce, Comparison of tests for mutagenicity or carcinogenicity using assays for sperm abnormalities, formation of micronuclei and mutations in Salmonella, in: "Origins of Human Cancer," J. J. Hiatt, ed., Cold Spring Harbor Laboratory, pp. 1549-1556 (1977).
44. N. K. Hooper, B. N. Ames, M. A. Saleh, and J. E. Casida, Toxaphene, a complex mixture of polychloroterpenes and a major insecticide, is mutagenic, Science, 205:591-593 (1979).
45. L. M. Hunt, W. F. Chamberlain, B. N. Gilbert, D. E. Hopkins, and A. R. Ginsrich, Absorption, excretion and metabolism of nitrofen by a sheep, J. Ag. Food Chem., 25:1062-1065 (1977).
46. P. H. Jellinck and J. H. Bowen, Metabolism of (14C) diethylstilboestrol epoxide by rat liver in vitro, Biochem. J., 185:129-137 (1980).
47. D. Jenssen and C. Ramel, The micronucleus test as part of a short-term mutagenicity test program for the prediction of carcinogenicity evaluated by 143 genes tested, Mutat. Res., 75:191-202 (1980).

48. T. Kada, M. Moriya, and Y. Shirasu, Screening of pesticides for DNA interactions by rec-assay and mutagenesis testing, and frameshift mutations detected, Mutat. Res., 26:243-248 (1974).
49. A. Kaletsky, R. Oyasu, and J. K. Reddy, Mutagenicity of the pyrrolizidine (Senecio) alkaloid, lasiocarpine in the Salmonella/microsome test, Lab. Invest., 38:352 (1978) Abstract.
50. T. Kawachi, et al., Cooperative program on short-term assays for carcinogenicity in Japan, IARC publ., 27:323-330 (1980).
51. E. LaVoie, L. Tulley, E. Fow, and D. Hoffmann, Mutagenicity of aminophenyl and nitrophenyl ethers, sulfides, and disulfides, Mutat. Res., 67:123-131 (1979).
52. T. Lawlor and S. R. Haworth, Evaluation of the genetic activity of nine chlorinated phenols, seven chlorinated benzenes, and three chlorinated hexanes, Env. Mut., 1:143 (1979) Abstract.
53. E. J. Lazear, J. G. Shaddock, P. R. Barren, and S. C. Louie, The mutagenicity of some of the proposed metabolites of Direct Black 38 and Pigment Yellow 2 in the Salmonella typhimurium assay system, Toxicol. Lett., 4:519-525 (1979).
54. A. Lemma and B. N. Ames, Screening of mutagenic activity of some molluscicides, Trans. R. Soc. Trop. Med. Hyg., 69:167-168 (1975).
55. G. Lofroth, The mutagenicity of dichloroacetaldehyde, Z. Naturforsch., 33:783-785 (1978).
56. F. de Lorenzo, N. Stalano, L. Silengo, and R. Cortese, Mutagenicity of diallate, sulfallate, and triallate and relationship between structure and mutagenic effects of carbamates widely used in agriculture, Cancer Res., 38:13-15 (1978).
57. D. Maron, J. Katzenellenbogen, and B. N. Ames, Compatibility of organic solvents with the Salmonella/microsome test, Mutat. Res., 88:343-350 (1981).
58. H. Marquardt and H. Marquardt, Induction of malignant transformation and mutagenesis in cell cultures by cancer chemotherapeutic agents, Cancer, 40:1930-1934 (1977).
59. T. C. Marshall, H. W. Dorough, and H. E. Swim, Screening of pesticides for mutagenic potential using Salmonella typhimurium mutants, J. Ag. Food Chem., 24:560-565 (1976).
60. H. B. Matthews and S. Kato, The metabolism and disposition of halogenated aromatics, ANYAS, 230:131-137 (1979).
61. J. McCann, E. Choi, E. Yamasaki, and B. N. Ames, Detection of carcinogens as mutagens in the Salmonella/microsome test: Assay of 300 chemicals, PNAS, 72:5135-5139 (1975).
62. E. C. McCoy, L. Burrows, and H. S. Rosenkranz, Genetic activity of allyl chloride, Mutat. Res., 57:11-15 (1978).
63. R. H. McKee and A. M. Tometsko, Inhibition of promutagen activation by the antioxidants butylated hydroxyanisole and butylated hydroxytoluene, JNCI, 63:473-477 (1979).
64. R. S. McMahon, J. C. Cline, and C. Z. Thompson, Assay of 855 test chemicals in ten tester strains using a new modification of the Ames test for bacterial mutagens, Cancer Res., 39:682-693 (1979).
65. C. deMeester, F. Poncelet, M. Roberfroid, and M. Merciers, Impact of microsomal enzymes on the mutagenicity of acrylonitrile, butadine, and styrene, Mutat. Res., 64:132 (1979) Abstract.
66. V. Minnich, M. E. Smith, D. Thompson, and S. Kornfeld, Detection of mutagenic activity in human urine using mutant strains of Salmonella typhimurium, Cancer, 38:1253-1258 (1976).
67. R. Montesano and H. Bartsch, Mutagenic and carcinogenic N-nitroso compounds: possible environmental hazards, Mutat. Res., 32:179-228 (1976).
68. B. S. Morse, M. Conlan, D. G. Giuliani, and M. Nussbaum, Mechanism of arsenic-induced inhibition of erythropoiesis in mice, Am. J. Hematol., 8:273-280 (1980).
69. J. M. Muzzall and W. L. Cook, Mutagenicity test of dyes used in cosmetics with the Salmonella/mammalian microsome test, Mutat. Res., 67:1-8 (1979).
70. M. Nagao, T. Yahagi, and T. Sugimura, Differences in effects of norharman with various classes of chemical mutagens and amounts of S-9, Bioch. Biophys. Res. Commun., 83:373-378 (1978).
71. E. R. Nestman, T. I. Matala, and D. J. Kowbel, Mutagenicity of rhodamine dyes in the Salmonella/microsome test, Env. Mut., 1:140 (1979) Abstract.
72. J. H. Peters, G. R. Gordon, V. F. Simmon, and W. Tanaka, Mutagenesis of dapsone and its derivatives in Salmonella typhimurium, Fed. Proc., 37:450 (1978) Abstract.

73. M. J. Prival, E. C. McCoy, B. Gutler, and H. S. Rosenkranz, Tris (2,3-Dibromyl-propyl) Phosphate; mutagenicity of a widely used flame retardant, Science, 195: 76-78 (1977).
74. U. Rannug, Genotoxic effects of 1,2-dichloroethane, Mutat. Res., 76:269-295 (1980).
75. O. Rannug, A. Sundvall, and C. Ramel, The mutagenic effect of 1,2-dichloroethane on Salmonella typhimurium, I. Activation through conjugation with glutathione in vitro, Chem. Biol. Interact., 20:1-16 (1978).
76. T. K. Rao, J. A. Young, W. Lijinsky, and J. L. Epler, Mutagenicity of aliphatic nitrosamines in Salmonella typhimurium, Mutat. Res., 66:1-7 (1979).
77. S. J. Rinkus and M. S. Legator, The need for both in vitro and in vivo systems in mutagenicity screening, in: "Chemical Mutagens, Principles, and Methods for the Detection, Vol. 6," F. de Serres, ed., pp. 365-473 (1980).
78. R. S. Schoeny, C. C. Smith, and J. C. Loper, Non-mutagenicity for Salmonella of the chlorinated hydrocarbons Arocolor 1254, 1,2,4-trichlorobenzene, mirex, and kepone, Mutat. Res., 68:125-132 (1979).
79. M. M. Shahin, A. Bugatit, and G. Kalopissis, Structure-activity relationship within a series of m-diaminobenzene derivatives, Mutat. Res., 78:25-31 (1980).
80. Y. Shirasu, M. Moriya, K. Kato, A. Furuhashi, and T. Kada, Mutagenicity screening of pesticides in the microbial system, Mutat. Res., 40:19-30 (1976).
81. V. F. Simmon, In vitro mutagenicity assays of chemical carcinogens with Salmonella typhimurium, JNCI, 62:893-899 (1979).
82. V. F. Simmon, K. Kauhanen, and R. G. Tardiff, Mutagenic activity of chemicals identified in drinking water, in: "Progress in Genetic Toxicology," D. Scott, ed., Elsevier, New York, p. 249-258 (1977).
83. V. F. Simmon, K. Kauhanen, and R. G. Tardiff, Mutagenic activity of chemicals identified in drinking water, Dev. Tox. Env. Sci., 2:249-258 (1977).
84. V. Simmon, D. C. Poole, and G. W. Newell, In vitro mutagenic studies of twenty pesticides, Tox. Appl. Pharm., 37:109 (1976) Abstract.
85. V. Simmon et al., In vitro mutagenicity and genotoxicity of 38 pesticides, Env. Mut., 1:142-143 (1979) Abstract.
86. A. K. Solt and S. Neale, Natulan, a bacterial mutagen requiring complex mammalian metabolic activation, Mutat. Res., 70:167-171 (1980).
87. S. J. Stolzenberg and C. H. Hine, Mutagenicity of 2- and 3- carbon halogenated compounds in the Salmonella/mammalian microsome test, Env. Mut., 2:59-66 (1980).
88. G. D. Storer and M. B. Shimkin, et al., Test for carcinogenicity of food additives and chemotherapeutic agents by the pulmonary tumor response in strain of mice, Cancer Res., 33:3069-3085 (1973).
89. T. Sumiura et al., Overlapping of Carcinogens and Mutagens in PN Magee, in: "Fundamentals of Cancer Prevention," Univ. Park Press, Baltimore, pp. 191-215 (1976).
90. G. Sundstrom, O. Hutzinger, S. Safe, and N. Platonow, The metabolism of p, p-DDE in the pig, in: "Fate of Pesticides in Large Animals," G. W. Ivie and H. W. Dorough, eds., Academic Press, New York, pp. 175-182.
91. N. Takemura and H. Shimizu, Mutagenicity of some aromatic amino- and nitro-compounds, Mutat. Res., 54:256-257 (1978) Abstract.
92. L. K. Tkeshelashvili, C. W. Shearman, R. A. Zakour, R. M. Koplitz, and L. A. Loeb, Effects of arsenic, selenium, and chromium on the fidelity of DNA synthesis, Cancer Res., 40:2455-2460 (1980).
93. A. M. Torracca, G. Cardamone, V. Ortali, A. Carrere, R. Raschetti, and G. Ricciardi, Mutagenicity of pesticides as pure compounds and after metabolite activation with rat liver microsomes, Atti Assoc. Genet. Ital., 21: (1976).
94. J. Tosk, I. Schmeltz, and D. Hoffman, Hydrazines as mutagens in a histidine-requiring auxotroph of Salmonella typhimurium, Mutat. Res., 66:247-252 (1979).
95. H. Uehlehe, T. Werner, H. Greim, and M. Kraemer, Metabolic activation of haloalkanes and tests in vitro for mutagenicity, Xenobiot., 7:393-400 (1977).
96. M. Vahter and H. Norin, Metabolism of arsenic-74-labeled trivalent and pentavalent inorganic arsenic in mice, Environ. Res., 21:446-457 (1980).
97. G. W. Ware, D. G. Crosby, and J. W. Giles, Photodecomposition of DNA, Arch. Env. Contam. Tox., 9:135-146 (1980).
98. L. Waskell, A study of the mutagenicity of anaesthetics and their metabolites, Mutat. Res., 57:141-153 (1978).

99. J. S. Wassom, J. E. Huff, and N. Loprieno, Review of the genetic toxicology of chlorinated dibenzo-p-dioxins, Mutat. Res., 47:141-160 (1978).
100. P. Wislocki and R. Gingell, Mutagenicity of several pancreatic carcinogenic derivatives of N-nitrosodipropylamine in the Ames assay, Mutat. Res., 77:215-21a (1980).
101. D. T. Witiak, H. J. Lee, R. W. Hart, and R. E. Gibson, Study of trans-cyclopropylbis (diketopiperazine) and chelating agents related to ICRF-159, J. Med. Chem., 20:630-635 (1977).
102. F. C. Wright and J. C. Riner, Biotransformation and deposition of residues of fenthion and oxidative metabolites in the fat of cattle, J. Ag. Food Chem., 27: 576-577 (1979).
103. C. Wyndham, J. Devenish, and S. Safe, In vitro metabolism, macromolecular binding and bacterial mutagenicity of 4-chlorobiphenyl, a model PCB substrate, Res. Commun. Chem. Path. Pharmacol., 15:563-570 (1976).
104. T. Yahagi, H. Shimizu, M. Nagao, N. Takemura, and T. Sugimura, Mutagenicity of 5-nitroacenaphthene in Salmonella, Gann., 66:581-582 (1975).
105. T. Yahagi et al., Mutagenicities of N-nitrosamines on Salmonella, Mutat. Res., 48:121-130 (1977).
106. H. Yamanaka, M. Nagao, and T. Sugimura, Mutagenicity of pyrrolizidine alkaloids in the Salmonella/mammalian-microsome test, Mutat. Res., 68:211-216 (1979).
107. G. Zetterberg, L. Busk, R. Elonson, V. Starec-Nordenhammar, and H. Ryttman, The influence of pH on the effect of 2,4-D on Saccharomyces cerevisiae and Salmonella typhimurium, Mutat. Res., 42:3-18 (1977).
108. D. Zimmer, J. Mazurek, G. Petzold, and B. K. Bhuyan, Bacterial mutagenicity and mammalian cell DNA damage by several substituted anilines, Mutat. Res., 77:317-326 (1980).

Table 2. IARC Carcinogens

Chemical Name (IARC Reference)	Chemical Class	Animal Ranking	References	Salmonella Mutagenicity
Acrylonitrile (19:73)	38	suff	28	pos 100, 1535 ± S9 (desiccator)
Arsenic and compounds (23:39)	39	inad	1,24,68,92,96	Neg
Asbestos (14:11)	39	suff	--	Neg
1,2-Bis(chloromethoxy) ethane (15:31)	25	suff	--	NT
1,4-Bis(chloromethoxymethyl) benzene (15:37)	25,12	suff	--	NT
Carbon tetrachloride (20:371)	25	suff	61,82	Neg
Chlordecone (Kepone) (20:67)	29	suff	38,60,78	Neg
Chloroform (20:401)	25	suff	95	0
Copper-8-hydroxyquinoline (15:103)	37	ltd	--	NT
C.I. Acid Blue 1 (Blue VRS) (16:163)	10,12,30	ltd	14	Neg
C.I. Acid Blue 9 (Brilliant Blue FCF, FD and C Blue No. 1) (16:171)	10,12,30	ltd	4,14	Neg
C.I. Acid Green 3 (Guinea Green B) (16:199)	10,12,30	suff	14	weakly pos 98 + S9
C.I. Acid Green 5 (Light Green SF, FD and C Green No. 2) (16:209)	10,12,30	ltd	14,17	weakly pos 98 + S9
C.I. Acid Violet 49 (Benzyl Violet 4B, FD and C Violet No. 1) (16:153)	10,12,30	suff	14,89	weakly pos 98 + S9
C.I. Food Green 3 (Fast Green FCF, FD and C Green No. 3) (16:187)	10,12,30	ltd	14,17	Neg
2,4-D (Dichlorophenoxyacetic acid) (15:111)	12	ltd	47,107	0
N,N'-Diacetylbenzidine (16:293)	10	suff	53	pos 1538 + S9
2,4-Diaminotoluene (16:83)	10	suff	79	pos 1538, 98 + S9
1,2-Dibromo-3-chloropropane (15:139)	25	suff	11	pos 100, 1535 + S9
1,2-Dibromoethane (ethylene dibromide) (15:195)	25	suff	74,75,87	pos 100, 1535 ± S9
3,3'-Dichloro-4,4'-diaminodiphenyl ether (16:309)	27,10	suff	91	0
Trans-1,4-Dichlorobutene (15:149)	28	suff	7	0
1,2-Dichloroethane (20:429)	25	suff	74	pos 100, 1535 ± S9
Diethylstilbestrol (6:55)	15	suff	33,46	Neg
Dimethoxane (15:177)	19	suff	--	NT

Table 2 (continued)

Chemical Name (IARC Reference)	Chemical Class	Animal Ranking	References	Salmonella Mutagenicity
Hexachlorobenzene (20:155)	12	suff	--	NT
Hexamethylphosphoramide (15:211)	10,32	suff	3	pos 100, 1535 + S9
Methyl iodide (15:245)	25	suff	61,82	pos 100, 1535 ± S9 (disc or desiccator)
Mirex (20:283)	29	suff	38,60,78	Neg
5-Nitroacenaphthene (16:319)	11	suff	104	pos 98, 100 ± S9
N-Nitroso-m-butylamine (17:51)	7	suff	7,47,67,89	pos 100, 1535 ± S9
N-Nitrosodiethanolamine (17:77)	7	suff	42,64	pos 100, 1535 ± S9
N-Nitrosodiethylamine (17:83)	7	suff	47,67,105	pos 100, 1535 ± S9
N-Nitrosodimethylamine (17:125)	7	suff	47,67,105	pos 100 + S9 (preincubation)
N-Nitrosodi-n-propylamine (17:177)	7	suff	7,105	pos 100, 1535 ± S9
N-Nitroso-N-ethylurea (17:191)	7,8	suff	7	pos 100, 1535 ± S9
N-Nitrosomethylethylamine (17:221)	7	suff	76,100	Neg
N-Nitroso-N-methylurea (17:227)	7,8	suff	7	pos 100, 1535 ± S9
N-Nitrosomethylvinylamine (17:257)	7	suff	--	NT
N-Nitrosomorpholine (17:263)	7	suff	7,100	pos 1535, 1537, 1538 + S9
N-Nitrosonornicotine (17:281)	7,24	suff	--	NT
N-Nitrosopiperidine (17:287)	7	suff	7,76	pos 100, 1535 + S9
N-Nitrosopyrrolidine (17:313)	7	suff	7,76	pos 1535, 1537, 1538 + S9
N-Nitrososarcosine (17:327)	7	suff	26	0
N-Phenyl-2-naphthylamine (16:325)	10,12	ltd	3,7,50	Neg
Polychlorinated biphenyls (18:43)	12	suff	78,103	Neg
para-Quinone (15:255)	24	suff	12	Neg
Rhodamine B (C.I. Basic Violet 10, FD and C Red No. 19)(16:221)	10,12,24,30	suff	35,69,71	Neg

Table 2. (continued)

Chemical Name (IARC Reference)	Chemical Class	Animal Ranking	References	Salmonella Mutagenicity
Rhodamine 6G (C.I. Basic Red 1) (16:223)	10,12,24,30	suff	71	pos 100 + S9
Streptozotocin (17:337)	7	suff	61,64	pos + S9
Styrene (19:231)	12	ltd		0
Succinic anhydride (15:265)	21	ltd	61,81	Neg
TCDD (15:41)	24,19	suff	99	probably Neg
4,4-Thiodianiline (16:343)	10	suff	51	pos 100, 98 + S9
2,4,5-Trichlorophenoxyacetic acid (15:273)	12	suff	47	0
Toxaphene (20:327)	29	suff	44	pos 100, 98 ± S9
1,2,3-Tris(chloromethoxy) propane (15:301)	25	suff	--	NT
Tris (2,3-dibromopropyl) phosphate (20:575)	25,32	suff	73	pos 100, 1535 ± S9
Vinyl bromide (19:367)	28	ltd	6,7	pos 100 + S9
Vinyl chloride (19:377)	28	suff	61,82	pos 100, 1535 + S9
Vinylidene chloride (19:439)	28	suff	6,7	pos 100 + S9 (desiccator)

Footnotes

a. See Table I

b. suff = sufficient evidence (multiple species or strains, multiple experiments or other clear indication of potency; see IARC Supplement 1)
ltd = limited evidence but suggestive of carcinogenic effect
inad = inadequate animal studies or experimental limitations (NOT to be interpreted as negative evidence)

Critique of the NCI Bioassay Program

Carcinogenesis Bioassays in general and the NCI Carcinogenesis Bioassay Program in particular have been adequately discussed with respect to guidelines, problems and drawbacks, (Page, 1977; IRLG, 1979; Smith, 1979). However, there are a number of points we wish to briefly highlight here concerning interpretation of the NCI reports.

The purity of the chemicals tested was in many instances approximately 90%; some impurities were identified, but many were not. In instances where no carcinogenic response was seen, these impurities apparently had no detrimental effect. However, in a lifetime study the total dose can be very large and impurities could be responsible for influencing a carcinogenic response (as known for dioxin in 2,4,5-T). For example, heptachlor (NCI-9) was tested using a technical grade product of 73% purity. 1,2-Dichloroethane (NCI-55) was also of technical grade and contained 11 contaminants. Nitrofen (NCI-184) was determined to have a melting point of 55-62 °C whereas the pure compound was reported in the literature as having a melting point of 71-72°C. Contaminants can also be very toxic and decrease the effective testing range of the chemical in question. Of course, use of technical grade material does more accurately reflect human exposure, and also eliminates the need for testing all the common impurities separately, while still picking up any positive direct, syngergisic or co-carcinogenic effect these impurities might have at these concentrations.

Another group of chemicals which vary in purity are the complex azo dyes. As a group their synthesis is complicated, and it is difficult to separate each product in a pure form. For example, the dyes tested in NCI Report 108 were Direct Brown 95 (72% pure), Direct Blue 6 (60% pure) and Direct Black 38 (87% pure). Each was found to be carcinogenic (placement in NCI Table 3 or strong evidence in one species). Each of these dyes were administered at 1500ppm and 3000ppm over the 2 year period, so impurities might have had considerable impact on the results.

There were at least two carcinogens whose mutagenicity in Salmonella was known to be due to an impurity: Rhodamine B and 2-aminoanthraquinone. Rhodamine B (IARC 16:221) was reviewed from experiments published in 1956, 1958 and 1961. Methods for analysis of Rhodamine were not published until 1967 to 1973, so purity of the compound in the earlier studies is questionable. Technical grade Rhodamine is 92% pure, with several impurities including heavy metals (FD and C certification, 1976), so earlier preparations could well have been even less pure. The contaminant responsible for in vitro mutagenicity has not been identified. (Nestman et al, 1979).

2-Aminoanthraquinone (NCI Report 9) is not mutagenic when pure, but a common contaminant, 1,2-diaminoanthraquinone is a direct-acting mutagen (Brown and Brown, 1976). Both compounds, however, may well be carcinogenic (see discussion on aniline below). Unfortunately, purity of 2-aminoanthraquinone tested in the Bioassay was not established. Two batches of apparently different composition were used during the bioassay, one with a melting point of 215 °C to 235 °C and the other of 255° to 292°C. The melting point reported in the literature is 303°C to 306°C. The infrared spectra agreed with that in the literature, but the UV spectra of each batch in chloroform did not agree with reference spectra. One of these batches was tested 5 years after the bioassay was begun. Furthermore, at the high dose, 2-aminoanthraquinone comprised 1% of the feed by weight for mice (slightly less for rats), so any impurity even at relatively low levels could have had considerable cumulative effect during lifetime feeding.

After the recommended time for the subchronic studies was extended to 90 days, prediction of long-term survival improved (Page 1977), there were still a few instances in which toxicity apparently was cumulative (especially with alkylating agents) such that there was little weight loss but delayed high mortality. In other instances there was substantial weight loss but no mortality. A structure-activity correlation with morbidity or mortality may allow prediction of cululative toxicity. This problem does not reflect inadequacy of experimental protocol.

However, there were many instances in which guidelines were not followed. For example, there were a number of bioassays in which the animals survived well without weight loss. In such cases where the chemical was administered at less than the maximum limit of 5% in the diet and no carcinogenicity was observed, there is not conclusive evidence of noncarcinogenicity. Of course, there will be some chemicals which are toxic but not carcinogenic, but these will only be apparent if the maximum tolerated chronic dose (MTD) is attained. In the bioassay for 1,1-dichloroethane (NCI Report 66) the MTD was not adequately determined, and in other cases the MTD was determined, but not used in the chronic study. In still other cases (e.g. 2,7-dichlorodibenzo-p-dioxin) the subchronic study was not done at all. In this instance, the high dose was set at 1% in the diet, not at 5%, even though the chemical was presumed to be nontoxic. On the other hand, clonitralid (NCI-91) was tested chronically at greater than the determined MTD, resulting in poor survival, and consequently inadequate statistics and "equivocal" evidence of carcinogenicity.

Another deviation from the NCI quidelines occurred with respect to the duration of exposure. The guidelines stipulate two-year exposure, yet some studies were conducted using half-lifetime (one year) or three-quarter lifetime exposures. Furthermore, one lab consistently used only one species, so their carcinogens automatically fall into Tables 3 or 5, or lower. In these cases, three dosages were used so that the Bonferroni inequality (see below) increases the incidence required for significance and thus actually lowers the statistical sensitivity.

There are also many problems with the interpretation of the bioassays. First, we will briefly discuss the use of historical controls. Arguments concerning whether or not historical controls should be used at all have appeared in the literature many times and will not be repeated here. We should, however, point out the inconsistency of the use of historical controls between contract labs, as well as variation in the control values reported by individual labs in different reports. We have generated tables of tumor incidences by compiling historical control values from the NCI reports. It is not possible to establish such a table by simply adding control incidences from each report because of the use of the same control group for several reports in an unspecified manner. This is permitted by the guidelines because of simultaneous testing of several chemicals in the same room, with one negative control group per dose per room. Our compilation of historical controls appear in Table 3; compilations by other authors have appeared (with varying degrees of completeness) in the literature (for instance Page, 1980; Festig, 1979; Baker et al, 1979). During this process, we noticed considerable variation in reported values not only between labs but also within the same lab at different times. There were also several instances of up to a two-fold difference in incidence of a particular tumor for the same total number of animals, reported in different reports but by the same lab. The reasons are unknown, perhaps due to mis-reporting, poor record keeping or to reevaluation by different pathologists. In our tables we used the latest reporting from each lab, with the ranges reported in parentheses. Of particular note is the extremely wide range at certain sites. Since the reasons for this are purely speculative, one cannot automatically assume that the entire control range represents a no-effect level, and individually high control values place the entire experiments in a questionable light (at least for that site). Lastly, the fewer the animals for which incidences have been reported, the greater is the difference in incidences between various published references.

It is obvious that certain strains are not suitable for the detection of tumors at certain sites because of high spontaneous incidence at these sites. For example, testicular cell tumors could not be detected in Fisher 344 rats unless, as with the lung adenoma system of strain A mice, latency is significantly shorter. However, NCI Bioassays are not designed to measure latency because the animals are studied for two years or until natural death if that occurs earlier. Latency or first appearance of early neoplasia must be detected by serial sacrifice before overt symptoms appear.

Table 3a. Historical Controls

B6C3F1 MICE

Site	average, male (range)	average, female (range)
hepatocellular adenoma or carcinoma or both	19% (0-58%)	4% (0-10%)
lymphoma/leukemia	7% (up to 50%)	10% (to 40%)
stomach-squamous cell papilloma or carcinoma	<1% (all < 1%)	1% (all < 1%)
lung-alveolar/bronchiolar adenoma and/or carcinoma	12% (to 22%)	5% (to 7%)
adenoma of lachrymal (Harderian) gland of the eye	≤2.4%	<1%
thyroid-follicular cell adenoma, carcinoma or other	1%	NR
sarcoma of myocardium	0	0
fibrosarcoma of subcutaneous tissue	5%	NR
squamous cell carcinoma or sebaceous adenocarcinoma of Zymbal's gland	NR	0
clitoral gland carcinoma	N/A	0
adenocarcinoma of uterus/endometrium	N/A	0
endometrial stromal polyps	N/A	0
mammary adenocarcinoma	NR	1%
hemangiosarcoma, all sites	4%	NR
kidney-tubular cell adenoma or adenocarcinoma or both	0	NR

NR= not reported

Table 3b. Historical Controls

FISHER 344 RATS

Site	average, male (range)	average, female (range)
mammary fibroadenoma	NR	19% (to 38%)
stomach-squamous cell papilloma or carcinoma	0	0
mouth-squamous cell papilloma or carcinoma	<1%	NR
colon-adenoma or adenocarcinoma	<1%	≤5%
peritoneum-sarcoma or fibrosarcoma	0	NR
liver-nodules or adenoma or carcinoma	2% (to 11%)	≤3%
lymphoma/leukemia "Fisher leukemia"	8% (to 35%)	8% (to 20%)
uterus-endometrial stromal polyps	N/A	16% (to 31%)
uterus-leimyosarcoma	N/A	<1%
uterus/endometrium-adenocarcinoma	N/A	<1%
testis-interstitial cells	79% (to 100%)	N/A
preputial gland	1%	N/A
thryoid-C-cell adenoma or carcinoma or other	NR	6% (to 7%)
pancreas-islet cell adenoma	7% (to 19%)	NR
brain-glioma or other	0	<1%
mesothelioma, all sites	≤3%	NR
ear-Zymbal's gland, ear canal, ear skin-any tumor	<1%	<1%
urinary bladder-transitional cell carcinoma	0	1%
fibrosarcoma		
cutaneous/subcutaneous	≤4%	NR
spleen/multiple organs	0	0
lung-alveolar/bronchiolar adenoma or carcinoma	1%	1%

Table 3b. (continued)

FISHER 344 RATS		
Site	average, male (range)	average, female (range)
pituitary-chromophobe adenoma or carcinoma or other	22% (to 42%)	19%
adrenal-pheochromocytoma	9% (to 26%)	6%
adrenal-ganglioneuroma	0	0

OSBORNE-MENDEL RATS		
Site	average, male (range)	average, female (range)
mammary adenocarcinoma	1%	3% (to 10%)
stomach-squamous cell carcinoma	0	<1%
thyroid-follicular cell adenoma or carcinoma	6%	2%
kidney-tubular cell adenoma	1%	0
pancreatic islet tumor	2% (to 22%)	
adrenal cortical adenoma and carcinoma	NR	1%

SPRAGUE-DAWLEY RATS		
Site	average, male (range)	average, female (range)
mammary fibroadenoma	3%	14%
uterine adenocarcinoma	N/A	0

In the reports themselves, historical controls are used inconsistently. For example, the appearance of a very rare tumor in numbers too low to be statistically significant may still be suggestive of a carcinogenic effect. Often this was the opinion of the report's pathologist, but this finding was omitted in the summary and sometimes also from the discussion. The rarity of these tumors, however, leaves this question open to statistical arguement (see below). Of more serious concern is a falsely negative conclusion based on the wide variation in some of the control incidences. As mentioned above, an incidence statistically increased over experimental control animals may not be statistically increased with respect to a historically maximum incidence. Apparently positive results were thus negated in a number of cases, and the summary reported "no conclusive evidence" of carcinogenicity. The very fact that historical ranges may be so large requires that only concurrent controls be used for statistical analysis.

The statistical issues surrounding the NCI bioassay program are very important and have been previously discussed to some extent by Gart et al. (1979). Among the major points put forward in their discussion are the low power (high Type II error) that is built into the experimental design, and the inappropriateness of criticism about multiple comparisons which are performed. We wish to address both of these issues in some detail.

Due to the binomial nature of the scoring procedures in the NCI bioassay program, the statistics are rather straight-forward. The variance of a given tumor is simply a function of the proportion p(1-p) and thus calculations involving needed samples sizes can easily be done. If one wishes to detect a five-fold increase in tumor incidence at a site which has a spontaneous background rate of 1%, and to detect that increase 90% of the time that it occurs, 312 animals per treatment group are needed. This number is simply a function of the background proportion, p, and the true treated proportion, p', and can be calculated by the following equation

$$N = \frac{(\sigma_1^2 + \sigma_2^2)(Z\alpha + Z\beta)^2}{\Delta^2}$$

where σ_1 and σ_2 are the variance of the control and treated populations (α_2^1 =p (1-p), α_2^2 =p'(1-p')), $Z\alpha$ is the Z value at α = .05, $Z\beta$ is the Z value at β=.1, Δ is the desired difference, p'-p, you wish to observe and N is the number of animals per treatment group.

Using this equation, the number of animals which are needed to observe various increases in tumor rates with a given Type II error rate are given in Table 4 for various background tumor rates. Important to note is the fact that if a Type II error rate of no more than 10% is deemed acceptable, then the NCI bioassay design is only

Table 4
Number of Animals Needed to Achieve Desired Type II Error Rate
With a Type I Error Rate of 0.5

Background Rate	for β=.01 Increase Detected 2-fold	5-fold	10-fold	Background Rate	for β=.05 Increase Detected 2-fold	5-fold	10-fold
.01	4,650	566	195	.01	3,193	389	134
.02	2,286	270	88	.02	1,570	186	60
.03	1,498	172	52	.03	1,029	118	36
.04	1,104	123	30	.04	758	84	21
.05	867	93	21	.05	596	64	14
.10	394	35	-	.10	271	23	-
.20	158	-	-	.20	109	-	-

Background Rate	for β=.10 Increase Detected 2-fold	5-fold	10-fold	Background Rate	for β=.20 Increase Detected 2-fold	5-fold	10-fold
.01	2,533	308	106	.01	1,825	222	77
.02	1,245	147	48	.02	897	106	35
.03	816	94	29	.03	588	68	21
.04	601	67	17	.04	433	48	12
.05	473	51	11	.05	341	37	8
.10	215	19	-	.10	155	14	-
.20	86	-	-	.20	62	-	-

sufficient for detecting ten-fold increases in tumors with a background frequency of 2% or greater and five-fold increases in tumors which have a background rate of greater than 5%. These factors become increasingly important considering the fact that 15 of 17 sites in male B6C3F1 mice have a background rate of less than 2% (for spontaneous tumors) and that 17 of 18 sites in female B6C3F1 mice have a background rate of less than 5% and 14 of 18 are less than 2%. From Gart et al. (1979), if a chemical indeed caused a five-fold increase in tumor incidence in any one of the 27 sites in male and female B6C3F1 mice (out of 30- 35 total sites) with a background rate of approximately 1%, the probability of concluding that that increase was due to the chemical is .0235.

To operate in this power vacuum, statistically speaking, demonstrates a desire to detect only the most carcinogenic of chemicals. Only those substances which cause greater than ten-fold increases in tumor rates will have a significant chance of being detected as a carcinogen, and in studies where less than 50 animals were used per treatment group, the situation is even more perturbed. One particular point to note is that in male mice, only one site occurs frequently enough spontaneously, that a five-fold increase in tumors at that site would be detected statistically. That site is the liver, and it is this very site about which questions have been raised as to the validity of the scoring of that endpoint. It could well be the case that the liver of the male B6C3F1 mouse is not biologically poised for neoplastic transformation, but rather, is the only site that the statistical power is such to <u>demonstrate</u> an effect once it has occurred.

Gart et al. (1979) defend multifactorial comparisons in the NCI bioassay program. The major consideration to be dealt with is the fact that binomial data are not continuous and thus the borderline values of p=.05 cannot be obtained. In fact, the first possible p-value which can be obtained and will lead to a conclusion of "significant difference" is p=.028, when a 50 control-, 50 treated-animal bioassay is done and no tumors are observed in the control group. Also, due to the fact that so many tissue sites have a very low incidence of occurrence, it is almost impossible to speak to the question of false positives at these sites. Statistically, in a 50 control, 50 treated animal study, 5 tumor bearing animals must be observed in the treated group and none in the control to obtain a p<.05. However, because the true historical values for the tumor incidence at various sites tells us that 27 of 35 sites in mice and 22 of 37 sites in F344 rats have a rate of about 1 per 100, the true probability of seeing 5 tumor-bearing animals in the treated group by chance and thus making a Type I error is approximately .000135. Thus any observation of 5 tumor-bearing animals in a treated group and 0 tumor-bearing animals in a control group must be viewed as almost certainly being indicative of an effect and not a potential false positive.

Even though this makes the use of multiple comparisons acceptable, the process must be extended to comparisons of different doses at a common site. For this approach, the NCI bioassay program has used the Bonferroni correction to assure an overall Type I error rate of .05. However, as previously discussed, the correction does not take into account the rare event nature of tumor induction. The use of the Bonferroni correction further stresses an experimental design in which the power is extremely low and the probability of committing a Type I error is much less than .05. Borderline p-values (<.10) should not be quickly overlooked, especially when the site involved is one which has a very low background rate of occurrence.

The final statistical problem is the overdependency on p-values. The automatic decision making approach used in the NCI bioassay program substitutes the subjective ability of the researchers and pathologists to an arbitrary number crunching system. There is not a tremendous amount of difference between p=.045 and p=.065 yet one is quickly labelled significant and the other is brushed off as insignificant. Once again, in a design where statistical power is unacceptably small and historical control values put a better perspective on potential false positive rates, it is unfortunate that decisions could not be made but instead mathematical equations superseded the authority of competent scientists.

One final point can be made concerning a number of reports which used 20 animals per group instead of 50. As can be seen in Table 4, there is only a marginal chance of detecting a 10-fold increase in incidence due to treatment and that is only if the background rates are 4 to 5% and a 10% type II error rate is considered acceptable.

SALMONELLA MUTAGENICITY

A computerized literature search was performed for each carcinogen. Our references are therefore largely limited to the information in the EMIC data base; such a search can never be absolutely complete, and newer references have since appeared for some chemicals. In order to evaluate degree of evidence for Salmonella mutagenicity, the quality and completeness of each report was determined. A positive mutagenic effect can, of course, be seen with minimal testing if the mutagen is potent and direct-acting, whereas a negative effect is more difficult to establish. The minimal criteria for non-mutagenicity is that the chemical be tested to toxicity, with and without liver microsomes, and with at least strains TA98 and TA100, but preferably TA1535, TA1537 and TA1538 also (Rinkus and Legator, 1980). If non-mutagenicity was not well-established, results were reported as incomplete ("0" in the Tables) (Brusick 1980). Special conditions were sometimes required to detect bacterial mutagenicity such as pre-incubation or the testing of volatile chemicals in a dessicator.

There are several criticisms of the Salmonella/microsome system that have been extensively discussed in the literature. We will mention some of these here briefly because they create difficulties in interpreting reported results. First, a decrease in the number of bacteria added per plate (due to toxicity or poor growth) may result in an apparent increase in mutation rate because the amount of histidine available per bacterium increases. Replica plating on histidine-free medium will distinguish between these and true histidine-independent revertants. Conversely, excess bacteria or bacteriolysis on the plate may release free histidine and allow growth of non-revertants.

Other factors causing inaccuracies include variations in liver microsome preparations (S9), and the occasional presence of mutagenic impurities which may account for a mutagenic effect when the carrier compound is added in high amounts. Complex metabolism involving several steps is often a detection - limiting factor in vitro (Rinkus and Legator, Cancer Res., in press). Differences in metabolic activation between Salmonella and the host and/or host flora are discussed below where information is available. These differences are often due to multiple steps required for activation or to activation in an oxidative or reductive milieu in vivo. The use of hamster S9, even though most of the assays to date have used rat or occasionally mouse S9, may improve Salmonella mutagenicity (e.g. p-rosaniline and phenacetin, Dunkel and Simmon, 1980). Finally, there are many instances in which mutagenic activity is due to an in vitro-generated metabolite different from the carcinogenic metabolite generated in vivo. Examples are discussed below, as appropriate.

CORRELATIONS OF MUTAGENICITY WITH CARCINOGENICITY

Correlations of carcinogenicity with Salmonella mutagenicity are given in Tables 5 through 10. As indicated above, many carcinogens have been inadequately tested or not tested at all; in fact of all the NCI carcinogens from NCI Tables 1 - 6, only 57/124 (46%) have been adequately tested in Salmonella, while 45/60 (75%) of IARC carcinogens have been adequately tested in Salmonella. The untested or poorly tested carcinogens clearly deserve priority in mutagenicity studies. The number of chemicals which have not been adequately tested stresses the need for complete testing, as defined above.

An overall success rate, i.e. the number of mutagenic carcinogens out of all carcinogens which have been adequately tested for Salmonella mutagenicity, can be calculated. The overall success rate of these carcinogens detected by Salmonella is 62% (33/57 or 57% for NCI carcinogens and 30/45 or 67% for IARC carcinogens; together

Table 5. Correlation of NCI Carcinogens with Mutagenicity in Salmonella

NCI Table	Salmonella positive	Salmonella negative	"O"	NT*	Total number of chemicals in Table	Pos/Neg
1	13	7	3	7	30	1.9
2	2	2	2	2	8	1.0
3	9	7	4	15	35	1.3
4	1	1	0	2	4	1.0
5	4	2	5	8	19	2.0
6	4	5	5	14	28	0.8
	33	24	19	48	124	

overall Pos/Neg = 1.4

*NT= not tested
"O" = incomplete testing

Table 6. Correlation of IARC Carcinogens with Mutagenicity in Salmonella

	Salmonella positive	Salmonella negative	"O"	NT	Pos/Neg
Sufficient animal evidence	28	10	5	7	2.8
Limited animal evidence	2	5	2	1	0.4
	30	15	7	8	

overall Pos/Neg = 2.0

"O" = incomplete testing
NT = not tested

Table 7. NCI Carcinogens not Mutagenic in Salmonella (by NCI-Table, or degree of evidence of carcinogenicity)

NCI-Table		NCI-Table	
1	chlordecone (Kepone)	3	cinnamylanthranilate
1	1,4-dioxane	3	dapsone
1	hydrazobenzene	3	p,p'-DDE
1	procarbazine	3	6-nitrobenzimidazole
1	nitrilotriacetic acid or trisodium salt	3	N-nitrosodiphenylamine
1	o-toluidine HCl	4	ICRF-159
1	reserpine	5	aldrin
2	2-aminoanthraquinone	5	ethyl tellurac
2	nitrofen	6	p-anisidine HCl
3	aniline HCl	6	Aroclor 1254
3	chlorobenzilate	6	p-chloroaniline
		6	fenthion
		6	styrene

Table 8. IARC Carcinogens not Mutagenic in Salmonella

Sufficient evidence of carcinogenicity

asbestos	N-notrosomethylethylamine
carbon tetrachloride	p-quinone
chlordecone*	PCB's (see Aroclor*)
diethyl stilbestrol	rhodamine B
mirex	TCDD

Limited evidence of carcinogenicity

arsenic and arsenic compounds (animal studies inadequate)

C.I. Acid blue 9 (Brilliant blue FCF)

C.I. Acid blue 1 (Blue VRS)

C.I. Food Green 3 (Fast green FCF)

N-phenyl-2-naphthylamine

succinic anhydride

*overlap with NCI carcinogens

Table 9. Salmonella Non-mutagens by Primary Chemical Class

Class*	#Pos/#Neg	Non-mutagens
6: hydrazine	0/2	hydrazobenzene procarbazine
7: nitroso	7/2	N-nitrosomethylethylamine N-nitrosodiphenylamine
8: carbamyl	1/1	ethyl tellurac
10: aromatic amine	17/9	see Table 10
11: nitroaromatic	6/2	nitrofen 6-nitrobenzimidazole
12: phenyl	11/4	PCB's, Aroclor p-quinone TCDD styrene
14: diphenylethane	0/2	p,p'-DDE (chloroethylene) chlorobenzilate
15: stilbenediol	0/1	DES
16: polyaromatic	2/2	2-aminoanthraquinone (Table 10) cinnamylanthranilate
18: oxirane	0/1	aldrin (chlorinated aliphatic)
21: anhydride	0/1	succinic anhydride
24: heteroaromatic	0/1	reserpine
25: halomethane, ethane	5/1	carbon tetrachloride
28: chloroethylene	6/1	p,p'-DDE
29: chlorinated aliphatic	2/3	chlordecone (kepone) aldrin mirex
32: alkyl phosphate	4/1	fenthion
38: other	--	ICRF-159
39: inorganic	0/2	asbestos arsenic

* Class numbers and designation taken from Rinkus and Legator, 1980.

Table 10. Aromatic Amines Tested in Salmonella

Salmonella mutagens	Source and degree of evidence
o-anisidine HCl	NCI-1
2,4-diaminoanisole SO_4	NCI-1
2,4-diaminotoluene	NCI-1
4,4'-methylene-bis-(N,N-dimethyl) benzeneamine	NCI-1
1,5-naphthylenediamine	NCI-1
4,4'-thiodianiline	NCI-1
2,4,5-trimethylaniline	NCI-1
4-amino-2-nitrophenol	NCI-3
2-amino-5-nitrothiazole	NCI-5
2-nitro-p-phenylenediamine	NCI-5
Acid green 3	IARC-suff.
Acid violet 4	IARC-suff.
N,N-diacetylbenzidine	IARC-suff.
hexamethylphosphoramide	IARC-suff.
rhodamine 6G	IARC-suff.

Acid green 5	IARC-limited
p-chloroaniline	NCI-6
Salmonella non-mutagens	
O-toluidine HCl	NCI-1
2-aminoanthraquinone	NCI-2
aniline HCl	NCI-3
dapsone	NCI-3
rhodamine B	IARC-suff.
--------	
p-anisidine HCl	NCI-6
Acid blue 1	IARC-limited
Acid blue 9	IARC-limited
Food green 3	IARC-limited
N-phenyl-2-naphthylamine	IARC-limited

63/102). This calculation is subjective in that our criteria for non-mutagenicity are stringent, though necessary. However, since positive mutagenicity is easier to establish than non-mutagenicity (with a few exceptions), the success rate would actually be an overestimate if the incompletely tested chemicals were proven to be non-mutagenic. Too few of these carcinogens have been tested in Salmonella to indicate any linear relationship between detection in Salmonella and degree of evidence of carcinogenicity or NCI-Table placement. Of primary concern are the carcinogens not detected by Salmonella; these are listed in Tables 7 and 8, according to evidence of carcinogenicity. Table 9 tabulates IARC and NCI carcinogens by chemical class, for which Salmonella data is available. Note that we are not discussing chemicals from NCI - Table 7 nor are we discussing the false - positives among the non-carcinogens.

Discussion of Carcinogens not Detected in Salmonella/Microsome Tests

a. Hydrazine

The hydrazine class in general has been discussed by Rinkus and Legator (1980). In the present study, two hydrazine carcinogens were non-mutagenic in Salmonella: procarbazine and hydrazobenzene.

Procarbazine (NCI - Table 1), an immunosuppressive and carcinostatic drug, has been extensively tested for mutagenicity, carcinogenicity and teratogenicity (reviewed in Lee, 1978). Procarbazine is generally negative with in vitro microbial test systems even in the presence of a source of mammalian metabolic activation (Solt and Neale, 1980). Two reports have appeared in which a positive dose-response was detected by E. coli (Solt and Neale, 1980) and Salmonella (Moriya et al, 1980); both of these reports were host-mediated assays. There are probably two contributing factors to the lack of in vitro mutagenicity. First, activation of procarbazine is relatively slow in vivo (90 minutes in mice, Solt and Neale, 11980) and complex (discussed in Moriya et al, 1980). Induction of liver microsomes by Aroclor 1254 greatly increased the mutagenicity of procarbazine in the host-mediated assay, and suggested an important role for cytochrome P-448 (Moriya et al,1980). A second factor concerning in vitro results is the ability of intestinal microflora to reduce azo groups (reviewed by Scheline, 1980); this is thought to contribute to carcinogenicity another hydrazine, dimethyl hydrazine (DMH). However, procarbazine and DMH also undergo oxidative metabolism (oxidation of the azo to azoxy to hydroxylated azoxy) (discussed in Moriya et al, 1980). Since the mutagenicity of procarbazine, but not of DMH, was increased by induction of host liver microsomes, the in vivo rate-limiting steps for activation may be reductive for DMH and oxidative for procarbazine.

Confusion also exists concerning the metabolism of hydrazobenzene

(NCI - Table 1), the other non-mutagenic hydrazine. Hydrazobenzene is the in vivo product of reductive metabolism of azobenzene by intestinal microflora (discussed in Rinkus and Legator, 1980). Recovery of aniline derivatives and benzidine as urinary metabolites (Elson and Warren, 1944) confirms this as a minor route of metabolism in vivo. However, azobenzene is clearly mutagenic with S9 activation in vitro, yet hydrazobenzene is clearly negative (Cotruvo et al, 1977; see Tables I and II). It would thus seem that azobenzene undergoes oxidative activation in vitro whereas hydrozobenzene must be metabolized to a non-reactive species. The only possible mechanism is metabolism at the azo/hydrazomoiety. Oxidation may also be an important reaction in vivo since hydroxylated derivatives are recovered in greater amounts from the urine than products of reduction. However, if the active intermediate is an arene oxide, one would expect azobenzene and hydrazobenzene to be equally mutagenic. Also, if non-enzymatic rearrangement were the major route of metabolism thus producing benzidine, then hydrazobenzene should be as mutagenic as benzidine, which it clearly is not.

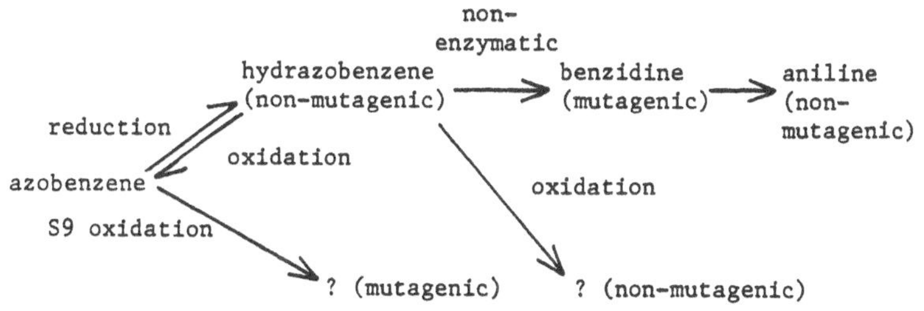

Figure 1. Azobenzene pathway

Further circumstantial evidence for different routes of metabolism can be derived from the difference in target organs of neoplasia. Azobenzene (NCI-Table 3) caused sarcomas of multiple sites in rats but caused no tumors in mice. A number of observations can be made concerning tumor sites (also discussed later). First, azobenzene is clearly not a mouse liver carcinogen (the most common tumor site in the mouse). It was also not a rat liver carcinogen, but the small incidence of liver tumors was suggestive of a dose-related trend, though not statistically significant. This may be related to the significant dose-related trends seen in other abdominal organs which is often the case when peritoneal sarcomas are the major tumors. Other chemicals causing rat peritoneal or spleen sarcomas but not liver tumors include o-toluidine (NCI-Table 1, administered in feed), phenoxybenzamine (NCI-Table 1, intraperitoneal), acronycine (NCI-Table 3, IP), aniline (NCI-Table 3, feed, <u>not</u> a bladder carcinogen in these reports), dapsone (NCI-Table 3, feed), and 3,3'-iminobis -1-propanoldimethanesulfonate (NCI -Table 5, IP). The three chemicals which were administered in feed all happen to be aromatic amines, but any hypothesis (whether they all behave like aniline and whether aniline will always cause peritoneal tumors in rats), is purely conjectural at this point.

Hydrazobenzene, administered in the same dose range as azobenzene (300-500 ppm) provided much more evidence of carcinogenicity despite the fact that this was a very poor study. Fortunately hydrazobenzene is a strong carcinogen, because doses varied and groups had to be restarted so linear trend- and dose related - statistics could not be calculted. It caused rat liver, Zymbal gland and mammary tumors, and mouse liver tumors. Rat liver and mammary gland are non-specific target sites: no predominance of any chemical class is particularly evident for either site. Zymbal gland (ear and ear canal) tumors are uncommon, but again there is nothing striking about the Zymbal gland carcinogens (see Griesemer and Cueto, 1980 for a concise listing of tumor sites for each chemical). One chemical, 5-nitroacenaphthene, caused both zymbal and mammary gland tumors in rats, as well as mouse liver tumors (and some other sites in addition) as did hydrazobenzene. We cannot say at this point if this relfects some active species or metabolism common to both compounds or if similar patterns of tumor incidence is simply coincidental.

b. Nitroso

Two of 9 nitroso compounds were not detected by Salmonella in vitro: N-nitrosomethylethylamine (NMEA) and N-nitrosodiphenylamine. Rao et al (1979) tested 17 carcinogenic nitrosamines in the Salmonella assay, and 9 of these, including NMEA, were not mutagenic in vitro. This included 6 rat-hepatocarcinogens, even though induced rat liver was used as the source of metabolic activation. Although not discussed by the authors, none of the unsymmetrical nitrosamine carcinogens were detected by Salmonella in vitro (but several symmetrical nitrosammines were also negative). Furthermore, at least 2 nitrosamines, dimethyl and diethylnitrosamine (DMN and DEN), as well as several dimethyltriazines and dimethylphenylazobenzenamines require liquid preincubation in order to be detected by Salmonella. The carcinogens tested by Rao et al were tested by the liquid preincubation test, which improved overall nitrosamine detection, but still left 9 undetected. As reviewed by Magee et al (1976) and Rinkus and Legator (1980), N-dealkylation may be deficient in S9 such that a higher ratio of S9 and chemical to bacteria (as provided by preincubation) may be necessary for detection in vitro. Unsymmetrical substitution may further influence activation. Thus even though only 2 of 9 carcinogenic nitrosamines in the present review were not mutagenic, there are several other non-mutagenic but carcinogenic nitrosamines known from the literature.

c. Carbamyl

Two carcinogenic carbamyls in this review have been tested in Salmonella: sulfallate (diethyl carbamodithioic acid 2-chloro-2-propenyl ester; positive) and ethyl tellurac (tellurium diethyl dithiocarbamate; negative). As a class, carcinogenic carbamyl and thiocarbamyls are poorly detected (Rinkus and Legator, 1980). Although sulfallate is chlorinated, the presence of chlorine is probably not responsible for mutagenicity since several non-chlorinated thiocarbamates are also mutagenic (Hedenstedt et al, 1979).

Mutagenicity of a series of dithiocarbamates was studied by Hedenstedt et al (1979), without regard to carcinogenicity. Zinc dimethyl dithiocarbamate was a potent mutagen while the copper congener was weakly mutagenic at high doses and relatively non-toxic. Increasing substituent length decreased mutagenicity (Zn diethyl congener) and then abolished activity altogether (Zn dibutyl congener). For the diethyl-substituted compounds, the Zn congener was again the most potent mutagen followed by cadmium (with a narrow non-toxic range) while tellurium (ethyl tellurac) was not mutagenic but fairly toxic. The authors proposed that the metal ion might affect the stability of the chelate formed; they did not discuss decreasing reactivity with increasing substituent length. They proposed a mixed anhydride reactive intermediate, analogous to the proposed parathion activation,

$$(R)_2 - N - \overset{\overset{O}{\|}}{C} - S - \overset{\overset{S}{\|}}{C} - N - (R)_2$$

following loss of a reactive sulfur by oxidative desulfuration. Since substituent length affects reactivity, however, dealkylation must also be involved, particularly since a dimethylcarbamoyl group is postulated to attach to nucleophilic sites.

d. Aromatic Amines

Seventeen of the carcinogenic aromatic amines from this review were detected by Salmonella, and 10 were not. Of the carcinogens detected in vitro, there was sufficient evidence of carcinogenicity for 15 of them, while 5 of the 11 non-mutagenic amines were equivocal carcinogens or had limited evidence of their carcinogenicity; these included 3 complex amine dyes.

Carcinogenicity of aromatic amines derives from (1) the type of ring system, (2) the position of the amine group, and (3) the substituents. The metabolism of aromatic amines is very complex since these compounds can undergo a variety of reactions (Kriek and Westra 1979; Kriek, 1979; Parris, 1980). Acetylation seems to be a major reaction in vivo, but N-oxidation is the first step in carcinogenic activation. The N-hydroxy derivatives may be further activated by several other reactions. Relatively stable N-glucuronides may be formed, but under conditions of low pH such as in acidic urine, hydrolysis to the arylhydroxylamine could occur and finally a reactive arylnitrenium ion resonance form may be produced. N-sulfates, formed by the action of liver sulfotransferase, have also been shown to be active metabolites, and there is evidence for the generation of nitroxide radicals during the metabolism of aminoazo dyes.

Loew et al (1979) made a series of theoretical calculations, and showed that the most mutagenic isomers have the highest potential for stable epoxide formation. Less mutagenic isomers may be epoxidated but quickly rearrange to the phenols. The presence of substituted chlorine decreases the probability of amine N-hydroxylation, and although epoxidation is possible, it would quickly rearrange to the phenol. Nitro substitution acts in the same manner as chlorine except that metabolism at the nitro group itself is probably responsible for the activiy of nitro-aromatic amines.

Garner and Nutman (1977) examined the mutagenicity of a series of substituted anilines and concluded that two positions must be substituted for the compound to be mutagenic. Two amino groups, 2 nitro groups or one of each were mutagenic, but aniline with substituted methyl or methoxy groups, or chlorine was not mutagenic (even through they may be fairly strong carcinogens). A third substitution by a nitro or amine group greatly increased mutagenicity. In general, when only amine groups were present on the ring, S9-mediated metabolism (probably N-hydroxylation) was required for mutagenic activity, while bacterial nitro-reductase activity eliminated the necessity for S9 when nitro substituents were present. This observation is confirmed by Table 10: di- and tri-substituted amines are detected by Salmonella.

As discussed earlier, mutagenicity reported in early studies of Rhodamine B and 2-amioanthraquinone was later found in each case to definitely be due to an impurity. 2-Aminoanthraquinone was non-mutagenic when pure, but its contaminant 1,2-diaminoanthraquinone was mutagenic, again consistent with the work of Garner and Nutman (1977). The carcinogenicity of these two compounds may thus need to be verified.

Finally the β-carboline compounds harman and norharman are known to alter the mutagenicity of several aromatic compounds. Both aniline and o-toluidine (but not m-toluidine or p-toluidine), are positive in Salmonella when assayed in the presence of norharman. The mutagenicity of 2-acetylaminofluorene, benzo(a) pyrene and other compounds is increased or decreased by the presence of norharmon depending on the amount of S9 present. While not mutagenic itself, norharman may alter the ratio of activation to inactivation pathways; specifically norharman is known to inhibit aryl hydrocarbon hydroxylase and monoamine oxidase (Nagao et al, 1978; Fujino et al, 1980). These observations, when considered with the number of pathways by which these chemicals can be metabolized as well as the number of cytochromes which have been identified support the known complexity of mammalian metabolism, and it is not surprising that current in vitro systems do not completely mimic mammalian metabolism.

e. Nitroaromatic

Of the carcinogenic nitroaromatic compounds tested in Salmonella, 2 out of 6 were not mutagenic. This would not have been expected from the review by Rinkus and Legator (1980) in which all of 32 carcinogenic nitroaromatics tested in Salmonella were positive. Of course, there always remains the possibility that further testing, perhaps using liquid preincubation, may provide some evidence of in vitro mutagenicity.

Nitrofen (NCI Table - 2) is an example of a chemical with at least 5 unidentified impurities. The reported melting point is 71 $^{\circ}$- 72°C, but that of the experimental lot (Report 26) was 53° - 62°C. In report 26, nitrofen caused tumors at multiple sites in rats and mice. This study was nevertheless repeated (report 84); in this report no tumors were seen in rats, and only liver tumors were seen in mice. Since different strains of rats were used, these reports are not directly comparable for the rat data. Nitrofen was a potent liver carcinogen in both mouse experiments, but slightly lower in the second report (different lab, different pathologist, some difference in terminology between the use of "carcinoma" vs. "carcinoma plus adenoma"). In report 26, liver tumor incidence in the high dose groups was 96% for males and 98% for females. In report 84, incidences were 83% and 60%.

Metabolites of nitrofen were measured in various tissues of sheep (Hunt et al, 1977). 30% was found as amino-nitrofen (converson of nitro to amino); other metabolites included 3% as the 5-hydroxy form, 2-6% as as 2,4-dichlorophenol, 4% as 2-chlorophenyl, 1% as azonitrofen, and glucuronide and sulfate conjugates. There were also 5 unknown metabolies, one of which was perhaps a catechol, and 2 of which were probably polymers. There was no evidence of chloride rearrangement (Hunt et al, 1977). Nitrofen and its major metabolite amino-nitrofen bear a resemblence to 4-aminobiphenyl and 4-nitrobiphenyl, both of which are mutagenic. If the ether linkage is broken in vitro as it is to a small extent in vivo, the resultant possible forms (nitrobenzene, chlorophenols etc.) are known not to be mutagenic. It seems likely that in vitro liver S9 does not accurately reflect the balance of metabolism pathways that occur in vivo, even though the target organ is the liver.

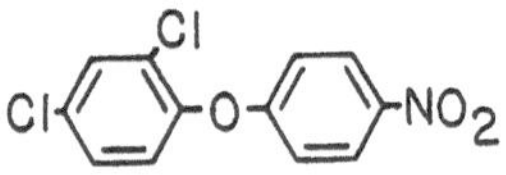

Nitrofen

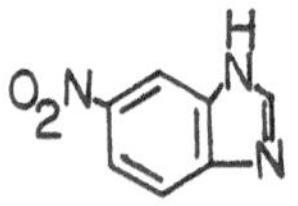

6-Nitrobenzimidazole

6-Nitrobenzimidazole, another liver carcinogen, presents much the same dilemma. Nitroimidazoles are uniformly mutagenic, but the nitrobenzene (non-mutagenic) portion of nitrobenzimidazole might account for the lack of mutagenic acitvity (Chiu et al, 1978).

f. Phenyl

Many chemicals are listed secondarily in the phenyl class on the basis of structure, even though their primary listings are in other classes. The only carcinogens whose primary listing is in the phenyl class are p-quinone and Aroclor or polychlorinated biphenyls. In general chlorinated hydrocarbons are at best weakly mutagenic but most of them cause tumors in mice during lifetime feeding studies, especially hepatocarcinomas (Burchfield and Storrs, 1977). Metabolism of polychlorinated biphenyls in mammals has been reviewed by Bedford (1977). Chlorinated biphenyls are hydroxylated, either by direct hydroxylation or via the arene oxide, and generally are not dehalogenated. 4-Chlorobiphenyl is hydroxylated at the 4' position (via arene epoxide) or at the 3' and 4' positions (direct hydroxylaton) (Burchfield and Storrs, 1977; Wyndham et al, 1976; Crawford and Safe, 1979; Ghiasuddin et al, 1976). Loew and Sudhindra (1979) have calculated that chlorine substitution deactives the ring to epoxidation and also decreases the activation of other substituents to mutagenic intermediates. Overall metabolism of PCB's in vitro by liver microsomes decreases quantitatively as the degree of chlorination increases (Ghiasuddin et al, 1976); chlorine was not removed. If hydroxylated products formed by S9 or by the bacteria in vitro are formed via the arene oxide, then this pathway would be expected to mutagenically active intermediates analogous to polyaromatics. This is not the case, however for 4-chlorobiphenyl which is not mutagenic in Salmonella (Wyndham et al, 1976), even though it is hydroxylated via the arene oxide.

In general, as the number of chlorines per molecule increase, lipid solubility increases so that more is stored in adipose tissue and thus is unavailable for metabolism. The source of PCB carciogenicity may be related in part to the ability to induce liver cytochromes, but the effect of chronic lifetime induction of liver

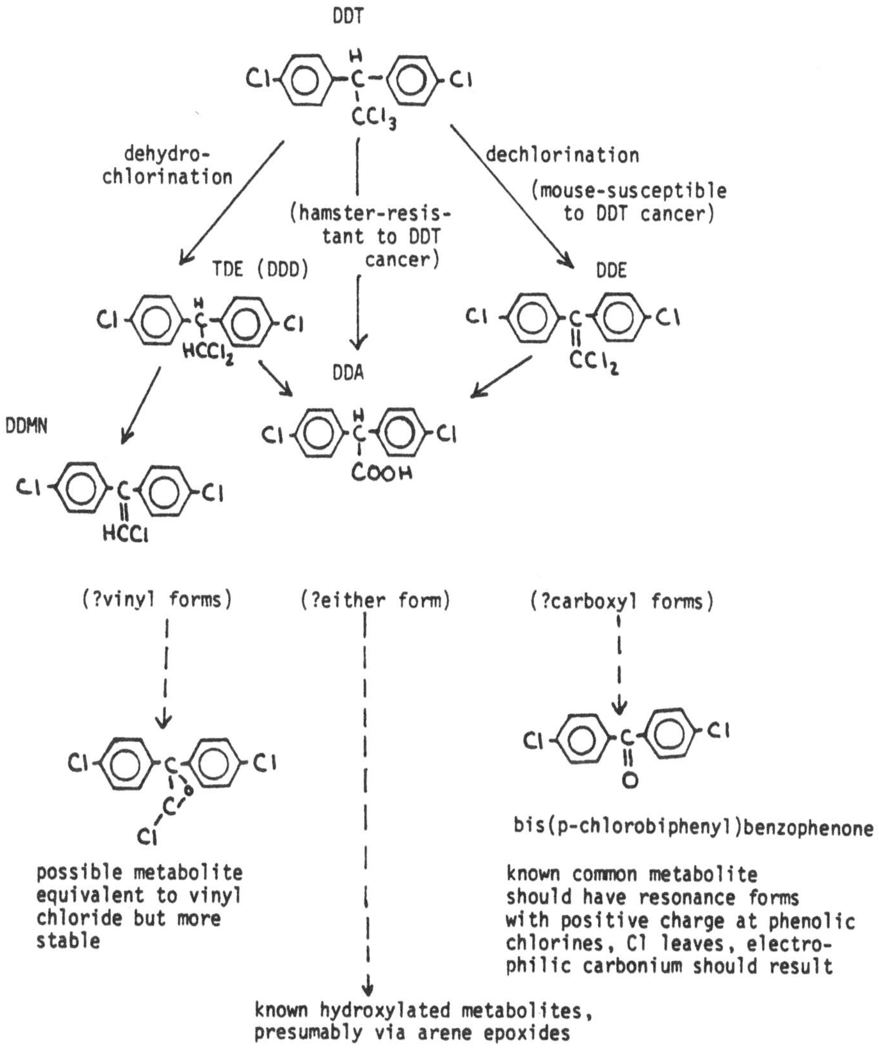

Figure 2. DDT Metabolites

enzymes has not been established. Since different PCB's induce different cytochromes depending on the position of the chlorine (Crawford and Safe, 1979), one might examine corresponding carcinogeniciy to test this theory.

g. Diphenylethane (and Chloroethylene)

The metabolism of DDT, its analogues and its metabolites have been reviewed (Bedford, 1977; Burchfield and Storrs, 1977). The two compounds in question here, p,p'-DDE and chlorobenzilate (an analog of DDT) both caused liver tumors in mice but not in rats. During daily feedings of DDT, mice excreted p,p'-DDE and p,p'-DDA, while hamsters excreted only p,p'-DDA in the urine. The feces of both contained p,p'DDD and p,p'DDT In pigs, DDT feeding produced p,p'-DDA and a small amount of 3-OH-p,p'-DDE in the urine but in the feces, only p,p'-DDE and nothing else was found (Sundstrom, 1977). In man, DDD, DDE and DDA have been identified as metabolites discussed in Bedford, 1977. It thus appears that species variation in routes of metabolism may account for the pattern of carcinogenicity between species. In fact, the mechanism of carcinogenicity in mice is unknown, although p,p'-DDE (non-toxic and the form stored in adipose tissue) is suspected as being close to the active metabolite. DDT and its analogs undergo a series of reductive dechlorinations or dehydrochlorinations of the alkyl group. It has been suggesed that the alkyl group in bis(p-chlorophenyl) benzophenone, a metabolite common to DDT, DDD and chlorobenzilate, can be completely dechlorinated and oxidized, creating positive charges at the para positions of the benzene rings (Burchfield and Storrs 1977). On the other hand, the detection of small amounts of hydroxylated p,p'-DDE in pigs and seals suggests that the chlorinated ring can be hydroxylated via the arene oxide in conjunction with chlorine rearrangemet (Sundstrom et al, 1975; Sundstrom, 1977). Either of these mechanisms could contribute to carcinogenicity and the weak mutagenicity which has occasionally been seen.

h. Stilbenediol

It is well-established that diethylstilbestrol (DES) is carcinogenic but not mutagenic. It is included for discussion here because of the structural similarity to recently identified hydroxylated products of p,p'-DDE. It has been suggested that this similarity accounts for estrogenic effects of the DDT series (Sundstrom, 1977). Metabolism and mutagenicity of DES has been studied by Jellinck and Bowen (1980) and Glatt et al (1979). A number of metabolic routes may be possible, but the first major reaction by rat liver microsomes is epoxidation of the ethylene group to form DES-3,4-oxide. This compound is not mutagenic but is a potent inducer of sister chromatid exchange. It is relatively stable and requires further microsomal activation, and is not a substrate for epoxide hydrase. Another metabolite, dienestrol, is formed from the 4,4''-semiquinone, and is also non-mutagenic but a potent inducer of sister chromatid exchange (Glatt et al, 1979). A third point of metabolism is epoxidation at the 2'-3' position on the aromatic ring. Thus, there are 2 arene oxides and one ethylene epoxide initially formed. The action of the arene oxides probably resembles those formed from benzene and perhaps phenol; both are basically non-mutagenic although they bind to DNA and are clastogens (Kinoshita et al, 1981).

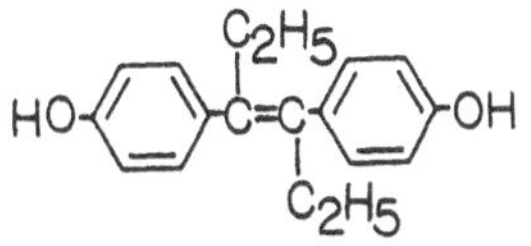

Diethylstilbestrol

i. Halomethane, Haloethane

Carbon tetrachloride (and chloroform, incompletely tested) are volatile halomethanes for which mutagenicity has proven difficult to demonstrate. Haloethanes and haloethylenes are base pair mutagens when completely tested, although being volatile, a desiccator system is often required. Methyl iodide is also mutagenic with a spot test or desiccator system. Alkyl iodides are more reactive with nucleophilic substrates than bromides and chlorides, respectively, and are more carcinogenic (Burchfield and Storrs, 1977). One halogen per molecule allows a general correlation between carcinogenicity and mutagenicity, at least in E. coli (Burchfield and Storrs, 1977; Simmon and Poirier, 1976). However, when two or more halogens are present on the same carbon atom, mutagenicity is not detected in conventional systems. The metabolism of halomethanes has been recently reviewed (Reynolds and Moslen, 1980; Ahmed et al, 1980). The cytotoxic effect of carbon tetrachloride is now considered to be due to its activation to a $\cdot CCl_3$ free radical; final metabolites include chloroform and CO_2. The free radical is generated by cytochrome P450 and is involved in lipid peroxidation (Recknagel et al, 1975; Recknagel et al, 1977; Ts'o et al, 1977; Vehleke, 1975). Another pathway with secondary importance to membrane toxicity involves the generation of phosgene (reviewed by Rinkus and Legator, 1980).

j. Chlorinated Cyclic

Of the chlorinated aliphatic carcinogens, two (toxaphene and chlordane) were mutagenic in Salmonella, three (chlordecone or kepone, aldrin/dieldrin and mirex) were not mutagenic, and one (heptachlor) has been incompletely tested. Chlordane was not mutagenic until tested in a desiccator; modified systems such as liquid preincubation or desiccator use may improve detection of this class. Chlordane undergoes reductive dechlorination, although in vitro and in vivo metabolites were not always identical (Brimfield and Street, 1979, 1981). Metabolism is probably to dichlorochlordene and then to oxychlordane (in vitro). The liver in vitro metabolizes very little chlordane; in vivo metabolites include the 1-chloro-2-hydroxy and 2-chloro-1-hydroxy forms, and eventually a compound similar to heptachlor is formed which possibly undergoes epoxidation similar to polyaromatics (Brimfield and Street, 1979, 1981).

Other non-mutagenic carcinogens of this group include mirex and kepone (chlordecone). Mirex is one of the most persistent pesticides in existence -- it is virtually inert to biological degradation (Matthews, 1979). It is stored in adipose tissue, and the half-life is longer than the experiments that have so far been conducted. In rats, the concentration of mirex declined only 40% 10 months after cessation of exposure (cited in Bedford). A small amount (5%) was excreted by Rhesus monkeys as the 9- or 10-monohydro product (Stein and Pitman, 1977; Weiner et al, 1976). Mirex is not degraded in soil, although anaerobic sewage sludge yields some monohydro products. It will also undergo photodecomposition at very low rates. Mechanism of carcinogenicity is unknown. Chlordecone (kepone NCI-Table 1) is a degradation product of mirex. It is more polar than mirex and therefore concentrates more in the liver and less in fat, but its metabolism is also unknown.

The last chlorinated aliphatics are aldrin and dieldrin (Ashwood-Smith, 1981). Aldrin is epoxidated by cytochrome P450 to dieldrin; after epoxidation of aldrin (and heptachlor), pentachlorodicarboxylic acids may be detected in vivo and in rat-liver homogenates in vitro, one chlorine having been removed. Dieldrin is excreted as hydroxylated products, with considerable variation between species and between organ systems.

The bioassay data for dieldrin were too limited to draw a conclusion as to its carcinogenicity, although EPA lists it as a suspect carcinogen. Aldrin and dieldrin were tested together in report 21, and dieldrin alone was tested again in report 22. For aldrin (Report 22) the subchronic test was inadequate, consequently during the chronic test groups had to be terminated and restarted, and/ or doses had to be reduced. Chronic exposure was approximately three-quarter-lifetime. The low-dose groups of rats had significant incidences of thyroid and adrenal tumors but the high-dose groups did not (no explanation given); this evidence was not sufficient to indicate a carcinogenic effect of aldrin in rats. Aldrin was therefore placed in NCI-Table 5 on the basis of statistically significant mouse hepatocarcinomas.

Dieldrin experiments (Report 2) had the same drawbacks as the aldrin experiments. Again in rats, the low dose groups frequently showed the highest incidence at several sites, such that there was a significant departure from linear trend, but only adrenal tumors in low-dose female rats were significant (p=.007). Female rats had thyroid (p=.043) and mammary (p=.041) tumors, but these were disregarded after the Bonferroni inequality was invoked.

The second study of dieldrin (Report 22) did not clarify matters. Only rats were tested, and a different strain was used. Group size was only 24 each, and three doses were used so that the Fisher probability was divided by 3 when the Bonferroni inequality was invoked. Also, the low dose was 1/5 the high dose, not 1/2 as mandated. Naturally nothing was significant even though there was a 5 1/2 -fold increase in leukemia in females. As seen in Table 4, for a β error of .20, 48 animals per group would be needed to detect a five-fold increase over a 4% control rate.

Leukemia incidence in female mice
(incidence/ number in group (% incidence))

matched control	low dose	mid-dose	high dose
1/24 (4%)	3/24 (13%)	5/24 (21%)	5/23 (22%)

k. Alkyl Phosphate

Of the 9 carcinogenic phosphates, 4 were positive in Salmonella, 4 were not tested completely and one, fenthion, was reported (in abstract form) to be non-mutagenic. The thioether of fenthion is metabolized by the FAD-dependent monoxygenase in hepatic microsomes to the sulfoxide, whereas parathion is oxidized by cytochrome P450. A study of fenthion metabolism in cattle showed that although 90% was unmetabolized, there was metabolism to the sulfoxide, sulfone and the oxygen analog (Hajjar and Hodgson, 1980; Wright and Riner, 1979). Fenthion is a weak carcinogen (mouse only) as are the other phosphates and thiophosphates, with the exception of tris (dibromopropyl) phosphate (NCI-Table 1) and trimethyl phosphate (NCI-Table 2). Table II lists organophosphates with the exception of the two (both mutagenic) just mentioned. On the whole, this class looks fairly innocuous as far as evidence of carcinogenicity is concerned. Even so, several have at least suggestive evidence (NCI-Table 6). No target site in particular was affected. Obviously toxicity varies tremendously, but is not consitently correlated with carcinogenicity.

There are marked strain differences (e.g. dioxathion) and sex differences (e.g. azinphosmethyl in the mouse: male MTD=60 ppm, female=125 ppm). Mutagenicity of this class as a whole has not been established, but more compounds may prove to be weakly mutagmnic with further testing.

Parathion, generally considered to be a much more potent and toxic analog of malathion, was placed in NCI-Table 6 although it probably could have been justifiably placed in Table 5 based on the total number of significant and suggestive incidences of tumors in rats.

Malathion, ten-fold less toxic than parathion, was tested twice yet still had to be placed in NCI-Table 7 as being neither positive nor negative. In Report 24, the incidence of female rat thyroid carcinoma showed a positive dose-related trend (Cochran-Armitage) but no group was significantly elevated (Fisher exact test). In male mice, hepatocarcinomas were significant at the p=.031 level, which was above the cutoff (p=.025) established by the Bonferroni inequality.

The second report 92 used a different strain of rats and no mice. Rat MTD's were set at 4000 ppm (male) and 2000 ppm (female) even though the subchronic studies suggested that 8000 ppm be used. Even at much less than the MTD, several tissues had 3-fold increased incidences (not statistically significant). Many of the control incidences were unusually high, particularly pituitary tumors in females. This particular site averages approximately 36% incidence, with a range from 8% (Report 22) to 73% Report 92.

1. Other

Four other carcinogens were found to be non-mutagenic: succinic anhydride, ICRF-159, asbestos and arsenic. Succinic anhydride is bactericial which hinders its testing in bacteria. ICRF-159 and related compounds have been tested in several assays (Witiak et al, 1977). ICRF-159, an acyclic diketopiperazine, blocks the cell cycle at G2 and inhibits DNA synthesis, is mutagenic to V79 cells and induces unscheduled DNA synthesis (UDS). The isopropyl connecting moiety, when cyclized to the cyclopropyl form, is not mutagenic to V79 cells but does induce UDS. Conversely, the analog trans-cycloprane-diamine tetraacetic acid blocks DNA synthesis and mutagenic to V79 but does not induce UDS. The latter analog is a strong chelator and may exert part of its affect in this way. A second undefined mechanism must also be in effect, and the authors pointed out that inhibition of DNA synthesis could lead to error-prone repair.

Table 11. Organophosphates

Chemical (NCI-Table)		MTD(ppm)* rat	mouse	Mutagenicity in Salmonella **
tetrachlorvinphos	(5)	16,000	16,000	0
fenthion	(6)			neg
dichlorvos	(6)	325	625	pos 100, 1535 ± S9
phosphamidon	(6)	160	145	NT
parathion	(6)	50	140	0
azinphosmethyl	(6)	140	90	0
malathion	(7)	8,500	16,000	pos? (conflicting results)
dimethoate	(7)	350	425	w. pos. 100 ± S9
methyl parathion	(7)	40	100	0
coumaphos	(7)	20	20	NT
malaoxon	(8)	1,000	1,000	NT
dioxathion	(7)	140	800	0

* approximate time-weighted average of both male and female high dose levels

** 0 = incomplete testing; NT= not tested ; w.pos. = weakly positive

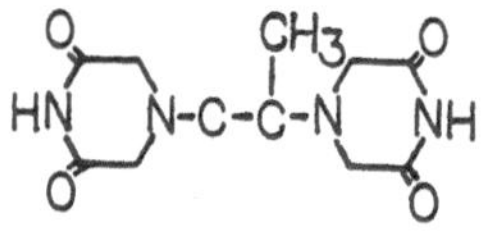

ICRF - 159

Inorganics are generally regarded as poor mutagens, although cadmium and chromium compounds have been detected in Salmonella (Rinkus and Legator, 1980). Arsenic and arsenic compounds have been designated as human carcinogens by the IARC. Arsenic exists in valence states of -3, 0, +3 (arsenite) and +5 (arsenate), most commonly as oxides but also as organic arsenicals. Metabolism of aresenic in mammals, including humans is by methylation: As(V) is methylated slower and eliminated faster thas As(III), which in humans is methylated to dimethylarsenic acid (Vahter and Norin, 1980). In the lobster, arsenite binds to protein sulfhydryl groups, being recovered as trimethylarsonium lactate or arsenobetaine (Cooney and Benson, 1980). Although arsenic has been reported not to affect the fidelity of DNA synthesis (Tkeshelashvili et al, 1980), it inhibits DNA synthesis in fetal liver nucleated erythroid cells and in man the presence of megaloblastosis implies aberrant DNA synthesis according to Morse et al (1980). Arsenic did not induce TK mutants in L5178Y cells (Amacher and Paillet, 1980), but did cause mutations in the *B. subtilis* rec assay, as well as in *E. coli* WP2 and WP2uvrA but not in *E. coli* CM571 carrying the rec A$^-$ allele. This suggests that arsenic causes non-excisable misrepair damage (Green and Muriel, 1979). Arsenic has recently been reviewed by Leonard and Lauwerys (1980).

m. Organohalogens in general

Many of the carcinogens considered in this report are chlorinated, especially in Tables I and III, and most of these are mouse liver carcinogens. The limited evidence available thus far suggests that many chlorinated hydrocarbons may not be mutagenic in vitro or in vivo, or at best may give limited evidence of weak mutagenicity. Many halogen fungicides are powerful biological alkylating agents, which is their mode of action as fungicides, because they contain halogen atoms activated by adjacent substituents (Burchfield and Storrs, 1977), but few are mutagenic in bacterial assays (Shirasu et al, 1976; Anderson et al, 1972; McCann et al, 1975). Chlorinated hydrocarbon insecticides are not strong alkylating agents but perhaps may be converted to alkylating agents by enzymatic dichlorination, dehydrochlorination, or epoxidation (Burchfield and Storrs, 1977).

Chlorines may be removed by either oxidative or reductive reactions (Ahlborg, 1980; Engst et al, 1979; Pal et al, 1980). Oxidative dechlorination can occur probably via cytochrome P450-dependent hydroxylation, followed by immediate covalent interactions with components of the membranes and destruction of the P450. Reductive dichlorination involves the action of two molecules of glutathione. DDT is reductively dechlorinated to DDD in vitro with microsomes if riboflavin is added. This reaction may also occur during the activation of CCl_4 to the free radical CC1 (Hutson, 1977). The controversy surrounding lindane metabolism stems largely from use/of anaerobic and aerobic systems: rapid anaerobic dehydrogenation (and loss of 2 chlorines) versus slower aerobic dehydrochlorination (one chlorine loss). Aryl hydroxylation via the arene oxide results in hydroxylation with or without loss of one chlorine, or with halogen migration (Engst et al, 1979).

Increasing chlorine content, for example in PCB's, increases lipid storage and decreases the amount available to the liver for metabolism and excretion. Peristence in tissues is not always correlated with carcinogenicity, however, or with other biological activity such as enzyme induction. Induction of particular liver enzymes by PCB's depends both on the amount and on the position of the chlorines. The presence of a chlorine may actually decrease carcinogenicity as in the case of 5-chloro-o-toluidine (NCI-Table 3) and o-toluidine (NCI-Table 1); and is consistent with ring deactivation (Garner and Nutman, 1977). O-Toluidine caused high incidences of spleen, bladder and mammary tumors, squamous fibromas and mesotheliomas in the rat, and hemangiosarcomas and hepatocarcinomas in the mouse. 5-Chloro-o-otoluidine given in the same dose range (3000-6000 ppm) caused no significant incidences in the rat, but still caused mouse hemangiosarcomas and hepatocarcinomas. The addition of a chlorine para to the amino group of aniline (p-chloroaniline) also decreases apparent carcinogenicity from NCI-Table 3 to NCI-Table 6. It is not really proper to make direct comparisons since NCI-Table placement refers to degree of evidence which in turn is at least partially dependent on toxicity and other factors.

As with the organophosphates, toxicity is not generally correlated with carcinogenicity in general. The 4 compounds dicofol, chlorobenzilate, DDT, and DDD all have a common metabolite (bis-p-chlorophenyl- benzophenone) (Burchfield and Storrs, 1977), and thus would be expected to have the same carcinogenic effect. The only site affected by clorobenzilate and dicofol was the mouse liver; DDD (or TDE) was weakly carcinogenic only to the rat thyroid. Chlorobenzilate was an order of magnitude less toxic than dicofol and thus could be tested at much higher doses, while DDD was approximately 10-fold less toxic than DDT. All 4 of these compounds were much less toxic and less carcinogenic to rats, but more toxic and more carcinogenic to

Table 12. Organochlorine Insecticides

Chemical (NCI-Table)		MTD (ppm)* rat	mouse	Mutagenicity in Salmonella
chlordecone (kepone)	(1)	25[a]	30[a]	neg
chlorobenzilate	(3)	7,000	3,000[a]	neg
DDE	(3)	700	290[a]	neg
chlordane	(3)	325[b]	60[a]	pos 100-desiccator
heptachlor	(3)	65	20[a]	0
toxaphene	(3)	1,000[b]	200 [a]	pos 100, 98 ± S9
dicofol	(5)	850	300 [a]	0
aldrin	(5)	60[b]	10 [a]	Neg
DDD (TDE)	(6)	3,000[b]	800 [a]	NT
methoxychlor	(7)	1,000	3,000	neg
lindane	(7)	400	160	neg
endosulfan	(7)	1,000	6	0
dieldrin	(7)	50	5	neg
endrin	(7)	5	3	neg
photodeildrin	(7)	7	0.6	NT
DDT	(7)	500	50-175	neg

* approximate time-weighted average of both male and female high-dose levels

[a] liver tumors only

[b] thyroid tumors, borderline significance

mice; this is contrast to the relationship between chlorobenzilate (less toxic but more carcinogenic) and dicofol.

In looking at organochlorines as a whole, one can see that the only site of tumors in mice was the liver; in addition to this some chemicals caused low levels of thyroid tumors in rats. The only exception to this was with chlordecone which caused high incidences of tumors in both rats and mice but in the livers only.

Some Comments on Structure-Activity Relationships

We have cautioned against using degree of evidence of carcinogenicity (NCI-Table placement) as a direct indication of carcinogenic potency. We will now ignore that caution and assume that degree of evidence per weight of chemical will give a rough indication of relative potency. Since almost two dozen tested chemicals were substituted anilines (Table 13), some general relationships might be suggested. Some chemicals (4-chloro-o-phenylenediamine, o-anisidine, p-cresidine) were non-toxic, therefore administered in high doses resulting in a high degree of evidence, in this case especially in reference to the bladder. Comparison of 2,4-diaminotoluene and 2,4-dinitrotoluene (both administered at fairly low doses) suggests that although some of the same sites were affected, the difference in apparent potency is due to the nature of the substituents. As disussed before, the addition of a chlorine to o-toluidine or aniline reduces apparent carcinogenicity. Positioning of the substituents is also of primary importance (compare o-anisidine, NCI-Table 1 to p-anisidine, NCI-Table 6). Other reports have considered these factors in more detail (Sontag, 1981; Garner and Nutman, 11977; Loew et al, 1979; Arcos and Argus, 1974; Clayson and Garner, 1976; Irving, 1979; Kriek, 1979; El-Bayoumy et al, 1981; Greene and Friedman, 1980; Zimmer et al, 1980).

In trying to determine relative potency, one might use the purely artificial gimmick of multiplying Table number x dose (Table 14). This calculation is similar to the "dose" x "response" = "potency" calculations used for risk evaluations (Crouch and Wilson, 1981). The smaller the number, the greater the potency, thus 2,4- diaminotoluene would have the greatest potency of chemicals in Table 13 and p-anisidine the least. It can be argued that a chemical with at least equivocal evidence (p-anisidine) could not be less potent than a chemical from NCI-Table 8 (2,5-toluenediamine), but p-anisidine was administered at a 5-fold higher dose. Likewise, non-toxic chemicals such as o-anisidine, although they are definitely carcinogens, may not be more carcinogenic per weight of chemical than more toxic chemicals which provided less evidence of carcinogenicity. Of course, more exposure to o-anisidine could be tolerated therefore it might indeed prove a greater risk in chronic exposure. We must await support of this kind of manipulation (evaluation of mutagenicity and other

Table 13.

	chemical(dose-rats,mice,ppm)	NCI-Table	tumor sites rat	 mouse
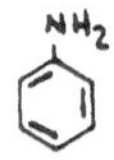	aniline (6,000; 12,000)	3	spleen peritoneum	none
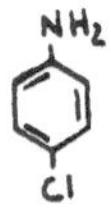	p-chloroaniline (- -)	6	spleen ±	hemangiosar- coma ±
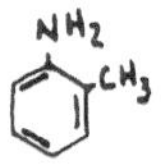	o-toluidine (6,000; 3,000)	1	liver peritoneal organs mammary bladder	hemangiosar- coma
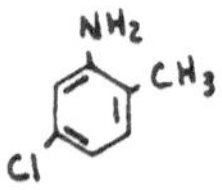	5-chloro-o-toluidine (5,000; 4,000)	3	none	liver hemangiosar- coma
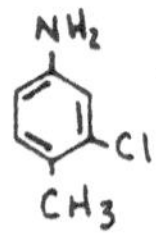	3-chloro-p-toluidine (3,300; 1,200)	7	none	none
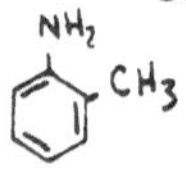	4-chloro-o-toluidine (- -)	3	none	hemangiosar- coma
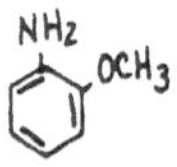	o-anisidine (10,000; 5,000)	1	bladder kidney thyroid	bladder
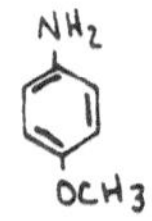	p-anisidine (6,000; 10,000)	6	preputial ±	none
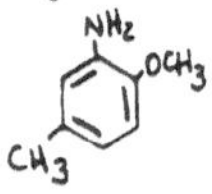	p-cresidine (5-methyl-o-anisidine) (10,000; 4,500)	1	liver nasal bladder	bladder
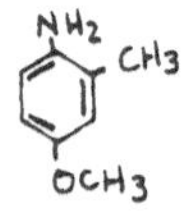	m-cresidine (2-methyl-p-anisidine) (gavage-not comparable: .16g/kg; .11g/kg)	3	bladder	none
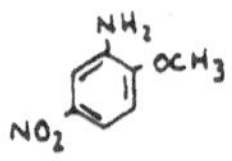	5-nitro-o-anisidine (8,000; 8,000)	2	skin Zymbal clitoral	liver

Table 13. (continued)

	chemical (dose-rats, mice, ppm)	NCI-Table	tumor sites rat	tumor sites mouse
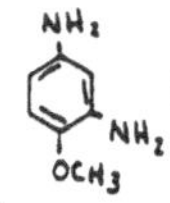	2,4-diaminoanisole sulfate (5,000; 2,400)	1	skin glands thyroid	thyroid
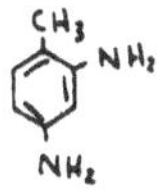	2,4-diaminotoluene (175; 200)	1	liver mammary squamous	liver lymphoma ±
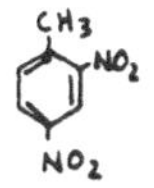	2,4-dinitrotoluene (200; 400)	5	skin, squamous mammary	none
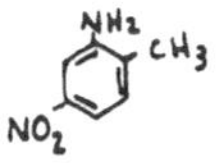	5-nitro-o-toluidine (100; 2,300)	3	none	hemangiosar-coma
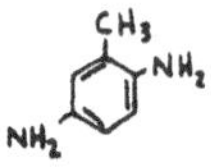	2,5-toluenediamine sulfate (2,000; 1,000)	8	none	none
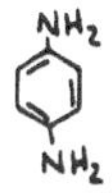	p-phenylenediamine (1,250; 1,250)	7	none	none
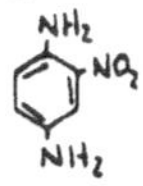	2-nitro-p-phenylenediamine (2,200; 4,400)	5	none	liver
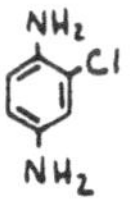	2-chloro-p-phenylenediamine (3,000; 6,000)	6	bladder ±	none
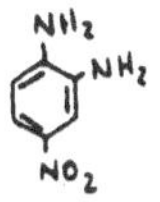	4-nitro-o-phenylenediamine (750; 7500)	7	none	none
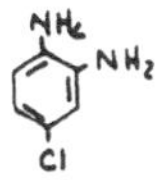	4-chloro-o-phenylenediamine (10,000; 14,000)	1	bladder forestomach	liver
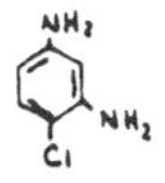	4-chloro-m-phenylenediamine (4,000; 1,400)	4	adrenal	liver
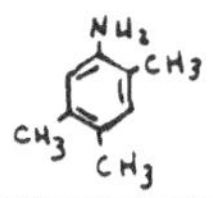	2,4,5-trimethylaniline (800; 100)	1	liver lung	liver

Table 14. Substituted Anilines

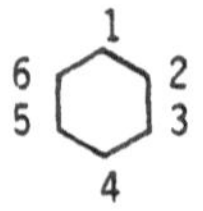

chemical	substituent at position 2	4	5	NCI-Table x high dose* rat	mouse
aniline	-	-	-	18,000	36,000
p- chloroaniline	-	Cl	-		
o-toluidine	CH_3	-	-	6,000	3,000
5-chloro-o-toluidine	CH_3	-	Cl	15,000	12,000
4-chloro-o-toluidine	CH_3	Cl	-		
2,4-diaminotoluene	CH_3	-	NH_2	175	200
2,4,5-trimethylaniline	CH_3	CH_3	CH_3	800	100
m-cresidine	CH_3	OCH_3	-	not comparable	
p-anisidine	-	OCH_3	-	36,000	60,000
o-anisidine	OCH_3	-	-	10,000	5,000
5-nitro-o-anisidine	OCH_3	-	NO_2	16,000	16,000
2,4-diaminoanisole	-	OCH_3	NH_2	5,000	2,400
p-cresidine	OCH_3	-	CH_3	10,000	4,500
3-chloro-p-toluidine	-	CH_3	Cl	23,100	8,400
5-nitro-o-toluidine	CH_3	-	NO_2	300	6,900
5-nitro-o-anisidine	OCH_3	-	NO_2	16,000	16,000
p-phenylenediamine	-	NH_2	-	8,750	8,750
2-nitro-p-phenylenediamine	NO_2	NH_2	-	11,000	22,000
2-chloro-p-phenylenediamine	Cl	NH_2	-	18,000	36,000
4-nitro-o-phenylenediamine	NH_2	Cl	-	10,000	14,000
4-chloro-m-phenylenediamine	-	Cl	NH_2	16,000	5,600
2,5-toluenediamine sulfate	NH_2	-	NH_2	16,000	8,000
2,4-dinitrotoluene 1=CH_3	NO_2	-	-	1,000	2,000

* NCI-Table number x high dose (ppm)

biological effects, calculation of ring activation by particular substituents) before this sort of numerical description of potency can be applied to one of the risk- estimate formulas. These issues are discussed in the new journal, "Risk Analysis" (Vol. 1, Number 1, March 1981, Plenum Press).

Extrapolation and Target Sites

There have been many arguments published concerning extrapolation from rodent to human, in particular concerning tumors with high spontaneous incidences in various strains of rodents. There will inevitably be some chemicals carcinogenic in rats but ineffective in mice (e.g. aflatoxin B) or vice versa, or human carcinogens not detected in rat experiments (e.g. 2-naphthylamine). There have similarly been extensive arguments concerning the basis for high spontaneous rates of pulmonary adenomas in Strain A mice or hepatomas in other strains of mice, ranging from genetically initiated lesions to differences in metabolism in target organs between species (Tomatis 1973, 1977; Ward, et al, 1975 and many others). Even though these differences exist, there is abundant justfication for accepting mouse hepatomas as evidence for potential human carcinogenicity, although not necessarily at the same site. For example, 2-napthylamine, benzidine and 4-aminobiphenyl are known human bladder carcinogens which cause hepatomas in mice (Shubik and Clayson, 1976). Species variation in metabolism, pharmacokinetics and pharmacogenetics, well-established for many pharmaceuticals, are increasingly being recognized in short-term mutagenicity tests. Specifically, for in vitro mutagenicity testing, a chemical is not well-tested currently unless liver microsomes from 2 to 3 species and with various pretreatments are used for bioactivation.

The liver is the target organ which has generated the most controversy, but which may be in fact the organ with the greatest statistical sensitivity as discussed earlier. Liver carcinogens for both rats and mice from NCI-Tables 1, 2 and 4 are listed in Table 15. Only NCI-Tables 1, 2 and 4 required that chemicals show evidence of carcinogenicity in two species; other liver carcinogens may be found in NCI- Tables 3 and 5, but the chemicals themselves are carcinogenic in one species only. Of 42 chemicals carcinogenic in both species, 15 were not liver carcinogens (carcinogenic at other sites only).

One chemical, chlordecone, was carcinogenic in both species only in the liver. One chemical, 1,2-dibromoethane, was a liver carcinogen in the rat but a non-liver carcinogen in the mouse (mouse lung and forestomach). Seven chemicals were not liver carcinogens in the rat but carcinogenic in the mouse only to the liver. Thus, with the exception of the 15 chemicals totally without effect on the liver of either species, mouse carcinogens were invariably mouse liver

Table 15. Liver Carcinogens

NCI-Table	Chemical	carcinogen* rat	mouse
1	3-amino-9-ethyl carbazole	+; yes	+; no
1	o-anisidine	non-liver only	
1	chlordecone	+; no	+; no
1	chloroform	-; yes	+; no
1	4-chloro-o-phenylenediamine	-; yes	+; no
1	p-cresidine	+; yes	+; yes
1	cupferron	+; yes	+; yes
1	2,4-diaminoanisole	non-liver only	
1	2,4-diaminotoluene	+; yes	+; possible
1	dibromochloropropane	non-liver only	
1	1,2-dibromoethane	+; yes	-; yes
1	1,2-dichloroethane	non-liver only	
1	1,4-dioxane	+; yes	+; no
1	hydrazobenzene	+; yes	+; no
1	4,4'-methylene-bis(N,N-dimethyl)benzeneamine	-; yes	+; no
1	Michler's ketone	+; no	+; yes
1	1,5-naphthylenediamine	-: yes	+; yes
1	5-nitroacenaphthene	-; yes	+; yes
1	nitrilotriacetic acid	non-liver only	
1	phenazopyridine	-; yes	+; no
1	phenoxybenzamine	non-liver only	
1	procarbazine	non-liver only	
1	reserpine	non-liver only	

Table 15. (continued)

NCI-Table	Chemical	rat	mouse
1	selenium sulfate	+; no	+; yes
1	sulfallate	non-liver only	
1	4,4'-thiodianiline	+; yes	+; yes
1	thio-TEPA	non-liver only	
1	o-toluidine	+; yes	+; yes
1	2,4,5-trimethylaniline	+; yes	+; no
1	Tris(2,3-dibromopropyl)phosphate	-; yes	+; yes

2	2-aminoanthraquinone	+; no	+; yes
2	1-amino-2-methylanthra-quinone	+; yes	+; possible
2	5-nitro-o-anisidine	non-liver only	
2	nitrofen	-; yes	+; yes
2	p-nitrosodiphenylamine	+; possible	+; no
2	phenestrin	non-liver only	
2	2,4,6-trichlorophenol	-; yes	+; no
2	trimethylphosphate	non-liver only	

4	4-chloro-m-phenylenediamine	-; yes	+; no
4	ICRF-159	non-liver only	
4	isophosphamide	non-liver only	
4	nithiazide	-; yes	+; no

* +; yes = liver carcinogen; other site ot sites also
+; no = liver carcinogen only; no other site
+; possible = liver carcinogen; possibly carcinogenic at other site also
-; yes = non-liver carcinogen only; no other site

carcinogens (except for DBE). Of the chemicals from NCI-Tables 3 and 5 which were carcinogenic in the mouse, only 8 of 32 were not liver carcinogens, including one mustard (mustards are generally non-liver carcinogens), captan (pH-dependent duodenal carcinogen), ethyl tellurac (see above) and 3,3'-iminobis-1-propanol dimethanesulfonate (injection site and local sarcomas only). Thus any mouse carcinogen is likely to be a liver carcinogen. This analogy cannot be made for rats: 16 chemicals caused cancer of the rat liver (among other sites) and 11 chemicals caused liver cancer in mice but not rats. These eleven chemicals plus 15 totally-non-liver carcinogens come to 26, or over half of the 43 total carcinogens from Table 13 were carcinogenic to rats at sites other than the liver.

Endless comparisons can be made between other target organs and chemicals or chemical classes, such as aromatic amine bladder carcinogens, carcinogens with hormonal-like actions, or sulfur-containing thyroid carcinogens. A few other chemical classes may have some consistency of target organs, particularly sites with rare incidences. The mustards were totally non-liver carcinogens, and two mustards (phenestrin and estradiol mustard) caused the only two significant incidences of heart sarcoma. However, other rare tumor sites such as Zymbal's gland or the Harderian gland do not have a readily apparent chemical- structural mechanism. It is hard to say how often an effect on rare sites is missed altogether strictly because of the unlikelihood of an effect there, or because such tissues are not routinely examined (see Page, 1980). Furthermore, different pathologists use slightly different terminology (e.g. fibrous sarcoma/fibroma) which make it a little difficult to compare incidences. For example, "sarcoma, multiple sites" includes peritoneal sarcomas and may also include sarcoma of peritoneal organs such as the spleen. Hydrazobenzene is reported as causing sarcoma of multiple sites only; aniline as causing sarcoma of multiple sites plus spleen sarcoma; acronycine and phenoxy benzamine as causing peritoneal sarcoma; dapsone as causing peritoneal plus spleen sarcomas, and o-toluidine as causing spleen sarcoma only. In this case, 3 of these chemicals were administered intraperitoneally (IPD, p. 19, acronycine and phenoxy benzamine), which must be taken into consideration.

A second data set available from the NCI reports are non-malignant endpoints (IRLG, 1979; Ward et al, 1979; Butler, 1979). Hyperplasia, for example, is considered the second step in the sequence: chronic inflammation-hyperplasia-nodules - adenomas-carcinomas. Since progression of this sequence is still open to controversy, these data are reported only as the pathologist's opinion, although the data could be statistically analyzed at some future date. Actually, the Interagency Regulatory Liason Group (1980) assume that preneoplastic lesions will become neoplastic. The malignant or benign response to a particular chemical is determined in part by genetics, and there is no known evidence for a different mechanism giving rise to benign versus malignant tumors. Also not considered statistically, although the raw data are presented, is total tumor incidence per test group or per animal. Total tumor burden might be increased without there being a significant increase at any particular site. This would only pertain to broad-spectrum carcinogens or promoters and not those with narrow target organ specificity or those which are so active that they act close to the point of entry. Indeed, known human carcinogens have been identified primarily by specific tumor incidences; only very large epidemiological studies have recently begun to pinpoint geographical cancer "hot spots" but even then the particular agent (or mixture of agents) cannot usually be determined.

CONCLUSION

Any report which attempts to correlate mutagenicity with carcinogenicity is dependent on the quality of data from two independent data sets, and on the selection of chemicals included in each set. It is logistically and theoretically, if not financially feasible to test large numbers of randomly-chosen chemicals for mutagenicity in the Salmonella/microsome assay, but it is completely impossible to do the same in lifetime animal bioassays. Thus, chemicals chosen for carcinogenicity testing are often at least suspected carcinogens, and not the random sampling of chemicals that a statistically-meaningful "correlation" requires. On a more limited level, we can calculate a "success rate", or the number of proven carcinogens which are mutagenic in the Salmonella assay. Of NCI carcinogens, 33 out of the 57 well-tested chemicals (57%) were mutagenic. If the incompletely- tested chemicals are indeed non-mutagenic, as they are often assumed to be, the success rate would then by 33 mutagens out of 82 carcinogens (40%). Of the more recent IARC carcinogens, there are 30 mutagens out of 45 well-tested carcinogens (67%) or 30 out of 52 well- plus incompletely-tested carcinogens (58%). As discussed above and by Rinkus and Legator (1980; in press), the selection of carcinogens could be varied such that a "success rate" could be very low (including inorganics, polymers, chlorinated aliphatics) or very high (alkylating agents, ultimate carcinogens).

The success rate is thus often predictable based on chemical class, nature and number substituents (e.g. aromatic amines) or metabolism. Several trends are suggested for non- mutagenic carcinogens: a) metabolism to an electrophile too short-lived to be mutagenic in vitro, b) too many sequential enzymatic steps required to produce an electrophile in vitro, c) several possible pathways of metabolism, only one or a few of which lead to an electrophile, d) the ratio of oxidative to reductive pathways in vivo and in vitro, and e) metabolism by host flora or other special conditions in the host.

The Salmonella/microsome assay has been fairly-well standardized, and is the most widely used mutagenicity assay. However, a number of chemicals have not been tested according to these standards (particularly in older reports), or have not been reported in readily-accessible literature. Furthermore, a large number of these carcinogens considered in this report have never been tested in the Salmonella assay and clearly deserve priority.

Bioassay reports in general are quite variable, and as with in vitro mutagenicity testing, often do not provide very strong evidence for a non-effect. For the chemicals which have a positive or suggestive effect, however, some indication of relative potency may be derived from a consideration of degree of evidence of carcinogenicity per weight of chemical in addition to mutagenicity, possible routes of metabolism and structure-activity relationships.

A major objective of all the various bioassay programs or reviews and of all the correlation- type studies is to provide some numerical factor for risk analysis (Pitot, 1980; Ashby, 1980; Shubik and Clayson, 1976). Of course, risk analysis itself is risky. One should ideally analyze for acute mortality and morbidity, although sometimes acute morbidity (or toxicity) is not recognized in humans or in animals as being caused by a particular agent because of non-specific clinical presentation, or anything short of death of a lab animal. Chronic morbidity and mortality from causes other than cancer (e.g. pneumoconioses) is even less readily visible. Equally difficult to measure is chronic morbidity and mortality due to mutations and/or cancer. There are many interrelated factors which have much more of an effect on the human situation than they have on inbred rodents in controlled environments, including the genetic basis of metabolism, induction of metabolizing enzymes, and tumor promotion. Other contributing factors or effects include variation in hyperplastic or inflammatory responses, compromised immunity (hypersensitivity or susceptibility to infection or autoimmunity), subclinical toxicity (weight loss and/or poor nutrition, subclinical neurological effects), sterility, interactions between multiple drugs and chemicals, and many others. Other effects of mutagens not related directly to cancer include the potential for increased birth defects, recessive mutations, and other theoretical effects of mutation such as viral reactivation or premature aging.

REFERENCES

1. Ahlborg, U. G. Dechlorination of pentachlorophenol in vivo and in vitro. In K. R. Rao, ed. Pentachlorophenol, Chemistry, Pharmacology and Environmental Toxicology, Plenum Press, New York, p. 115-130 (1980).
2. Ahmed, A. E., Kubic, V. L., Stevens, J. L. and Anders, M. W.

Halogenated methanes: metabolism and toxicity. Fed. Proc. 39: 90-95 (1980).

3. Amacher, D. E., and Paillet, S. C. Induction of trifluoro-thymidine-resistant mutants by metal ions in L5178Y/Tk cells. Mutat. Res. 78: 279-288 (1980).
4. Andersen, K. J., Leighty, E. G. and Takahashi, M. T. Evaluation of herbicides for possible mutagenic properties. J. Ag Food Chem. 20: 649-656 (1972).
5. Arcos, J. C. and Argus, M. F. Chemical Induction of Cancer-Structural Bases and Biological Mechanisms. Academic Press, N.Y. (1974).
6. Ashby. J. The significance and interpretation of in vitro carcinogenicity assay results. in K. H. Norpoth and R. C. Garner, Eds. Short-term Test Systems for detecting Carcinogens, Springer- Verlag, New York, p. 74-93 (1980).
7. Ashwood-Smith, M. J. The genetic toxicology of aldrin and dieldrin. Mutat. Res. 86: 137-154 (1981).
8. Baker, H. J., Lindsey, J. R. and Weisbroth, S. H. The Laboratory rat. Volume I. Biology and Diseases. Academic Press, (1979).
9. Bedford, C. T. Agricultural and Industrial chemicals; miscellaneous organis. in D. E. Hathaway, ed. Foreign Compound Metabolism in Mammals, Volume 4, The Chemical Society, London, p. 193-258 (1977).
10. Brimfield, A. A. and Street, J. C. Mammalian biotransformation of Chlordane: in vivo and primary hepatic consideration. ANYAS 320: 247-256 (1979).
11. Brimfield, A. A. and Street, J. C. Microsomal activation of chlordane isomers to derivatives that irreversibly interact with cellular macromolecules. J. Tox. Env. Health 7: 193-206 (1981).
12. Brown, J. P. and Brown, R. J. Mutagenesis by 9,10-anthraquinone derivatives and related compounds in Salmonella typhimurium. Mutat. Res 40: 203-224 (1976).
13. Brusick, D. Principles of Genetic Toxicology Plenum Press, N.Y. (1980).
14. Burchfield, H. P. and Storrs, E. E. Organohalogen carcinogens, in H. F. Kraybill and M. A. Mehlman, eds. Advances in Modern Toxicology, Volume 3, Environmental Cancer, John Wiley and Sons, New York, p. 319-371 (1977).
15. Butler, W. H. Pesticide related lesions of the liver and their interpretation. in P. Emmelot and E. Kriek, eds. Environmental Carcinogenesis, Elsevier Press, Amsterdam, p. 193-201 (1979).
16. Chiu, C. W., Lee, L. H. Wang, C. Y. and Bryan, G. T. Mutagenicity of some commercially available nitro compounds for Salmonella typhimurium. Mutat Res. 58: 11-22 (1978).
17. Clayson, D. B. and Garner, R. C. Carcinogenic aromatic amines and related compounds. in C. E. Searle, ed, Chemical

Carcinogens ACS Monograph 173, p. 366-461 (1976).
18. Cotruvo, J. A., Simmon, V. F. and Spanggard, R. J. Investigation of mutagenic effects of products of ozonation reactions in water. ANYAS 298: 124-140 (1977).
19. Crawford, A. and Safe, S. 4-Chlorobiphenyl metabolism: The effects of chemical inducers. Gen. Pharmacol 10: 227-231 (1979).
20. Crouch, E. and Wilson, R. Regulation of carcinogens. Risk Analysis 1: 47-58 (1981).
21. Dunkel, V. C. and Simmon, Y. F. Mutagenic activity of chemicals previously tested for carcinogenicity in the National Cancer Institute Bioassay Program. in R. Montesano, ed. Molecular and Cellular Aspects of Carcinogen Screening Tests. 1ARC, Lyon, p. 283-302 (1980).
22. El-Bayoumy, K., Lavoie, E. J., Hecht, S. S., Fow, E. A. and Hoffmann, D. The influence of methyl substitution on the mutagenicity of nitronaphthalenes and nitrobiphenyls. Mutat. Res, 81: 143-153 (1981).
23. Elson, L. A. and Warren, F. L. The metabolism of azo compounds. Biochem. J. 38: 217-220 (1944).
24. Engst, R., Macholz, R. M. and Kujawa, M. Recent state of bindane metabolism. Resid. Rev. 72: 71-95 (1979).
25. Festing, M.F.W., Inbred strains in Biomedical Research Oxford University Press, New York (1979).
26. Fujino, T., Matsuyama, A. Nagoa, M. and Sugimura. T. Inhibition by norharman of metabolism of benzo((a)pyrene by the microsomal mixed function oxidase or rat liver. Chem-Biol. Interact 32: 1-12 (1980).
27. Garner, R. C. and Nutman, C. A. Testing of some azo dyes and their reduction products for mutagenicity using Salmonella typhimurium TA1538. Mutat. Res. 44: 9-19 (1977).
28. Gart, J. J., Chu, K. C. and Tarone, R. E. Statistical issues in interpretation of chronic bioassay tests for carcinogenicity. JNCI 62: 957-974 (1979).
29. Ghiasuddin, S. M., Menzer, R. E. and Nelson, J. O. Metagolism of 2,5,2,5'- pentachlorobiphenyl in rat hepatic microsomal systems. Toxicol. App. Pharmacol. 36: 187-194 (1976).
30. Glatt, H. R., Metzler, M., and Oesch, F. Diethylstilbestrol and 11 derivatives. A mutagenicity study with Salmonella typhimurium. Mutat Res. 67: 113-121 (1979).
31. Greene, E. J. and Friedman, M. A., In vitro cell transformation screening of 4 toluene diamine isomers. Mutat. Res. 79: 363-375 (1980).
32. Green, M. and Muriel, W. J. Mutagen testing using trp reversion in Escherichia coli. in B. J. Kilbey, ed. Handbook of Mutagenicity Test Procedures, Elsevier, N.Y. (1979) pp. 65-94.
33. Griesemer, R. A. and Culto, C. Toward a classification scheme

for degrees of experimental evidence for the carcinogenicity of chemicals for animals. in R. Montesano, ed. Molecular and cellular aspects of carcinogen screening tests, IARC, Lyon, p. 259-281 (1980).

34. Hajjar, N. P. and Hodgson, E. Flavin adenine dinucleotide-dependent monooxygenase: its role in the sulfoxidation of pesticides in mammals. Science 209: 1134-1136 (1980).

35. Hedenstedt, A., Rannug, U., Ramel, C. and Wachimeister, C. A. Mutagenicity and metabolism studies on 12 thiouram and dithiocarbamate compounds used as accelerators in the Swedish rubber industry. Mutat. Res. 68: 313-325 (1979).

36. Hunt, L. M., Chamberlain, W. F., Gilbert, B. N., Hopkins, D. E. and Finsrich, A. R. Absorption, excretion and metabolism of nitrofen by a sheep. J. Ag. Food Chem 25: 1062-1065 (1970.

37. Hutson, D. A. Mechanisms of Biotransformation, in D. E. Hathaway, ed. Foreign Compound Metabolism in Mammals, Volume 4. The Chemical Society, London, p. 259-346 (1977).

38. Interagency Regulatory Liason Group, Scientific bases for identification of potential carcinogens and estimation of risks. JNCI 63: 242-268 (1979).

39. Irving, C. C. Species and tissue variations in the metabolic activation of aromatic amines in A. C. Griffen, ed., Carcinogens: Identification and Mechanisms of Action Raven Press, N.Y. (1979). pp. 211-227

40. Jellinck, P. H. and Bowen, J. H. Metabolism of 14 diethylstilboestral epoxide by rat liver in vitro. Biochem J. 185: 129-137 (1980).

41. Kinoshita, R., Santella, R., Pulkerabek, P. and Jeffrey, A. M. Benzene oxide: Genetic Toxicity. Mutat. Res. 91: 99-102 (1981).

42. Kriek, E., Aromatic amines and related compounds as carcinogenic hazards to man. in P. Emmelot and E. Kriek, eds. Environmental Carcinogenesis, Elsevier Press, Amsterdam, p. 143-164 (1979).

43. Kriek, E. and Westra, J. G. Metabolic activation of aromatic amines and amides and interactions with nucleic acids. in P. L. Grover, ed. Chemical Carcinogens and DNA Vol. II, CRC press, p. 1-28 (1979).

44. Lee, I. P., and Dixon, R. L. Mutagenicity, Carcinogenicity and Teratogenicity of procarbazine. Mutat. Res. 55: 1-14 (1978).

45. Leonard, A. and Lauwerys, R. R. Carcinogenicity, Teratogenicity and Mutagenicity of arsenic. Mutat. Res. 75: 49-62 (1980)

46. Loew, G. H., Sudhindra, B. S., Walker, J. M. Sigman, C. C. and Johnson, H. L. Correlation of calculated electronic parameters of fifteen aniline derivatives with their

mutagenic potencies. J. Env. Path. Tox. 2: 1069-1078 (1979).
47. Magee, P. N., Montesano, R. and Preussmann, R. N-nitroso compounds and related carcinogens. in C. E. Searle, Ed., Chemical Carcinogens ACS Monograph 173, p. 491-625 (1976).
48. Matthew, H. B. and Kato, S. The metabolism and disposition of halogenated aromatics. Annals N.Y. Acad. Sci. 320: 131-137 (1980).
49. McCann, J., Choi, E., Yamasaki, E., and Ames, B. N. Detection of carcinogens as mutagens in the Salmonella/microsome test: Assay of 300 chemicals. PNAS 72: 5135-5139 (1975).
50. Moriya, M., Watanabe, K., Ohta, T., and Shirasu, Y. Detection of mutagenicity of procarbazine by the host-mediated assay with polychlorinated biphenyl (Aroclor 1254) as enzyme inducer. Mutat. Res. 79: 107-114 (1980).
51. Morse, B. S., Conlan, M., Guiliani, D. G., and Ussbaum, M. N. Mechanism of arsenic-induced inhibition of erythropoiesis in mice. Am. J. Hematol. 8: 273-280 (1980).
52. Nagao, M., Yahagi, T. and Sugimura, T. Differences in effects of norharman with various classes of chemical mutagens and amounts of S-9. Bioch. Biophys. Res. Commun. 83: 373-378 (1978).
53. Nestman, E. R., Matula, T. L. and Kowbel, D. J. Mutagenicity of rhodamine dyes in the Salmonella/ microsome test. Env. Mut. 1: 140 (1979).
54. Page, N. P. Concepts of a bioassay program in environmental carcinogenesis. in H. F. Kraybill and M. A. Mehlman, eds: Advances in Modern Toxicology volume 3: Environmental Cancer. John Wiley and Sons, New York p. 87-171 (1977).
55. Pal, D., Wever, J. B. and Overcash, M. R. Fate of polychlorinated biphenyls (PCB's) in soil-plant systems. Residue Rev. 74: 45-98 (1980).
56. Parris. G. E. Environmental and metabolic transformations of primary aromatic amines and related comounds. Residue Rev. 76: 1-30 (1980).
57. Pitot. H. C. Relationships of bioassay data on chemicals to their toxic and carcinogenic risk for humans. J. Env. Path. Toxicol 3: 431-450 (1980).
58. Rao, T. K., Young, J. A., Lijinsky, W. and Epler, J. L. Mutagenicity of aliphatic nitrosamines in Salmonella typhimurium. Mutat. Res 66: 1-7 (1979).
59. Recknagel, R. D., Glende, E. A., and Hruszkewycz, A. M. Chemical mechanisms in carbon tetrachloride toxicity. in W. A. Pryor, ed. Free Radicals in Biology, Volume III. Academic Press, New York, p. 97-132 (1977).
60. Recknagel, R. O., Glende, E. A. and Hruszkewycz, A. M. New data supporting an obligatory role for lipid peroxidation in carbon tetrachloride-induced loss of aminopyurine demethylase, cytochrome P450 and glucose-6-phosphate. in D.

J. Jollow, ed. Biological Reactive Intermediates. Plenum Press, New York p. 417-428 (1975).

61. Reynolds, E. S. and Moslen, M. T. Environmental Liver injury: halogenated hydrocarbons. in E. Farber and M. M. Fisher, eds. Toxic Injury of the Liver, Marcel Dekker, New York, p. 541-596 (1980).

62. Rinkus. S. J., and Legator, M. S. The need for both in vitro and in vivo systems in mutagenicity screening. in F. de Serres, ed. Chemical Mutagens, Principles and Methods for their Detection Vol. 6, p. 365-473 (1980).

63. Scheline. R. R. Drug metabolism by the gastrointestinal microflora. in T. E. Gram,, ed., Extrahepatic Metabolism of Drugs and Other Foreign Compounds. S. P. Medical and Scientific Books, New York, pp. 551-580 (1980).

64. Shirasu, Y., Oriya, M., Kato, K. and Furuhashi, A. and Kada, T. Mutagenicity screening of pesticides in the microbial system. Mutat. Res. 40: 19-30 (1976).

65. Shubik, P. and Clayson, D. B. Application of the results of carcinogen bioassays to man. in ANSERM, 52: 241-252 (1976).

66. Smith, R. J. NCI Bioassays yield a trail of blunders. Science 204: 1287-1292 (1979).

67. Solt, A. K. and Neale, S. Natulan, a bacterial mutagen requiring complex mammalian metabolic activation. Mutat. Res. 70: 167-171 (1980).

68. Sontag, J. M. Carcinogenicity of substituted-benzene diamines (phynylenediamines) in rats and mice. JNCI 66: 591-602 (1981).

69. Stein, V. B. and Pitman, K. A. Identification of a mirex metabolite from monkeys. Bull. Env. Contam. Toxicol. 18: 425-427 (1977).

70. Sundstrom, G., Hutxinger, O., Safe, S. and Platonow, N. The metabolism of P,P'- DDE in the pig. In G. W. Ivie and H. W. Dorough, eds. Fate of Pesticides in Large Animals. Academic Press, New York, p. 175-182 (1977).

71. Tkeshelashvili, L. K. and Shearman, C. W., Zakour, R. A., Koplity, R. M. and Loeb, L. A. Effects of arsenic, selenium and chromium on the fidelity of DNA synthesis. Cancer Res. 40: 2455-2460 (1980).

72. Tomatis, L. The value of long-term testing for the implementation of primary prevention. in H. H. Hiatt, ed. Origins of Human Cancer, Volume 4, Cold Spring Harbor Laboratory, p. 1339-1357 (1977).

73. Tomatis, L., Partensky, C. and Montesano, R. The predictive value of mouse liver tumor induction in carcinogenicity testing - a literature survey. Int. J. Cancer 12:1 (1973).

74. Ts'o, P. O., Caspary, W. J. and Lorentzen, R. J. The involvement of free radicals in chemical carcinogenesis. in W. A. Pryor, ed. Free Radicals in Biology, Vol III.

Academic Press, New York, p. 251-303 (1977).
75. Uehleke, h. Binding of haloalkanes to liver microsomes. in D. J. Jollow, ed. Biological Reactive Intermediates. Plenum Press, New York, p. 431-445 (1975).
76. Vahter, M. and Norin, H. Metabolism of arsenic-74- labeled trivalent and pentavalent inorganic arsenic in mice. Environ Res. 21: 446-457 (1980).
77. Ward, M., Goodman, D. G., Squire, R. A. Chu, K. C. and Linhart, M. S. Neoplastic and non-neoplastic lesions in aging C57BL/6N x C3H/HeN (B6C3F) JNCI 63: 849-854 (1979).
78. Ward, J. M., Griesemer, R. A. and Weisburger, E. K. The mouse liver tumor as an endpoint in carcinogenesis tests. Toxicol Appl. Pharmacol. 5: 389-397 (1979).
79. Weiner, M., Pittman, K. A. and Stein, V., Mirex kinetics in the rhesus monkey. I. Disposition and excretion. Drug Metab. Dispos. 4: 281-287 (1976).
80. Witiak, D. T., Lee, H. j. Hart, R. W. and Gibson, R. E. Study of trans-cyclopropylbis (diketopiperazine) and chelating agents related to ICRF-159. J. Med. Chem. 20: 630-635 (1970.
81. Wright, F. C. and Riner, J. C. Biotransformation and deposition of residues of fenthion and oxidative metabolites in the fat of cattle. J. Ag. Food Chem,. 27: 576-577 (1979).
82. Wyndham, C. and Devenish, J. and Safe, S. In vitro metabolism, macromolecular binding and bacterial mutagenicity of 4-chlorobiphenyl, a model PCB substrate. Res. Commun. Chem. Path Pharmacol 15: 563-570 (1976).
83. Zimmer, D., Mazurek, J. Pezold, F. and Bhuyan., B. K. Bacterial mutagenicity and mammalian cell DNA damage by several substituted anilines. Mutat. Res. 77: 317-326 (1980).

A REVIEW AND EVALUATION OF HUMAN GENETIC BIOASSAY DATA FOR SOME KNOWN OR SUSPECTED HUMAN CARCINOGENS

Michael D. Waters,[a] Neil E. Garrett,[b]
Christine M. Covone-de Serres,[c] Barry E. Howard,[a]
and H. Frank Stack[b]

[a]Genetic Toxicology Division,
Health Effects Research Laboratory
U.S. Environmental Protection Agency
Research Triangle Park, NC 27711

[b]Northrop Services, Inc. - Environmental Sciences
Research Triangle Park, NC 27709

[c]Genetics Curriculum
University of North Carolina
Chapel Hill, NC 27514

INTRODUCTION

The purpose of this paper is to review and to evaluate a subset of the data base described by Waters et al.[1] This data subset deals specifically with the application of genetic bioassays utilizing human cells, tissues, and body fluids, to 13 of the 24 known or suspected human carcinogens cited in the larger data base.

METHODS

The procedure for collecting published papers has been described.[1] A selection of bioassay systems was made from the approximately 100 bioassays represented in the data base. The bioassays selected were those that 1) utilize human cells or tissues or 2) have been directly applied to body fluids or tissues from exposed human beings. The agents evaluated in either of the two bioassay system types were then selected by computer search from the larger data base. Papers dealing with combined chemical exposures were excluded as were reports concerning chemically induced sperm count depression or altered sperm morphology.

RESULTS

The results of the computer-assisted selection may be seen in Table 1. A matrix was printed by the computer which consisted of 13 compounds for which there were qualitative data in 1 or more of 12 different bioassay systems. The bioassay data retrieved are presented in this section according to bioassay group. The five bioassay groups are those which:

1) provide a measure of primary damage to the DNA of human cells by either a) monitoring the non-S phase incorporation of radiolabeled [^{3}H]-thymidine into DNA, so-called unscheduled DNA synthesis (UDS), or b) determining the extent of DNA strand breakage in human cells

2) measure the potential of an agent to inhibit the normal replicative synthesis of DNA in human cells in culture

3) determine the frequency of sister-chromatid exchange (SCE) formation in human cells exposed *in vitro* or *in vivo*

4) examine and quantitate gross chromosomal aberrations in human cells under *in vitro* or *in vivo* conditions

5) assess exposure to a genotoxic agent by use of an indicator organism (such as *S. typhimurium*) to detect mutagens in human body fluids or tissues.

Bioassays Measuring Primary Damage to Human Cell DNA (Bioassay Group 1)

Whiting et al.[2] have performed a comprehensive study on the effects of chromium salts on UDS and on DNA fragmentation as measured by alkaline sucrose gradient sedimentation. Hexavalent chromium, but not a chromic glycine complex, caused significant cytotoxicity, DNA damage, and DNA repair in cultured human cells. The specificity of chromium (VI) for SCE and aberrations was also reported by the same research group in a companion paper.[3] The ranges of concentration of chromate in which effects were detected in human skin fibroblasts are shown in Table 2. The lower limit for detection of genetic damage in the various assays spanned four

Table 1. Human Cell and Tissue Test Systems: Summary of Bioassay Results and Article Citations[a]

		Bioassay System												
			Higher Eukaryotic Primary DNA Damage						Sister Chromatid Exchange		Chromosome Aberrations			
		Body Fluid, Urine	(UDL)[b]	UDH	(UDX)	(UDB)	(IDL)	(DBH)	SCF	SCL	CYL	(CYX)	CYH	
Compound	Ref.	A B	A B	A B	A B	A B	A B	A B	A B	A B	A B	A B	A B	Ref.
Aflatoxin B1 (1162-65-8)	4		0/+											4
	6			(+)/+										6
	7			(+)/+	0/+							(+)/+		7
	10						-/+							10
	11						-/+							11
	12									+/0			+/0	12
	13									+/+				13
Arsenic, pentavalent (17428-41-0)	14									+/0			+/0	14
	31												+/0	31
Arsenic, trivalent (22541-54-4)	23									+/0	-/0			23
	30												+/0	30
	31												+/0	31
	43										+/0			43
Benzene (71-43-2)	15									-/0			-/0	15
	16									(+)/(+)				16
	17									-/0				17
	32												+/0	32
	48										+/0			48
	51										+/0			51
	52										+/0			52
	53										±/0			53
Benzidine (92-87-5)	4		0/+											4
	10						+/0							10
	11						+/0							11
Chloramphenicol (56-75-7)	33										+/0			33
Chromium compounds	2			+/0				+/0						2
	3								+/0					3
	34												+/0	34

(continued)

Table 1. (Continued)

		Bioassay System												
			Higher Eukaryotic Primary DNA Damage						Sister Chromatid Exchange		Chromosome Aberrations			
		Body Fluid, Urine	(UDL)[b]	UDH	(UDX)	(UDB)	(IDL)	(DBH)	SCF	SCL	CYL	(CYX)	CYH	
Compound	Ref.	A B	A B	A B	A B	A B	A B	A B	A B	A B	A B	A B	A B	Ref.
Cyclophosphamide (50-18-0)	4		0/+											4
	9							-/+						9
	10						-/+							10
	11						-/+							11
	18									±/0				18
	26									-/0				26
	35												-/0	35
	36												0/+	36
	37												(+)/0	37
	54										+/0			54
	55										+/0			55
	56										+/0			56
	57										+/0			57
	58										+/0			58
	70	+/+												70
	71	+/0												71
Diethylstilbestrol (56-53-1)	4		0/+											4
	19								+/0					19
	38												-/0	38
Epichlorohydrin (106-89-8)	20									+/+				20
	21									+/0			+/0	21
	39												+/0	39
	40												+/0	40
	59										+/0			59
	60												+/0	60
	73	+/0												73

Table 1. (Continued)

Compound	Ref.	Body Fluid, Urine	(UDL)[b]	UDH	(UDX)	(UDB)	(IDL)	(DBH)	SCF	SCL	CYL	(CYX)	CYH	Ref.
		Bioassay System												
			Higher Eukaryotic Primary DNA Damage						Sister Chromatid Exchange		Chromosome Aberrations			
		A B	A B	A B	A B	A B	A B	A B	A B	A B	A B	A B	A B	
Ethylene oxide (75-21-8)	22								+/0					22
	24									+/0				24
Melphalan (148-82-3)	8					+/0								8
	9							+/0						9
	26									+/0				26
	70	-/0												70
Phenytoin (57-41-0)	41												-/0	41
Vinyl chloride (75-01-4)	27									-/0				27
	28									-/+	+/0			28
	29										+/0			29
	61										+/0			61
	63										+/0			63
	64										+/0			64
	65										-/0			65
	66										-/0			66
	68										±/0			68
	69									-/0	-/0			69
	72	-/-												72

[a]Abbreviations used: UDL, unscheduled DNA synthesis in mammals--HeLa cells; UDH, unscheduled DNA synthesis in mammals--human diploid fibroblasts; UDX, unscheduled DNA synthesis in mammals--*Xeroderma pigmentosum* cells; UDB, unscheduled DNA synthesis in mammals--human bone marrow; IDL, inhibition of DNA synthesis--HeLa cells; DBH, DNA strand break--human; SCF, sister chromatid exchange--human fibroblasts, normal; SCL, sister chromatid exchange--human lymphocytes; CYL, mammalian cytogenetics *in vivo* and *in vitro* lymphocyte or leukocyte studies--all animals; CYX, mammalian cytogenetics, *in vitro* cell culture--*Xeroderma pigmentosum* cells; CYH, mammalian cytogenetics *in vitro* lymphocytes--human; A, no metabolic activation; B, with metabolic activation; 0, not tested; +, positive; (+), weak positive; -, negative.

[b]Parentheses indicate codes not specified by the EPA GENE-TOX Program.

Table 2. Ranges of Concentration of Chromate in Which Effects Were Detected in Cultured Human Skin Fibroblasts[a]

Effect	Concentration Limits (M) for Detection of Effect	
	Lower	Upper
Sister chromatid exchanges[b]	$3 \cdot 10^{-8}$	10^{-6}
Inhibition of colony formation		
chronic exposure	10^{-7}	-
acute exposure	$5 \cdot 10^{-6}$	-
Chromosomal aberrations[b]	$8 \cdot 10^{-7}$	$2 \cdot 10^{-6}$
DNA repair	10^{-6}	$3 \cdot 10^{-3}$
DNA fragmentation	$5 \cdot 10^{-4}$	-

[a]Taken from Whiting et al.[2]
[b]Data from MacRae et al.[3]

orders of magnitude. Increases in SCE's were observed at low concentrations without apparent toxicity, but maximum frequencies of SCE and gross aberrations were limited by the toxic effects of chromate. DNA repair and fragmentation were observed at concentrations and times for which colony formation from single cells was inhibited. The techniques used with the various assays differed to some extent, but the concentrations shown in Table 2 were thought to provide a reasonable estimate of the relative sensitivities of the assays to chromate.

Unscheduled DNA synthesis in human cells in culture (Bioassay Group 1a). HeLa cells. Among 51 compounds that Martin et al.[4] tested for induction of UDS in HeLa cells, the following results were obtained for 4 agents included in the data base. Aflatoxin B1 was active over the dose range 10^{-8} to 10^{-4} M in the presence of phenobarbital-induced S-9. Exposure was carried out for 2.5 h. Benzidine, cyclophosphamide, and diethylstilbestrol (DES) were active under the same conditions of metabolic activation--the former compounds over the ranges of 10^{-7} to 10^{-3} M and 10^{-7} to 10^{-4} M, respectively, and the latter compound at the single concentration tested of 10^{-6} M. Insufficient data were presented to permit definitive comparison of the relative biological activity of the four compounds in the system. However, the relative activities of aflatoxin B1 and benzidine observed in the UDS assay clearly do not reflect the substantial differences in activity observed in the Ames test or in rodent carcinogenesis bioassays that were reported by Meselson and Russell[5] (Fig. 1).

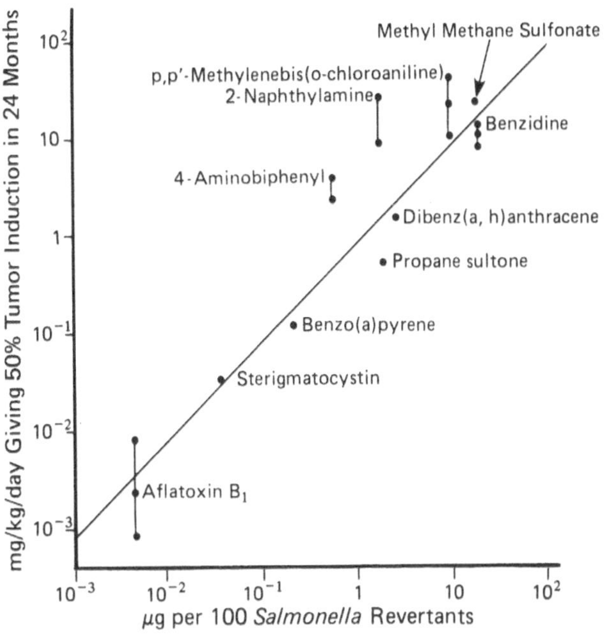

Fig. 1. Relation between mutagenic and carcinogenic potency. Used with permission of Meselson and Russell.[5]

Human skin fibroblasts. Among 64 compounds, San and Stich[6] examined the effect of aflatoxin B1 on the induction of UDS in diploid human skin fibroblasts. They observed [^{3}H]-thymidine uptake between approximately 10^{-5} and 5×10^{-4} M after a 30-min exposure to the compound in the presence of exogenous metabolic activation. Stich and Laishes[7] examined the possible specificity of exogenous metabolic activation systems from liver, lung, and kidneys of various animals for aflatoxin B1; they found no significant difference, although the carcinogenic effect of aflatoxin B1 differs greatly for the species used. In the same paper, Stich and Laishes compared the relative sensitivity of normal and Xeroderma pigmentosum (XP-E) fibroblasts with respect to the induction of UDS after exposure to aflatoxin B1 (2×10^{-4} M), and they found about 20 to 25% less UDS in the XP-E fibroblasts. However, the XP-E cells were more sensitive than normals to chromosome-damaging and lethal effects of aflatoxin B1.

Human bone marrow cells. The Swedish team of Lewensohn and Ringborg[8] examined the effect of the bifunctional alkylating agent melphalan on UDS in human bone marrow cells and in peripheral leukocytes. After a 30-min exposure to 10^{-6} to 10^{-3} M melphalan, UDS increased in the absence of an exogenous activation system. The various types of bone marrow cells were examined individually for their UDS levels, and UDS was generally greatest in the blast cells, i.e., myeloblasts (and promyelocytes) and erythroblasts.

DNA strand breaks in human skin fibroblasts (Bioassay Group 1b). Nordenskjold et al.[9] have described a procedure for studying DNA strand breaks using alkaline denaturation followed by hydroxylapatite column chromatography. The bifunctional alkylating agents cyclophosphamide and melphalan were tested in the system. In agreement with previous information, melphalan was direct acting, while cyclophosphamide required rat liver S-9 metabolic activation to induce DNA strand breakage in the normal human fibroblasts. Fig. 2 shows the time-related and concentration-related DNA strand breaks after exposure to melphalan at 10^{-5}, 10^{-4}, and 10^{-3} M. After removal of the drug at 0.5 h, DNA strand

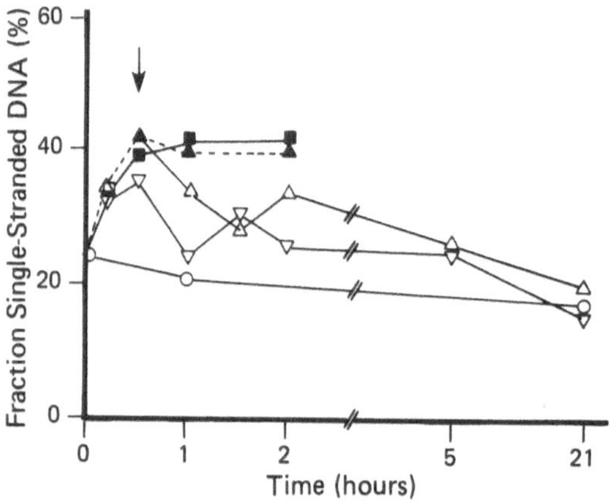

Fig. 2. Induction of DNA strand breaks in human fibroblasts by melphalan. Cells were incubated at 37°C in complete medium without melphalan (o) or with melphalan at 1 x 10^{-5} M (▽), 1 x 10^{-4} M (Δ), and 1 x 10^{-3} M (■) concentrations. Open symbols indicate incubations from which the drug was omitted after 30 min of incubation (arrow). Solid symbols indicate incubations in which the drug was present throughout the incubation. Used with permission of Nordenskjold et al.[9]

breaks decreased to background levels during a 21-h period, indicating DNA repair. The results for cyclophosphamide at 5 x 10^{-5}, 5 x 10^{-4}, and 5 x 10^{-3} M are shown in Fig. 3. In contrast with the results for melphalan, the DNA strand breakage level did not decrease within 21 h after removal of cyclophosphamide at 60 min. According to the authors, the initial decrease in single-stranded DNA eluted suggests the presence of interstrand crosslinks. This follows, since after a certain amount of chain breakage has occurred, crosslinks will result in an increase in the DNA fraction eluted as double stranded from hydroxylapatite. Thus, an apparently lower rate of DNA strand breaks will be recorded.

Inhibition of DNA Synthesis (Bioassay Group 2)

Inhibition of DNA synthesis in HeLa cells. In 1978, Painter[10] described a model which measures inhibition of incorporation of [^{3}H]-thymidine. After controls and treated cultures are prelabeled with ^{14}C-thymidine, $^3H/^{14}C$ ratios of treated cells are

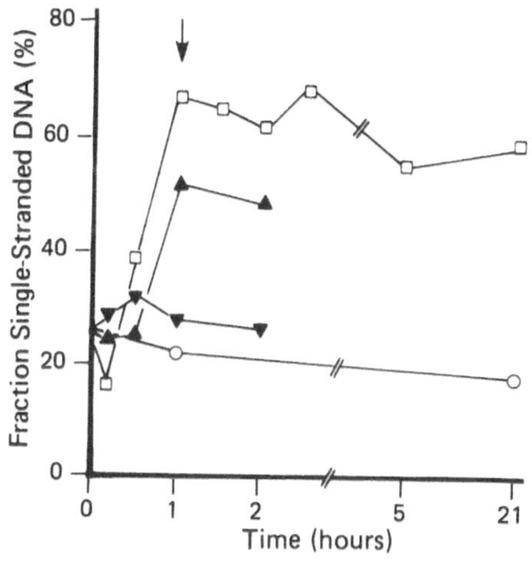

Fig. 3. Induction of DNA strand breaks in human fibroblasts by cyclophosphamide at 0 (o), 5 x 10^{-5} M (▼), 5 x 10^{-4} M (▲), and 5 x 10^{-3} M (□) concentrations. Cells were incubated with liver microsomes (0.7 mg protein/ml) from phenobarbital-treated rats, an NADPH-generating system, and cyclophosphamide. Open symbols indicate incubations from which the drug was omitted after 60 min of incubation (arrow). Solid symbols indicate incubation in which the drug was present throughout the incubation. Used with permission of Nordenskjold et al.[9]

divided by the $^3H/^{14}C$ ratios of controls, and the data are plotted as percentages of control incorporation into DNA. Aflatoxin B1, benzidine, and cyclophosphamide have been evaluated in this system, and the results have been compared with those of the Ames test.[11] The concentration that inhibited HeLa cell DNA synthesis by 40% within 2.5 h after removal of the agent from the cells, i.e., the "effective molarity," was plotted against the yield of mutants (in units of revertants per nanomole) in the Salmonella system. The results obtained are illustrated in Fig. 4. Aflatoxin B1 was effective at 5×10^{-8} M in the presence of S-9. Benzidine was directly active at an effective molarity of 6×10^{-4} M, and cyclophosphamide was effective at 6×10^{-4} M in the presence of

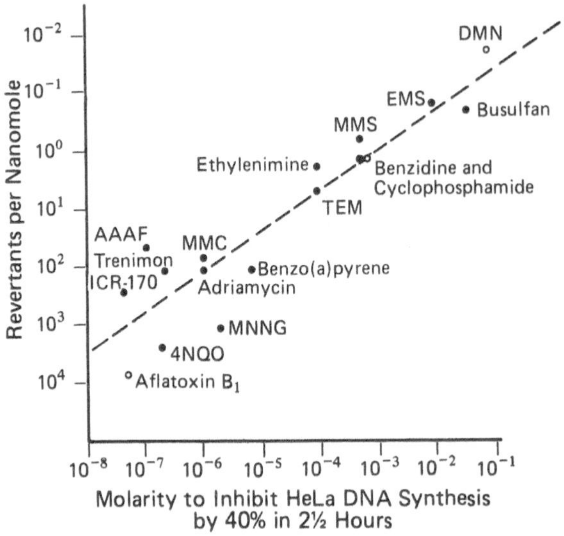

Fig. 4. A comparison of the relative effectiveness of various chemicals to inhibit HeLa DNA synthesis and to form revertants of mutants of Salmonella typhimurium: ●, Agents that did not require metabolic activation with S-9; o, agents that did require activation with S-9. The dashed line represents the best fit for the 17 points on the graph but does not imply statistical significance. Abbreviations: DMN, dimethylnitrosamine; EMS, ethyl methanesulfonate; MMS, methyl methanesulfonate; TEM, triethylenemelamine; MMC, mitomycin C; MNNG, N-methyl-N'-nitro-N-nitrosoguanidine; AAAF, N-acetoxy-2-acetyl-aminofluorene; 4NQO, 4-nitroquinoline-1-oxide. Used with permission of Painter and Howard.[11]

S-9.[10] These relative activity values compare favorably with those determined for the same compounds in the Ames test.[11]

Sister-Chromatid Exchange in Human Cells (Bioassay Group 3)

Data from SCE studies are presented below in two categories: *in vitro* studies and *in vivo* exposure. Also, because in most cases SCE studies were performed using human lymphocytes, these results are organized alphabetically by compound.

In vitro SCE. Aflatoxin B1. Elevated SCE frequencies were observed in human peripheral lymphocytes from healthy donors in an Egyptian study[12] at 72 h following exposure to aflatoxin B1 *in vitro* at concentrations of 0.01 and 0.05 μg/ml (3.2×10^{-5} and 1.6×10^{-4} M) in the medium. Nonrandom chromosome breaks and interchanges were also reported. In an additional study by Thomson and Evans,[13] SCE's were induced in human lymphocyte cultures after 1 h at aflatoxin concentrations of 10^{-3} to 10^{-7} M. Analysis of the dose-response curves generated showed that the addition of an S-9 mixture approximately doubled the SCE response. The results of these studies imply that human lymphocytes possess some ability to metabolically activate aflatoxin.

Arsenic. Zanzoni and Jung[14] of West Germany reported that inorganic pentavalent arsenic (Na_2HAsO_4), 10^{-6} M and 2×10^{-6} M, present for 72 h in cultures of normal human lymphocytes, induced a dose dependent increase in SCE per cell, which was significantly different from untreated controls at the higher concentration. Cell survival remained high at these concentrations. Chromosome aberrations recorded as breaks and pulverized chromosomes were observed at concentrations of 2×10^{-6} M to 2×10^{-5} M, which coincided with reduced cell survival.

Benzene. According to a 1978 paper by Gerner-Smidt and Friedrich,[15] benzene failed to change the SCE rate or number of chromosomal aberrations, compared to controls, when presented to human lymphocytes *in vitro* at 15.2 μg/ml or 1.52 mg/ml (1.9×10^{-4} M or 1.9×10^{-2} M) for 72 h in the absence of an exogenous metabolic activation system. Benzene did not inhibit cell growth at these concentrations.

An Argentinian group reported[16] in abstract form in 1979 that human lymphocyte cultures exposed to benzene in the presence of rat liver microsomes for 1 h or in the absence of exogenous activation for the first 24 h of culture exhibited elevated SCE/cell observed at 72 h. Exposure to benzene without exogenous activation for the last 48 or 18 h of culture inhibited SCE. Exposure concentrations were not provided.

Morimoto and Wolff[17] reported the results of a study on benzene and three of its metabolites--phenol, catechol, and hydroquinone--in human lymphocyte cultures. The study examined SCE and cell cycle kinetics. Shown in Table 3 are the estimated concentrations of benzene and its metabolites required to induce cytogenetic and cytotoxic effects. Exposure was for 72 h in the absence of exogenous metabolic activation. Benzene did not increase SCE nor delay cell turnover, in contrast with its metabolites. Catechol was the most toxic of the metabolites, and phenol was the least toxic. The SCE frequency in cells exposed to benzene, phenol, hydroquinone, or catechol as a function of exposure concentration is shown in Fig. 5. Elevated SCE frequencies were observed with benzene metabolites only at concentrations sufficient to cause significant (50% or greater) reduction in the mitotic index.

Cyclophosphamide. Raposa[18] tested several cytostatic drugs for their *in vitro* effect on SCE frequency. Cyclophosphamide did not induce SCE at 0.01 μg/ml (3.8×10^{-8} M) in phytohemagglutinin-stimulated lymphocytes exposed for 21 h *in vitro*.

Diethylstilbestrol. A study was reported by Rudiger and colleagues[19] in West Germany on SCE induction in human skin fibroblasts by diethylstilbestrol (DES) and two of the DES metabolites, DES-α,β-oxide and β-dienestrol (Fig. 6). The former metabolite results from oxidation of the olefinic α,β-double bond and is an electrophilically active epoxide. The latter metabolite is formed by peroxidases, probably via highly reactive semiquinones and quinones. It can be further oxidized to ω-hydroxy-β-dienestrol, which can form reactive esters. A third metabolic

Table 3. Estimated Concentration (M) of Benzene and its Metabolites Required to Induce Cytogenetic and Cytotoxic Effects[a]

Effect	Catechol	Hydro-quinone	Phenol	Benzene
SCE doubling	3×10^{-5}	9×10^{-5}		
12 h delay of cell cycle	2×10^{-5}	1×10^{-4}	5×10^{-4}	
50% reduction in mitotic index	3×10^{-5}	4×10^{-5}	7×10^{-4}	8×10^{-4}

[a]Taken from Morimoto and Wolff.[17]

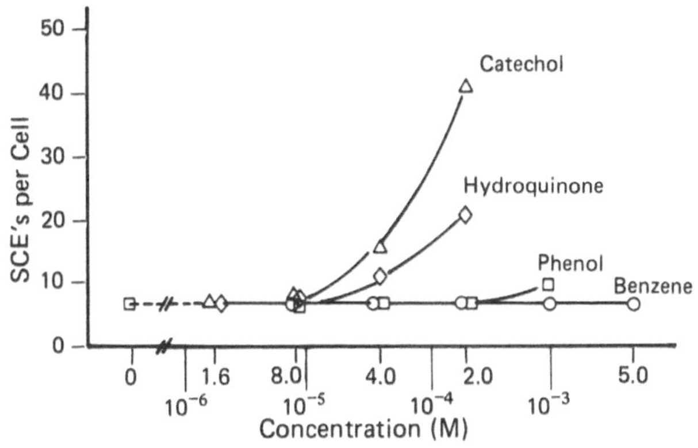

Fig. 5. The SCE frequency in cells exposed to benzene or one of its metabolites. The standard error of the mean is not shown, because it is less than 6% of the mean at each point. Used with permission of Morimoto and Wolff.[17]

pathway involves orthohydroxylation relative to the phenolic hydroxyl groups, leading to highly reactive catechols. With the two metabolites tested, DES-α,β-oxide and dienestrol, SCE frequency was increased at lower concentrations than with DES (Fig. 7), suggesting that the induction of SCE by DES required metabolic activation. In the presence of α-naphthoflavone, a cytochrome P-450 monooxygenase inhibitor, the induction of SCE by DES and β-dienestrol were markedly inhibited, suggesting that both these compounds require metabolic activation by monooxygenase(s) for induction of SCE.

Epichlorohydrin. Epichlorohydrin was evaluated for its ability to induce SCE in human lymphocytes in vitro in a study by White.[20] The compound induced SCE in a concentration-dependent fashion after a 2-h exposure at 2 x 10^{-4} M (twofold increase over control) and at 4 x 10^{-4} M (threefold increase over control). As would be expected for a direct-acting mutagen, the presence of rat liver S-9 reduced the apparent activity. The concentrations required to produce a threefold increase in SCE yield over control was raised from 4 x 10^{-4} M without activation to 10^{-3} M with activation (Fig. 8).

Norppa et al.[21] demonstrated an eightfold increase in SCE's in human lymphocytes exposed to epichlorohydrin for 48 h at a concentration of 0.4 mM. The compound significantly elevated ($P < 0.05$) the SCE level at concentrations of 0.05 mM. Other substituted epoxides (styrene-7,8-oxide, 1,1,1-trichloropropane-

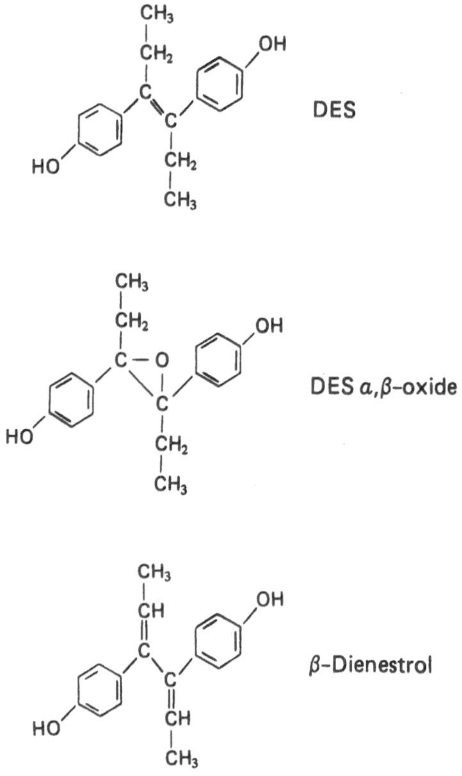

Fig. 6. Chemical structure of diethylstilbestrol (DES) and two metabolites used for SCE induction. Used with permission of Rudiger et al.[19]

2,3-oxide, and glycidol) enhanced SCE in a dose-dependent fashion and over the same concentration range as epichlorohydrin.

Ethylene oxide. The effects of ethylene oxide on SCE in human skin fibroblast cultures were studied by Star.[22] Concentrations of 360 ppm in the liquid medium caused total cell destruction, but at 36 ppm the cells remained alive, and SCE frequency rose from 12.53 to 16. Endotracheal tubes containing residual ethylene oxide at 200 to 600 ppm also caused elevated SCE.

<u>In vivo SCE</u>. Arsenic. Burgdorf et al.[23] in 1977 described an elevated SCE frequency in lymphocytes of six patients treated with trivalent arsenic (as Fowler's solution, 1% $KAsO_2$ in H_2O). All

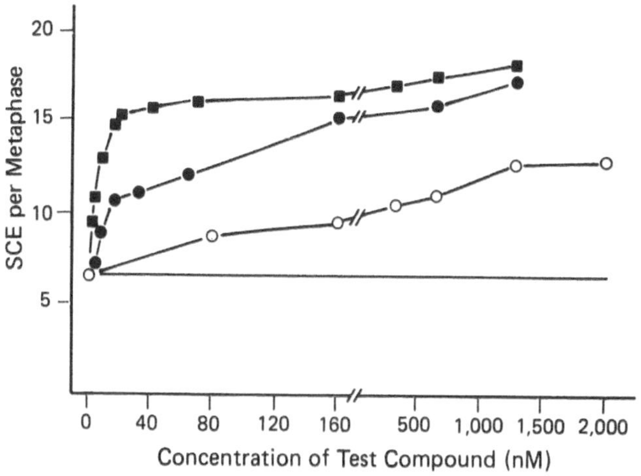

Fig. 7. SCE induction by DES (o) DES-α,β-oxide (●), and β-dienestrol (■). Used with permission of Rudiger et al.[19]

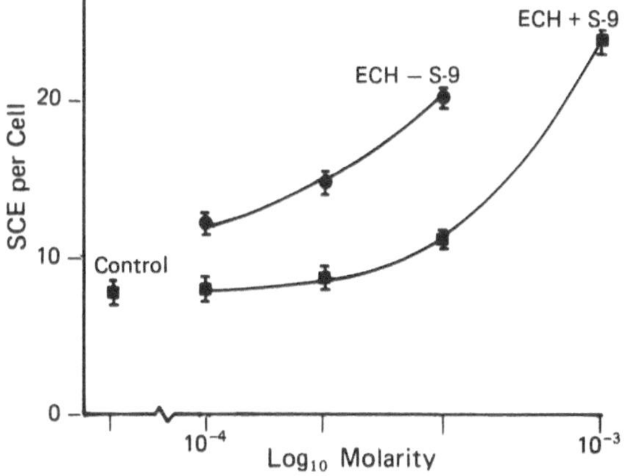

Fig. 8. The yield of SCE per cell induced in lymphocytes after exposure to epichlorohydrin for 2 h with and without metabolic activation. Used with permission of White.[20]

patients had stigmata (keratosis or diffuse pigmentary changes) from arsenic use as well as biopsy-proven skin cancers. The 6 arsenic-exposed patients had a mean of 14.00 (SD 3.12) SCE/mitosis, whereas 44 normal controls had a mean of 5.8 (SD 2.27) SCE/mitosis. There was no difference in chromosomal breakage between the two groups. The characteristics of the six patients exposed to arsenic are shown in Table 4; noteworthy is the latency period that was generally >25 years. The authors conclude that arsenic is implicated in the etiology of multiple cutaneous malignancies in the six patients and suggest that the significantly elevated SCE in cultured lymphocytes from these patients may be related to arsenical carcinogenesis.

Table 4. Characteristics of the Six Patients Exposed to Arsenic[a]

Patient	Age	Sex	Reason for As Admin.	Duration of As Rx (Years)	Interval Since Rx (Years)	Skin Cancer	Comments
1	45	M	asthma	2	26	+	
2	53	M	asthma	0.33	26	+	
3	41	F	psoriasis	2	24	+	
4	70	M	anxiety	0.50	56	+	400 rad to squamous cell carcinoma 1967
5	84	M	asthma	27	1	+	inoperable lung carcinoma; 5000 rad to skin metastasis 1975
6	72	F	asthma	1	33	+	fluoroscopy 2 x wk during As admin.

[a]Taken from Burgdorf et al.[23]

Cyclophosphamide. Clinical data were obtained in a study by Raposa[18] of SCE induction in lymphocytes after administration of cyclophosphamide or of cyclophosphamide in combination with other cytostatic drugs. A patient was given 100 mg cyclophosphamide daily for 22 days. After 13 days of therapy, the SCE frequency was greater than 20 SCE's/cell, and 3 weeks after cessation of chemotherapy, the SCE level was reduced to the spontaneous level (less than or equal to 10 SCE's/cell). SCE did not increase in all cells, and this observation was attributed to differing sensitivities of subpopulations of circulating lymphocytes.

Ethylene oxide. Twelve hospital workers involved in chemical sterilization using ethylene oxide were examined for elevated SCE in a study by Garry et al.[24] Peripheral lymphocytes from four exposed workers who complained of upper respiratory tract irritation displayed significantly elevated SCE frequencies, as compared to controls, 3 weeks after the last exposure to the gas. The same group of four individuals maintained significantly elevated SCE frequencies (10.3 ±1.8) relative to controls (6.37 ±0.47) as long as 8 weeks postexposure. Eight other individuals also displayed significantly elevated SCE frequencies between the eighth and ninth week after exposure. Controls consisted of 12 individuals who worked in an adjacent operating room area, who were considered unexposed or incidentally exposed to ethylene oxide. Infrared spectroscopy showed an ambient concentration of 36 ppm ethylene oxide in the hospital sterilization room during the purge/exhaust phase of the sterilization cycle. The open drain from the sterilizer unit showed a concentration in excess of 1500 ppm during the purge phase. The prolonged elevation of SCE in lymphocytes of employees after they had left the working environment was considered unusual by the authors, but this prolonged SCE elevation has been reported for animals exposed to mitomycin C in studies by Stetka and Wolff.[25]

Melphalan and cyclophosphamide. In another clinical study reported in abstract form, Lambert et al.[26] described elevated SCE frequency in peripheral lymphocytes from one cancer patient 2 weeks after melphalan treatment (SCE frequency 24.8 ±7.7 SCE/cell per individual, as compared to a frequency of 13.1 ±2.9 for nonsmokers and 16.2 ±3.6 for smokers). Cyclophosphamide-treated patients exhibited SCE frequencies just below the upper limit of control.

Vinyl chloride. Cytogenetic studies were performed on workers at a polyvinyl chloride factory in Norway.[27] Exposure had not exceeded 1 ppm in the past 2 years, and SCE frequencies did not differ from matched controls. For 16 workers, the mean SCE frequency per cell was 7.6, with a range of 4.7 to 10.5. The matched-control mean frequency was 7.5, with a range of 5.2 to 11.6.

In a more recent study concerning 21 workers exposed to vinyl chloride, Anderson et al.[28] found a slight increase in SCE frequency, but this effect was not statistically significant as compared to controls. The 21 workers comprised the second sampling from exposed workers and controls first examined 18 months earlier.[29] Chromosome aberrations in the exposed workers remained significantly elevated, suggesting that chromosomal aberrations may be more sensitive than sister chromatid exchange as an indicator of exposure to vinyl chloride.

Chromosomal Aberration (Bioassay Group 4)

Since aberration studies were frequently carried out in more than one *in vitro* test system, all such studies are grouped alphabetically by compound. Chromosomal aberration *in vivo* exposure studies are also organized alphabetically by compound.

Chromosomal aberration in vitro. Arsenic. Oppenheim and Fishbein[30] studied chromosomal aberrations in peripheral lymphocytes exposed to potassium arsenite. Cells were exposed for 48 or 72 h. Potassium arsenite at 1 μM produced chromosome gaps and breaks, translocations, dicentrics, and rings. The authors concluded that interference with oxidative phosphorylation or energy depletion can produce chromosomal breaks and rearrangements.

In a study reported in 1981 by Nakamuro and Sayato[31], the comparative cytogenetic effects of trivalent and pentavalent arsenic were investigated. Cultures were treated with arsenicals after 24 h and were harvested after 72 h. This protocol is preferred, since it avoids potential problems associated with blastogenic transformation in the presence of phytohemagglutinin. The number of chromosome breaks in human leukocytes was significantly higher for the compounds of trivalent arsenic ($NaAsO_2$, $AsCl_3$, and As_2O_3) than those of pentavalent arsenic (Na_2HAsO_4, H_3AsO_4, and As_2O_5). On an equimolar basis ($\sim 2 \times 10^{-6}$ M), the efficiency in inducing chromosomal aberration was in the order $As_2O_3 > AsCl_3$, $NaAsO_2 \gg Na_2HAsO_4 > H_3AsO_4$, As_2O_5. Trivalent arsenic was about 5 times more efficient than pentavalent arsenic in damaging chromosomes. The activity of the compounds with cultured human skin fibroblasts was similar to that observed in leukocyte cultures. An evaluation of colony-forming capacity after exposure to arsenicals indicated that trivalent arsenic was more toxic than pentavalent arsenic. It was also reported that arsenite (III) was more effective than arsenate (V) in inhibiting incorporation of [^{3}H]-thymidine and [^{14}C]-leucine into leukocytes.

Benzene. Koizumi et al.[32] of Japan reported in 1974 that exposure of human leukocytes to benzene in the concentration range of 2.2×10^{-5} to 2.2×10^{-3} M caused dose dependent breaks and gaps. Also, the higher the exposure concentration, the greater the percentage of hypo- and hyperploid cells. It should be noted that benzene did not induce SCE's in human lymphocytes in vitro at concentrations up to 1.9×10^{-2} M in one study[15] and 5×10^{-3} M in another.[17]

Chloramphenicol. Goh[33] reported that chloramphenicol, at a concentration of 80 µg/ml (2.4×10^{-2} M), added to lymphocyte cultures at 0, 24, 68, or 71 h produced chromosomal abnormalities (analyzed as vacuoles, dissociations, and translocations) in excess of those observed in controls. No increase in chromosomal breaks was observed. The highest incidence of abnormalities was seen when the compound was added at the G_0 phase of the cell cycle. Results were consistent with the known ability of chloramphenicol to inhibit protein synthesis.

Chromium. Nakamuro et al.[34] investigated the effects of chromium compounds on chromosomal aberrations, breaks, and exchanges. The compounds were added to lymphocyte cultures at various concentrations 24 h before treatment with colchicine. Compounds containing hexavalent chromium were much more effective than trivalent compounds in producing chromosomal damage. The efficiency of inducing chromosomal aberration was in the order $K_2Cr_2O_7 > K_2CrO_4 >> Cr(CH_3COO)_3 > Cr(NO_3)_3$, $CrCl_3$. K_2CrO_7 produced significant damage ($P < 0.01$) at 0.5×10^{-6} M, whereas 1.6×10^{-5} M $Cr(CH_3COO)_3$ was required to obtain the same level of statistical significance. These observations are consistent with other data[1] demonstrating that the hexavalent compounds are more effective inducers of gene mutation, primary DNA damage, and chromosomal effects.

Cyclophosphamide. Several reports were recovered on the cytogenetic evaluation of cyclophosphamide in human peripheral lymphocytes in vitro. The first of these by Chebotarev et al.[35] recognized the requirement for metabolic activation and treated cultures of human lymphocytes with the blood serum of mice injected intraperitoneally with aqueous cyclophosphamide solutions of 200 to 1000 mg/kg. Dilutions of active metabolites in the serum were estimated at ten-, fifteen-, or twentyfold in the lymphocyte cultures and were present for 1 h after 32 h of cultivation. Colchicine was added for 2 h prior to fixation at 56 h. A dose dependent increase in chromosome breaks and chromatid exchange figures was observed. An additional report by Madle et al.[36] in 1978 described: 1) the perfusion of rat liver in situ with cyclophosphamide and the direct addition of the perfusate to human whole blood cultures and (2) activation of cyclophosphamide with a crude homogenate of mouse liver and its addition to the cultures by means of dialysis bags. The former technique led to dose dependent suppression of mitotic indices and to the induction of chromatid translocations. The latter technique produced similar results when cofactors (NADP and glucose-6-phosphate) were added to the homogenate in a buffered salt solution. A report by Morad and El-Zawahri[37] described an incidence of chromatid breaks of 2, 5.33, and 6% at cyclophosphamide concentrations of 10, 100, and 1000 μg/ml of culture medium (3.8×10^{-5} M → 3.8×10^{-3} M), respectively. No exogenous activation was provided for the in vitro experiments. Because of the indirect method for applying the test agent reported by Chebotarev et al. and by Madle et al. and because of the relatively high concentration of test agent employed by Morad and El-Zawahri, these reports were not considered for comparative analysis.

Diethylstilbestrol. An abstract by Bishun et al.[38] indicated that DES was inactive in KB carcinoma cells and human peripheral blood leukocytes at concentrations ranging from 5 to 20 μg/ml (1.9 to 7.4×10^{-5} M). No additional details were provided. This report is in contrast with the report by Rudiger et al.[19] concerning induction of SCE in human skin fibroblasts by DES and two of its metabolites.

Epichlorohydrin. Sram et al.[39] reported that epichlorohydrin induced dose dependent chromosomal abnormalities in human peripheral lymphocytes in vitro at concentrations of 10^{-7} to 10^{-5} M. In that study, lymphocytes were cultured for 56 h, and epichlorohydrin was added 24 h prior to fixation; as a result, 28 aberrant cells were detected among 360 examined at the highest concentration.

Kucerova and Polivkova[40] studied the effect of a 24-h exposure of 10^{-6} M epichlorohydrin on human peripheral blood samples. Cells were examined by conventional cytogenetic and by banding techniques. Cells exposed in the G phase of the cell cycle demonstrated 2.5% aberrations by classical methods and 6% by the banding technique. When determined by the banding method, the number of aberrations increased to 18% if the cells were exposed in the G_1S or G_2 phase. Many aberrations escaped cytogenetic detection when only conventional techniques were utilized.

Norppa et al.[21] also studied chromosome aberration in PHA-stimulated human lymphocytes 24 h after epichlorohydrin treatment. However, the concentrations employed were much higher (0.05 to 0.4 mM). Aberrations were detected in 2% of the cells when exposed to the compound at 0.05 mM and in 6% at 0.2 mM.

Phenytoin. In a 1976 report by Alving et al.,[41] phenytoin was studied in 72 h cultures of human peripheral lymphocytes at concentrations of 10, 50, and 100 mg/ml in the culture medium. The compound was added 4, 24, and 48 h prior to harvest and fixation.

In 300 cells counted at each concentration, no significant chromosomal effects were observed, as compared to 300 control cells. These results conflict with the results of Muniz et al.,[42] who reported that phenytoin caused chromosomal damage under identical conditions.

Chromosomal aberration in vivo. Arsenic. A cytogenetic study on arsenic-exposed individuals was reported by Petres et al.[43] Chromosomal aberrations were observed in peripheral lymphocytes of 31 patients who had a history of arsenic exposure--14 psoriasis patients and 17 vine-growers. All displayed typical arsenic hyperkeratosis on the palms of their hands and the soles of their feet. Several of the patients had had arsenic-induced skin carcinomas excised. The control group consisted of 14 psoriasis patients and 17 healthy volunteers. The frequency of aberrations among the arsenic-exposed subjects was significantly elevated in comparison to controls (Table 5). Of interest was the observed aneuploidy, evidenced as chromosome "deficiency," in the arsenic-exposed population. Although the information contained in this report is incomplete, it provides human data which substantiate the in vitro chromosomal studies[31] and in vitro[14] and in vivo[23] SCE studies described in previous sections of this report.

Benzene. A number of reports have appeared in the literature linking chromosome damage in human lymphocytes to benzene exposure. Pollini and coworkers[44,45,46] published a series of papers describing chromosome damage in men that was related to blood disorders believed to be caused by benzene exposure. Vigliani and Saita[47] also described the clinical and laboratory details relating

Table 5. Number of Chromosome Aberrations in 31 Chronic Arsenic Patients and 31 Healthy Subjects[a]

Type of Abnormality	Arsenical Exposure Group	Control Group
Secondary constrictions	52	13
Achromatic lesions	29	3
Gaps	58	9
Chromatid breaks	34	1
Acentric fragments	39	2
Dicentric chromosomes	3	0
Number of mitoses	1121	1247

[a]Taken from Petres et al.[43]

benzene exposure and leukemia in six individuals. In 1965, Tough and Court Brown[48] reported that individuals exposed to benzene, but who have no blood disorders, may show chromosome aberrations in cultured peripheral lymphocytes. Forni[49] in 1966 described cytogenic studies of patients who had recovered from benzene-induced blood disorders and of individuals exposed to benzene but who did not show signs of toxicity. In both cases a slight increase in chromosome aberrations was demonstrated. In 1970, Tough et al.[50] published a report on individuals exposed to benzene in three different factories. In two of these groups, the percentage of lymphocytes with unstable chromosome aberrations (e.g., rings, dicentrics, and fragments) was higher than in the general population. However, the observed effects could not be attributed entirely to benzene exposure.

In a study from West Germany by Khan and Khan,[51] cytogenetic evaluation was performed using peripheral blood lymphocytes from 14 controls and 15 workers exposed chronically to benzene. Chromosome studies were performed on bone marrow preparations from four benzene-exposed workers and two controls. For each experimental subject or control, 50 lymphocyte mitoses were analyzed, and a smaller number (number not given) of bone marrow mitoses was scored. The aberrations were classified as chromatid type or chromosome type, and the latter included a) unstable changes, e.g., rings, dicentrics, or fragments, and b) stable monocentric anomalies, e.g., deletions, translocations, and trisomics.

In a more recent study by Picciano,[52] 52 workers exposed to benzene at less than 10 ppm were examined for cytogenetic damage in their peripheral lymphocytes. The controls for the study were 44 individuals seen in preemployment examinations, but these control individuals tended to be younger than the exposed workers. Table 6 summarizes the overall cytogenetic data obtained. Picciano scored 200 cells per individual for the presence of chromatid breaks (deletions), chromosome breaks (deletions), marker chromosomes (rings, dicentrics, translocations, and exchange figures), and total abnormal cells. Although there appeared to be no difference in the presence of chromatid breaks and total abnormal cells between the two groups, the benzene-exposed workers had twice the percentage of chromosomal breaks and three times the percentage of marker chromosomes.

The workers were divided into two groups according to the length of benzene exposure. Group I included 7 men with 11 to 20 years' exposure; Group II consisted of 8 men with 2 to 5 years' exposure. The percentage of chromatid-type aberrations in lymphocytes was 18.2 in Exposure Group I, 15.0 in Exposure Group II, and 13.2 in controls. Percentages of unstable chromosome

Table 6. Cytogenetic Summary of 44 Nonexposed Individuals and 52 Workers Exposed to Benzene[a]

Cell Characteristic	Nonexposed Individuals (8800 Cells)	Workers (10,400 Cells)
Chromatid breaks	1.1%	1.0%
Chromosomal breaks	0.35%	0.67%[b]
Marker chromosomes[c]	0.06%	0.19%[d]
Abnormal cells	1.4%	1.6%

[a]Taken from Picciano.[52]
[b]$t = 2.54$, $P = 0.01$.
[c]Rings, dicentrics, translocations, and exchange figures.
[d]$t = 2.18$, $P = 0.03$.

anomalies (e.g., rings, dicentrics, and fragments) in Groups I and II (2.3 and 2.2, respectively) were significantly higher than the control percentage (0.3). The percent stable chromosome anomalies (e.g. deletions, translocations, and trisomics) in Groups I and II (2.8 and 1.8, respectively) was also considerably higher than in controls (0.2). The chromosomal analysis of bone marrow cells showed similar changes. The relatively increased rate of aberrations in Group I was attributed to a 58-year-old male with benzene myelopathy, who had 30% chromatid-type and 14% chromosome-type anomalies.

A study of 65 persons exposed occupationally to benzene was reported by Fredga et al.[53] The study included truck drivers carrying gasoline, crew members of coastal tankers, employees at filling stations, and workers at industrial gasworks exposed to benzene. A moderate increase in chromosome aberrations was found in truck drivers and industrial workers who were exposed to the compound but not in the ship tanker crews or filling station staff. The authors concluded, however, that the truck drivers delivering gasoline did not have a higher number of aberrations than drivers carrying milk. The highest benzene exposure was a time-weighted average of 5 to 10 ppm for the industrial workers, and the corresponding frequency of chromosome breaks was approximately 3%.

Cyclophosphamide. Cytogenetic effects attributed to cyclophosphamide (aneuploidy and structural changes) were reported frequently in the 1960's. Unfortunately, many of these studies were performed in patients with malignant tumors, precluding a determination of whether these aberrations were caused by cyclophosphamide or were a result of neoplasia. Dobos et al.[54] reviewed the earlier studies and demonstrated in nontumorous children undergoing therapy with cyclophosphamide that the agent caused increased breaks (by 18.6%, including chromatid and chromosomal breaks and fragments) after as little as 4 weeks of therapy. This relatively high frequency of breaks was detectable during treatment and for 6 weeks afterwards. After 6 months, chromosomal aberrations returned to almost normal levels.

In a 1962 study by Arrighi et al.[55] of a patient with a sarcoma, examination of blood samples showed 0.17 abnormalities per lymphocyte (0.01 for the control) after the patient had received a total dose of 250 mg/day of cyclophosphamide for 20 days. Schmid and Bauchinger[56] found that in 13 patients with gynecological tumors who had received cyclophosphamide, 13.4% of the lymphocytes had chromosomal aberrations. This result was similar to a study by Bauchinger and Schmid[57] in which 19 patients with ovarian tumors showed 15 to 20% chromosomal defects in their lymphocytes. The number of abnormalities increased with the dose and the number of infusions of cyclophosphamide.

In a study by Schmid and Bauchinger[58] of 20 women with ovarian carcinoma, chromosomal analyses were carried out on peripheral lymphocytes. These patients received cyclophosphamide in doses of 15 to 30 mg/kg body weight and total doses of 1.2 to 18.2 g during an interval of 6 to 8 weeks. Structural chromosome aberrations were found in 16% of all cells compared with 1.9% for the controls. These patients also exhibited 13 times more chromosome breaks in their lymphocytes.

Epichlorohydrin. Thirty-five workers occupationally exposed to epichlorohydrin were examined in a 1977 study by Kucerova et al.[59] As a control measure, blood samples were collected before the opening of a new plant for production of the chemical. After 2 years of exposure to epichlorohydrin (0.5 to 5 mg/m^3) and of no exposure to radiation or drugs, workers were generally healthy. Four slides were prepared for each blood sample, and, if possible, 50 cells per slide were scored blind by 2 separate laboratories. Chromosomal aberrations were scored as chromatid breaks, chromatid exchanges, chromosomal breaks, and chromosomal exchanges. Gaps were scored separately and were not included in the number of cells with aberrations. Results of cytogenetic analyses from the two laboratories were not significantly different and were pooled. The average percentage of aberrant cells found in blood samples prior to exposure was 1.37; this number increased to 1.91 at the end of the first year of exposure and to 2.69 at the end of the second year. These postexposure numbers were significantly different from the preexposure value, with $P = 0.025$ and $P < 0.0001$, respectively. Chromatid and chromosomal breaks made up most of the increasing number of aberrant cells; chromatid and chromosome exchanges were rare. This study confirmed previous findings with epichlorohydrin in human lymphocytes _in vitro_.[60]

Vinyl Chloride. Purchase and colleagues[61,62] reported in 1975 and 1976 on effects of vinyl chloride. Of the 80 workers studied, 56 had been working in the manufacure of polyvinyl chloride and, therefore, were exposed to vinyl chloride monomer (VCM); the remainder were working in plants and laboratories where exposure to the monomer did not occur. The exposed group consisted of autoclave workers, maintenance workers, and workers involved with the manufacture of vinyl chloride; however, no estimates of exposure levels were provided (but see subsequent report by Purchase et al.[29]).

In Table 7 it may be seen that in the exposed workers there was a significantly increased ($p < 0.05$) percentage of cells with chromatid or chromosomal breaks (B cells) and of cells with aberrant chromosomes, both stable and unstable. These results confirm other findings[63,64] and demonstrate that vinyl chloride monomer at sufficent dosage has an effect on chromosomal aberrations in man.

In a study by Leonard et al.,[65] 11 male workers employed in the polymerization department of a vinyl chloride factory, 7 people from a laboratory of another vinyl chloride plant, and 10 controls from outside the factory environment were examined for the presence of chromatid and chromosomal aberrations in peripheral lymphocytes.

Table 7. B Cells[a] and Cells with Chromosomal Aberrations in Vinyl Chloride-Exposed Workers and in Controls[b]

Workers			Cells with Aberrant Chromosomes	
Category	No.	B cells (%)	Unstable (%)	Stable (%)
Exposed	56	6.30	1.45	0.38
Nonexposed	24	3.63	0.46	0.09

[a]B cells are cells with chromatid or chromosome breaks.
[b]Taken from Purchase et al.[61]

Although no chromatid aberrations were observed, chromosomal anomalies including fragments, rings, translocations, and dicentrics were seen in lymphocytes from most of the workers from the polymerization department of the vinyl chloride factory. However, it was not possible to determine if the observed chromosomal anomalies resulted from vinyl chloride exposure, since the medical histories of these workers showed that they had received frequent radiographs.

In 1977 Picciano et al.[66] described cytogenetic evaluations of a group of 209 workers employed for up to 28 years in the manufacture of VCM. The findings were compared to results from examination of 295 individuals given preemployment examinations. On a group basis, no statistical difference was found between the two groups when they were compared for chromatid aberrations, chromosome aberrations, and proportion of abnormal cells. A comparison of these results with previous reports suggests that the level of cytogenetic aberrations in vinyl chloride workers is probably related to the length and level of exposure. Results are shown in Table 8.

Based upon a 1973-1974 study, a 1978 report by Purchase et al.[29] documented the chromosomal morphology in peripheral lymphocytes of 57 men engaged in manufacturing vinyl chloride or polyvinyl chloride. The control group was composed of 19 on-site individuals and 5 off-site individuals who, for experimental purposes, did not differ significantly. Subjects with recent exposure to x-rays, viral infections, or prolonged drug therapy were excluded from the study. A significant increase in chromosomal abnormalities was observed in peripheral lymphocytes of exposed workers when compared to the combined controls. Greatest statistical significance was observed for the increase in total

Table 8. Cytogenetic Study of Effects of Vinyl Chloride on 209 Workers in Comparison to 295 Controls[a]

Cell Characteristic	Workers (10,483 cells)	Controls (14,761 cells)
Chromatid breaks	2.4%	3.6%
Chromosome breaks	1.0%	1.1%
Rings, dicentrics, and exchanges	0.4%	0.2%
Abnormal cells	3.7%	4.5%

[a]Taken from Picciano et al.[66]

number of chromatid breaks, chromatid gaps, or chromosome gaps, and in total cells having increased chromosomal abnormalities, both stable and unstable. This increase occurred in autoclave workers who were considered to be exposed to the highest average levels of vinyl chloride. Estimates of exposure (Table 9) were slightly lower than those reported by Hansteen et al. in 1978.[68] (See below.)

Of five other groups having lower average exposure, maintenance workers displayed the greatest increase in total cells with chromosomal abnormalities, as compared to controls; and a miscellaneous worker group (laboratory workers and managers) showed the smallest increase, with only chromatid gaps occurring significantly more frequently than in controls.

Workers with a history of exposure to excursion levels of VCM exhibited a higher percentage of abnormal cells. Further analysis indicated that a recent exposure to excursion levels and length of employment were both significantly correlated with chromatid gaps, total C cells, and fragments.

Cytogenetic studies were performed in 1974 by Hansteen and colleagues[68] on 39 workers from a Norwegian polyvinyl chloride plant. Sixteen healthy men not associated with the plant were chosen as controls. The cytogenetic study was repeated 2 to 2.5 years later for 37 of the 39 workers. According to the authors, during this time interval, the workers had minimal exposure to VCM. There was a substantial reduction in the estimated exposure to vinyl chloride from 1950 to 1975, as shown in Table 10. This repeated study was performed using 32 matched controls from the office employees in the factory. Using 48-h lymphocyte cultures, the breaks, gaps, and stable rearrangements were scored in 100 metaphases per person. In the first

Table 9. Estimated Average Operator Exposure to VCM in PVC Plants[a]

Time Periods	Approximate VCM Concentration (ppm)
1945-1955	1000
1955-1960	400-500
1960-1970	300-400
Mid 1973	15
1975	5

[a]Taken from Purchase et al.[29] Estimates of Barnes.[67]

Table 10. Air Concentration of VCM in the PVC Plant[a,b]

Time Periods		VCM Concentration (ppm)
1950-1954		2000
1955-1959		1000
1960-1967		500
1968-1972		100
1972-1974		80
1974	Measured	25
1975-		1

[a]Taken from Hansteen et al.[68]
[b]Estimates are based upon the level of production, and the number and types of autoclaves used in the respective time periods.

cytogenetics study, the mean chromosome breakage frequency for the workers (3.41%) was significantly higher than for the controls (1.79%). Bone marrow preparations from four workers were studied in the first investigation. The frequency of mean chromosome breaks was higher (4.2%) in the bone marrows of these four workers than that reported by the authors for normal bone marrows (0.2, 0.4, 1.7%; reference not provided), and higher than for the corresponding lymphocyte cultures. In the repeated lymphocyte study, however, no difference was found in the mean frequency of chromosome breakages between the workers and matched controls. Also, there was no difference between these breakage frequencies and the breakage frequency for the previous control group. The results suggested a relationship between the reduction in exposure to VCM and the normalized chromosome breakage frequency. SCE's were studied for 16 workers and 16 matched controls, and a mean of 7.6 SCE's per cell was found for workers and for controls.

In a separate study reported in abstract form by Hansteen[69] in 1978, two young Norwegian workers who had not previously been exposed to any chemical were exposed to 1000 to 3000 ppm VCM for 5 min. Blood samples were taken from the workers and one control individual at 4 h, 28 h, and 7 days after exposure. Lymphocyte cultures were prepared and harvested after 53 h. Breaks, gaps, and rearrangements were scored in 100 cells per person. The total breakage frequency varied in each of the exposed individuals from 0 to 4% for each of the time intervals tested. There was no difference in the frequencies of gaps and rearrangements between the workers and the control. To study SCE's, fresh blood samples and 1-day-old samples stored at 4°C were cultured for 69 and 72 h.

The last 48 h of the culture period was in the presence of 3 μg/ml BrdU. SCE frequencies were within the normal range of 7.3 to 10.4 exchanges per cell for both 69- and 72-h cultures of fresh and stored blood for each of the times tested. The authors concluded that high exposure of 1000 to 3000 ppm for the short time of 5 min had no chromosome-damaging effect on blood samples taken 4 h, 28 h, and 7 days after exposure. This study argues against the attribution of any significant chromosomal effects immediately resulting from exposure to vinyl chloride monomer.

The Screening of Human Body Fluids for Mutagenic Activity (Bioassay Group 5)

One of the best sources of information concerning mutagenic activity in human body fluids is from clinical studies of patients receiving chemotherapeutic agents. A study by Minnich et al.[70] showed that 8 mg of oral melphalan did not increase the mutagenic activity of urine detected using *S. typhimurium* strain TA1535. However, patients receiving cyclophosphamide showed high mutagenic activity in their urine with TA1535. No difference in mutagenic activity with cyclophosphamide was observed when the urine was tested with and without S-9. The urine but not the ascitic fluid of a patient receiving a 0.4-g dose of cyclophosphamide induced mitotic gene conversion in *S. cerevisiae*.[71] The patient received 0.2 g of cyclophosphamide on 2 successive days, and samples of urine and ascitic fluid were collected after 2, 4, and 8 h. Mutagenicity of urine was also evaluated in 20 people working in a vinyl chloride-producing plant,[72] but no activity was observed using *S. typhimurium* TA100 as the indicator strain. An abstract by Kilian et al.[73] described direct testing of epichlorohydrin in *S. typhimurium* strain TA1535 with positive results. The report indicated that an analysis of the urine of six workers exposed to 0.8 to 4.0 ppm epichlorohydrin failed to reveal any activity, even in pooled and concentrated samples. However, in the urine of two workers who were inadvertently exposed to a concentration in excess of 25 ppm, mutagenic activity was detected as a conjugate. Mutagenic activity also was reported in the urine of mice after oral administration of epichlorohydrin at 200 to 400 mg/kg.

DISCUSSION

The relatively small number of papers recovered in the present data base subset precludes extensive comparison and discussion of findings. However, Tables 11 and 12 reflect our effort to organize information relative to exposure concentration (dose) and response obtained in several genetic bioassays. These bioassays represent four of the five categories of systems mentioned earlier: unscheduled DNA synthesis, DNA strand breaks, inhibition of DNA

Table 11. Concentrations Required of Selected Compounds to Induce DNA Damage or Inhibition of DNA Synthesis *In Vitro*[a]

Compound	Unscheduled DNA Synthesis in HeLa Cells (E = 2.5 h)[b]	Unscheduled DNA Synthesis in Human Skin Fibroblasts and Human Bone Marrow Cells (E = 0.5 h)	Inhibition of DNA Synthesis in HeLa Cells (E = 0.5 h -S-9, E = 1 h +S-9)	DNA Strand Breaks in Human Skin Fibroblasts
Aflatoxin B1	$10^{-8} \rightarrow 10^{-4}$ M max[c] 10^{-4} M 0/+[d] (Martin et al.[4])	$10^{-5} \rightarrow 5 \times 10^{-4}$ M (+)/+ (San and Stich[6])	5×10^{-8} M[e] -/+ (Painter[10])	
Benzidine	$10^{-7} \rightarrow 10^{-3}$ M max[c] 10^{-6} M 0/+ (Martin et al.[4])		6×10^{-4} M[e] +/0 (Painter[10])	
Cyclo-phosphamide	10^{-6} M max[c] 10^{-6} M 0/+ (Martin et al.[4])		6×10^{-4} M[e] -/+ (Painter[10])	$5 \times 10^{-5} \rightarrow 5 \times 10^{-3}$ M max[f] 5×10^{-3} M E = 1 h -/+ (Nordenskjold et al.[9])
Diethyl-stilbestrol	10^{-6} M max[c] 10^{-6} M 0/+ (Martin et al.[4])			
Melphalan		$10^{-6} \rightarrow 10^{-3}$ M max[g] 10^{-3} M +/0 (Lewensohn & Ringborg[8])		$10^{-5} \rightarrow 10^{-3}$ M max[f] 10^{-4} M E = 0.5 h +/0 (Nordenskjold et al.[9])

[a] Appropriate researchers are cited for producing the data retrieved.
[b] E, exposure time.
[c] Maximum dpm/μg DNA above background.
[d] Without S-9/with S-9: 0, not tested; +, positive results; -, negative results.
[e] Effective molarity, concentration that inhibited DNA synthesis by 40% within 2.5 h after removal of agent.
[f] Maximum fraction of single-stranded DNA.
[g] Maximum net grain count per nucleus.

Table 12. Concentrations Required of Selected Compounds to Induce Sister Chromatid Exchange and Chromosome Aberrations in Human Lymphocytes[a]

Compound	Sister Chromatid Exchange In Vitro	Sister Chromatid Exchange In Vivo	Chromosome Aberration In Vitro	Chromosome Aberration In Vivo
Aflatoxin B1	$10^{-7} \rightarrow 10^{-3}$ M E^b = 1 h +/+[c] (Thomson & Evans[13])		$3.2 \times 10^{-7} \rightarrow 3.2 \times 10^{-8}$ M E = 24, 48, 72 +/0 (El-Zawahri et al.[12])	
Arsenic	10^{-6} M & 2×10^{-6} M E^b = 72 h +/0 (Zanzoni & Jung[14])	Unknown concentration +/0 (Burgdorf et al.[23])	$6 \times 10^{-7} \rightarrow 7.2 \times 10^{-6}$ M E = 24 h +/0 (Nakamuro & Sayato[31])	Unknown concentration +/0 (Petres et al.[43])
			10^{-6} M E = 48, 72 h +/0 (Oppenheim & Fishbein[30])	
Benzene	1.9×10^{-4} or 1.9×10^{-2} M E = 3 days -/0 (Gerner-Smidt & Friedrich[15])		$2.2 \times 10^{-5} \rightarrow 2.2 \times 10^{-3}$ M E = 24 h +/0 (Koizumi et al.[32])	< 10 ppm +/0 (Picciano[52])
	$8 \times 10^{-4} \rightarrow 5 \times 10^{-3}$ M E = 72 h -/0 (Morimoto & Wolff[17])		$1.9 \times 10^{-4} \rightarrow 1.9 \times 10^{-2}$ M E = 3 days -/0 (Gerner-Smidt & Friedrich[15])	≤ 10 ppm ±/0 (Fredga et al.[53])
				Unknown concentration E = 1 → 20 years +/0 (Tough & Court Brown[48])
				Unknown concentration E = 2 → 20 years +/0 (Khan & Khan[51])

(continued)

Table 12. (Continued)

Compound	Sister Chromatid Exchange In Vitro	Sister Chromatid Exchange In Vivo	Chromosome Aberration In Vitro	Chromosome Aberration In Vivo
Cyclophosphamide	3.8×10^{-8} M E = 21 h -/0 (Raposa[18])	100 mg/day E = 22 days +/0 (Raposa[18])	$5 \times 10^{-5} \rightarrow 5.7 \times 10^{-3}$ M E = 3 h 0/+ (Madle et al.[36])	1.5 → 1.7 g (total) E unknown +/0 (Schmid & Bauchinger[56])
				250 mg/day E = 20 days +/0 (Arrighi et al.[55])
				1.2 → 18.2 g (total) E = 6 → 8 weeks +/0 (Schmid & Bauchinger[58])
				1.5 → 18.8 g (total) E = variable +/0 (Bauchinger & Schmid[57])
				3 → 5 mg/day E = 6 → 8 months +/0 (Dobos et al.[54])
Diethylstilbestrol	$8 \times 10^{-8} \rightarrow 2 \times 10^{-6}$ M E = 72 h +/0 (Rudiger et al.[19])		$1.9 \rightarrow 7.4 \times 10^{-5}$ M E unknown -/0 (Bishun et al.[38])	
Epichlorohydrin	2×10^{-4}, 4×10^{-4}, & 10^{-3} M E = 2 h +/+ (White[20])		$10^{-7} \rightarrow 10^{-5}$ M E = 24 h +/0 (Sram et al.[39])	0.5 → 5.0 mg/m^3 E = 1 → 2 years +/0 (Kucerova et al.[59])
	$5 \times 10^{-5} \rightarrow 4 \times 10^{-4}$ M E = 48 h +/0 (Norppa et al.[21])		10^{-6} M E = 24 h +/0 (Kucerova & Polivkova[40])	
			$5 \times 10^{-5} \rightarrow 4 \times 10^{-4}$ M E = 24 h +/0 (Norppa et al.[21])	

(continued)

Table 12. (Continued)

Compound	Sister Chromatid Exchange *In Vitro*	Sister Chromatid Exchange *In Vivo*	Chromosome Aberration *In Vitro*	Chromosome Aberration *In Vivo*
Ethylene oxide	36 ppm E = 24 h +/0 (Star[22])	~36 ppm E unknown +/0 (Garry et al.[24])		
Vinyl chloride monomer	10 → 100% E = 3 h -/+ (Anderson et al.[28])	<1 ppm -/0 (Hansteen[27]) 1000 → 3000 ppm E = 5 min -/0 (Hansteen[69])		~1 → 5 ppm -/0 (Picciano et al.[66]) ~15 ppm +/0 (Purchase et al.[29]) ~25 ppm +/0 (Hansteen et al.[68] original study) Unknown concentration (possibly >500 ppm) E = 4 → 28 years +/0 (Ducatman et al.[64]) 1000 → 3000 ppm E = 5 min -/0 (Hansteen[69]) ~20 → 30 ppm E = 9 → 29 years +/0 (Funes-Cravioto et al.[63])

[a]Appropriate researchers are cited for producing the data retrieved.
[b]E, exposure time.
[c]Without S-9/with S-9: 0, not tested; +, positive results; -, negative results.

synthesis, sister chromatid exchange, and chromosomal aberration. The tables include only those compounds for which at least two published reports contained quantitative data for an assay involving human material. Forty-three publications from the total of sixty-one contained in the data base subset are represented in the tables. Table 11 provides comparative data for aflatoxin B1, benzidine, cyclophosphamide, and melphalan. Information on diethylstilbestrol, evaluated for unscheduled DNA synthesis, is also shown and may be compared to other data for the same compound shown in Table 12.

It may be seen in Table 11 that aflatoxin B1 effectively inhibits DNA synthesis (see Footnote c, Table 11) in HeLa cells after a 1-h exposure at only 5 x 10^{-8} M in the presence of S-9 metabolic activation.[10] Higher concentrations, by three to four orders of magnitude, are required to induce maximal levels of UDS in HeLa cells[4] or in human skin fibroblasts.[6] In the case of benzidine, however, a higher concentration (6 x 10^{-4} M) was required to effectively inhibit DNA synthesis in HeLa cells in the absence of S-9 metabolic activation[10] than was needed to maximally induce UDS (10^{-6} M) in HeLa cells in the presence of S-9.[4] Similarly, with cyclophosphamide a higher concentration (6 x 10^{-4} M) was required to effectively inhibit DNA synthesis in HeLa cells[10] or to cause maximal levels of single-strand breaks in DNA (5 x 10^{-3} M) of human skin fibroblasts[9] than to induce maximum UDS. It should be noted that a longer exposure time, 2.5 h, was employed with the UDS assay[4] than was used with the DNA-synthesis-inhibition assay[10] or the DNA-strand-breakage assay.[9] Painter[10] used 0.5 h in the absence of S-9 and 1 h in the presence of S-9, whereas Nordenskjold et al.[9] exposed the cells to the chemical for 1 h. In the case of melphalan, the same exposure time (0.5 h) was employed with UDS assays[8] and with DNA-strand-break assays[9] in human skin fibroblasts. Neither type of assay required S-9 activation. A positive response was obtained over a similar concentration range in the two test systems: 10^{-6} to 10^{-3} M with the UDS assay,[8] and 10^{-5} to 10^{-3} M in the DNA strand break assay.[9]

Carefully controlled experiments employing similar conditions of metabolic activation and exposure time in similar experimental systems must be conducted before more definitive comparisons can be made.

In Table 12, comparative data on SCE and chromosomal aberrations may be seen for aflatoxin B1, arsenic, benzene, cyclophosphamide, diethylstilbestrol, epichlorohydrin, ethylene oxide, and vinyl chloride monomer. For the <u>in vitro</u> systems represented in Table 12, the exposure periods are generally longer

(24 to 72 h) than with the DNA damage or inhibition assays (0.5 to 2.5 h) discussed in Table 11.

If the results of in vitro human lymphocyte assays for SCE and chromosomal aberrations in Table 12 are compared, it may be seen that the qualitative results of the assays were in agreement for studies of aflatoxin B1,[12,13] arsenic,[14,30,31] and epichlorohydrin,[20,21,39,40] and disagreed in part for studies of benzene[15,17,32] and DES.[19,38] In vivo results for SCE and chromosomal aberrations are concordant for arsenic[23,43] and cyclophosphamide.[18,54,55,56,57,58] However, several in vivo chromosomal aberration studies for vinyl chloride are discordant.[27,29,63,64,66,68,69]

Aflatoxin B1 induced chromosomal aberrations in vitro at a concentration of 3.2 x 10^{-8} M,[12] a dosage comparable to that required for induction of SCE (10^{-7} M).[13] It should be noted, however, that the exposure period used was longer for chromosomal aberrations.

The approximate concentration of arsenic required to induce SCE in vitro (1 μM)[14] was equal to that required to produce chromosomal aberrations in vitro.[30,31] The exposure times were also similar. Human in vivo lymphocyte assays for exposure to arsenic compounds were positive for SCE[23] and for chromosomal aberrations.[43] No quantitative estimates of arsenic exposure were provided.

Benzene was negative in two SCE studies in vitro wherein quantitative information was reported,[15,17] but positive[32] and negative[15] results were reported for chromosomal aberrations in vitro. Chromosomal damage to human lymphocytes in vivo has been documented in several reports.[48,51,52,53]

Although cyclophosphamide gave negative results in one SCE study at a low concentration (3.8 x 10^{-8} M),[18] the compound gave positive results for SCE induction in vivo[18] and for chromosomal aberration in vitro[36] and in vivo.[54,55,56,57,58] It should be noted, however, that the total dose of cyclophosphamide administered to patients in some cases exceeded 10 g.[57,58]

Diethylstilbestrol was positive in an in vitro SCE assay[19] but negative for chromosomal aberration in vitro.[38]

Epichlorohydrin gave positive results in all in vitro assays for SCE and chromosomal aberration[20,21,39,40] over a concentration range of 10^{-4} - 10^{-7} M. An additional alkylating agent, ethylene oxide, gave positive results at 36 ppm in SCE assays in vitro[22] and in vivo.[24]

In vivo lymphocyte assays on individuals exposed to VCM at low levels were negative (<1 ppm) for SCE[27] and were negative (1-5 ppm) for chromosomal aberrations.[66] SCE and chromosomal aberration assays were also negative in *in vivo* studies at high levels (1000-3000 ppm) for short exposure periods (5 min).[69] Exposure to VCM at higher concentrations (~15 → ~30 ppm) resulted in chromosomal aberrations in lymphocytes of workers.[29,63,68]

It is apparent that much more work needs to be done in the application of genetic bioassays involving the use of human cells and tissues both *in vitro* and *in vivo*. However, it must be emphasized that the chemicals which have been considered in this report and in the previous one (Waters et al.[1]) are among the few for which there is evidence of human carcinogenic potential. For this reason, the completion of the present human genetic bioassay data base is suggested as a research objective for scientists involved in the development and application of such systems. Additional efforts to fill data gaps in the larger data base[1] should enhance the utility of the information for purposes of developmental research and quantitative risk assessment.

REFERENCES

1. M. D. Waters, N. E. Garrett, C. M. Covone-de Serres, B. E. Howard, and H. F. Stack, 1982, Genetic bioassay data on some known or suspected human carcinogens, *in*: "The Use of Human Cells for the Assessment of Risk from Physical and Chemical Agents," A. Castellani, ed., Plenum Press, New York.
2. R. F. Whiting, H. F. Stich, and D. J. Koropatnick, 1979, DNA damage and DNA repair in cultured human cells exposed to chromate, *Chem-Biol. Interactions* 26:267.
3. W. D. MacRae, R. F. Whiting, and H. F. Stich, 1979, Sister chromatid exchanges induced in cultured mammalian cells by chromate, *Chem-Biol. Interactions* 26:281.
4. C. N. Martin, A. C. McDermid, and R. C. Garner, 1978, Testing of known carcinogens and noncarcinogens for their ability to induce unscheduled DNA synthesis in HeLa cells, *Cancer Res.* 38:2621.
5. M. Meselson and K. Russell, 1977, Comparisons of carcinogenic and mutagenic potency, *in*: "Origins of Human Cancer," H. H. Hiatt, J. D. Watson, and J. A. Winsten, eds., Cold Spring Harbor Conferences on Cell Proliferation, 4:1473, Cold Spring Harbor Laboratory, New York.
6. R. H. C. San and H. F. Stich, 1975, DNA repair synthesis of cultured human cells as a rapid bioassay for chemical carcinogens, *Int. J. Cancer* 16(2):284.

7. H. F. Stich and B. A. Laishes, 1975, The Response of Xeroderma pigmentosum cells and controls to the activated mycotoxins, aflatoxins, and sterigmatocystin, Int. J. Cancer 16(2):266.
8. R. Lewensohn and U. Ringborg, 1979, Induction of unscheduled DNA synthesis in human bone marrow cells by bifunctional alkylating agents, Blood 54:1320.
9. M. Nordenskjold, S. Soderhall, and P. Moldeus, 1979, Studies of DNA-strand breaks induced in human fibroblasts by chemical mutagens/carcinogens, Mutation Res. 63:393.
10. R. B. Painter, 1978, DNA synthesis inhibition in HeLa cells as a simple test for agents that damage human DNA, J. Environ. Pathol. Toxicol. 2(1):65.
11. R. B. Painter and R. Howard, 1978, A comparison of the HeLa DNA-synthesis inhibition test and the Ames test for screening of mutagenic carcinogens, Mutation Res. 54:113.
12. M. El-Zawahri, A. Moubasher, M. Morad, and I. El-Kady, 1977, Mutagenic effect of aflatoxin B_1, Ann. Nutr. Alim. 31:859.
13. V. E. Thomson and H. J. Evans, 1979, Induction of sister-chromatid exchanges in human lymphocytes and Chinese hamster cells exposed to aflatoxin B1 and N-methyl-N-nitrosourea, Mutation Res. 67:47.
14. F. Zanzoni and E. G. Jung, 1980, Arsenic elevates the sister chromatid exchange (SCE) rate in human lymphocytes in vitro, Arch. Dermatol. Res. 267(1):91.
15. P. Gerner-Smidt, U. Friedrich, 1978, The mutagenic effect of benzene, toluene and xylene studied by the SCE technique, Mutation Res. 58:313.
16. M. Diaz, N. Fijtman, V. Carricarte, L. Braier and J. Diez, 1979, Effect of benzene and its metabolites on SCE in human lymphocytes cultures, In Vitro 15(3):172.
17. K. Morimoto and S. Wolff, 1980, Increase of sister chromatid exchanges and perturbations of cell division kinetics in human lymphocytes by benzene metabolites, Cancer Res. 40(4):1189.
18. T. Raposa, 1978, Sister chromatid exchange studies for monitoring DNA damage and repair capacity after cytostatics in vitro and in lymphocytes of leukaemic patients under cytostatic therapy, Mutation Res. 57:241.
19. H. W. Rudiger, F. Haenisch, M. Metzler, F. Oesch, and H. R. Glatt, 1979, Metabolites of diethylstilboestrol induce sister chromatid exchange in human cultured fibroblasts, Nature 281:392.
20. A. D. White, 1980, In vitro induction of SCE in human lymphocytes by epichlorohydrin with and without metabolic activation, Mutation Res. 78(2):171.
21. H. Norppa, K. Hemminki, M. Sorsa, and H. Vainio, 1981, Effect of Monosubstituted epoxides on chromosome aberrations and SCE in cultured human lymphocytes, Mutation Res. 91:243.

22. E. G. Star, 1980, Mutagene und zytotoxische Wirkung von Athylenoxid auf menschliche Zellkulturen, Zbl. Bakt. Hyg. I. Abt. Orig. B170:548.
23. W. Burgdorf, K. Kurvink, and J. Cervenka, 1977, Elevated sister chromatid exchange rate in lymphocytes of subjects treated with arsenic, Hum. Genet. 36:69.
24. V. F. Garry, J. Hozier, D. Jacobs, R. L. Wade, and D. G. Gray, 1979, Ethylene oxide: Evidence of human chromosomal effects. Environ. Mutagenesis 1:375.
25. D. G. Stetka and S. Wolff, 1976, Sister chromatid exchange as an assay for genetic damage induced by mutagen-carcinogens. I. In vivo test for compounds requiring metabolic activation. Mutation Res. 41:333.
26. B. Lambert, U. Ringborg, A. Lindblad, E. Harper, M. Nordenskjold, and B. Werelius, 1979, Sister-chromatid exchanges in smoking and non-smoking control subjects, patients receiving cancer chemotherapy and laboratory workers exposed to organic solvents, Mutation Res. 64:138.
27. I-L. Hansteen, 1979, A follow-up study of the PVC workers two years after exposure. Preliminary results using sister chromatid exchange frequency as an assay of genetic damage, in: "Genetic Damage in Man Caused by Environmental Agents," K. Berg., ed., Academic Press, New York, p. 279.
28. D. Anderson, C. R. Richardson, I. F. H. Purchase, H. J. Evans, and M. L. O'Riordan, 1981, Chromosomal analysis in vinyl chloride exposed workers: comparison of the standard technique with the sister-chromatid exchange technique, Mutation Res. 83:137.
29. I. F. H. Purchase, C. R. Richardson, D. Anderson, G. M. Paddle, and W. G. F. Adams, 1978, Chromosomal analyses in vinyl chloride-exposed workers, Mutation Res. 57:325.
30. J. J. Oppenheim and W. N. Fishbein, 1965, Induction of chromosome breaks in cultured normal human leukocytes by potassium arsenite, hydroxyurea and related compounds, Cancer Res. 25:980.
31. K. Nakamuro and Y. Sayato, 1981, Comparative studies of chromosomal aberration induced by trivalent and pentavalent arsenic, Mutation Res. 88(1):73.
32. A. Koizumi, Y. Dobashi, Y. Tachibana, K. Tsuda, and H. Katsunuma, 1974, Cytokinetic and cytogenetic changes in cultured human leucocytes and HeLa cells induced by benzene, Ind. Health 12:23.
33. K. Goh, 1979, Chloramphenicol and chromosomal morphology, J. Med., 10(3):159.
34. K. Nakamuro, K. Yoshikawa, Y. Sayato, and H. Kurata, 1978, Comparative studies of chromosomal aberration and mutagenicity of trivalent and hexavalent chromium, Mutation Res. 58:175.

35. A. N. Chebotarev, L. Y. Telegin, and E. M. Derzhavets, 1976, Cytogenetic effect of cyclophosphamide in a culture of human lymphocytes after its activation in the mouse organism, Genetika 12(11):151.
36. S. Madle, D. Westphal, V. Hilbig, and G. Obe, 1978, Testing in vitro of an indirect mutagen (cyclophosphamide) with human leukocyte cultures. Activation by liver perfusion and by incubation with crude liver homogenate, Mutation Res. 54:95.
37. M. Morad and M. El-Zawahri, 1977, Non-random distribution of cyclophosphamide-induced chromosome breaks, Mutation Res. 42:125.
38. N. P. Bishun, N. Smith, H. Eddie, and D. C. Williams, 1977, Cytogenetic studies and diethyl stilboestrol, Mutation Res. 46:211.
39. R. J. Sram, M. Cerna, and M. Kucerova, 1976, The genetic risk of epichlorohydrin as related to the occupational exposure, Biol. Zbl. 95:451.
40. M. Kucerova and Z. Polivkova, 1976, Banding technique used for the detection of chromosomal aberrations induced by radiation and alkylating agents TEPA and epichlorohydrin, Mutation Res. 34:279.
41. J. Alving, M. K. Jensen, and H. Meyer, 1976, Diphenylhydantoin and chromosome morphology in man and rat: A negative report, Mutation Res. 40:173.
42. F. Muniz, E. Houston, R. Schneider, and M. Nusyowitz, 1969, Chromosomal effects of diphenylhydantoins, Clin. Res. 17:28.
43. J. Petres, D. Baron, and M. Hagedorn, 1977, Effects of arsenic cell metabolism and cell proliferation: Cytogenetic and biochemical studies, Environ. Health Perspect. 19:223.
44. G. Pollini and R. Colombi, 1964a, Il danno cromosomico midollare nell'anemia aplastic benzolica, Med. Lavoro 55:241.
45. G. Pollini and R. Colombi, 1964b, Il danno cromosomico dei linfociti nell'emopatia benzenica, Med. Lavoro 55:641.
46. G. Pollini, E. Stroselli, and R. Colombi, 1964, Sui rapporti fra alterazioni cromosomiche delle cellule emiche e gravita' dell-emopatia benzenica, Med. Lavoro 55:735.
47. E. C. Vigliani and G. Saita, 1964, Benzene and leukemia. New England J. Med. 271(17):872.
48. I. M. Tough and W. M. Court Brown, 1965, Chromosome aberrations and exposure to ambient benzene, Lancet 1:684.
49. A. Forni, 1966, Chromosome changes due to chronic exposure to benzene, in: "Proceedings of the 15th International Congress on Occupational Health, Vienna, October 1966," Wiener Medizinishe Akademie, Vienna, Vol. 2, part 1, pp. 437-439.

50. I. M. Tough, P. G. Smith, W. M. Court Brown, and D. G. Harnden, 1970, Chromosome studies of workers exposed to atmospheric benzene. The possible influence of age, Eur. J. Cancer 6:49.
51. H. Khan and M. H. Khan, 1973, Cytogenetische untersuchungen bei chronischer benzolexposition, Arch. Toxikol. 31:39.
52. D. Picciano, 1979, Cytogenetic study of workers exposed to benzene, Environ. Res. 19:33.
53. K. Fredga, J. Reitalu, and M. Berlin, 1979, Chromosome studies in workers exposed to benzene, in: "Genetic Damage in Man Caused by Environmental Agents," K. Berg, ed., Academic Press, New York, p. 187.
54. M. Dobos, D. Schuler, and G. Fekete, 1974, Cyclophosphamide-induced chromosomal aberrations in nontumorous patients, Humangenetik 22:221.
55. F. E. Arrighi, T. C. Hsu, and D. E. Bergsagel, 1962, Chromosome damage in murine and human cells following cytoxan therapy, Tex. Rep. Biol. Med. 20:545.
56. E. Schmid and M. Bauchinger, 1968, Chromosomenaberrationen in menschlichen peripheren lymphozyten nach endoxan-stosstherapie gynakologischer tumoren, Deutsche Medizinische Wochenschrift 93(23):1149.
57. M. Bauchinger and E. Schmid, 1969, Cytogenetische veranderungen in weissen blutzellen nach cyclophosphamidtherapie, Z. Krebsforsch. 72:77.
58. E. Schmid and M. Bauchinger, 1973, Comparison of the chromosome damage induced by radiation and cytoxan therapy in lymphocytes of patients with gynaecological tumours, Mutation Res. 21:271.
59. M. Kucerova, V. S. Zhurkov, Z. Polivkova, and J. E. Ivanova, 1977, Mutagenic effect of epichlorohydrin. II. Analysis of chromosomal aberrations in lymphocytes of persons occupationally exposed to epichlorohydrin. Mutation Res. 48:355.
60. M. Kucerova, Z. Polivkova, R. Sram, and V. Matousek, 1976, Mutagenic effect of epichlorohydrin I. Testing on human lymphocytes in vitro in comparison with TEPA, Mutation Res. 34:271.
61. I. F. H. Purchase, C. R. Richardson, and D. Anderson, 1975, Chromosomal and dominant lethal effects of vinyl chloride, Lancet 2:410.
62. I. F. H. Purchase, C. R. Richardson, and D. Anderson, 1976, Chromosomal effects in peripheral lymphocytes, Proc. Roy. Soc. Med. 69:290.
63. F. Funes-Cravioto, B. Lambert, J. Lindsten, L. Ehrenberg, A. T. Natarajan, and S. Osterman-Golkar, 1975, Chromosome aberrations in workers exposed to vinyl chloride, Lancet 1:459.

64. A. Ducatman, K. Hirschhorn, I. J. Selikoff, 1975, Vinyl chloride exposure and human chromosome aberrations, Mutation Res. 31:163.
65. A. Leonard, G. Decat, E. D. Leonard, M. J. Lefevre, L. J. Decuyper, and C. Nicaise, 1977, Cytogenetic investigations on lymphocytes from workers exposed to vinyl chloride, J. Toxicol. Environ. Health 2(5):1135.
66. D. J. Picciano, R. E. Flake, P. C. Gay, and D. J. Kilian, 1977, Vinyl chloride cytogenetics, J. Occup. Med. 19(8):527.
67. A. W. Barnes, 1976, Vinyl chloride and the production of PVC, Proc. Roy. Soc. Med. 69:277.
68. I-L. Hansteen, L. Hillestad, E. Thiis-Evensen, and S. S. Heldaas, 1978, Effects of vinyl chloride in man: A cytogenetic follow-up study, Mutation Res. 51(2):271.
69. I-L. Hansteen, 1978, Acute exposure to VCM: A cytogenetic study of two workers, Mutation Res. 53:196.
70. V. Minnich, M. E. Smith, D. Thompson, and S. Kornfeld, 1976, Detection of mutagenic activity in human urine using mutant strains of Salmonella typhimurium, Cancer 38:1253.
71. D. Siebert and U. Simon, 1973, Genetic activity of metabolites in the ascitic fluid and in the urine of a human patient treated with cyclophosphamide: Induction of mitotic gene conversion in Saccharomyces cerevisiae, Mutation Res. 21:257.
72. I. E. Mattern and W. B. van der Zwaan, 1977, Mutagenicity testing of urine from vinylchloride (VCM) treated rats using the Salmonella test system, Mutation Res. 46:230.
73. D. J. Kilian, T. G. Pullin, T. H. Connor, M. S. Legator, and H. N. Edwards, 1978, Mutagenicity of epichlorohydrin in the bacterial assay system: Evaluation by direct in vitro activity and in vivo activity of urine from exposed humans and mice, Mutation Res. 53:72.

FROM BACTERIA TO MAN, THE EVOLUTION OF MUTAGENICITY TESTING

Marvin S. Legator and Barbara L. Harper

Department of Preventive Medicine and Community Health
University of Texas Medical Branch
Galveston, Texas 77550

> "Radiation risk resembles the risk we undergo when involved in automobile traffic: The enhanced rate can be estimated approximately, and adequate precautions are to a certain extent possible. The risk due to chemical mutagens on the other hand, resembles the risk involved in a walk through the jungle at night. Hear a crackling in the underbush, there an unexplained sound may signal unknown hidden dangers". (Gruneberg et al., 1979).

In a little over a decade the field of toxicology has seen an unprecendented growth in the sub-area known as Genetic Toxicology or Molecular Toxicology. In the early development of this field, a great deal of optimism was generated as a result of identification of mutagen-carcinogenic agents in simple bacterial tester strains. This optimism has slowly given way to a more realistic understanding of the area, and the realization of a need for more complex studies that can be conducted with microorganisms. In recent years, the need to evaluate the effects of chemicals on the complex organization of DNA in mammalian systems, and the necessity of intact animal studies, where pharmacokinetic effects and relevant host metabolic pathways can be taken into account, is generally accepted as a pre-requisite for chemical evaluation. In addition to animal procedures, we now have the unique capability of detecting potential carcinogens in man by a variety of short-term procedures. The unique contribution of this field to the fundamental understanding of the modification of the genetic process by chemicals and its potential for alleviating some of the major afflictions occuring in man, however, remains unchallenged.

In this analysis of the field, I will address (a) problems of short term mutagenicity testing, (b) the optimum tests for identifying mutagenic agents, (c) our inability to do quantitative human risk assessment from presently available procedures, and (d) a non-quantitative approach to risk assessment.

A. PROBLEMS IN *IN VITRO* BACTERIAL MUTAGENICITY TESTING

The salmonella/microsome mutagenicity assay (Ames et al., 1973; McCann et al., 1975) is currently the most widely used in mutagenicity test. This assay uses several strains of *Salmonella typhimurium,* (all of which are histidine auxotrophs) and detects reversion or backmutation to histidine prototrophy. The particular strains most widely used were specially designed and include various combinations of a lipopolysaccharide deletion to facilitate absorption of chemicals, a repair deficiency and a plasmid which greatly increases sensitivity to mutation. Chemicals are tested with and without a mammalian liver homogenate (S9) to provide metabolic activation; generally rat liver mixed function oxidases are induced by pretreatment of the animal with Aroclor 1254, phenobarbital or 3-methylcholanthrene.

One of two original underlying hypotheses of this assay was that all mutagens may be carcinogenic, therefore bacterial mutagenicity was proposed as a screen for carcinogenicity. This immediately led to controversies concerning "validation" or "correlation" between mutagens and carcinogens, as well as to discussions of sources of variability within the assay. Validation estimates (percentage of known carcinogens which are mutagenic in the Salmonella/microsome assay) range from 63% to 93%. As pointed out by Rinkus and Legator (1980), calculations of "validation", "correlation", "specificity" and so on, should really be termed "success rates" since each one pertains to a different set of chemicals. Known carcinogens do not represent a random sampling of present and yet-to-be synthesized chemical compounds. Human carcinogenic chemicals have been detected because they are either very potent, site-specific, or in very wide usage. Animal carcinogens are known because they were suspected highly enough to warrant extensive and expensive bioassays. Thus, the denominator of specificity calculations in general is not "all carcinogens" but "all carcinogens known to date". Furthermore, the figure used for each individual success rate dose not really include "all known carcinogens" but only the particular subset of carcinogens considered in each report (Purchase, 1980; Bartsch, 1980; Ashby, 1980; Kawachi et al., 1980; Simmon, 1979; Anderson and Styles, 1980) and earlier studies cited in these references).

Evidence for mutagenicity, as derived from the literature, has also proven somewhat troublesome. Earlier reports were published before the most sensitive tester strains were designed, or before a source of metabolic activation was included. Many early non-mutagens are now detected as mutagens, many other chemicals, however, have never been retested so their status remains incomplete.

Many recent publications have dealt with sources of variability inherent in the assay itself. These discussions give us an overall impression of fairly high reproducibility when procedures are rigidly standardized (Belser et al., 1981; Chu et al., 1981; Brusick, 1979; Dunkel, 1979; Bartsch, 1980; Salmeen and Durisin, 1981, among others). Particular factors concerning the assay itself include the use of the most sensitive tester strains, chemical lot and preparation, numbers and growth phase of the bacteria, differences between batches of media, concentration of growth factors, sterilization procedures of petri plates, and similar factors which might be expected to affect background reversion rates as well as growth of colonies which are not true revertants. When these factors are controlled, variation between laboratories can be greatly reduced, but not completely eliminated (Rosenkranz et al., 1980; Grafe et al., 1981).

The second underlying hypothesis for bacterial mutagenicity testing was that _in vitro_ metabolism by mammalian enzymes adequately relected _in vivo_ metabolism. The most controversial source of variation in detection occurs during metabolic activation of proximate carcinogens to reactive intermediates or ultimate carcinogens. Many or most chemicals must be activated, usually to an electrophilic species, in order to be mutagenic. Most of our current concerns about bacterial mutagenicity testing center on metabolic activation.

In trying to determine why up to 40% of known carcingens are not mutagenic in Salmonella, the first logical step is to chemically categorize these "non-mutagens ". It immediately becomes apparent that not all carcinogens would be expected to be mutagenic, or dependent on bacterial repair systems (Hartman, 1980). There are several types of interaction with DNA other than the intercalation or adduct formation which most bacterial mutagens have in common. Thus, some carcinogens crosslink DNA (pyrrolizidine alkaloids, psoralens), bind noncovalently to DNA (mycotoxins), are mitotic poisons, have antireplication effects, or are acylating agents (anhydrides, perhaps carbamates) (see Legator and Rinkus, 1981; Bartsch, 1980). Other carcinogenic agents may be hormonal (DES), immunosuppressive, cocarcinogens or promoters.

Additionally, some chemical classes are not well detected as salmonella mutagens (Rinkus and Legator, 1980; Kawachi et al., 1980; Clayson, 1980; Bartsch, 1980). These classes include organohalogens, hydrazines, metals and nitrosamines, among others. Knowing mutagenic characteristics of particular chemicals or chemical classes, it is possible to design a test that is 0% predictive or 100% predictive (Ashby, 1980).

We have recently reviewed the chemicals tested in the National Cancer Institute Bioassay program, and correlated carcinogenicity with their Salmonella mutagenicity (Harper et al., this volume). Out of 124 chemicals determined to be carcinogens, 33 were mutagenic in Salmonella, 24 were non-mutagenic, 19 were incompletely tested and 48 were not tested. Out of 60 carcinogens reviewed in recent IARC monographs, 30 were mutagenic, 15 were non-mutagenic and 15 were incompletely or not tested. Thus, out of 184 carcinogens from both programs, 102 have been adequately tested in Salmonella. Of these 102 carcinogens, 63 were mutagenic, giving an overall success rate of 62%. Many of these non-mutagenic carcinogens fall into predictable chemical classes: chlorinated aliphatics and monosubstituted or complex aromatic amines.

Several aspects of in vitro activation systems contribute to false negative (non-mutagenic) carcinogens. Besides non-genotoxic mechanisms of carcinogenesis, metabolic trends include complex metabolism, reductive or oxidative activation by enzymes other than cytochrome P450, activation by host intestinal flora, the source and concentration of the in vitro activating enzymes (S9), volatility or instability or lipophilicity of the chemical, generation of a reactive metabolite that is too short-lived to act in the bacterial assay, and the ratio of activating to detoxifying pathways of metabolism.

Some of these factors may be overcome by modifications of the assay, for example by the testing of volatile chemicals in closed systems, or by incubating the chemical, S9, and bacteria together before dilution onto the growth medium (Rosenkranz, 1980; Bartsch, 1980). The mutagenicity of some chemicals has been enhanced by the addition of cofactors required by particular reactions; this presupposes knowledge of the chemical class under consideration. For example, ATP or NADH enhance the mutagenicity of dimethylaminoazobenzene; riboflavin a cofactor for azoreductase, increases mutagenicity of azo and diazo compounds and may decerease mutagenicity of other chemicals; norharman enhances (e.g. aniline) or suppresses mutagenicity depending on its concentration; glycosidase enhances the mutagenicity of glycosides such as cycasin (Matsushima et al., 1980).

Several examples of differences in metabolic activation will illustrate some of the points mentioned above. The most widely cited example of in vivo / in vitro differences in metabolism are the polyaromatic hydrocarbons, benzo(a)pyrene and

7,12-dimethylbenzanthracene. The primary mutagenic metabolite of benzo(a)pyrene *in vitro* is the K-region expoxide (benzo(a)pyrene-5,6-oxide), whereas the metabolite found in DNA adducts after *in vivo* administration is an adduct of the bay region diol epoxide, benzo(a)pyrene 7,8-diol-9,10-oxide (Selkirk, 1977; King, et al., 1979). The balance of these two reactive species depends on the relative amounts of cytochrome P450 and P448, respectively (Selkirk, 1980), and which in turn basically depends on the source and pretreatment of the activating system, whether *in vivo* or *in vitro* . A similar phenomenon has been reported for 7,12-dimethylbenzanthracene (Bigger et al., 1978, 1980) and 7-methylbenzanthracene (Thompson et al., 1976).

A second example of *in vivo* / *in vitro* differences in metabolites is 2-acetylaminofluorene (2-AAF) (Brouns et al., 1981). Mutagenesis by 2-AAF can be almost completely blocked by inhibiting the de-acetylase reaction whereas induction of DNA excision repair by 2-AAF was prevented by blocking the sulfation reaction. This suggests that these genotoxic effects are caused by different reactive metabolites. There does not appear to be a consistent relationship between the ability of the liver to activate metabolites *in vivo* and the formation of mutagenic products *in vitro* (Irving, 1979).

The *in vivo* metabolism of chlordane appears to be considerably different from *in vitro* metabolism; even though heptachlor (oxychlordane) may be recovered *in vivo* and *in vitro* , other pathways are active as well (Brimfield and Street, 1979).

One final difference between *in vivo* and *in vitro* metabolism is that metabolism may occur in a reductive or anaerobic situation, especially with reference to anaerobic intestinal bacteria. Azo benzene (a strong carcinogen NCI Boiassay #154) can be reduced *in vivo* to hydrazobenzene (a more potent carcinogen, NCI Bioassay #92) as evidenced by the recovery of reductive metabolites (aniline and benzidine) from the urine.

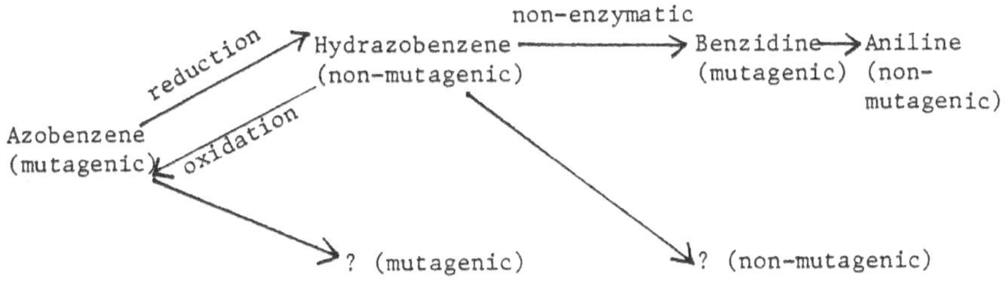

A greater total amount of hydroxylated products are also recovered in the urine, indicating that oxidative metabolism is the major type of metabolism in vivo. However, azobenzene is mutagenic in vitro while hydrazobenzene is not. The reductive products (aniline and benzidine) are thought to arise from hydrazobenzene by nonenzymatic rearrangement in reductive conditions. This apparently does not occur in vitro since benzidine would be detected as a mutagen if it were produced. Since hydrazobenzene can also be hydroxylated, either this does not occur in vitro or the hydroxylated products are non-mutagenic.

It is generally accepted that although there is a rough correlation between mutagenic and carcinogenic potency, this is not quantitative to the extent that a constant mutation rate per weight of chemical can be calculated. A general idea of mutagenic potency can be gained, however, and certain chemicals (diethylnitrosamine, for example), are seen to be very poor mutagens for their given carcinogenic potency (Bartsch et al., 1980). This is intuitively known, of course, for the carcinogens which are poor or non-mutagens in bacterial assays, although they may cause chromosomal damage or have some other effect in short term in vitro testing.

Even though certain chemical classes predictably tend to be non-mutagenic carcinogens, other classes show no apparent correlation between mutagenic and carcinogenic potency. Glatt et al., (1980) tested 49 closely related heterocyclics and found that there was no relation between mutagenicity and carcinogenicity even though they were all structurally similar. Furthermore, 15 "non-carcinogens" were mutagenic. It is harder to prove non-mutagenicity than mutagenicity, even harder to prove carcinogenicity, and hardest of all to prove non-carcinogenicity. The study by Glatt et al. is a logical approach to the question of how mutagenicity and carcinogenicity should be compared.

In conclusion, the Salmonella/microsome assay has proven to be a valuable screen for mutagens, and should continue to be used for this purpose. One must remember, however, that up to 40% of the carcinogens known to date are not mutagenic in this assay, and a small number of carcinogens in addition to this are mutagenic only in a modified test system.

B. THE OPTIMUM TESTS FOR DETERMINING MUTAGEN ACTIVITY

The evaluation of a chemical for mutagenic activity is essentially a two-phase process. First, there is the qualitative identification of the mutagenic activity; the testing in this phase is designed primarily to answer the question whether a chemical is mutagenic or a potential carcinogen. The preceding section discussed some of the problems associated with using only non-mammalian systems for this qualitative assessment. Subsequently, qualitative mutagens are to be assessed quantitatively, with the ultimate goal of understanding the potential risk to user population. In a recent publication (Legator and Rinkus, 1981) the basic prerequisite for qualitative mutagen testing was described. The qualitative testing should be capable of detecting the entire spectrum of mutagenic events; it should account for the importance of metabolism in activating and deactivating mutagens, it should produce no false negatives unnecessarily and only a nominal amount of false positives and it should provide reproducible results within any given laboratory and among different laboratories. Obviously, this last criterion necessitates the use of standardized protocols in order to judge reproducibility. Also, from a regulatory agency's viewpoint, standardized protocols for testing would be essential to the evaluation process. Finally, it would be desirable if not essential, that the qualitative testing make use of short term test procedures as opposed to long-term animal studies. Fortunately, almost all practical mutagenicity procedures are short term and can be completed in days or weeks.

It is now generally accepted that no single test procedure can satisfy these criteria, and, consequently, a battery of test procedures will be necessary. However, there are still differences of opinion over the exact prescription of test procedures that should make up the qualitative testing.

That the qualitative testing for mutagens of the sophistication required cannot be accomplished by any battery of in vitro test procedures is best illustrated by reviewing the complexity of mammalian mutagenicity. The phenomenon of inducing mammalian mutagenicity is depicted schematically in Figure 1 as having three levels of complexity: the mammalian chromosomal organization, mammalian metabolism and the mammalian membrane. The induction of a genetic lesion and the subsequent development into cells phenotypically altered from the parental population is contingent upon the interplay of a number of factors including the unique characteristics of the chemical under investigation. As we become cognizant of these various factors, it becomes apparent that classifying compounds as mutagens solely on the basis of direct interaction with DNA in a non-animal system is overly simplistic (see preceeding section).

A comprehensive discussion of the complexity of chemical mutagens as related to cell metabolism, chromosomal organization and the cell membrane was presented by Legator and Rinkus, 1981. Given the complexities of the mutagenesis process, any battery of tests should rely primarily on <u>in vivo</u> procedures. This approach

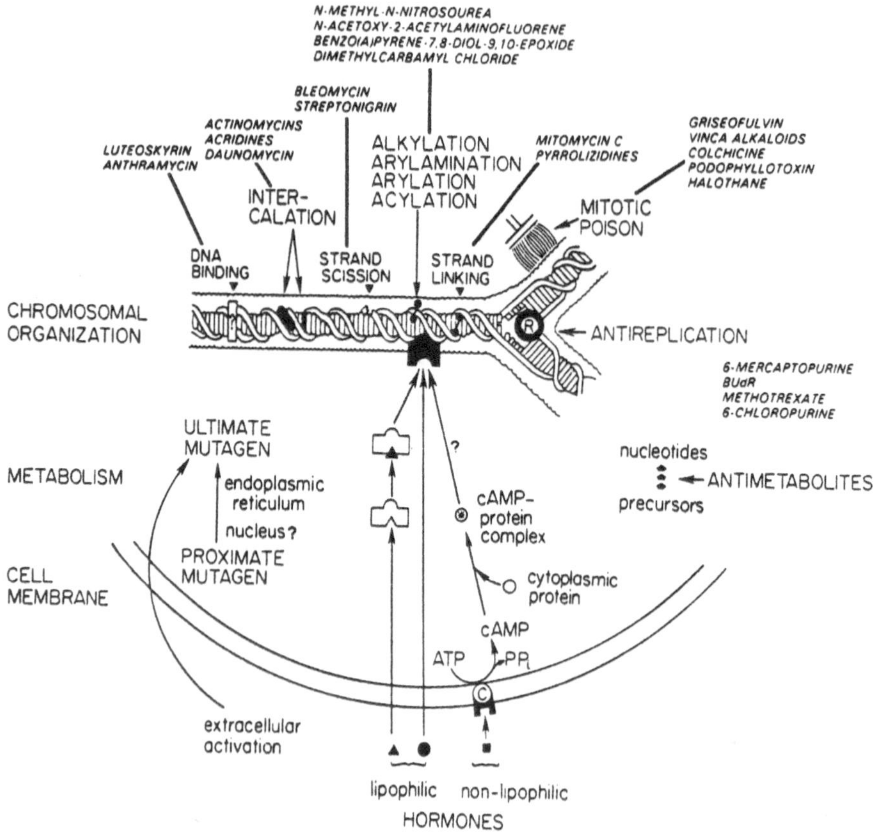

Figure 1. Complexity of chemical mutagenesis in a mammalian system. Chromosomal organization, intracellular and extracellular metabolism, and the cell membrane are three levels of complexity in chemical mutagenesis. Known or assumed modes of action by which mutagens can be classified are illustrated in the diagram of a replicating chromosome ("R", DNA-replicating enzyme). Examples of chemicals that are presumably active in these manners are also shown. Three aspects of mammalian metabolism that may be important in chemical mutagenesis are the activation of proximate mutagens by mixed-function oxidases embedded in the endoplasmic reticulum and the nucleus, excessive stimulation by lipophilic and possibly nonlipophilic hormones or their analogues ("C", adenyl cyclase), and interference with the proper production of nucleotide pools or competition by nucleic acid analogues during replication (anti-replication). The cell membrane becomes a consideration when test systems that are nonmammalian are used to predict chemical mutagenesis in a mammalian setting. Modified after Figure 5.1 in Gale et al. (1972) with permission.

is in direct opposition to the tier or hierarchal approach where microbial tests are used as an initial primary screen and, if positive, then more advanced tests are performed. It is interesting to note that the initial presentation of the tier approach was, in reality, a battery approach, in which sequential testing was recommended only with a chemical of low volume where microbial screens were deemed sufficient in the initial testing phase (Bridges 1973).

In the selection of test procedures, due emphasis should be placed on the cytogenetic endpoint. Almost every known mutagen-carcinogen induces chromosomal abnormalities. The occurrence of a mutagen with a specificity for inducing gene mutations but not inducing chromosomal abnormalities is an exceedingly rare occurrence. There is little documentation in the literature for this mutagenic classification. In the studies of Vogel and Soebels 1976 and, Vogel 1977 with drosophila, it was shown that some mutagenic chemicals do not break chromosomes (dominant lethal test); for those that do break chromosomes, the chromosomal effect occurs at concentrations substantially higher than those that induce gene mutations (recessive lethals). These tests in drosophila clearly show a difference in sensitivity between dominant lethal tests and the recessive lethal test. With mammalian systems however, the inactive chemicals in the chromosome test (dominant lethal) in drosophila are known to produce extensive cytogenetic damage (see Table I). In fact, the most potent clastogenic agents in mammals are either negative or weakly positive in the drosophila chromosome (dominant lethal) study . These findings may indicate significant differences between the genetic lesions induced by the same chemical in drosophila and mammalian cells. Although chemicals that induce point mutations, with rare exception, induce chromosome damage, the reverse seems not to be the case. In fact, several carcinogens which have proven negative in gene mutation assays, are active cytogenetically, e.g. asbestos (Sincock, 1977), benzene (Hite et al., 1980) hexachlorocyclohexane, ethinyl estradiol, testosterone-propionate (Shimazu et al., 1976) diethylstilbesterol (Sawada and Ishidate, 1978) and urethane (Wild, 1978). From presently available information, it may well be that <u>in vivo</u> cytogenetic studies comprise the single most important procedure in any battery of mutagenic tests. Most chemicals that induce gene mutations also cause chromosome aberrations; additionally, there is a large group of chemicals active only at the chromosomal level.

A suggested core battery of tests in which most of the procedures satisfy the aforementioned criteria will include the following, (Wodicka et al., 1980):

1. Assay for induction of point mutations by microbial cell

Table I.
Comparison of Mutagenic Activity in Drosophila with Mammalian Cytogenetics[a]

Chemical	Drosophila[b]		Mammalian cytogenetics		
			In vivo		
	Recessive lethals	Dominant lethals	Somatic	Gametic	In vitro
Procarbazine	+	(+)	+.MNT (Wild, 1978	+.DL (Ehling, 1974)	
Diethylnitrosamine	+	0	0.MNT[c] (Wild, 1978)	0.DL (Propping et al., 1972)	+.MA (with S9 activation) (Matsuoka et al., 1979)
1-(2,4,6-Trichlorophenyl)-3,3-dimethyltriazene	+	(+)	+.MNT (Wild, 1978)		
1-(3-Pyridyl)-3,3-dimethyl-triazene	+	0	+.MNT (Wild, 1978)		
Cyclophosphamide	+	0	+.MNT (Wild, 1978)	+.DL (Propping et al., 1972)	+.MA (with S9 activation) (Benedict et al., 1978)
			+.MA. human (Musilova et. al., 1979)		+.MA (rat-liver cells) (Dean and Hodson-Walker, 1979)
Trofosfamide	+	0	+.MNT (Wild, 1978)		
Ifosfamide	+	0	+.MNT (Wild, 1978)		
Vinyl chloride	+	0	+.MA. human (Purchase et al., 1976)	0.DL[d] (Purchase et al., 1976)	
Hycanthone	+	0	+.MNT (Weber et al., 1975)	(+), DL (Russell, 1975)	+.MA (Benedict et al., 1977a)

[a]Symbols: +, positive response; 0, negative response; (+), marginal increase over control values. Abbrevations: DL, dominant lethal test; MA, metaphase spread analysis; MNT, micronucleus test.

[b]From Vogel and Sobels, 1976; Vogel, 1977.

[c]Karyotypic changes in liver cells isolated from rats treated with diethylnitrosamine has been reported(Grover&Fischer,1971).

[d]Excessive miscarriages have been noted in wives of male workers exposed to vinyl chloride in the workplace(Infante et.al., 1976).

systems incoporating *in vitro* activating systems.

2. Assay for induction of point mutations in cultured mammalian cells incorporating a mammalian activating system.

3. Assay for induction of chromosomal changes *in vitro* in cultured mammalian cells.

4. Tests for induction of chromosomal changes *in vivo* by direct cytogenetic analysis of metaphase and/or micronucleus test.

5. Testing of body fluids of treated mammals using microbial indicator systems.

6. Assay for cell transformation using appropriate *in vitro* mammalian cultures or human cell lines.

As an adjunct to this core battery, it may be desirable initially to add a test for sex-linked recessive lethals in drosophila and an assay for primary non-specific damage to DNA such as induction of unscheduled DNA synthesis and/or DNA repair in mammalian cells.

If further exploration is to be undertaken to establish categories of concern for potential mutagenic risk of the chemical in man, additional investigations should include:

1. A dominant lethal test;

2. A test for induction of point mutations by a host-mediated assay using microbial or mammalian cells as indicator systems;

3. Cytogenetic studies in germinal cells;

4. Heritable translocation test.

To summarize, the essential data base for detecting mutagenic activity should include *in vitro* microbial and somatic cell tests for point mutations with *and without* metabolic activation, indirect *in vivo* tests for gene mutations (body fluid analysis), and tests for chromosomal aberrations in intact mammals. The determination of the occurrence of chromosomal changes might require further exploration by a dominant lethal study, scoring for sperm abnormalities or for chromosomal aberrations in mammalian testicular cells, or a heritable translocation test.

C. DETERMINATION OF RISK TO MAN

In the preceeding section we discussed the optimal procedures that can be used to identify a compound as being carcinogenic and mutagenic. In all of the systems outlined, a dose-response curve should be generated. After it has been determined that a compound is a mutagen and potential carcinogen, there is a need to determine potential risk to man. It should be obvious that the systems most suited to estimate risk to man would be those that utilize responses in the intact animal. Even with animal procedures however, there are serious reservations concerning our ability to do quantitative risk assessment. Prior to discussing the problems of quantifying the data and extrapolating mutagenic risk to man, it may be worthwhile to review the methodology employed to estimate risk in the field of carcinogenicity where the information for animal studies is routinely used in predicting the actual risk to man. With the majority of known animal carcingoens, no human data are available for risk estimate and, therefore, it is necessary to make both low dose and inter-species extrapolations from measured responses in animals to potential human risk. This is also true with mutagenicity data where we do not have any direct method for measuring effects in man. With a known animal carcinogen, in attempting to estimate risk to man, there are certain factors that must be considered in making such risk assessment. These factors include long term feeding, testing at several doses, and complete pathology. It should be obvious that risk estimates should only be attempted when meaningful data is generated from well-conducted studies. The extrapolation to man is based on a mathematical model that should reflect the biological information and should correctly reflect the animal data. Not only should the selected mathematical model take into account our understanding of biological processes leading to tumor induction but the model should also be sufficiently conservative to compensate for areas of uncertainty, thus providing maximum protection from exposure to carcinogenic agents. In almost all cases, a linear function is found between incidence of tumor formation and dose. The major problem is the selection of the most suitable model to best approximate the response at low-dose for which no data are available. In a recent publication of the Office of Technology Assessment (1981) a stylized dose response curve and various extrapolated curves are presented (see Figure 2). It can be seen from the figure that the model one selects for extrapolation at low dose regions has a profound effect upon the final risk estimate. Although there is a reluctance among certain scientists to accept a no- threshold model, the fact is that we can neither prove or disprove the threshold concept. The repair of genetic lesions is often given as a reason for believing that a threshold effect may occur, below which DNA repair can occur. It should be emphasized however, that the successful repair of genetic lesions may not be accomplished by repair processes and, in fact, even may be amplified by the error-prone post- replication repair process. Even if repair were to be accomplished correctly in animals, thus leading to a

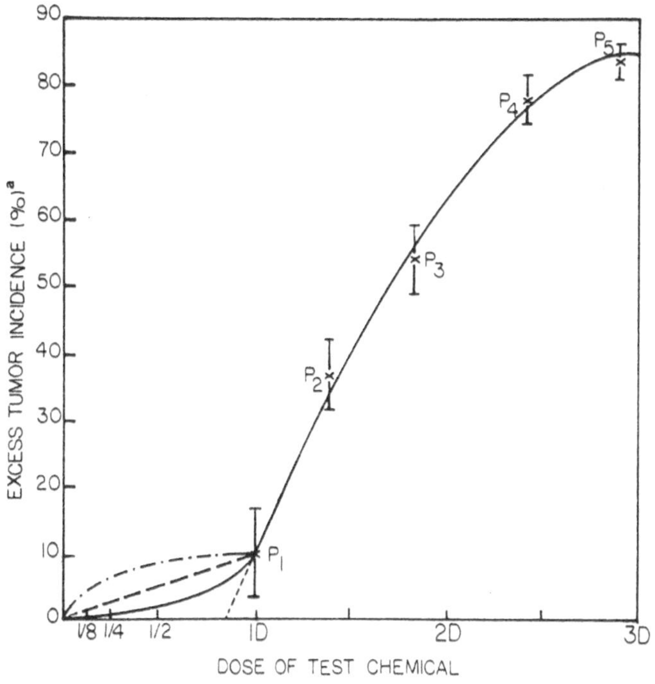

Figure 2. A Stylized Dose-Response Curve and Some Extrapolated Curves.

[a]Excess Tumor Incidence (%) is defined as:

$$\frac{\text{tumors in exposed population}}{\text{number of exposed population}} - \frac{\text{tumors in control population}}{\text{number of exposed population}} \times 100$$

Taken from: Office of Technology Assessment, Assessment of technologies for determining cancer risks from the environment, 1981.

threshold effect, its relevance to humans may be questionable. Crump (1981), in advocating the use of a linear dose-response at low doses, presented the argument that in man new carcinogenic agents would probably interact additively with agents already present in the environment. The multiple exposure to environmental agents in man is distinctly different than in laboratory animal testing in which, generally, exposures occur. In fact, in the few evaluated cases in man of multiple exposure, a syngergistic rather than an additive response often seems to occur. This synergistic effect has been noted between asbestos and smoking as well as smoking and occupational exposure of uranium miners (Hammond et al., 1968 and Archer et al., 1972). It may well be that since since most carcinogens are both initiators as well as promoters, the promoting activity would tend to yield more than an additive response between chemicals affecting the same target organ. Given all available data it seems reasonable, in the field of carcinogenicity and, indeed, mutagenicity to reject a model that would indicate a threshold effect. Another feature of most models is to select a confidence limit (usually 95%) for each observed responses when extrapolating to the low dose area. This upper confidence limit adds another safety factor for risk estimate calculations. At the present time, there are several models that can be used for evaluating risk to humans by extrapolation from animal data. In most instances, these models are compatible with the data in the observed range. The choice of models therefore, is dependent upon the degree of conservatism one wishes to build into risk estimates. At one extreme, mathematical models could essentially eliminate compounds that are positive at any concentration in any animal test from being used commercially (i.e., The Delaney Amendment), while at the other extreme we could treat the induction of cancer as a trivial toxicological endpoint. In addition to all of these confounding factors that make extrapolation from animal data to man difficult, we have a problem of organ specificity. Although there are numerous examples where a carcinogen in both animals and man acts at the same site, there are also examples where site specifity does not hold such as aromatic amines which produce hepatomas in rodents and bladder tumors in dogs and man. It is, thus, difficult to derive a meaningful figure where we do not have the same target organ involved in both animals and man. The careful evaluation of all of the variable factors involved in quantitative risk estimates for carcinogens in man, leads to the inescapable conclusion that based on animal data, specific numbers derived may be so innaccurate as to be almost meaningless. Acknowledgingly the limitations of mathematical models in deriving a specific figure for for estimating risk, there is however a need to derive a reasonable estimate of carcinogenic potency in man from animal data. Thus, though quantitative extrapolation on the basis of animal data may not be scientifically justified, certainly there are large valid differences between chemicals such as aflatoxin, vinyl chloride, nitrites and saccharin which must be taken into account.

In a recent report, an approach to deriving potency estimates from animal experiments to man was presented (Squire, 1981). In this report the animal carcinogens are ranked semi-quantitatively. The proposed system is based on the weight of evidence derived from animal tests. The author assumes that animal carcinogens have been identified by testing, using multiple doses in at least two species, and with an approved cancer bioassay protocol. On the basis of the cancer bioassay testing, six factors are proposed for ranking the chemicals. These factors include, (1) the number of different species affected, (2) the number of histogenetically different types of induced neoplasms in one or more species, (3) the spontaneous incidence in the appropriate control group relative to the neoplasms induced in exposed group, (4) the dose response relationship, (5) the classification of the induced neoplasm ranging from greater than 50% malignant to non malignant and (6) the genotoxicity of the chemical. On the basis of the various factors a score is derived and carcinogens are placed in the appropriate class, ranging from one to five. Table II illustrates the use of this system in ranking the animal carcinogen, dibromochloropropane. The use of categories for determining relative risk to man, rather than from mathematical models may be a more realistic approach that takes into account the present state of the art with the known uncertainties in this area.

D. RISK ASSESSMENT FOR MUTAGENIC AGENTS

Given our inability to assess accurately the risk to humans by utilizing animal data on carcinogenicity, is it possible to conduct risk assessment for heritable genetic damage? The long latent (generations or more) before phenotypic expression of the chemically induced genetic lesion as well as the high background rate of genetic diseases in our population, make associations between effects seen in animals being confirmed in man highly unlikely. Therefore reliance on human risk estimate from animal data becomes, for all intensive purposes, the only feasible approach for estimating the final expression of heritable genetic damage. The suggested battery approach should identify compounds that induce mutations and, if it is known that the chemical reached the germinal cells, it is logical to presume that the chemical has the potential to induce heritable genetic damage. With the present state of the art, is it possible to move beyond the qualitative identification of a mutagen? One major approach to quantify the mutagenic response is to determine the reaction of the chemical with DNA. A large number of genotoxic agents possess electrophilic reactivity and are converted in vivo to reactive chemicals. Most, but not all, of these chemicals are alkylating agents. There is

Table II. Use of the Squire System for Ranking Dibromochloropropane (DBCP) (Squire, 1981)

Factors	Points	DBCP Points
A. Number of different species affected		
Two or more	15	15
One	5	
B. Number of histogenetically different types of neoplasms in one or more species		
Three or more	15	15
Two	10	
One	5	
C. Spontaneous incidence in appropriate control groups of neoplasms induced in treated groups		
Less than 1 percent	15	15
1 to 10 percent	10	
10 to 20 percent	5	
More than 20 percent	1	
D. Dose-response relationships (cummulative oral dose equivalent per kilogram of body weight per day for 2 years)		
Less than 1 microgram	15	
1 microgram to 1 milligram	10	10*
1 milligram to 1 gram	5	
More than 1 gram	1	
E. Malignancy of induced neoplasms		
More than 50 percent	15	15
25 to 50 percent	10	
Less than 25 percent	5	
No malignancy	1	
F. Genotoxicity, measured in an appropriate battery of tests		
Positive	25	25
Incompletely positive	10	
Negative	0	
Total	100	95

* Based on dose and brief latency.

considerable experimental data to indicate that the mutagenic-carcinogenic process is initiated by reaction with certain sites on DNA. The single largest group of known genotoxic agents forms adducts with DNA, although there are significant classes of agents which produce DNA alterations by other mechanisms (see preceeding section). Examples of non-adduct forming chemicals include non-reactive intercalating agents which bind reversibly to the DNA bases (Van der Waal forces) producing frameshift mutations. Also, several chemicals act by interfering with nucleic acid synthesis such as by forming base analogues. There is a group of chemicals, the C-mitotic poisons, and chemicals such as halothane that effect spindle mechanisms of the cell. Thus, risk assessments which depends on chemical reaction with DNA are not applicable to a significant number of potential mutagens. Even where adduct formation occurs, serious errors could be introduced since available information indicates that certain sites have far more importance for inducing mutations than others. As a distinction is made between alkylation at various sites, the amount of DNA available from in vivo studies may be a limiting factor, in deriving a correct and accurate measure, since DNA constitutes one tenth of the mass of the cell. A further confounding factor is the fact that a single chemical may produce a variety of different adducts, and the initial adduct measured may not reflect, either qualitatively or quantitatively, the important DNA reactions. Although in certain instances, risk estimates may be made by determining the reaction of the chemical with DNA using intact animals, it is probably of limited value as a routine procedure for estimating potential risk to man. Estimate of adduct formation using drosophila and cultured mammalian cells will be even less accurate than for rodents.

In cancer bioassays we are measuring the final toxicological endpoint, that is the induction of a neoplasm. In mutagenicity studies, even with intact animals, we are frequently using indirect measurements (testing urine for the presence of mutagens with bacterial tester strains), or measuring an intermediate stage of the genetic process. (cytogenetic damage as opposed to a final heritable outcome). Our use of indirect measures compromises our ability to do meaningful risk estimate on mutagens. If meaningful numbers cannot be predicted from animal studies in terms of carcinogenic risk, one would certianly question our ability to do risk estimates from routine mutagenicity studies. The most realistic approach may be to acknowledge the limitations existing in short-term tests for mutagenicity as applied to risk estimate. An alternative approach for risk estimate for potential mutagens would be the use of categories of concern based on experimental animal data as has been suggested for carcinogens. For mutagenicity assessment, one could take into acount the results from a variety of genetic endpoints including the dose-response curves from these tests, in order to establish appropriate categories. A landmark document in genetic toxicology proposed this type of non-quantitative risk assessment based on information derived from an initial testing battery (Wodicka, 1980).

For categorizing mutagenic risk, in addition to the biological information derived from the suggested test battery (see previous section) the essential requisites are information on biochemical and pharmacokinetic behavior of the compound and evidence of its reaching the germ cells. The following three categories could be established:

Category A
Chemicals can be placed into this category, based upon the recommended battery, if multiple tests including *in vitro* tests in pro-and eukaryotic systems as well as more than one *in vivo* test are positive with adequate evidence of dose response relationship.

Category B
Positive outcome in any *in vitro* test for either point mutations or chromosomal abnormalities and any single positive result of *in vivo* tests by established criteria, including a clear dose response relationship. To confirm that the chemical is in Category B the following additional tests should be conducted and be negative: dominant lethal test, germ cell cytogenetics, heritable translocation. If any of these additional tests is positive the chemical falls into Category A.

Category C
1. Positive *in vitro* findings in prokaryotic and eukaryotic systems only.

2. Marginal but statistically significant activity at high concentrations as the outcome in only one of the *in vivo* tests which include the additional tests mentioned under Category B, and where a dose/response relationship cannot be established.

The position of Genetic Toxicology in safety assessment is presented in Figure 3. As depicted here, the results of genetic toxicology studies can lead either to the rejection or acceptance of a test substance. Mutagenicity test studies are carried out concurrently with metabolic and pharmacokinetic studies. If a substance is accepted or rejected at this point in the decision tree, we are acknowledging the relationship between mutagenicity and carcinogenicity and indicating that it is highly unlikely that a carcinogenic agent would not be detected by these studies. To further ensure that the decision is correct to accept the substance based on mutagenicity studies , there is an additional stipulation that metabolites of the compound under study be known and safe.

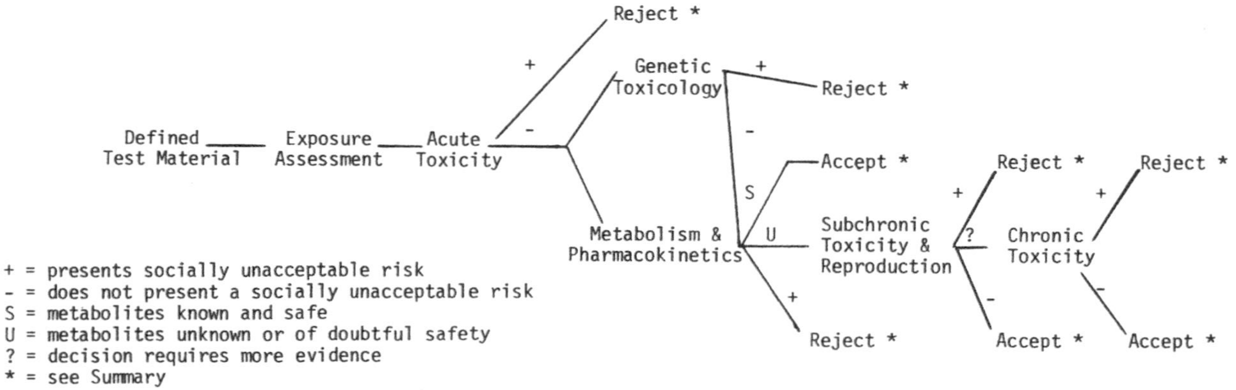

Figure 3. Safety decision tree.

Figure 4 indicates how categorizing of the chemical as a potential risk is used in the safety decision process. Cases 1 and 2 in the figure indicate clear-cut results, either negative or positive, that would allow us to "accept" (negative in all tests) or "reject" (positive in multiple tests with dose response relationship) the chemical. For intermediate categories, as 3 and 4, compound can either be rejected or tested further depending on the need for the product.

CONCLUSION

In a recent publication (Legator and Rinkus, 1981) the growth of the field of genetic toxicology and possible future developments of this area were presented. In the 1960's and early 1970's the concept of proximate carcinogens was developed using the polcyclic hydrocarbons and nitrosamines as examples. The realization that mammalian cells can metabolize chemically unreactive chemicals to electrophiles which could react with intracellular nuclophiles, including DNA provided the logical theoretical basis for the relationship between carcinogens and mutagens. The concept of promutagens and/or pro-carcinogens being metabolically activated to an active electrophile lead to the development of microbial and mammalian cell mutagenicity assays which employ cellular homogenates of mammalian liver or fractions thereof to stimulate <u>in vitro</u> metabolic activation. The use of the host -mediated assay where a indicator organism was placed in an intact animal treated with a potential pro-mutagen-carcinogen was yet another attempt to detect active metabolites of pro-mutagens-carcinogens. The early success of this experimental approach is clearly optomized by the near 90% of correlation between chemical carcinogens and mutagens that was. soon being quoted by many in the mid 1970's. These results were so impressive that a high level of optimism was generated that these <u>in vitro</u> assays would suffice in themselves as an efficient means to identify potential genotoxins. However, by the late 1970's it became apparent that <u>in vitro</u> systems for mutagenicity testing have critical shortcomings that detract from their efficiency as general screening assays. Firstly the activation of some chemicals to electrophiles is more complex than just one or two P-450-mediated oxidations, and this complexity does not lend itself easily to <u>in vitro</u> simulation. Secondly, with regard to the popular microbial systems, their phylogenetic unsimilarity to mammalian organisms poses at least two other problems; their inability to detect the entire spectrum of mutational events; and differences in passages of some chemicals a cross microbial versus mammalian cell membranes. Consequently, the 1970's closed with a growing consensus that a battery of <u>in vitro</u> and <u>in vivo</u> sytems would be the best strategy for screening genotoxic chemicals. There is still however, a tendency to discuss the detection of gentotoxic agents by a battery of <u>in vitro</u>

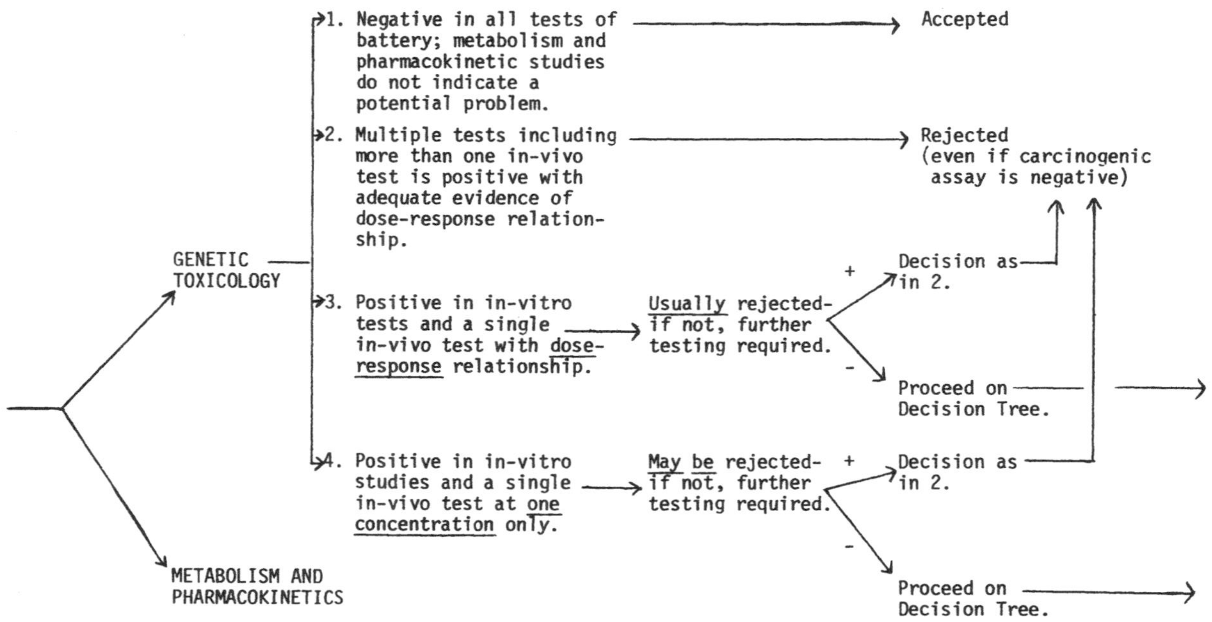

Figure 4. Expansion of safety decision tree to indicate possible outcomes from mutagenicity screening.

procedures (Weisburger and Williams, 1981). This battery approach as the initial screen although somewhat more definitive than a microbial screening program (similiar membrane and chromosomal organization as in intact mammal) will fail to detect a significant number of genetically toxic agents. There is a group of chemicals for example that are activated by the intestinal flora of experimental animals in man, such as cycasin and certain anti-schistosomal agents which would not be detected in an in vitro approach. Also, are a group of chemicals where the metabolite are unique in that the active chemicals have only been found in man or intact experimental animals such as metranidazol; and there are a number of chemicals where activity has not been demonstrated for undetermined reasons in vitro sytems but are active in vivo such as benzene. It should also be emphasized that a great deal of our mutagenicity testing in the last two decades has involved standard agents with known and predictable biological activity. As we look at unique untested chemicals, we will no doubt find unusual activity that will necesitate, to even a greater extent the use of whole animal studies. From available data with intact animals, a likely assumption is that the cytogenetic endpoint will be increasingly more important in definitive mutagenicity studies. The use of a cytogenetic endpoint would seem to detect almost all chemicals that induce point mutations as well as detecting a number of chemical that produce chromosomal anomalies where point mutations have not been demonstrated. Although several attempts have been made to quantitate and extrapolate the results of mutagenicity carcinogenicity studies, from animal and non-animal studies to man, the uncertainties of these approaches may be so great that we will have to rely on semi-quantitative procedures such as discussed in this article where broad categories are used to determine potential risk to man.

In the 1980's one can expect renewed emphasis will be placed on in vivo studies and this may result in new levels of testing sophistication. Emphasis will be placed on two areas; animal studies that measure both specific genetic alterations and their accompanying phenotypic manifestations, e.g. histocompatability studies and behavioral effects; and new procedures for monitoring high risk populations for chemical mutagenesis. In high risk populations we may see the initiation of studies using non-invasive procedures such as cytogenetic studies, body fluid analysis, YFF test and sperm morphology. These procedures should detect individuals who are being exposed to potential mutagens and carcinogens. There also will be a shift in the perception of the magnitude of the problem of mutagenesis in the human community. This increased awareness will be in response to further identification of chemicals producing a variety of effect in progeny following parental exposure in both animal and human populations. Recent findings have shown increased spontaneous abortions after male exposure to chemicals (in man); and behavioral anomalies in animals and brain tumors following parental exposure in both animals and man has only recently been reported (Corbett, 1979; Tomatis, 1981; Peters et al, 1981, Adams et al, 1981). It can only be hoped that our ability to detect and eliminate chemicals that induce heritable damage will keep pace with our concern.

REFERENCES

1. Adams, P.M., Fabricant, J.D., Legator, M.S. Cyclophosphamide-induced spermatogenic effects detected in the F generation by behavioral testing. Science 211: 80-82 (1980).
2. Ames, B.N., Lee, F.D. and Durston, W.E. An improved bacterial test system for the detection and classification of mutagens and carcinogens. Proc. Natl. Acad. Sci. 70: 782-786 (1973).
3. Anderson, D. and Styles, J.A. An evaluation of 6 short-term test for detecting organic chemical carcinogens. Appendix 2. The bacterial mutation test. Br. J. Cancer 37: 924-930 (1978).
4. Archer, V.E., Wagonner, J.K. and Lundin, F.E. Jr. Uranium mining and cigarette smoking effects on man. J. Occup. Med. 15: 204 (1972).
5. Ashby. J. The significance and interpretation of _in vitro_ carcinogenicity assay results. in: K. H. Norpoth and R. C. Garner, eds. _Short-term tests systems for detecting carcinogens_. Springer-Verlag, New York, pp. 74-93 (1980).
6. Bartsch, H., Malaveille, C. Camus, A.M., Brun, G., and Hautefeville, A. Validity of bacterial short-term tests for the detection of chemical carcinogens in K. H. Norpoth and R. C. Garner, eds. _Short-term tests systems for detecting carcinogens_. Springer-Verlag, New York, pp. 58-73. (1980).
7. Belser, W. L., Shaffer, S. D., Bliss, R. D., Hynds, P.M., Yamamoto, L., Phihs, J.N. and Winer, J.A., A standardized procedure for quantification of the Ames Salmonella/mammalian-microsome mutagenicity test. Env. Mut. 3: 123-139 (1981).
8. Bigger, C.A.H., Tomaszewski, J.E. and Dipple, A. Differences between products of binding 7,12-dimethylben(a)anthracene to DNA in mouse skin and in a rat liver microsomal system. Biochem. Biophys. Res. Commun. 80: 229-235 (1978).
9. Bigger, C.A.H., Tomaszewski, J.E., Andrews, A.W., and Dipple, A. Evaluation of metabolic activation of 7,12-dimethylben(a)anthracene _in vitro_ by Aroclor

1254-induced rat liver S-9 fractions. Cancer Res. 40: 655-661 (1980).

10. Bridges, B.A. Some general principles of mutagenicity testing and a positive framework for testing procedures. Environ. Health Perspec. 6: 221-227 (1973).

11. Brimfield, A.A., and Street, J.C. Mammalian bistransformation of chlordane: in vivo and primary hepatic considerations. A.N.Y.A.S. 320: 247-256 (1979).

12. Brouns, R.M.E., van Doorn, R., Bos, R.P. Mulleners, L.J.S. , and Henderson, P.T. Metabolic activation of 2-aminofluorene by isolated rat liver cells through different pathways leading to hepatocellular DNA-repair and bacterial mutagenesis. Toxicol. 19: 67-75 (1981).

13. Brusick, D.J., Observations and recommendations regarding routine use of bacterial mutagenesis assays as indicators of potential chemical carcinogens. in B. E. Butterworth, ed. Strategies for Short-term Testing for Mutagens/Carcinogens. CRC Press, New York, pp. 3-12 (1980).

14. Chu, K.C., Cueto, C. and Ward, J.M. Factors in the evaluation of 200 National Cancer Institute Carcinogen bioassays. J. Tox. Env. Health 8: 251- 280 (1981).

15. Clayson, D.B., Comparison between in vitro and in vivo tests for carcinogenicity. Mutat. Res 75: 205-213 (1980).

16. Corbett, T.H., Cornell, R. G., Endres, J.L. and Lieding, K. Birth defects among children of nurse-anesthetists. Anest. 41: 341-344 (1975).

17. Crump, K.S., Hoel, D.G., Langley, C.H. and Peto, R. Fundamental carcinogenic processes and their implication for low dose risk assessment. Cancer Res. 36: 2973-2979 (1976).

18. Dunkel, V.C., Collaborative studies on the Salmonella/microsome mutagenicity assay. J. Assoc. Off. Anal. Chem. 62: 874-882 (1979).

19. Glatt, H.R., Schwind, H., Schectman, L.M., Beard, S., Kouri, R.E., Zajdela, F., Croisy, A., Perin, F., Jacquignon, P.C., and Oesch, F., Mutagenicity of closely related carcinogenic and noncarcinogenic compounds using various metabolizing systems and target cells. in: K.H. Norpoth and R. C. Garner. Short-term tests systems for detecting carcinogens. Springer-Verlag. New York, pp. 103-126 (1980).

20. Grafe, A., Mattern, I.E. and Green, M. A European collaborative study of the Ames assay. I. Results and general interpretation. Mutat. Res 85: 391-410 (1981).

21. Gruneberg, H. Das problem der mutations belastung. In: Geuetik and Gessel Schaft. G. G. Wendt (ed.), pp. 72-77, Stuttgart: Wisenschaft liche Verlagsanstalt (1979).

22. Hammond, E.C. and Selikoff, I.J. Relation of cigarette smoking to risk of death of asbestos associated disease among insulation workers in the Unites States. In: Biological Effects of Asbestos , P. Bogovski, et al., eds. Scientific Publication No. 8 (Lyon France: Int. agency Res. Cancer, 1973) pp. 312-317.
23. Harper, B.L., Rinkus, S.J., Scott, M. Ammenhauser, M., Bang, K.M., Lowery, M. and Legator, M.S., Correlation of NCI and IARC carcinogens with their mutagenicity in Salmonella. This volume.
24. Hartman, P.E., Bacterial mutagenesis: review of new insights. Env. Mut. 2: 3-16 (1980).
25. Hite, M., Pechamo, M., Smith, I. and Thornton, S. The effect of benzene in the micronucleus test. Mutat. Res. 77: 149-155 (1980).
26. Irving, C.C. Species and tissue variations in the metabolic activation of aromatic amines. in: A.C. Griffin and C.R. Shaw, eds. Carcinogens: Identification and Mechanisms of Action. Raven Press, New York, pp. 211-227 (1979).
27. Kawachi, T., Yahagi, T., Kada, T., Tazima, Y., Ishidate, M., Sasaki, M., and Sugiyama, T., Cooperative programme on short-term assays for carcinogenicity in Japan. in: R. Montesano, ed. Molecular and cellular aspects of carcinogen screening tests. IARC Publ. No 27, Lyon, pp. 323-330 (1980).
28. King, H.W.S., Thompson, M.H. and Brooks, P. The benzo(a)pyrene deoxyribonucleoside products isolated from DNA after metabolism of benzo(a)pyrene by rat liver microsomes in the presence of DNA. Cancer Res. 35: 1263-1269 (1975).
29. Legator, M.S., and Rinkus, S.J., Mutagenicity testing: problems in application. in: H.F. Stich and R.H.C. San. Short-term tests for Chemicals Carcinogens. Springer-Verlag, New York. pp. 483-504 (1981).
30. Matsushima, T., Sugimura, T., Nagao, M. Yahagi, T. Shirai, A., and Sawamura, M. Factors modulating mutagenicity in microbial tests in: K.H. Norpoth and R.C. Garner, eds. Short-term test systems for detecting carcingogens Springer-Verlag, New York, pp. 273-285 (1980).
31. McCann, J., Choi, E., Yamasaki, E., and Ames, B.N. Detection of carcinogens as mutagens in the Salmonella/microsome test: assay of 300 chemicals. Proc. Nat. Acad. Sci. 72: 5135-5139 (1975).
32. Office Technology Assessment. Assessment of technologies for determining cancer risks from the environment. U.S. Government Printing Office, 1981.
33. Peters, J.M., Preston-Martin, S. and Yer, M.C. Science 213: 235-237 (1981).

34. Purchase, I.F.H., Procedure for Screening chemicals for carcinogenesis. Br. J. Indus. Med. 37: 1-10 (1980).
35. Rinkus, S. J. and Legator, M.S. The need for both in vitro and in vivo systems in mutagenicity screening. in F.J. de Serres and A. Hollaender, eds. Chemical Mutagens, vol. 6. Plenum Pub. Co., New York, pp. 365-473 (1980).
36. Rosenkranz, H.S., Karpinsky, G., and McCoy, E.C. Microbial assays: evaluation and application to the elucidation of the etiology of colon cancer. in K. H. Norpoth and R.C. Garner, eds. Short-term test systems for detecting carcinogens. Springer-Verlag, New York, pp. 19-57 (1980).
37. Salmeen, I., and Durisin, A.M. Some effects of bacteria population on quantitation of Ames salmonella-histidine reversion mutagenesis assays. Mutat. Res. 85: 109-118 (1981).
38. Sawada, M. and Ishidate, M., Jr. Colchicine-like effect of diethyl-stilbesteros (DES) on mammalian cells in-vitro. Mutat. Res. 57: 175-182 (1978).
39. Selkirk, J.A., Comparison of epoxide and free-radical methods for activation of benzo(a)pyrene by Sprague-Dawley rat liver microsomes. JNCI 64: 771-774 (1980).
40. Selkirk, J.A. Divergence of metabolic activation systems for short-term mutagenesis assays. Nature 270: 601-608 (1977).
41. Shimazu, H., Shiraishy, N., Akenatsu, T., Veda, N. and Sugiyama, T. Carcinogenicity screening tests on induction of chromosomal aberrations in rat bone marrow cells in vivo. Mutat. Res. 38: 347 (1976).
42. Simmon, V.F. In vitro mutagenicity assays of chemical carcinogens and related compounds with Salmonella typhimurium. JNCI 62: 893-899 (1979).
43. Sincock, A.M. Preliminary studies of the in vitro cellular effects of asbestos and fine class dust. In: Origins of Human Cancer , Book A., H.H. Hiatt, J.D. Watson and J.A. Winsten (eds.), New York: Cold Spring Harbor Laboratory, pp. 941-954 (1977).
44. Squire, R.A. Ranking animal carcinogens: a proposed regulatory approach. Science 214: 877-880 (1981).
45. Thompson, M.H., Osborne, M.R., King, H.W.S. and Brookes, P. the 7-methylbenz(a) antracene deoxyribonucleoside products isolated from DNA after metabolism of the carcinogen by rat liver microsomes in the presence of DNA. Chem.-Biol. Interact. 14: 13-19 (1976).
46. Tomatis, L., Cabral, J.R.P., Likhhachev, A.J. and Ponomarkovv, M. Int. J. Cancer 27: 465-478 (1981).
47. Vogel, E., Soebels, F.H. The function of drosophila in genetic toxicology testing. In: Chemical Mutagens:

Principles and Methods for Their Detection , A. Hollaender (ed.), New York: Plenum Press, pp. 93-142 (1976).

48. Vogel, E. Identification of carcinogens by mutagen testing in drosophila: The relative reliability for the kinds of genetic damage measured. In: Origins of Human Cancer Book C, H.H. Hiatt, J.D. Watson and W.A. Winsten (eds)., New York: Cold Spring Harbor Laboratory, pp. 1483-1497 (1977).

49. Weisburger, J.H. and Williams, G.M. The decision point approach for systematic carcinogen testing. Food Cosmet. Toxic. 19: 561-566 (1981).

50. Wild, D. Cytogenetic effects in the mouse of 17 chemical mutagens and carcinogens evaluated by the micronucleus test. Mutat. Res 56: 319-327 (1978).

51. Wodicka, V.E., Golberg, L. and Carr, C.J., eds. Proposed System for Food Safety Assessment. Food Safety Council, Washington, D.C. (1980).

GENETIC BIOASSAY DATA ON SOME KNOWN OR SUSPECTED HUMAN CARCINOGENS

Michael D. Waters,[a] Neil E. Garrett,[b]
Christine M. Covone-de Serres,[c] Barry E. Howard,[a]
and H. Frank Stack[b]

[a]Genetic Toxicology Division
Health Effects Research Laboratory
U.S. Environmental Protection Agency
Research Triangle Park, NC 27711

[b]Northrop Services, Inc. - Environmental Sciences
Research Triangle Park, NC 27709

[c]Genetics Curriculum
University of North Carolina
Chapel Hill, NC 27514

INTRODUCTION

The purpose of this report is to summarize the currently available qualitative information, obtained from genetic and related bioassay systems, on 24 agents or groups of agents. These agents have been classified by the International Agency for Research on Cancer (IARC) as (1) known human carcinogens, (2) probable human carcinogens, or (3) unclassified carcinogens.[1,2] The intent is to examine the performance of genetic bioassay systems in the detection and evaluation of compounds for which there is some evidence of human carcinogenic potential. These compounds are of particular interest, in a retrospective sense, for purposes of relating evidence of carcinogenic effects in man and in experimental animals with the qualitative data base being assembled using short-term genetic bioassays. Ideally, it would be important to determine the quantitative response of genetic bioassays as a function of chemical dose and to relate these responses to quantitative evidence of carcinogenic and mutagenic effects in experimental animals. Such a quantitative evaluation is essential if we are to properly select from among the many chemicals active in short-term genetic bioassays those that should be subjected to further evaluation. Ultimately, quantitative evaluations of genetically mediated effects must be coupled with accurate estimates of dose to the DNA, since this combination of information forms the basis of all current models for quantitative risk assessment.

The present report considers the qualitative aspects of the overall assessment problem described above. A computerized data base on 24 agents or groups of agents was assembled following an examination of more than 600 published reports available as of June 1, 1981. The qualitative information on these 24 agents as compiled and evaluated in the U.S. Environmental Protection Agency (EPA) GENE-TOX Program[3,4] was used by permission. These qualitative data bases were applied in combination to generate an overall summary of the genetic bioassay data that are available for each agent.

CHEMICAL SELECTION

The 24 agents or groups of agents were selected for evaluation by reference to Supplement I of the IARC Monographs on the Evaluation of Carcinogenic Risk of Chemicals to Humans.[1] Fifty-six agents, groups of agents, or industrial processes are discussed in the Supplement. The IARC Working Group concluded that the first 18 of these agents (Group 1) are carcinogenic for humans. This category was used only when sufficient evidence was found to support a causal association between exposure to the agent and cancer. The next 18 agents (Group 2) were considered "probably carcinogenic for humans." This category included chemicals for which the evidence of human carcinogenicity was almost "sufficient," i.e., the evidence suggested a causal association between exposure and human cancer. The Group 2 chemicals were divided into those with higher (Group 2A) or lower (Group 2B) degrees of evidence. Experimental animal studies were important in assigning agents to Group 2, especially Group 2B. The third group of 18 agents could not be classified by the IARC Working Group as to carcinogenicity for humans.

Table 1 gives alphabetical listings by IARC classification of the agents evaluated in this report. The following section describes the process of collating and evaluating the literature.

METHOD OF LITERATURE REVIEW

A search of the major computer-based bibliographic systems was performed by the EPA Library at Research Triangle Park, NC. Toxline

Table 1. IARC Classification of Agents in the Present Data Base

Group	Classification	Agents
1	carcinogenic for humans	4-aminobiphenyl arsenic and certain arsenic compounds[a] asbestos benzene benzidine N,N-bis(2-chloroethyl)-2-naphthylamine (chlornaphazine) bis(chloromethyl) ether and technical grade chloromethyl methyl ether chromium and certain chromium compounds[a] diethylstilbestrol melphalan mustard gas 2-naphthylamine vinyl chloride
2A	higher degree of evidence for probable human carcinogenicity	aflatoxins cadmium and certain cadmium compounds[a] cyclophosphamide nickel and certain nickel compounds[a]
2B	lower degree of evidence for probable human carcinogenicity	acrylonitrile auramine ethylene oxide oxymetholone
3	not classified	chloramphenicol epichlorohydrin phenytoin

[a]"The specific compound(s) which may be responsible for carcinogenic effect in humans cannot be specified precisely."[1]

was used as the primary source of literature citations for the following reasons: (1) comprehensiveness (includes Biological Abstracts, Chemical Abstracts, Index Medicus, Pesticide Abstracts, the Environmental Mutagen Information Center, the Environmental Teratology Information Center, Research Projects in Toxicology--Smithsonian Science Information Exchange), (2) inclusion of abstracts, (3) use of registry numbers for reliable retrieval of specific chemical substances, and (4) the cost is significantly less than that of accessing individual sources directly.

The search process also included Cancerlit, the National Technical Information Service file (government reports), and Excerpta Medica (a European biomedical file that is particularly strong in chemical and drug toxicity information).

From each report the reviewers abstracted information for any of the 24 agents evaluated in this study. The overall test result was recorded together with an appropriate assay code and publication identification number. The use of an exogenous metabolic activation system was indicated. Each report was evaluated a second time by a different reviewer for assurance of completeness and accuracy.

The data were coded on data entry forms, keypunched, and verified before entry into a data base maintained at the EPA Univac 1110 Data Center at Research Triangle Park, NC. These data were processed through the use of a System 2000 (Intel Corp., Austin, TX) data management software package. Results are retrieved through a data selection program written in COBOL that allows reports to be generated in matrix format on the basis of chemical name, Chemical Abstracts Service number, and/or assay code.

RESULTS

Published reports on the 24 agents under consideration represented approximately 100 different genetic and related bioassay systems. This fact necessitated codification of bioassay system names. For purposes of standardization with similar literature evaluations, the three-character EPA GENE-TOX bioassay codes were used when applicable; other three-character codes were assigned as needed. The bioassay codes used in this report are listed and defined in Table 2. Codes not specified by GENE-TOX appear in parentheses.

To evaluate the qualitative information in the detailed data base, it was necessary to organize the bioassay data according to classes of genetic or related activity and, where applicable, to subdivide the classes of activity according to the phylogenetic level of organization of the indicator organism (prokaryote or eukaryote). A condensation of the bioassay data was achieved by

Table 2. Definitions of Bioassay Codes

Code[a]	Definition
ARM	*Arabidopsis* mutation
(BSD)	dog urine, *Salmonella typhimurium*
(BSH)	human urine, *Salmonella typhimurium*
(BSM)	mouse urine, *Salmonella typhimurium*
(BSR)	rat urine, *Salmonella typhimurium*
(BWH)	human urine, WI-38 cells in culture
(BYH)	human urine, yeast
(BYM)	mouse urine, yeast
(BYR)	rat urine, yeast
(CHL)	Chinese hamster lung cells in culture
CHO	Chinese hamster ovary (CHO) cells in culture
CT7	cell transformation, SA-7/SHE cells
CTB	cell transformation, BALB/c3T3 cells
CTC	Syrian hamster embryo, clonal assay
CTF	Syrian hamster embryo, focus assay
CTH	cell transformation, C3H10T1/2 cells
CTK	cell transformation, AKR/ME cells
CTL	cell transformation, established cell lines
CTR	cell transformation, RLV/Fischer rat embryo cells
CTS	Syrian hamster embryo, transformation strains
CYB	mammalian cytogenetics, *in vivo* bone marrow studies, all animals
CYC	mammalian cytogenetics, *in vitro* cell culture, all cell types
CYG	mammalian cytogenetics, spermatogonial stem cells treated, spermatocytes observed
CYH	mammalian cytogenetics, *in vitro* lymphocytes, human
CYL	mammalian cytogenetics, *in vivo* and *in vitro* lymphocyte or leukocyte studies, all animals
CYO	mammalian cytogenetics, *in vivo* oocyte or early embryo studies
CYS	mammalian cytogenetics, *in vivo* studies, spermatogonia treated, spermatogonia observed
CYT	mammalian cytogenetics, *in vivo* studies, differentiating spermatogonia or spermatocytes treated, differentiating spermatocytes observed
CYU	mammalian cytogenetics, *in vitro* cell culture, Chinese hamster ovary (CHO) cells
CYV	mammalian cytogenetics, *in vitro* cell culture, Syrian golden hamster

(continued)

Table 2. (continued)

Code[a]	Definition
(CYX)	mammalian cytogenetics, *in vitro* cell culture, *Xeroderma pigmentosum* cells
CYY	mammalian cytogenetics, *in vitro* cell culture, mouse
CYZ	mammalian cytogenetics, *in vitro* cell culture, human
DAC	*Drosophila melanogaster* aneuploidy, whole sex chromosome loss
DAP	*Drosophila melanogaster* aneuploidy, partial sex chromosome loss
(DBH)	DNA strand break, human
DHT	heritable (reciprocal) translocation, *Drosophila melanogaster*
(DLD)	dominant lethal test, *Drosophila melanogaster*
DLM	dominant lethal test, mouse
DLR	dominant lethal test, rat
(ECO)	*Escherichia coli* differential toxicity, miscellaneous strains
HMA	host-mediated assay
HOC	*Hordeum* cytogenetics
(IDL)	inhibition of DNA synthesis, HeLa cells
(IDP)	inhibition of DNA synthesis, rat primary hepatocytes
(IDR)	inhibition of DNA synthesis, rat
L5T	mouse lymphoma (L5178Y) cells in culture, TK locus
(MHT)	heritable (reciprocal) translocation, mouse
(MNC)	micronucleus test, *in vitro*
(MNH)	micronucleus test, hamster
(MNM)	micronucleus test, mouse
(MNR)	micronucleus test, rat
MST	mouse spot test
NEF	*Neurospora crassa*, forward mutation
NEN	*Neurospora crassa*, aneuploidy
NER	*Neurospora crassa*, reversion test
REC	DNA repair-deficient bacteria tests
REP	*Escherichia coli* Pol A (*W3110-P3478), spot test
RER	*Escherichia coli* Pol A (*W3110-P3478), spot test, well
RET	*Escherichia coli* Pol A (*W3110-P3478), liquid suspension test
REW	*Bacillus subtilis* rec (*H17-M45), spot test

(continued)

Table 2. (continued)

Code[a]	Definition
SA0	*Salmonella typhimurium* (histidine reversion test), strain TA100
SA5	*Salmonella typhimurium* (histidine reversion test), strain TA1535
SA7	*Salmonella typhimurium* (histidine reversion test), strain TA1537
SA8	*Salmonella typhimurium* (histidine reversion test), strain TA1538
SA9	*Salmonella typhimurium* (histidine reversion test), strain TA98
SC2	sister chromatid exchange, *in vitro*, all animals except human
SC3	sister chromatid exchange, *in vivo*, all animals except human
SC4	sister chromatid exchange, *in vivo*, human cells
SCC	sister chromatid exchange, Chinese hamster ovary (CHO) cells, transformed
SCF	sister chromatid exchange, human fibroblasts, normal
SCL	sister chromatid exchange, human lymphocytes
SCP	sister chromatid exchange, Chinese hamster fibroblasts, transformed
SCV	sister chromatid exchange, Chinese hamster lung fibroblasts (V-79 cells), transformed
SLP	mouse specific locus test, postspermatogonial stages
SLT	mouse specific locus test, all
SPA	effects on mammalian sperm, rat
SPF	effects on mammalian sperm, mouse, F_1 assay
SPH	effects on mammalian sperm, human
SPI	effects on mammalian sperm, mouse
SPR	effects on mammalian sperm, rabbit
SPS	effects on mammalian sperm, sheep
SRL	*Drosophila melanogaster* sex-linked recessive lethal test
TRC	*Tradescantia* cytogenetics
TRM	*Tradescantia* mutation
(UDB)	unscheduled DNA synthesis in mammals, human bone marrow
UDH	unscheduled DNA synthesis in mammals, human diploid fibroblasts

(continued)

Table 2. (continued)

Code[a]	Definition
(UDL)	unscheduled DNA synthesis in mammals, HeLa cells
(UDM)	unscheduled DNA synthesis, mouse, *in vivo*
UDP	unscheduled DNA synthesis in mammals, rat primary hepatocytes
UDS	unscheduled DNA synthesis in mammals, all cell types, *in vitro*
(UDX)	unscheduled DNA synthesis in mammals, *Xeroderma pigmentosum* cells
V7H	Chinese hamster lung (V-79) cells in culture, HGPRT locus
V7O	Chinese hamster lung (V-79) cells in culture, ouabain locus
WP2	*Escherichia coli* WP2, reverse mutation
(WPR)	*Escherichia coli* WP100 uvrA$^-$ rec$^-$ or other rec$^-$ strains
WPU	*Escherichia coli* WP2 uvrA, reverse mutation
YEC	*Saccharomyces cerevisiae*, gene conversion
YEF	*Saccharomyces cerevisiae*, forward mutation
YEH	*Saccharomyces cerevisiae*, homozygosis (through recombination or gene conversion)
YER	*Saccharomyces cerevisiae*, reversion test
YEY	*Schizosaccharomyces pombe*, forward mutation
YEZ	*Schizosaccharomyces pombe*, reversion test

[a]Parentheses indicate codes not specified by the EPA GENE-TOX Program.

combining similar bioassay systems and tester strains. In a few cases different systems and/or different genetic end points were combined. This was done only when the concordance in data permitted such a combination. The resulting groupings of bioassay systems are shown in Table 3. Reading Table 3 from left to right illustrates the sequence of genetic bioassays as they are considered in the subsequent discussion of published results for each agent. In grouping assay systems or strains, generally the third letter of the three-letter code is left blank and is used to identify specific systems or strains.

Table 4 represents the total data base in its condensed form as it is discussed in subsequent sections. The bioassays are grouped as described in Table 3. In Table 4, where systems or

Table 3. Combined Groupings of Bioassay Systems[a]

POINT/GENE MUTATION ASSAYS

Prokaryotic Point/Gene Mutation Assays

SA_					WP_	
SA5	SA7	SA8	SA9	SA0	WP2	WPU

Lower Eukaryotic Gene Mutation and Body Fluid Assays

YE_				NE_		(B__)							
YEF	YER	YEY	YEZ	NEF	NER	(BSD)	(BSH)	(BSM)	(BSR)	(BWH)	(BYH)	(BYM)	(BYR)

Higher Eukaryotic *In Vitro* Gene Mutation Assays

CH_		V7_		L5T
(CHL)	CHO	V7H	V70	

Higher Eukaryotic *In Vivo* Gene Mutation Assays

_RM		SRL	MST	SL_		HMA
ARM	TRM			SLP	SLT	

PRIMARY DNA DAMAGE ASSAYS

Prokaryotic Primary DNA Damage Assays

RE_					(WPR)	(ECO)
REP	RER	RET	REW	REC		

(continued)

Table 3. (continued)

Lower Eukaryotic Primary DNA Damage Assays

YE_

YEC YEH

Higher Eukaryotic Primary DNA Damage Assays *In Vitro* and *In Vivo*

UD_   UDP (UDM)   (ID_)   (DBH)

(UDB) UDH (UDL) UDS (UDX)   (IDL) (IDP) (IDR)

CHROMOSOMAL EFFECTS ASSAYS

Sister Chromatid Exchange *In Vitro* and *In Vivo*   Aneuploidy

SC_   SCL   SC_   NEN   DA_

SCC SCF SCP SCV   SC2 SC3 SC4   DAC DAP

Chromosomal Aberrations *In Vitro*

CY_   CYH   (CYX)

CYU CYV CYY CYZ CYC

Chromosomal Aberrations *In Vivo*

CY_   CYG   CY_   _C

CYB CYL   CYO CYS CYT   HOC TRC

(continued)

Table 3. (continued)

Micronuclei *In Vitro*			
(MNC)			

Micronuclei *In Vivo*		
(MN_)		
(MNH)	(MNM)	(MNR)

Chromosomal Damage *In Vivo*				
(DLD)	DLM	DLR	DHT	(MHT)

CELLULAR TRANSFORMATION ASSAYS

CT_			CT_			CT_		CT7
CTC	CTF	CTS	CTB	CTH	CTL	CTK	CTR	

STUDIES INVOLVING SPERM

SP_					SPF
SPA	SPH	SPI	SPR	SPS	

[a]Bioassay codes are defined in Table 2.

strains are combined under a specific column, the letter(s) in the three-character code appropriate to a specific entry in the body of the table appear immediately above the test result(s).

The detailed data base used to construct Table 4 was derived from a review of approximately 600 published reports. Each entry is keyed to a specific literature citation. This detailed data base could not be reproduced here but is available from the first author.

Table 4. Condensed Data Base[a]

Compound	Point/Gene Mutation Assays													Primary DNA Damage Assays			
System:	SA_	WP_	YE_	NE_	(B__)	CH_	V7_	L5T	_RM	SRL	MST	SL_	HMA	RE_	(WPR)	(ECO)	YE_
Test/Strain:	57890	2U	FRYZ	FR	SWY DHMR	(L)O	HO		AT			PT		PRTWC			CH
acrylonitrile	5890 -/+	2U +/+			S MR +/+												
aflatoxin B1	7890 ±/+		F +/0	F +/+	S R -/+		HO -/+			+/0			+/0	PW +/+	-/+	+/+	CH -/+
4-aminobiphenyl	7890 -/+	2U -/-			S R ±/+		H 0/-						-/0	T 0/+			H +/+
arsenic compounds	5780 -/-	2U ±/-						+/+		±/0				W +/0	+/0	-/0	H +/+
asbestiform minerals	58 -/-	2U -/-				(L) +/+											
auramine	57890 -/-							0/-					-/0	PT +/0			H +/+
benzene	57890 -/-								T +/0	-/0				C -/-			H -/-
benzidine	57890 -/+				S R -/+					+/0					-/+		H -/-

(continued)

Table 4. (coutinued)

Compound	Primary DNA Damage Assays					Chromosomal Effects Assays													
System:	UD_	UDP	(UDM)	(ID_)	(DBH)	SC_	SCL	SC_	NEN	DA_	CY_	CYH	(CYX)	CY_	CYG	CY_	__C	(MNC)	(MN_)
Test/Strain:	(B)H(L)S(X)			LPR		CFPV		234		CP	UVYZC			BL		OST	HO TR		HMR
acrylonitrile														B -/0					
aflatoxin B1	H(L)S +/+	+/0		LR ±/+		CV ±/+	+/+	3 ±/0			UZC +/+	+/0		B +/0	-/0			+/+	HMR ±/0
4-aminobiphenyl	H -/0	+/0																	R -/0
arsenic compounds	H -/-						+/0			CP ±/0	Z +/0	+/0		BL +/0				-/0	
asbestiform minerals											UVC +/0	+/0		B -/0					M -/0
auramine																			M -/0
benzene				R +/0			±/+	3 +/0				±/0		BL ±/0		S -/0			M +/0
benzidine	(L) 0/+	+/0		L +/0															MR ±/0

(continued)

Table 4. (continued)

Compound	Chromosomal Effects Assays					Cellular Transformation Assays				Sperm Assays	
System:	(DLD)	DLM	DLR	DHT	(MHT)	CT_	CT_	CT_	CT7	SP_	SPF
Test/Strain:						CFS	BHL	KR		AHIRS	
acrylonitrile						F +/0			+/0		
aflatoxin B1						CF +/0	B +/0		+/0	AI -/0	
4-aminobiphenyl						C +/0		KR +/0			
arsenic compounds		-/0				C +/0			+/0		
asbestiform minerals							B +/0				
auramine						C -/+					
benzene									-/0	I +/0	
benzidine						C +/0		KR +/0	+/0	I -/0	

(continued)

Table 4. (continued)

Compound	Point/Gene Mutation Assays													Primary DNA Damage Assays			
System:	SA_	WP_	YE_	NE_	(B__)	CH_	V7_	L5T	_RM	SRL	MST	SL_	HMA	RE_	(WPR)	(ECO)	YE_
Test/Strain:	57890	2U	FRYZ	FR	SWY DHMR	(L)O	HO		AT			PT		PRTWC			CH
bis(chloromethyl) ether	0 0/+																
cadmium compounds	790 -/-					O +/0								W +/0			
chloramphenicol	58 -/0	2 -/0							A -/0	-/0				PRTW -/0		-/0	
chlornaphazine	0 +/+									+/0							
chloromethyl methyl ether																	
chromium compounds	7890 ±/±	2U +/0	Y +/0								+/0			PW ±/0		+/0	H +/+
cyclophosphamide	5890 -/+	2U ±/-	F +/0		SY HMR +/0		O +/0	-/+	A -/0	+/0	+/0	P +/0	+/0	PT 0/+			CH ±/+
diethylstilbestrol	57890 -/-	2U -/-					HO -/-	+/+								-/0	

(continued)

Table 4. (continued)

Compound	Primary DNA Damage Assays					Chromosomal Effects Assays													
System:	UD_	UDP	(UDM)	(ID_)	(DBH)	SC_	SCL	SC_	NEN	DA_	CY_	CYH	(CYX)	CY_	CYG	CY_	__C	(MNC)	(MN_)
Test/Strain:	(B)H(L)S(X)			LPR		CFPV		234		CP	UVYZC			BL		OST	HO TR		HMR
bis(chloromethyl) ether																			
cadmium compounds						C -/0					U +/0								M -/0
chloramphenicol														BL +/0					
chlornaphazine																			
chloromethyl methyl ether																			
chromium compounds	HS +/0				+/0	CF ±/0					UVYZ +/0	+/0						±/0	M +/0
cyclophosphamide	(L) 0/+		+/0	L -/+	-/+	CFP ±/+	-/0	234 +/0		CP -/0	UZC ±/+	-/+		BL +/0	+/0	OS +/0			HMR +/0
diethylstilbestrol	(L) 0/+					FP ±/0		3 -/0	-/0		C ±/0	-/0		B ±/0					M ±/0

(continued)

Table 4. (continued)

Compound	Chromosomal Effects Assays					Cellular Transformation Assays				Sperm Assays	
System:	(DLD)	DLM	DLR	DHT	(MHT)	CT_	CT_	CT_	CT7	SP_	SPF
Test/Strain:						CFS	BHL	KR		AHIRS	
bis(chloromethyl) ether											
cadmium compounds		±/0	-/0		-/0	C +/0			+/0	I -/0	
chloramphenicol	-/0	+/0									
chlornaphazine									+/0		
chloromethyl methyl ether									+/0		
chromium compounds						C +/0	B +/0	R +/0	+/0		
cyclophosphamide	-/0	+/0	+/0		±/0	C +/0	BHL -/+	R +/0		AHIS +/0	-/0
diethylstilbestrol						C +/0	B -/0	R +/0		HI ±/0	

(continued)

Table 4. (continued)

Compound	Point/Gene Mutation Assays													Primary DNA Damage Assays			
System:	SA_	WP_	YE_	NE_	(B__)	CH_	V7_	L5T	_RM	SRL	MST	SL_	HMA	RE_	(WPR)	(ECO)	YE_
Test/Strain:	57890	2U	FRYZ	FR	SWY DHMR	(L)O	HO		AT			PT		PRTWC			CH
epichlorohydrin	50 +/0	2U +/0	RZ +/0	F +/0	S HM +/0					+/0				TWC ±/±			CH +/0
ethylene oxide	50 +/+			R +/0				+/0		+/0							
melphalan	5 +/+				S H -/0			+/+		+/0				PR -/+			
mustard gas		U +/0		R +/0						+/0			+/0			+/0	
2-naphthylamine	5890 -/+		F +/0	F +/0	S R -/+		H 0/-			±/0			+/0	TC -/+	-/+	-/0	CH ±/±
nickel compounds		2 -/0				O +/0							-/0	W -/0			
phenytoin																	
vinyl chloride	50 ±/+		RY -/+	FR -/-	S HR -/-	O -/+	HO -/+		T +/0	+/0	-/0		+/0	PTC -/+			CH -/+

Table 4. (continued)

Compound	Primary DNA Damage Assays					Chromosomal Effects Assays													
System:	UD_	UDP	(UDM)	(ID_)	(DBH)	SC_	SCL	SC_	NEN	DA_	CY_	CYH	(CYX)	CY_	CYG	CY_	__C	(MNC)	(MN_)
Test/Strain:	(B)H(L)S(X)			LPR		CFPV		234		CP	UVYZC			BL		OST	HO TR		HMR
epichlorohydrin							+/+					+/0		BL +/0					M -/0
ethylene oxide			+/0			F +/0	+/0							BL +/0			HO TR +/0		MR +/0
melphalan	(B) +/0				+/0		+/0	2 +/0			C +/0								
mustard gas										CP +/0	C +/0								
2-naphthylamine	H +/0																		MR ±/0
nickel compounds											YC +/0								
phenytoin												-/0		B -/0					
vinyl chloride							-/+	34 ±/0		CP -/0				BL ±/0					M +/0

(continued)

Table 4. (continued)

Compound	Chromosomal Effects Assays					Cellular Transformation Assays				Sperm Assays	
System:	(DLD)	DLM	DLR	DHT	(MHT)	CT_	CT_	CT_	CT7	SP_	SPF
Test/Strain:						CFS	BHL	KR		AHIRS	
epichlorohydrin		-/0								I -/0	
ethylene oxide		+/0	+/0	+/0	+/0						
melphalan							H +/0				
mustard gas	+/0			+/0							
2-naphthylamine						C +/0		KR +/0	+/0	I -/0	
nickel compounds						CFS +/0			+/0		
phenytoin										I +/0	
vinyl chloride	-/0	-/0	-/0	-/0							

[a]System and test/strain codes are defined in Table 2. Test results are shown without metabolic activation/with metabolic activation and are expressed as follows: + = positive; − = negative; ± = different results in two or more tests; 0 = no result entered. In results from whole-animal systems, the 0 entry for "with metabolic activation" indicates that exogenous metabolic activation is not required.

DISCUSSION

To facilitate an integrated discussion of the condensed data base, the agents under investigation are grouped by target organ specificity. Chemical structures and IARC classifications are provided for each group. Since the genetic bioassay results have been condensed, not all citations pertinent to each statement regarding a qualitative response are provided. Instead, an appropriate reference that supports the statement is given.

Human Respiratory Tract Carcinogens

Ten compounds examined in this study are either volatile or undergo condensation on the surfaces of respirable particles and enter the human respiratory tract. Three of these compounds are highly volatile alkylating agents: bis(chloromethyl) ether, chloromethyl methyl ether, and mustard gas. Two others are highly reactive substituted alkenes: acrylonitrile and vinyl chloride. (The results of the literature review for vinyl chloride are presented in a later section, "Human Liver Carcinogens.") Four metals (arsenic, cadmium, chromium, and nickel) and the group of particulate minerals considered collectively as "asbestos" complete this group of agents that appear to induce cancer of the human respiratory tract. The chemical structures and IARC classifications of these agents are shown in Fig. 1.

Bis(chloromethyl) Ether and Chloromethyl Methyl Ether. Background Information. Bis(chloromethyl) ether (BCME) or dichloromethyl ether is a highly volatile compound sold as a laboratory chemical and used as a chloromethylating reaction mixture in the preparation of ion exchange resins.[5] Thiess et al. reported in 1973 on 6 cases of lung cancer in 18 testing laboratory workers who used BCME.[6,7] Five of these 6 men were moderate smokers. However, of the total cancers reported, the majority were oat-cell carcinomas, a tumor type not usually seen in smokers.

Chloromethyl methyl ether (CMME) also is highly volatile and frequently is contaminated with BCME. CMME is also used in the preparation of ion exchange resins. One study reported an increased risk of lung cancer for workers exposed to CMME.[8] Fourteen men developed lung cancer and 12 of these had oat-cell carcinomas.

Genetic Bioassay Results. BCME gives positive results in *Salmonella* strain TA100 in the presence of S-9 activation.[9] No other point/gene mutation, primary DNA damage, or chromosomal effects data are reported.

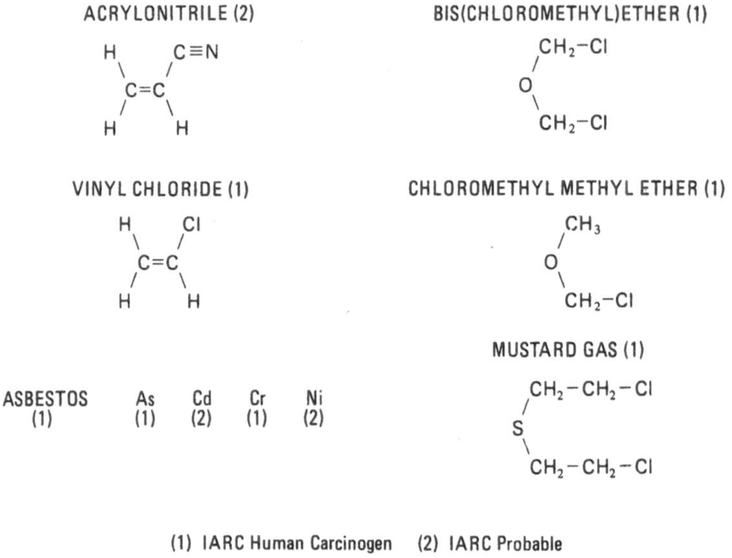

Fig. 1. Human respiratory tract carcinogens

Cell transformation assays have been performed with CMME. The compound enhances viral transformation of Syrian hamster embryo (SHE) cells in the absence of exogenous activation.[10]

BCME and CMME have not been studied extensively for genetic activity in short-term tests. This may be because of case reports indicating that these compounds are exceedingly dangerous, with a high percentage of oat-cell carcinomas developing in exposed workers. The paucity of data precludes consideration of the relevance of specific genetic bioassay systems for these compounds.

Mustard Gas. Background Information. Mustard gas or sulfur mustard is a deadly vesicant that has been used as a war gas. The compound causes conjunctivitis and blindness in man. It is an important model compound in biological studies requiring the use of direct-acting alkylating agents.

Wada et al. reported that factory workers engaged in the manufacture of mustard gas had an elevated incidence of respiratory neoplasia.[11] In this study, 33 deaths resulted from neoplasia of the respiratory tract. Thirty of these were histologically confirmed. Only 0.9 deaths were expected. A study of World War I veterans indicated that the risk of death from lung cancer for men gassed with the compound was significantly increased above that of the controls.[12] A similar study by Case and Lea indicated that persons exposed to mustard gas also suffered from chronic bronchitis.[13] These authors indicated that an increased risk of lung and pleural cancer appeared to be associated with the chronic bronchitis.

Genetic Bioassay Results. Mustard gas gives positive results in *E. coli* WP2 uvrA⁻ and in a host-mediated assay using L5178Y cells in mice in the absence of S-9.[14] The gas also produces reverse mutations in *Neurospora*[15] and sex-linked recessive lethality in *Drosophila*.[16]

In assays for primary DNA damage, mustard gas is more toxic to repair-deficient *E. coli* strains than to the corresponding competent strains.[17]

In assays for chromosomal effects, mustard gas produces positive responses in mammalian cells *in vitro*[18] and in the *Drosophila* aneuploidy,[19] dominant lethal,[16] and heritable translocation[19] tests.

The genetic toxicology data base indicates that exogenous metabolic activation is not required to produce point mutations, primary DNA damage, or chromosomal effects. Although only a portion of the test reports overlap, the data for mustard gas are consistent with those for two other direct-acting alkylating agents evaluated in this report, ethylene oxide and epichlorohydrin.

Acrylonitrile. Background Information. Acrylonitrile is an important industrial chemical used in the production of synthetic fibers. Its chemical structure resembles that of the known human carcinogen vinyl chloride. The copolymer consisting of acrylonitrile, butadiene, and styrene, the so-called "ABS plastic," is a particularly important chemical complex,[20] and acrylonitrile polymers are used frequently in food packaging materials.[21]

An increased risk of both lung and large intestine cancers for workers in fiber production plants has been reported.[22] A preliminary study by the U.S. Occupational Safety and Health Administration showed that persons exposed to acrylonitrile in the workplace are at a greater risk of developing cancer of the lung and large intestine.[23] Another study[24] consisted of 1,343 male workers who were exposed to acrylonitrile in a textile plant during the years 1950 to 1967. Eight cancer deaths were reported when only 4 were expected and 16 cases of cancer were diagnosed when only 5.8 were expected. Analysis of lymphocytes of the workers showed no evidence of chromosomal damage. More recent industrial epidemiological studies also indicate that acrylonitrile is a human carcinogen.[25,26]

Genetic Bioassay Results. Acrylonitrile has been tested as a gas in Salmonella and gives positive results in strains TA1535, TA1538, TA98, and TA100 in the presence of S-9 metabolic activation.[27] Interestingly, results are also positive in E. coli WP2 and WP2 uvrA$^-$ in the presence and absence of metabolic activation.[28] These strains of bacteria, except TA1538 and TA98, usually respond to chemicals which cause base-pair substitution reactions.

With reference to bioassays that may be useful for human monitoring, urine concentrates from the rat and from the mouse give positive results in Salmonella with and without metabolic activation. These positive results are enhanced when the urine is treated with appropriate deconjugating enzymes.[29]

With respect to chromosomal effects, acrylonitrile gives negative results in in vivo cytogenetic assays using bone marrow.[21]

In cellular transformation assays. acrylonitrile transforms SHE fibroblasts in a mass focus assay and enhances transformation of the same cells in the presence of SA-7 virus.[30]

In summary, although results from numerous assay systems suggest that acrylonitrile causes genetic damage, adequate data are available for only two bacterial systems. The other test results require confirmation. The lack of a sufficient number of test results precludes any recommendations concerning the appropriateness of specific test systems for further evaluation of acrylonitrile.

Arsenic Compounds. Background Information. Arsenic is used in metal alloys, in semiconductor devices, and in manufacture of certain types of glass. The compound has been used medically in the treatment of infections and various types of skin disorders. Arsenic is also used as a pesticide and in agricultural processes.

Hutchinson (1887-1888) first called attention to the relationship between certain arsenic-containing drugs and skin cancer.[31] Subsequently, a variety of reports appeared concerning arsenic-containing drugs and skin cancer. For example, in 1913 Pye-Smith reported 31 such cases, 24 apparently of medical origin.[32] Neubauer reviewed the reports of cancer resulting from arsenic.[33] Three major categories are of interest: (1) cancer resulting from arsenic-containing drugs, (2) cancer caused by arsenic in drinking water, and (3) cancer caused by occupational exposure to arsenic.

A study of occupational lung cancer presumably due to arsenic was reported by Kuratsune and coworkers.[34] The only significant difference between a studied group of cancer patients and the control group was that 11 of 19 who died from lung cancer had been employed as smelters in a local copper refinery where they had received heavy exposure to arsenic trioxide. Recently arsenic was found to be concentrated seven-fold in the lung tissue of smelter workers.[35] Other studies of occupational exposure in mines and smelters have been catalogued.[36]

Arsenic released into the environment by various industrial processes may contribute to the total cancer burden.[37] One area of concern is air pollution. Mortality rates from lung cancer are significantly increased in counties in which copper, lead, or zinc smelting or refining industries contribute to atmospheric arsenic.[38] Residents of an area near a pesticide plant that has produced arsenic-containing materials since the early 1900's were reported to have a significantly increased incidence of lung cancer.[39]

Genetic Bioassay Results. The trivalent arsenic compounds as a group give uniformly negative results in the standard *Salmonella* tester strains in the absence of S-9 metabolic activation.[40] Other reports of tests in *Salmonella* in the presence of metabolic activation are also negative. Trivalent arsenic compounds induce reverse mutations in *E. coli* WP2 and WP2 uvrA$^-$ in the absence of exogenous metabolic activation.[41] Trivalent arsenic induces forward mutations at the thymidine kinase (TK) locus in the mouse lymphoma system.[40] The trivalent compound causes sex-linked recessive lethality in *Drosophila*,[42] but the pentavalent compound does not.[43]

With regard to primary DNA damage, trivalent and pentavalent arsenic give positive results in relative toxicity assays in *B. subtilis* rec$^-$ strains.[41] Pentavalent arsenic induces enhanced mitotic recombination or gene conversion in *S. cerevisiae* with or without metabolic activation.[44] The compound does not induce unscheduled DNA synthesis (UDS) in human embryonic lung fibroblasts with or without activation.[44] Trivalent arsenic induces sister chromatid exchanges (SCEs) in lymphocytes of patients treated with the compound.[45] Arsenic also produces chromosome aberrations in bone marrow of mice,[46] in lymphocytes of exposed patients,[47] and in cultured human lymphocytes and fibroblasts.[48] Micronuclei are not induced *in vitro*.[49]

A cell transformation clonal assay in SHE cells is reported to be positive.[50] In addition, trivalent arsenic, among other metals, enhances viral transformation of cells in culture.[51]

In summary, the most convincing positive results indicate primary DNA damage and chromosomal effects in mammalian cells *in* vitro and in vivo. Results of cell transformation assays also are positive.

Cadmium Compounds. Background Information. Cadmium is used in semiconductors, in the manufacture of alloys and glass, in storage battery electrodes, as a nematocide, as a catalyst in various organic reactions, in electroplating, and as a stabilizer for plastics. Cadmium compounds are found in the natural environment in trace quantities in coals and oils. A substantial amount of cadmium is found in ambient air. Smelting operations are reported to account for 87% of emissions into the atmosphere.[52]

Cadmium oxide fumes are toxic, and extensive inhalation exposure may result in fatal pulmonary edema. Occupational exposure is associated with an increased risk of prostate cancer and respiratory tract cancer.[53,54] Potts reported a study of 70 men who were exposed to cadmium oxide dust while producing alkaline batteries. Eight deaths were reported, 3 from prostate cancer and 2 from other forms of cancer.[55] An epidemiological study of 248 workers indicated a total of 4 cases of prostate cancer.[56] A study of 292 smelter workers exposed to cadmium oxide dust and fumes showed increased incidences of prostate cancer and respiratory tract cancer.[57] Another report showed an association of renal cancer with cadmium exposure; the interpretation favored a synergistic effect between this exposure and smoking.[58]

Genetic Bioassay Results. Cadmium chloride fails to induce reverse mutations in S. typhimurium in the presence or absence of S-9 metabolic activation.[59] However, the compound is mutagenic in Chinese hamster ovary (CHO) cells at the hypoxanthineguanine phosphoribosyltransferase (HGPRT) locus.[60] Cadmium displays toxicity in B. subtilis rec$^-$ strains.[61]

Cadmium fails to induce SCEs in CHO cells at concentrations of up to 0.4 μM.[62] The metal does, however, cause chromosome aberrations in CHO cells at a concentration of ~1 μM.[62] The results of two micronucleus tests in the mouse are negative[59] and mixed positive and negative results are reported for a dominant lethal assay in the mouse.[63] Cadmium chloride gives negative results in the mouse heritable translocation test.[64] Cadmium does not induce dominant lethality or teratogenicity in the rat.[65]

Cadmium transforms SHE cells in a clonal assay[50] and enhances the viral transformation of SHE cells.[51] The metal does not, however, alter sperm morphology in the mouse.[59]

In summary, the data base consists of 15 reports and includes positive and negative responses.

Chromium Compounds. Background Information. Chromium compounds are used in the dyeing and tanning industries to improve the stability and affinity of dyes to textiles and various polymers. Chromium compounds are also used in coloring and hardening marble, in polishing metals, in coloring glass, and in printing fabrics. Several of the compounds, including chromic sulfate and chromium trioxide, are used in chrome plating. Chromium is used in the manufacture of chrome steel, chrome nickel steel alloys, and stainless steel.

Chromium compounds are strong nasal and pulmonary irritants and have been reported to cause bronchiogenic carcinoma. They may also cause gastrointestinal irritation and renal injury. Chromium is the only one of the essential trace metals that is retained in insoluble form in the lung.[66] Cancer of the lung in German chromate workers was first reported in 1911 and 1912.[67,68] The duration of exposure was often quite long, sometimes 40 years, and the time between the beginning of the exposure and onset of cancer was often 30 to 40 years. In 1948 Machle and Gregorius reported that almost 22% of all deaths in the United States chromate industry were due to cancer of the respiratory system.[69] This was 16 times the expected rate. The death rate for cancer of the lung in various plants was increased over normal values by as much as a factor of 50. A report on the bichromate production industry in Great Britain corroborated the findings pertaining to the health hazards involved in that industry in Germany and the United States.[70] More recently, a follow-up study of 2715 workers in chromate production factories showed an increased risk of lung cancer.[71] Lung cancer in Japanese chromate workers also has been reported.[72]

Genetic Bioassay Results. Hexavalent chromium compounds have been tested in all five standard *Salmonella* tester strains and the results are largely positive in the presence or absence of S-9.[73,74] Potassium dichromate induces forward mutation and gene conversion in *S. pombe*.[75] Hexavalent chromium and stainless steel welding fume particles containing chromium compounds give positive results in the mouse coat color spot test, a somatic tissue assay.[76]

Results of primary DNA damage assays in repair-deficient strains of *E. coli* Pol A and *B. subtilis* rec are mixed.[41,74] Chromium enhances homozygosis in *S. cerevisiae* with and without metabolic activation.[74] Hexavalent chromium compounds induce UDS in primary mouse cells[77] and in human diploid fibroblasts[78] in culture in the absence of exogenous activation.

SCEs are induced in CHO cells and in human fibroblasts after exposure to low levels of hexavalent chromium in the absence of exogenous metabolic activation.[79] Trivalent chromium does not induce SCEs in CHO cells.[79] *In vitro* cytogenetic assays in CHO cells, mouse cells, Syrian hamster cells, and human fibroblasts show positive results without exogenous metabolic activation.[79-81] Hexavalent chromium produces aberrations in metaphases of human cells at a concentration of 2 μM.[79] Mixed results are obtained in micronucleus assays in cells in culture.[82] Hexavalent chromium induces micronuclei in the mouse *in vivo*.[83]

In cell transformation assays, chromium gives positive results without exogenous metabolic activation using primary SHE cells[50] and established cell lines.[77] Positive results are also reported for the SA-7 viral enhancement assay.[10]

The genetic toxicology data base consists of mostly positive results for hexavalent chromium compounds and mixed results for trivalent chromium compounds. With hexavalent compounds, independent and concurring positive responses are reported for induction of reverse mutations in the *Salmonella* system, for SCEs, and for chromosome abnormalities in CHO and mouse cells. In *E. coli* reverse mutation and *B. subtilis* differential toxicity assays, in SCE assays in CHO cells *in vitro*, and in chromosomal aberration assays in mouse and Chinese hamster cells *in vitro*, the hexavalent compounds are positive while the trivalent compounds are negative.

Nickel Compounds. Background Information. Nickel is used in nickel plating and in the manufacture of coins, storage batteries, and machinery parts. It is used extensively in the manufacture of stainless steels and nickel-chrome resistant wires. Nickel occurs naturally in asbestos.[84] The metal enters the atmosphere from nickel production plants and from the combustion of fossil fuels.

Sunderman reviewed the carcinogenesis of nickel.[85] Cancer of the lung and nose in industrial settings was first brought to attention by case reports. Doll investigated the incidence of respiratory tract cancer among nickel workers in the years 1938-1947 and 1948-1956.[86] His study revealed that, of 187 deaths among workers in a Welsh nickel refinery during 1948-56, 48 deaths resulted from lung cancer. The expected number of deaths from lung cancer was 9.9. Thus, the risk to nickel workers of death from lung cancer was approximately 5 times normal. During the same interval there were 13 deaths due to cancer of the nose. Less than 0.1 deaths were expected, indicating a risk of death from nasal cancer that was 150 times normal. A later study indicated that, for men employed before 1925 in a Welsh nickel refinery, deaths from nasal cancer varied from 100 to 900 times the expected number.[87] Similar statistics for lung and nasal cancer in Norwegian nickel workers were reported.[88] In Canada, during the period 1948 to 1968, there were 24 cases of nasal cancer and 92 cases of lung cancer among nickel refinery workers.[89] Other case reports have been catalogued.[90,91] A recent study of nickel workers exposed to nickel and nickel oxide in the form of fine particles showed no evidence of any occupational hazard.[92] Statistically, risks were only 0.5 to 2.2 times normal.

Nickel subsulfide, nickel oxide, and metallic nickel dust have been suspected as the principal respiratory carcinogens.[93,94] Sunderman[85] indicated that the latent period for respiratory lung cancer in nickel workers averages 27 years. For nasal cancer, the latent period averages 23 years.

Genetic Bioassay Results. Negative results are obtained for reverse mutation in *E. coli* WP2 without metabolic activation.[95] Soluble nickel compounds give weakly positive results without S-9 in the CHO cell forward mutation assay.[60] Negative results are reported for a host-mediated assay using *Salmonella*.[96] Negative results are obtained in the *Bacillus subtilis* rec differential toxicity assay in the absence of S-9.[41] Chromosomal aberrations are observed in mouse[97] and rat embryo[98] cells after exposure to soluble nickel *in vitro*. These aberrations occur after recovery from the metal's acute toxic effects. The agent also causes cell transformation[50] and virus-enhanced transformation of SHE cells.[51]

In summary, the present data base on genotoxic effects consists of only 17 reports. Most of these reports show positive results, including several positive responses in *in vitro* mammalian cytogenetic assays. Although nickel data are present for only a few bioassay categories, the pattern of the response is consistent with that for chromium compounds, which are also lung carcinogens.

Asbestiform Minerals. Background Information. Although asbestos occurs naturally, mining operations introduce asbestos as a pollutant in both water and air. Also, asbestos fibers have been used to make filters and are thus introduced inadvertently in the manufacture of processed food, beverages, and drugs.

An association between respiratory exposure to asbestos and lung cancer was reported as early as 1935.[99,100] Doll presented evidence from an epidemiological study showing a ten-fold excess risk of lung cancer for asbestos textile workers.[101] In 1960, Wagner and coworkers reported on the occurrence of mesothelioma in asbestos mine workers and in non-mining populations close to the mines.[102] Selikoff et al. reported other studies of the association between asbestos exposure and neoplasia.[103] In a study population of 632 insulation workers, 45 died of cancer of the lung pleura when only 6.6 such deaths were expected. Twenty-nine men died of cancer of the stomach, colon, and rectum when only 9.4 such deaths were expected. Hammond and coworkers, reporting on cancer among insulation workers, noted a significantly increased incidence of intraabdominal neoplasias.[104] The occurrence of gastrointestinal cancer was also reported by Kleinfeld et al.[105] Gerber reported on asbestos exposure in neoplastic disorders of the hematopoietic system.[106] Many additional epidemiological studies on asbestos and lung cancer have been summarized.[107] Studies of workers in asbestos manufacture, insulation, and shipyards have provided the most concrete evidence for the association of asbestos with lung cancer. Several authors have reported on the synergistic effects of smoking and occupational exposure to asbestos in the induction of neoplasia. Selikoff et al. concluded that asbestos workers who smoke have 8 times the risk of developing lung cancer when compared with all other smokers, and 92 times the risk when compared with nonsmokers who do not work with asbestos.[108]

Genetic Bioassay Results. For the purpose of assessing qualitative genetic and related bioassay data, the results reported for amosite, chrysotile, and crocidolite were grouped under the category "Asbestiform Minerals."

Particulate samples of these minerals do not enter bacteria; hence, results in *Salmonella* strains TA1535 and TA1538 are negative both without and with S-9 activation.[109] Results in *E. coli* strain WP2 and WP2 uvrA$^-$ are also negative both without and with S-9 activation.[109] The CHL strain of Chinese hamster lung cells responds to this class of agents to exhibit forward mutation at the HGPRT locus[110]; however, the observed mutation frequency is low and may result via a clastogenic mechanism.

The results of *in vitro* cytogenetic assays without S-9 metabolic activation in SHE cells,[111] Chinese hamster cells,[112,113] and human lymphocytes[114] are positive. Oral or intraperitoneal administration of chrysotile asbestos does not induce micronuclei in the mouse.[111]

Foci of multilayered growth indicative of cell transformation are observed in the BALB/c3T3 assay in the absence of exogenous metabolic activation.[115]

In summary, nearly half of the bioassay results are negative. Positive responses have been confirmed only in independent investigations of cytogenetic abnormalities in mammalian cells in culture. Possibly because of their particulate nature, these materials are largely refractory to analysis by *in vitro* genetic bioassay systems.

Human Hematolymphopoietic System Carcinogens

Five of the agents examined in this report produce cancer of the bone marrow or of the lymphopoietic system. Three of these compounds (benzene, ethylene oxide, and melphalan) are alkylating agents or are believed to be metabolized to reactive intermediates that can alkylate. The two other agents, chloramphenicol and phenytoin, are structurally dissimilar and are IARC Unclassified Carcinogens. The structures and IARC classifications of these compounds are shown in Fig. 2. The group is characterized by single ring structures, in two cases heterocyclic. That hematolymphopoietic tissue is the common target of these compounds is especially interesting in view of the different routes of human exposure.

Benzene. Background Information. The major source of benzene in the United States is petroleum. Gasolines contain small quantities of benzene, usually less than 5%, although special motor fuels may contain up to 30%. Benzene has been heavily utilized in the manufacture of rubber, paint, and dry-cleaning fluids. The compound has also been used as the basis for fast-drying inks and in the manufacture of plastics. Currently about 87% of benzene is used in the chemical industry for synthesis of compounds such as styrene, phenol, and cyclohexane.[116] Environmental exposures to benzene occur from coke-oven emissions, automotive emissions, and at gas stations.[117]

Benzene is a bone marrow poison that has been used to treat leukemia, polycythemia vera, and malignant lymphoma.[118] Benzene resembles chloramphenicol, another agent evaluated in this report, in that it causes aplastic anemia and, in some cases, acute leukemia.[119] As early as 1928, Delore and Borgomano described a case of benzene leukemia.[120] Since then, approximately 150 cases have been identified.[121]

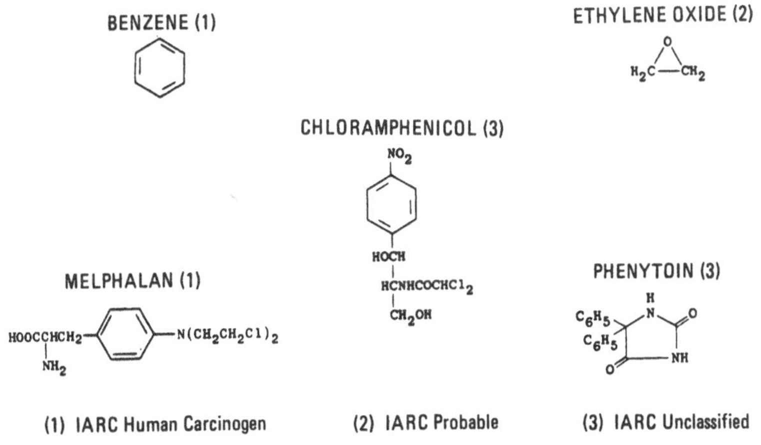

Fig. 2. Human hematolymphopoietic system carcinogens

In 1976 Vigliani and Forni reviewed the relationship between benzene and leukemia.[122] The relationship is strengthened by the major epidemiological study of Ishimaru et al.[123] Benzene exposure and leukemia also are discussed in a recent case-control study of leukemia in the United States rubber industry.[124]

The development of leukemia from benzene exposure generally results from chronic benzene poisoning. Numerous outbreaks of benzene poisoning have occurred and these have led to the prohibition of the use of benzene as a solvent in certain industries and in some materials such as inks and glues. In one study of shoe-industry workers in which the average exposure period was 9.7 years, 26 of approximately 28,500 employees developed pre-leukemia or leukemia.[125] A follow-up study of this population showed that 6 of 44 pancytopenic patients developed leukemia after chronic exposure to benzene.[126]

There is considerable interest in monitoring for chromosomal changes in workers exposed to benzene.[127] Dean, in a review of the genetic toxicology of benzene and related compounds, reported that the interpretation of chromosome monitoring studies is complicated by a lack of quantitative data on the amount of benzene exposure.[128] This is less of a problem when the clinical syndromes are present. The metabolism of benzene in vivo and in vitro has been the subject of extensive research and recently was reviewed by Snyder and Kocsis.[129]

Genetic Bioassay Results. Benzene gives negative results for reverse mutation in the five standard Salmonella tester strains both in the absence and in the presence of S-9 activation.[130] The compound causes forward mutation in the Tradescantia stamen hair assay, a somatic tissue assay.[131] However, when fed to Drosophila larvae, benzene does not cause sex-linked recessive lethality.[132]

In primary DNA damage assays in bacteria, benzene gives negative results in the absence and in the presence of S-9.[133] The compound does not cause enhanced mitotic recombination in yeast strain D3 in either the absence or presence of S-9.[130]

Both positive and negative results are reported in assays for SCEs after in vitro or in vivo exposure; however, there are more reports of negative results. According to one report, exogenous metabolic activation is not required for the induction of SCEs in human peripheral lymphocytes in vitro.[134] Both positive[135] and negative[136] results are obtained in cytogenetic studies following exposure of human lymphocytes to benzene in vitro; millimolar concentrations are necessary for positive effects. Positive[137] and negative[138] results are obtained in in vivo studies on bone marrow, and results from in vivo cytogenetic studies of lymphocytes are mostly positive.[139] Benzene induces micronuclei in the mouse[140] and alters the morphology of mouse sperm.[141]

Benzene fails to enhance the viral transformation of SHE cells.[142]

In summary, the results in the present data base are mixed. Although there is considerable interest in monitoring human subjects for benzene poisoning, the results of studies of chromosomal effects are discordant. Both positive and negative results are reported in SCE studies and in classical cytogenetic evaluations. The data base does contain five positive reports of induction of micronuclei in the mouse. Thus, this test may be a valuable indicator of benzene damage to the hematopoietic system.

Ethylene Oxide. Background Information. Ethylene oxide is used in organic synthesis in the production of ethylene glycol. The compound is also employed as a starting material for the production of acrylonitrile. Ethylene oxide is used in the sterilization of surgical instruments and foodstuffs and in agriculture as a fungicide.[143]

The compound is highly irritating to the eyes and mucous membranes, and in high concentrations can cause pulmonary edema.[144] Ethylene oxide has been used as a model epoxide to investigate the mechanism of mutagenesis by alkylating agents.[145] Early studies indicated that epoxides are toxic to living cells.[146,147] Only recently have studies indicated that ethylene oxide may be carcinogenic in man. Three cases of leukemia were reported in a small group of Swedish workers exposed to the compound; only 0.2 cases were expected.[148]

Genetic Bioassay Results. Ethylene oxide induces reverse mutations in *Salmonella* strains TA1535 and TA100 with and without S-9.[149] The compound also induces reverse mutations in *Neurospora*[150] and forward mutations in L5178Y mouse lymphoma cells.[151] Ethylene oxide produces sex-linked recessive lethality in *Drosophila*: the compound is effective when fed to larvae, when used in the form of an aerosol, or when injected into adult males.[152]

With respect to primary DNA damage, ethylene oxide causes UDS in the mouse.[153] The compound produces SCEs in human diploid fibroblasts[154] and in peripheral lymphocytes of exposed workers.[155] The results of *in vivo* bone marrow[156] and lymphocyte[157] cytogenetic assays in the rat are positive. Also, the results of micronucleus[158] and dominant lethal tests in the mouse[159] and rat[145] are positive. The results of heritable translocation tests in the mouse[159] and in *Drosophila*[160,161] are positive.

No cell transformation assays are reported.

In summary, results are positive in all test categories for which data are reported. The data for ethylene oxide are generally consistent with those for epichlorohydrin, with the exception that the latter compound gives negative results in the mouse micronucleus and dominant lethal tests.

Melphalan. Background Information. Melphalan, an alkylating nitrogen mustard, is phenylalanine-substituted mechlorethamine. The compound is used therapeutically in the treatment of multiple myeloma.

Several reports indicate that melphalan is a leukemogen.[162-164] These investigators detail five case studies and summarize a larger number of cases in which patients developed leukemia during therapy for multiple myeloma. These case studies indicate a causal relationship between the development of leukemia and therapeutic treatment with the alkylating agent. However, a number of questions have been raised concerning this relationship, such as whether the leukemia developed independently or was merely an unrecognized aspect of multiple myeloma.[165] Patients with a variety of disorders who were treated with alkylating agents including melphalan have developed acute leukemia.[166] The incidence of leukemia after melphalan treatment is low. Case studies of cancer induction after melphalan treatment have been reviewed.[167]

Genetic Bioassay Results. Melphalan gives positive results in *Salmonella* strain TA1535 with and without S-9.[168] Urine from exposed humans is not mutagenic in *Salmonella*.[169] The compound induces forward mutations in L5178Y cells without exogenous activation.[170] The compound is also active in the *Drosophila* sex-linked recessive lethal test.[171]

S-9 metabolic activation is necessary to elicit DNA damage in DNA polymerase mutants of *E. coli*.[172] UDS is observed in human bone marrow cells without activation.[173]

Human lymphocytes from an exposed patient are reported to show a weak positive SCE response.[174] A strong positive response is obtained in A(T_1)Cl-3 cloned hamster cells.[175] Fibroblasts cultured *in vitro* exhibit gross chromosomal aberrations[176] and DNA strand breaks[177] when exposed to melphalan in the absence of exogenous activation.

Melphalan transforms C3H10T1/2 cells exposed in the absence of an exogenous activation system.[176]

In summary, most of the results are positive. Independent and corroborative results exist in only a few cases. Sufficient data do not exist to compare adequately the pattern of responses obtained for melphalan and the other leukemogens. The data are unlike those for benzene and chloramphenicol in that melphalan causes point/gene mutation.

Chloramphenicol. Background Information. Chloramphenicol is a broad spectrum antibiotic. The antibiotic action results from binding of the compound to bacterial ribosomes, preventing peptide chain elongation.

Chloramphenicol produces toxic effects in man by damaging the bone marrow.[178] The risk of developing some type of blood disorder from chloramphenicol therapy is estimated at 1 in 24,500.[179] Patients can develop aplastic or hypoplastic anemia or a generalized cytopenia. An association is apparent between aplastic anemia and myeloblastic leukemia. Chloramphenicol is one agent that produces these effects; others include benzene and radiation. Fatal aplastic anemia is a rare disorder that occurs in 2 per million population each year.[179] A 1957 study indicated that, out of a sample of 138 deaths attributed to aplastic anemia, 30 of the patients had received treatment with chloramphenicol.[180]

Genetic Bioassay Results. Chloramphenicol gives negative results in Salmonella strains TA1535 and TA1538[181] and negative results in E. coli WP2[182] in the absence of S-9. The results of in vivo gene mutation assays in Arabidopsis are negative.[183] Chloramphenicol does not induce dominant lethality or sex-linked recessive lethality in Drosophila.[184]

The results of DNA damage assays in repair-proficient and -deficient strains of E. coli are negative without S-9.[74,185]

The results of in vivo cytogenetic assays are positive. The compound induces chromosomal aberrations in human lymphocytes[186] and in the bone marrow of mice given a human dose equivalent.[187] Chloramphenicol gives positive results in the mouse dominant lethal test.[188]

No cell transformation assays are reported.

In summary, chloramphenicol resembles benzene in its toxic and carcinogenic effects. A similarity in genotoxic effects is also apparent in the genetic bioassay data base. Although only a portion of test reports overlap, chloramphenicol, like benzene, gives negative results in the Salmonella reverse mutation, Drosophila sex-linked recessive lethality, and E. coli relative toxicity test systems. Both compounds induce chromosome aberrations in bone marrow and lymphocytes following in vivo exposure. Thus, for the overlapping test systems, identical responses are obtained for these two leukemogens.

Phenytoin. Background Information. Phenytoin (diphenylhydantoin or Dilantin) is used medically as an anticonvulsant and antiepileptic. The agent may be both a teratogen and a carcinogen. An enhanced rate of congenital malformation was reported for mothers who took phenytoin regularly during the first four months of pregnancy.[189] Other reports on the teratogenic effect of phenytoin have been reviewed.[190]

Relative to carcinogenic effect, an excessive risk (2 to 3 times) of malignant lymphoma for patients treated with the drug was reported.[191] However, a follow-up study of epilepsy patients, some of whom had been treated with phenytoin, showed no excess incidence of lymphomas.[192] Phenytoin causes a variety of hematological reactions, including megaloblastic anemia.[193] The fact that the compound alters folate absorption and metabolism in anemia is especially interesting in that it appears to induce neoplasia in the blood-forming organs.

Genetic Bioassay Results. Only two reports of genetic bioassays are found. The compound gives negative results in the rat bone marrow assay and in an in vitro lymphocyte cytogenetic assay.[194] A positive response is reported for an assay of mouse sperm morphology.[195]

Human Bladder Carcinogens

Of the human bladder carcinogens considered, four are aromatic amines (4-aminobiphenyl, benzidine, auramine, and 2-naphthylamine) and two are nitrogen mustards (chlornaphazine and cyclophosphamide). The latter two compounds are used in cancer chemotherapy and, in fact, chlornaphazine is a derivative of 2-naphthylamine. The chemical structures and IARC classifications of these compounds are shown in Fig. 3. In contrast to the respiratory tract and hematolymphopoietic system carcinogens, five of the six bladder carcinogens are multi-ring structures.

4-Aminobiphenyl. Background Information. 4-Aminobiphenyl is structurally similar to benzidine. Recent information suggests that 4-aminobiphenyl is no longer commercially produced.[196]

One of the first occupational studies of human bladder cancer concerned 4-aminobiphenyl.[197] This study of 171 male workers revealed 19 cases (11.1%) of bladder tumors. A more recent study[198]

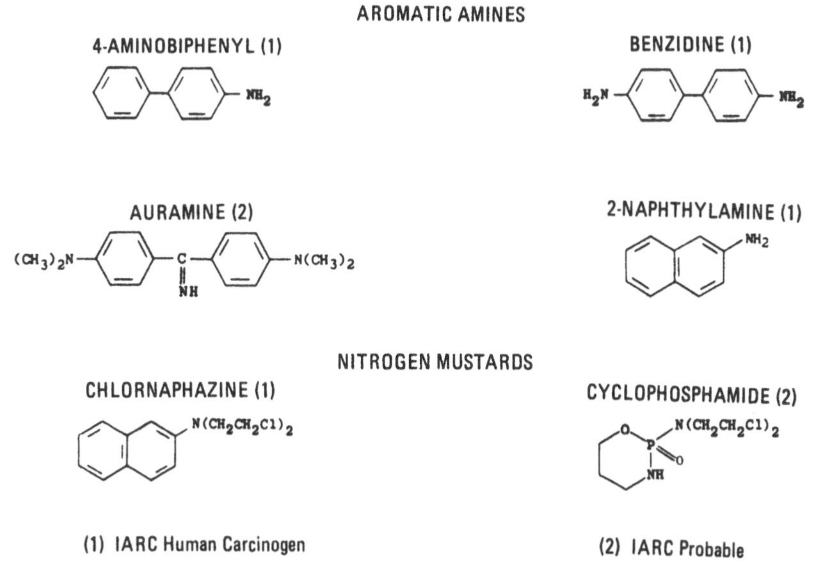

Fig. 3. Human bladder carcinogens

expanded the study population to 315 male workers. Of these, 53 (16.8%) were found to have bladder tumors.

Genetic Bioassay Results. 4-Aminobiphenyl has not been well tested in genetic bioassay systems. For those systems in which it has been examined, the profile of biological activity resembles that of the structurally similar compound benzidine.

In the presence of S-9 metabolic activation, 4-aminobiphenyl gives positive results in the standard *Salmonella* tester strains.[199] Without metabolic activation, results are negative.[200] The compound is not mutagenic at the HGPRT locus in V-79 Chinese hamster lung cells in the presence of activation.[201] A body fluid analysis using *Salmonella* to detect mutagens in urine of rats exposed to 4-aminobiphenyl shows positive results with S-9 activation and negative results without activation.[202] In another study, activation was not required for positive results.[200] One host-mediated assay shows negative results.[203]

In primary DNA damage assays using repair-proficient and -deficient strains of *E. coli*, 4-aminobiphenyl gives positive results in the presence of S-9 metabolic activation.[204] 4-Aminobiphenyl enhances mitotic recombination in strain D3 of *S. cerevisiae* in the absence and in the presence of S-9 metabolic activation.[205] Exogenous metabolic activation is not required for induction of UDS in primary rat hepatocytes.[206] Thus it appears that 4-aminobiphenyl causes genetic damage in prokaryotic and eukaryotic *in vitro* systems.

No chromosomal aberration assays are reported. However, micronucleus tests in the rat give negative results.[207]

Several cell transformation assays show positive results in the absence of exogenous metabolic activation. These include SHE cells in a clonal assay[208] and mouse[209] and rat[210] embryo cultures. The mouse and rat embryo cells were infected with the AKR leukemia and Rauscher leukemia viruses, respectively.

In summary, the results of the genetic tests reveal a response pattern similar to that for benzidine. Most of the test results are positive. 4-aminobiphenyl has been extensively tested in the *Salmonella* test and clearly causes point mutations in the presence of metabolic activation. In addition, several of the cell transformation tests exhibit positive results.

Benzidine. Background Information. Unlike 4-aminobiphenyl, benzidine is currently an important industrial chemical; 1.5 million pounds were produced in the United States in 1972.[211] More than 250 dyes are derived from benzidine.[212]

Benzidine produces kidney damage and can cause bladder tumors. The relationship between dyes and the induction of bladder tumors has been known since 1895.[213] In 1954 Case et al. reported on the relative frequency of bladder tumors among workers in the British dye industry.[214] Workers exposed to benzidine were 19 times as likely to develop bladder tumors as control workers not exposed. Haley reviewed the literature concerning the specific problems associated with benzidine use.[215] Scott and Williams described the prevalence of bladder tumors in industrial settings involving benzidine exposure.[216] They found the latency period for development of bladder cancer in workers to be approximately 16 years. Several outbreaks of bladder cancer in industrial settings have been reported. A typical report was provided by Zavon et al.[217] A series of cases were detected in 1958 in one manufacturing firm. One case of bladder cancer was noted after more than 25 years of benzidine manufacture. After the first case was detected, further study revealed that 25 of 35 exposed men eventually developed tumors. The route of exposure was thought to be the respiratory system. Presumably exposure of the bladder occurs via the urine: free benzidine was detected following acid hydrolysis of urine from workers who weighed benzidine-derived dyes.[218] Hueper reported other incidences of benzidine-induced bladder cancer in several countries.[219]

Genetic Bioassay Results. In the five standard Salmonella tester strains, benzidine gives positive results in the presence of S-9 metabolic activation and negative results without S-9.[220,221] Urine from rats exposed to the compound also gives positive results in Salmonella in the presence of S-9.[202] The results of the sex-linked recessive lethal test in Drosophila are positive.[222]

Benzidine does not induce enhanced mitotic recombination in S. cerevisiae D3 with or without S-9 activation.[223] The compound induces UDS in rat primary hepatocytes[206] in the absence of exogenous metabolic activation, and in HeLa cells[224] with activation. Benzidine also inhibits DNA synthesis in HeLa cell cultures in the absence of an added metabolic activation system.[225]

Conflicting positive and negative results are obtained in the rat micronucleus test.[207,226]

Results from several kinds of cell transformation assays are reported. The SHE cell clonal assay shows positive results without exogenous activation,[227] as do the AKR/ME mouse embryo cell system[209] and the Fisher RLV rat embryo cell system.[228] Benzidine also enhances the viral transformation of SHE cells in culture.[142]

Benzidine fails to alter the morphology of mouse sperm.[141]

In summary, more than half of the findings in the genetic toxicology data base are derived from the Salmonella test system, in which benzidine gives positive results when an exogenous source of metabolic activation is supplied. Consistently positive responses are obtained for effects relating directly to DNA synthesis and cell transformation. Although many of these results have not been confirmed in independent studies, the data suggest that short-term in vitro genetic bioassays are useful for evaluating benzidine-like compounds, including the closely related analogue 4-aminobiphenyl.

Auramine. Background Information. Auramine is used as an antiseptic and in the coloring of paper, cardboard, textiles, and leather.[229] A 1933 report described two cases of bladder cancer in men involved in the manufacture of auramine.[230] Case and Pearson reported other cases of bladder tumors caused by auramine.[231] There were 6 deaths when only 0.13 were expected. The latency period was determined to be 19.3 years. A similar latency has been reported for benzidine.

Genetic Bioassay Results. Auramine gives negative results in the five standard Salmonella tester strains both in the absence and in the presence of S-9.[199] The compound gives negative results with S-9 in the L5178Y mouse lymphoma assay.[232] The results of a host-mediated assay using yeast as the indicator organism are similarly negative.[203]

Repair-proficient and -deficient Pol A strains of E. coli exhibit DNA damage following exposure to auramine in the absence of S-9.[204] Enhanced mitotic recombination is observed in S. cerevisiae with and without metabolic activation.[205]

Auramine fails to induce micronuclei in the mouse.[233]

Auramine transforms SHE cells in the presence of exogenous metabolic activation.[208] Cryopreserved primary SHE cells are not transformed.[227]

In summary, auramine gives consistently negative results in Salmonella but independent and concurring positive responses in relative toxicity DNA damage assays in bacteria. The results of cell transformation assays are positive in the presence of exogenous metabolic activation. Although the test reports are meager, the pattern of the responses appears similar to that for 4-aminobiphenyl, which is also a bladder carcinogen.

2-Naphthylamine. Background Information. 2-Naphthylamine is an intermediate in the manufacture of dyes and antioxidants; it is also present in coal tar.[234]

The compound is recognized as a cause of malignant tumors of the bladder.[235] There are several case reports on the association of 2-naphthylamine with bladder cancer in workmen.[236,237] Goldwater et al. presented the startling finding that 12 out of 48 workmen exposed to 2-naphthylamine developed bladder cancers.[238] Dye industry workers exposed to 2-naphthylamine were reported to be 61 times as likely as control workers to develop bladder tumors.[214]

Genetic Bioassay Results. In Salmonella strains TA1535, TA1538, TA98, and TA100, 2-naphthylamine gives negative results in the absence of S-9 but positive results in the presence of S-9.[199,239] Similar results are obtained in E. coli rec$^-$.[240] Salmonella mutagenicity tests on urine of rats exposed to the compound give positive results with exogenous metabolic activation.[202] 2-Naphthylamine induces forward mutations in S. cerevisiae in the presence of an enzyme-free hydroxylation system.[241] Resting conidia of Neurospora crassa require microsomal activation to show a positive response, while growing conidia apparently have the ability to metabolize the compound endogenously.[242] V-79 Chinese hamster lung cells do not respond to 2-naphthylamine in the presence of S-9 metabolic activation.[201] A host-mediated assay using Salmonella gives positive results without S-9 activation.[203]

Repair-deficient bacteria require S-9 metabolic activation to exhibit a differential toxic response as compared to the wild-type strains.[133,204] Primary DNA damage as evidenced by enhanced mitotic recombination[243] or gene conversion[244] can be observed in yeast, although the reported results are not consistent.[205] UDS is obtained in human diploid fibroblasts without S-9.[245]

No gross chromosomal aberration assays are reported. Micronucleus tests in the mouse and rat show largely negative results,[207,246] although one positive result is reported for the mouse system.[247]

Cell transformation is observed in SHE cells,[227] in AKR/ME mouse embryo cells,[209] and in RLV/1706 Fischer rat embryo cells[210] in the absence of exogenous activation. Enhancement of viral transformation is observed in SHE cells infected with SA-7 virus in the absence of exogenous metabolic activation.[10]

2-Naphthylamine does not alter the morphology of mouse sperm.[59]

In summary, the present genetic bioassay data base consists of approximately 62 reports. Nearly half of the findings are derived from the Salmonella test system, in which the compound produces base-pair substitution reactions. Eleven test results are presented for a single Salmonella tester strain (TA100). The data are not as substantial for the other test systems, and many of the results must be confirmed. Overall, the pattern of test responses for 2-naphthylamine is very similar to that for benzidine and 4-aminobiphenyl. All three compounds are associated with increased incidence of carcinoma of the bladder.

Chlornaphazine. Background Information. Chlornaphazine or dichloroethyl-β-naphthylamine has been used as a chemotherapeutic agent in the treatment of leukemia.[248] The cytostatic activity of the compound resides in the bis-(2-chloroethyl) reactive group. The compound was the first cytostatic drug shown to be carcinogenic in man.[249] It has been used therapeutically for control of polycythemia vera because it inhibits hematopoiesis.[250] Presently, however, the compound does not have wide therapeutic usage.

Chlornaphazine is a derivative of β-naphthylamine, a well-known bladder carcinogen. Several reports have indicated that patients treated with chlornaphazine can develop the type of bladder cancer seen in workers exposed to β-naphthylamine. In 26 patients treated with high doses of chlornaphazine for polycythemia vera, there were 2 cases of bladder carcinoma and 1 of renal carcinoma.[251] In another study, 10 cases of bladder tumors were observed among 61 patients treated with chlornaphazine.[252]

Other case studies of the association between chlornaphazine use and bladder cancer have been catalogued.[253]

Genetic Bioassay Results. The present data base consists of a positive response in Salmonella strain TA100[168] and positive responses for sex-linked recessive lethality in Drosophila[254] and enhancement of viral transformation of SHE cells in culture.[10] These meager results preclude any assessment of the agent's activity in genetic bioassay systems.

Cyclophosphamide. Background Information. Cyclophosphamide is an alkylating nitrogen mustard and a derivative of mechlorethamine. Cyclophosphamide's reactive moiety is the bis-(2-chloroethyl) group also found in chlornaphazine. The compound is widely used clinically for treatment of Hodgkins disease. Cylophosphamide is also used as an antineoplastic agent in the treatment of a variety of diseases including malignant lymphomas and leukemias, neuroblastoma, and carcinoma of the breast. The agent is used as an immunosuppressant in a variety of nonmalignant diseases. These include rheumatoid arthritis, nephrotic syndrome in children, and chronic hepatitis.

Wall and Clausen[255] described five patients who received large doses of cyclophosphamide over a relatively long period of time and subsequently developed carcinomas of the urinary bladder. The tumors were fatal in four of the five patients. The occurrence of secondary cancers in certain patients from the pre-chemotherapy era makes it difficult to attribute secondary tumors directly to drug therapy. However, other cases have been reported in which cyclophosphamide was administered for nonmalignant diseases and malignant tumors developed.[256] There have been at least 10 cases of primary malignant tumors arising from cyclophosphamide treatment and 16 reports of secondary tumors. Several authors have expressed concern over the widespread use of cyclophosphamide in nonneoplastic diseases.[255,257]

Genetic Bioassay Results. Cyclophosphamide gives positive results in Salmonella strains TA1535,[170] TA1538,[9] TA98,[59] and TA100[258] in the presence of S-9 metabolic activation but not in its absence. In contrast, cyclophosphamide is direct-acting in forward mutation assays in S. cerevisiae.[259] Urine from mice, rats, and humans exposed to cyclophosphamide gives positive results in Salmonella or yeast test systems without exogenous activation.[169,260-263] There are additional reports of positive results in host-mediated systems.[264,265] Positive results are obtained in the L5178Y mammalian cell mutagenesis assay in the presence of S-9; weakly positive results are obtained without S-9.[266] Positive results are also obtained without S-9 in Chinese hamster lung cells at the ouabain locus.[265] Cyclophosphamide gives negative results in the *in vivo Arabidopsis* assay[183] and positive results in the sex-linked recessive lethal test in *Drosophila*.[267] Results of the mouse spot test[76] and the mouse specific locus test[268] also are positive.

The results of primary DNA damage assays in repair-deficient bacteria are positive,[185] and results for UDS in HeLa cells are positive when S-9 is added to the test system.[224] UDS is also observed in male germ cells of mice after exposure to cyclophosphamide.[269] Primarily positive results are obtained for mitotic recombination[259] and gene conversion[244] in yeast.

Cyclophosphamide induces SCEs with and without S-9 in cells in culture[270] and in various animal cell types after exposure *in vivo*.[271] Cytogenetic changes are observed *in vitro* in mammalian and human cells[272] and *in vivo* in bone marrow,[46] human lymphocytes,[273,274] oocytes,[275] and spermatogonia and spermatocytes.[276] The compound induces micronuclei in the mouse,[59] rat,[207] and Chinese hamster.[277] Positive results are also obtained in dominant lethal tests in the mouse[46] and rat.[278] Positive[279] and negative[280] results are reported for the heritable translocation test in the mouse. Negative results are obtained in the *Drosophila* dominant lethal test.[281]

Cell transformation is observed in the C3H10T1/2 cell line after treatment in the presence of S-9.[270] S-9 is not required for transformation of SHE cells[282] or RLV/1706 Fischer rat embryo cells.[283]

Altered sperm morphology is observed in the mouse,[59] rat,[278,284] sheep,[285] and man[286]; however, an assay for altered sperm morphology in the F_1 generation in mice is reported to give negative results.[287]

In summary, the present data base consists of 193 test results, 31 of which are from the *Salmonella* system. Results are positive in more than 82% of the reported tests, and positive responses are reported for each of the major categories of genetic damage. If prokaryotic gene mutation is not considered, 88% of the results are positive. Many of these responses have been confirmed by independent investigations.

Human Liver Carcinogens

The chemical structures and IARC classifications of aflatoxin B1, oxymetholone, and vinyl chloride are shown in Fig. 4.

Aflatoxin B1. Background Information. Aflatoxins are mycotoxins produced by the common molds *Aspergillus* and *Penicillium*,

AFLATOXIN B1 (1)

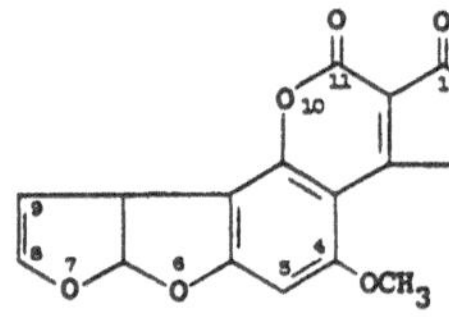

OXYMETHOLONE (2)

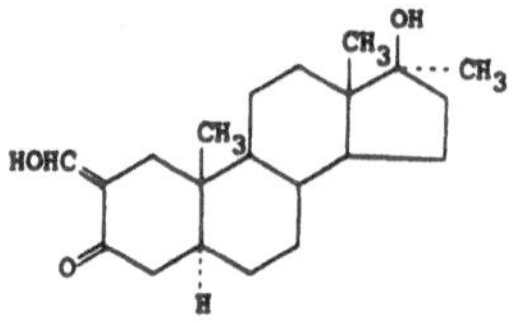

VINYL CHLORIDE (1)

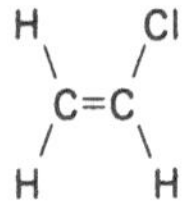

(1) IARC Human Carcinogen (2) IARC Probable

Fig. 4. Human liver carcinogens

which occasionally contaminate agricultural products. A variety of mycotoxins have been shown to cause DNA damage; aflatoxin B1 is the most extensively studied compound. An important series of papers by Shank et al. provides extensive epidemiological evidence in support of the relationship between aflatoxin consumption and the incidence of human liver cancer in Thailand.[288-291] Other reports consider aflatoxin intake and liver cancer in several areas of Africa.[292-295] Colon carcinoma also may be correlated with aflatoxin exposure.[296] Campbell and Stoloff reviewed the subject of mycotoxins and human health.[297] Their data were used as a basis for estimating the human health risk of these compounds. Campbell and coworkers presented an interesting report on the carcinogenic materials present in urine of humans consuming aflatoxins.[298]

Genetic Bioassay Results. Aflatoxin B1 is one of the most thoroughly tested human carcinogens; results are positive in a large proportion of genetic tests. Alfatoxin B1 gives positive results with S-9 metabolic activation and negative or weakly positive results without S-9 in each of the standard *Salmonella* tester strains except TA1535.[59,199] Aflatoxin B1 produces forward mutations without exogenous metabolic activation in *S. cerevisiae*[299] and in growing cultures of *N. crassa*.[300] However, metabolic activation is required for forward mutation in V-79 Chinese hamster lung cells.[301] Results of the sex-linked recessive lethal test in *Drosophila* are positive.[302] Positive responses are obtained in host-mediated assays that employ bacteria or yeast as indicator organisms for point/gene mutations.[203]

The results of primary DNA damage assays are uniformly positive with S-9 metabolic activation and, in many cases, without metabolic activation as well. These assays include relative toxicity in repair-proficient and -deficient strains of bacteria[240,303]; mitotic recombination[304] and gene conversion[305] in *S. cerevisiae*; and UDS in a variety of mammalian cell types including rat liver primary cells,[306] HeLa cells,[307] and human cells.[308,309] Results are positive in the prophage inductest[310] and in the test for inhibition of DNA synthesis in HeLa cells[225] when S-9 metabolic activation is added in each case.

Metabolic activation apparently is not required for the induction of SCEs in CHO cells[311] or in human lymphoblastoid cells *in vitro*.[312] Interestingly, the compound induces SCEs in the mouse *in vivo*[313] but not in the Chinese hamster treated *in vivo* by oral intubation.[271] Chromosomal aberrations are observed after *in vitro* treatment of mammalian and human cells with[308] and without[312] S-9 metabolic activation. Cytogenetic changes in bone marrow cells of hamsters administered aflatoxin B1 are reported.[314] Results of the micronucleus test are positive in mice[315] and rats[207] but negative in hamsters.[315]

Aflatoxin B1 transforms SHE cells in the clonal assay,[227] the mass focus assay,[316] and the viral enhancement assay[317] without metabolic activation. It also transforms BALB/c3T3 cells without metabolic activation.[318]

The morphology of sperm from mice[59] and rats[319] treated with aflatoxin B1 is not altered in comparison to controls.

In summary, the data base for aflatoxin B1 includes 46 test results in the *Salmonella* test system alone. The results are consistent when metabolic activation is employed. Aflatoxin is a mutagen in lower and in higher eukaryotic test systems. Independent results corroborating aflatoxin's genetic activity are obtained in test systems that measure DNA damage. Although data are not as substantial for chromosomal effects, most of the reported results are positive. In transformation tests all results are positive without exogenous metabolic activation.

Oxymetholone. Background Information. Oxymetholone is a synthetic androgenic steroid hormone. The agent is used in the treatment of anemias caused by deficient red cell production, such as congenital aplastic anemia and hypoplastic anemia.

Oxymetholone causes a variety of morphological and functional changes in the liver. Approximately 10 cases of liver cell tumors in young patients treated with oxymetholone have been reported[320];

still, a causal relationship has not been established. Farrell et al.[321] and Johnson et al.[322] reported on the effect of steroid therapy on development of hepatocellular carcinoma. Johnson indicated that use of the agent may cause liver cell damage, thereby predisposing tissues to subsequent malignant change.

Genetic Bioassay Results. The literature search produced no papers that report bioassays of oxymetholone.

Vinyl Chloride. Background Information. Over 90% of vinyl chloride monomer is used in the production of vinyl chloride homopolymer and copolymer resins used in the building and construction industries.

Workers exposed to vinyl chloride monomer have developed a variety of medical disorders.[323,324] Creech and Johnson first reported four fatal cases of angiosarcoma of the liver among men who worked in the manufacture of polyvinyl chloride and copolymers.[325] Spirtas and Kaminski reviewed 64 cases of angiosarcoma associated with vinyl chloride.[326] Monson et al. analyzed 161 deaths among workers at plants using vinyl chlorides and found an increase of 50% in cancer deaths.[327] These included cancers of the liver, biliary tract, lung, and brain. However, other investigators reported that the increased incidence of vinyl-chloride-induced cancer is much less.[328] Waxweiler et al. studied 1,294 individuals to determine the neoplastic risk to workers exposed to vinyl chloride.[329] For all malignant cancers the standard mortality ratio was 184. An excess of cancer was found in four organ systems: the brain and central nervous system, the respiratory system, the hepatic system, and the hematolymphopoietic system. In 14 cases involving biliary and liver cancer, the cancer was angiosarcomic in form. Extensive epidemiological studies of workers exposed to vinyl chloride monomer have been undertaken.[330,331] An increased fetal mortality was observed for the wives of workers who had been exposed to the compound.[324] Other studies indicated an increased risk of birth defects in children of parents residing in the vicinity of vinyl chloride production and polymerization plants.[323,324]

Genetic Bioassay Results. Vinyl chloride has been examined repeatedly in the Salmonella reverse mutation test. The gaseous agent returns mixed results in Salmonella strains TA1535 and TA100 in the absence of S-9 metabolic activation but generally positive responses in the same strains in the presence of S-9.[332] The results of reverse mutation assays in S. cerevisiae are negative[333]; however, the results of forward mutation assays in S. pombe are positive in the presence of S-9 and negative in its absence.[334] Negative results are obtained in Neurospora mutation tests.[335] Urine from exposed rats and humans gives negative results in

Salmonella.[336] Positive results are obtained with S-9 in CHO cells at the HGPRT locus[337] and in V-79 cells at the HGPRT and adenosine-triphosphatase loci.[338] The results of *in vivo* gene mutation assays are positive in *Tradescantia* (weak positive response in the stamen hair assay)[131] and in *Drosophila* (sex-linked recessive lethal test).[339] However, vinyl chloride apparently does not induce somatic gene mutation in mammals: negative results are reported for a coat color spot test in mice.[340] Results are positive in host-mediated activation systems using yeast as the indicator.[334]

Negative results are obtained in bacterial primary DNA damage assays in the absence of S-9[341]; in the presence of S-9, results are positive.[185] Tests for enhanced mitotic recombination[333] or gene conversion[334] in yeast show negative results without S-9 and positive results with S-9.

Vinyl chloride fails to induce SCEs in cultured human lymphocytes from exposed workers.[342,343] *In vitro* studies using the same cell type show positive results in the presence of S-9.[343] SCEs are induced in the bone marrow cells of Chinese hamsters after *in vivo* exposure at high concentrations (1.25% v/v).[344] Negative responses are reported for a *Drosophila* aneuploidy test.[339] Cytogenetic abnormalities are produced in bone marrow of hamsters[344]; mixed results are obtained in human lymphocytes.[345,342] Micronuclei are produced in the mouse *in vivo*.[346] Results are negative in dominant lethal tests in the rat[347] and mouse[348] and in *Drosophila*.[339] Results of the heritable translocation test in *Drosophila* are also negative.[339]

In summary, vinyl chloride clearly produces gene mutations and primary DNA damage when metabolic activation is employed. The compound induces SCEs, gross chromosomal aberrations, and micronuclei *in vivo*. Overall, approximately half of the test results in the data base are positive. Unfortunately many of the reports present conflicting results.

Other Human Carcinogens or Suspected Human Carcinogens

Two agents, diethylstilbestrol and epichlorohydrin, could not be assigned to one of the four target organ/system categories already discussed. The structures and IARC classifications of these compounds are shown in Fig. 5.

Diethylstilbestrol. Background Information. Diethylstilbestrol (DES) is used in human medicine to produce the physiological effects of the natural estrogens. The compound is also used as a growth promoter for cattle and sheep, although under restricted conditions.[349]

DIETHYLSTILBESTROL (1)

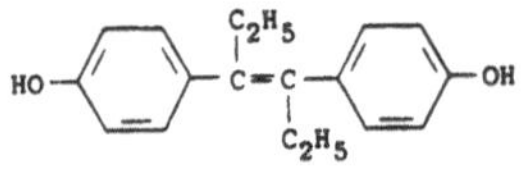

(1) IARC Human Carcinogen

EPICHLOROHYDRIN (3)

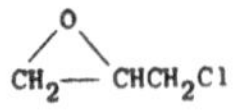

(3) IARC Unclassified

Fig. 5. Other human carcinogens

Herbst and colleagues originally reported the consequences of intrauterine exposure to DES.[350] Intrauterine exposure causes clear cell adenocarcinoma--an exceedingly rare tumor of the vagina. However, between 1966 and 1969, seven young women of 15 to 22 years of age were diagnosed with adenocarcinoma of the vagina. The most significant aspect of the study was that the patients' mothers had been treated with DES starting during the first trimester of pregnancy. Presently over 300 cases have been recorded in the registry of clear cell adenocarcinoma of the vaginal tract of young females.[351,352] Clear cell adenocarcinoma can be detected cytologically. Nonneoplastic changes of the female vaginal tract are also associated with prenatal exposure to DES.[351] Transitional changes between the nonneoplastic and fully developed cancers have not been carefully investigated. Herbst et al. estimated the risk to exposed female subjects at about 1 in 1,000 to 1 in 10,000.[352] These authors indicated that the development of tumors is more rare than previously assumed and is extremely rare even among DES-exposed individuals.

In summary, the available information suggests that cancer may occur in the vaginal tract of the human female exposed _in utero_ to DES, but that such occurrences are very rare.[353]

Genetic Bioassay Results. DES gives negative results in the five standard _Salmonella_ tester strains,[9] in _E. coli_ WP2 and WP2 uvrA$^-$,[258] and in V-79 Chinese hamster lung cells _in vitro_.[354] The compound is mutagenic, however, at the TK locus in L5178Y mouse lymphoma cells with and without metabolic activation.[266]

DES induces UDS in HeLa cells in the presence of activation.[224]

In assays for SCE, positive results are obtained in human fibroblasts[355] and negative results are obtained in Chinese hamster cells[356] exposed _in vitro_. Negative results are reported for SCE in the mouse _in vivo_.[357] The results of an assay for induction of aneuploidy in _Neurospora_ are negative.[358] Conflicting results are obtained in in vitro and in vivo cytogenetic assays.[359,360] Conflicting results are obtained in the mouse micronucleus assay.[361,246]

With regard to cell transformation, results are positive in the SHE cell clonal assay[362] and in the RLV/1706 Fischer rat embryo cell system[283] in the absence of exogenous metabolic activation. Results are negative using BALB/c3T3 cells in the absence of activation.[283]

Both positive and negative effects on sperm morphology are observed in the mouse[363,364] and in man.[365,366]

In contrast with many of the other agents examined in this report, DES elicits predominantly negative responses. All results from tests in Salmonella are negative. Most of the other test results have not been confirmed by independent studies. This variety of test results is consistent with the fact that DES only rarely is causally associated with tumor incidence in the human female.

Epichlorohydrin. Background Information. Epichlorohydrin or γ-chloropropylene oxide is used as a solvent in the manufacture of synthetic resins and gums, pharmaceutical products, insecticides, and agricultural and textile chemicals. The compound is also used in paints, varnishes, and as a raw material for the manufacture of epoxy resins. In the United States, a large amount of epichlorohydrin is used in the production of synthetic glycerin. The compound is a strong skin irritant, and chronic exposure can cause kidney injury.[367]

No epidemiological, clinical, or occupational data are presently available to indicate a significantly increased risk of carcinogenesis due to epichlorohydrin.[368]

Genetic Bioassay Results. Epichlorohydrin induces reverse mutation presumably through base-pair substitution in Salmonella strains TA1535 and TA100 without addition of S-9.[369] The urine of exposed humans and mice also gives positive results in Salmonella without further metabolic activation.[370] Reverse mutations are produced in E. coli WP2 and WP2 uvrA$^-$[371,372] and in S. cerevisiae[373] and S. pombe[374] without metabolic activation. Forward mutations are produced in Neurospora in the absence of exogenous activation.[375] Epichlorohydrin causes sex-linked recessive lethality in Drosophila.[267]

Primary DNA damage tests using repair-proficient and -deficient bacteria show largely positive results in the absence of activation[185] and weakly positive results in the presence of activation.[376] Epichlorohydrin causes mitotic crossing over and gene conversion in *S. cerevisiae*.[373]

SCEs are observed in human lymphocytes exposed to epichlorohydrin *in vitro*.[377] The compound produces chromosomal abnormalities in bone marrow cells[378] and in human lymphocytes *in vitro* and *in vivo*.[379]

The results of dominant lethal[378] and micronucleus[247] tests in the mouse are negative.

Epichlorohydrin does not alter the morphology of mouse sperm.[141]

In summary, although epichlorohydrin is not a demonstrated human carcinogen, the available genetic bioassay data indicate activity in most *in vitro* systems and in an *in vivo* assay for gene mutation (*Drosophila*). Epichlorohydrin does not require exogenous metabolic activation to produce point mutations, primary DNA damage, or chromosomal effects *in vitro*.

SUMMARY AND CONCLUSIONS

This study examined the genetic and related bioassay data available for 24 agents or groups of agents known or suspected to have human carcinogenic potential. To facilitate an examination of the available information, agents were divided into four major categories based on the target organ or system affected: (1) respiratory tract, (2) hematolymphopoietic system, (3) bladder, (4) liver. The examination of bioassay data followed this classification. Two other compounds, diethylstilbestrol and epichlorohydrin, could not be assigned to one of these four categories.

A search of the genetic bioassay literature identified approximately 600 citations for these 24 agents. Most of the data have been developed in relatively few screening tests, and most of those involve the use of microorganisms. The data base for known and suspected human carcinogens is not unlike the genetic toxicological data base as a whole. The preponderance of information concerns a limited number of compounds that have been evaluated in relatively few test systems.

To maximize the utility of genetic bioassay systems and of the overall genetic toxicological data base, it is important that information be developed on reference compounds. It is toward that end that the present data base on known and suspected human carcinogens was established. One important measure of the validity of a genetic bioassay is the strength of the correlation between the test results and the evidence for carcinogenicity of the compound or similar compounds in man. While the number of compounds for which there exist such human carcinogenicity data is small, these agents represent a diversity of chemical classes and hence a valuable resource for comparative mutagenesis assessment and test system validation. It is important to make the best possible use of the human exposure and effects information on these compounds and to exploit every opportunity to gather additional information. Simultaneously, efforts must be undertaken to complete the genetic bioassay data base for these and other known and suspected human carcinogens. These laboratory investigations should be carefully planned so that it will be possible to assess quantitatively the molecular dose-response relationships among the test systems employed. It is hoped that the present data base, which is so often incomplete, will serve as an impetus to stimulate further study of the known and suspected human carcinogens. Careful development of such reference information will assist ultimately in the identification and quantitative evaluation of additional agents that may pose a threat to human health.

ACKNOWLEDGEMENTS

The authors gratefully acknowledge the many hours spent in literature search by Libby Smith and Libby Evans and staff at the EPA Library in Research Triangle Park, NC, and the countless photocopies provided by Rose Thorn and her assistants at the Library. The authors further acknowledge the outstanding cooperation of John Wassom and the staff of the Environmental Mutagen Information Center, Oak Ridge National Laboratory, Oak Ridge, TN, in identifying and obtaining references contained in the GENE-TOX data base. Finally, the authors are indebted to Frederick J. de Serres, who reviewed the manuscript and offered many constructive comments.

REFERENCES

1. IARC, "Chemicals and Industrial Processes Associated with Cancer in Humans," Supplement I to Vols. 1-20 of IARC Monographs, IARC, Lyon, France (1979).
2. IARC Working Group, An evaluation of chemicals and industrial processes associated with cancer in humans based on human and animal data: IARC Monographs 1 to 20, Cancer Res. 40:1 (1980).
3. S. Green and A. Auletta, Editorial introduction to the reports of "The Gene-Tox Program." An evaluation of bioassays in genetic toxicology, Mutat. Res. 76:165 (1980).

4. M. D. Waters and A. Auletta, The GENE-TOX Program: Genetic activity evaluation, J. Chem. Inf. Comput. Sci. 21:35 (1981).
5. B. S. Pasternack, R. E. Shore, and R. E. Albert, Occupational exposure to chloromethyl ethers, J. Occup. Med. 19:741 (1977).
6. A. M. Thiess, W. Hey, and H. Zeller, Zur toxikologie von dichlordimethylather--Verdacht auf kanzerogene wirkung auch beim menschen, Zbl. Arbeitsmed. 23:97 (1973).
7. IARC Monographs, Vol. 4, IARC, Lyon, France (1974), pp. 231-245.
8. W. G. Figueroa, R. Raszkowski, and W. Weiss, Lung cancer in chloromethyl methyl ether workers, New England J. Med. 288: 1096 (1973).
9. D. Anderson and J. A. Styles, An evaluation of 6 short-term tests for detecting organic chemical carcinogens. Appendix II. The bacterial mutation test, Br. J. Cancer 37:924 (1978).
10. B. C. Casto, Detection of chemical carcinogens and mutagens in hamster cells by enhancement of adenovirus transformation, in: "Mammalian Cell Transformation by Chemical Carcinogens," N. Mishra, V. Dunkel, and M. Mehlman, eds., Advances in Modern Environmental Toxicology, Vol. 1, Princeton Junction, NJ (1981), p. 241.
11. S. Wada, M. Miyanish, Y. Nishimoto, S. Kambe, and R. W. Miller, Mustard gas as a cause of respiratory neoplasia in man, Lancet 1:1161 (1968).
12. J. E. Norman, Lung cancer mortality in World War I veterans with mustard-gas injury: 1919-1965, JNCI 54:311 (1975).
13. R. A. Case and A. J. Lea, Mustard gas poisoning, chronic bronchitis and lung cancer: Investigation into the possibility that poisoning by mustard gas in 1914-18 war might be a factor in production of neoplasia, Br. J. Prev. Soc. Med. 9:62 (1955).
14. R. L. Capizzi, B. Papirmeister, J. M. Mullins, and E. Cheng, The detection of chemical mutagens using the L5178Y/Asn murine leukemia in vitro and in a host-mediated assay, Cancer Res. 34:3073 (1974).
15. C. M. Stevens and A. Mylroie, Biological action of 'mustard gas' compounds. Mutagenic activity of beta-chloroalkyl amines and sulphides, Nature 166:1019 (1950).
16. C. Auerbach and J. M. Robson, The production of mutations by chemical substances, Proc. Royal Soc. Edinburgh Sect. B 62:271 (1947).
17. P. D. Lawley and P. Brookes, Cytotoxicity of alkylating agents towards sensitive and resistant strains of Escherichia coli in relation to extent and mode of alkylation of cellular macromolecules and repair of alkylation lesions in deoxyribonucleic acids, Biochem. J. 109:433 (1968).

18. D. Scott, M. Fox, and B. W. Fox, The relationship between chromosomal aberrations, survival and DNA repair in tumour cell lines of differential sensitivity to X-rays and sulphur mustard, Mutat. Res. 22:207 (1974).
19. I. I. Oster, Interactions between ionizing radiation and chemical mutagens, Z. Indukt. Abstamm. Vererbungsl. 89:1 (1958).
20. P. Milvy and M. Wolff, Mutagenic studies with acrylonitrile, Mutat. Res. 48:271 (1977).
21. M. N. Rabello-Gay and A. E. Ahmed, Acrylonitrile: In vivo cytogenetic studies in mice and rats, Mutat. Res. 79:249 (1980).
22. Pestic. Toxic Chem. News 5:21 (1977).
23. National Institute for Occupational Safety and Health, "A Recommended Standard for Occupational Exposure to Acrylonitrile," Publication 78-116, Department of Health, Education and Welfare, Cincinnati, OH (1978).
24. A. M. Thiess and I. Fleig, Analysis of chromosomes of workers exposed to acrylonitrile, Arch. Toxicol. 41:149 (1978).
25. M. T. O'Berg, Epidemiologic study of workers exposed to acrylonitrile, J. Occup. Med. 22:245 (1980).
26. J. B. Werner and J. T. Carter, Mortality of United Kingdom acrylonitrile polymerization workers, Br. J. Ind. Med. 38:247 (1981).
27. C. de Meester, F. Poncelet, M. Roberfroid, and M. Mercier, Mutagenicity of acrylonitrile, Toxicology 11:19 (1978).
28. S. Venitt, C. T. Bushell, and M. Osborne, Mutagenicity of acrylonitrile (cyanoethylene) in Escherichia coli, Mutat. Res. 45:283 (1977).
29. M. Lambotte-Vandepaer, M. Duverger-van Bogaert, C. de Meester, F. Poncelet, and M. Mercier, Mutagenicity of urine from rats and mice treated with acrylonitrile, Toxicology 16:67 (1980).
30. R. A. Parent and B. C. Casto, Effect of acrylonitrile on primary Syrian golden hamster embryo cells in culture: Transformation and DNA fragmentation, JNCI 62:1025 (1979).
31. J. Hutchinson, Br. Med. J. 11:1280 (1887); J. Hutchinson, Trans. Path. Soc. London 39:352 (1888).
32. R. J. Pye-Smith, Proc. Royal Soc. Med. Clin. Sect. 6:229 (1913).
33. O. Neubauer, Arsenical cancer: A review, Br. J. Cancer 1:192 (1947).
34. M. Kuratsune, S. Tokudome, T. Shirakusa, M. Yoshida, Y. Tokumitsu, T. Hayano, and M. Seita, Occupational lung cancer among copper smelters, Int. J. Cancer 13:552 (1974).
35. P. O. Wester, D. Brune, and G. Nordberg, Arsenic and selenium in lung, liver, and kidney tissue from dead smelter workers, Br. J. Ind. Med. 38:179 (1981).
36. IARC Monographs, Vol. 23, IARC, Lyon, France (1980), pp. 39-141.

37. A. Leonard and R. R. Lauwerys, Carcinogenicity, teratogenicity and mutagenicity of arsenic, Mutat. Res. 75:49 (1980).
38. W. J. Blot and J. F. Fraumeni, Jr., Arsenical air pollution and lung cancer, Lancet 2:142 (1975).
39. G. M. Matanoski, E. Landau, and J. Seifter, "Cancer Mortality in an Industrial Area of Baltimore," U.S. Environmental Protection Agency (in press).
40. C. E. Piper, N. E. McCarroll, and T. J. Oberly, Mutagenic activity of an organic arsenical compound detected with L5178Y mouse lymphoma cells, Environ. Mutagen. 1:165 (1978).
41. H. Nishioka, Mutagenic activities of metal compounds in bacteria, Mutat. Res. 31:185 (1975).
42. G. Dugatova, S. Podstavkova, and M. Trebaticka, Influence of arsenic on Drosophila melanogaster. II. Test on recessive lethal and other mutations affecting vitality and located in X chromosome and on the occurrence of chromosome aberations, Acta F.R.N. Univ. Comend. Genetica 9:79 (1978).
43. R. Valencia, "Mutagenesis Screening of Pesticides Using Drosophila" (unpublished).
44. V. F. Simmon, A. D. Mitchell, and T. A. Jorgenson, "Evaluation of Selected Pesticides as Chemical Mutagens: In Vitro and In Vivo Studies," EPA-600/1-77-028, U.S. Environmental Protection Agency (1977).
45. W. Burgdorf, K. Kurvink, and J. Cervenka, Elevated sister-chromatid exchange rate in lymphocytes of subjects treated with arsenic, Hum. Genet. 36:69 (1977).
46. R. J. Sram, Relationship between acute and chronic exposures in mutagenicity studies in mice, Mutat. Res. 41:25 (1976).
47. J. Petres, D. Baron, and M. Hagedorn, Effects of arsenic cell metabolism and cell proliferation: Cytogenetic and biochemical studies, Environ. Health Perspect. 19:223 (1977).
48. K. Nakamuro and Y. Sayato, Comparative studies of chromosomal aberration induced by trivalent and pentavalent arsenic, Mutat. Res. 88:73 (1981).
49. M. De Brabander, R. Van deVeire, F. Aerts, S. Geuens, and J. Hoebeke, A new culture model facilitating rapid quantitative testing of mitotic spindle inhibition in mammalian cells, JNCI 56:357 (1976).
50. J. A. DiPaolo and B. C. Casto, Quantitative studies of in vitro morphological transformation of Syrian hamster cells by inorganic metal salts, Cancer Res. 39:1008 (1979).
51. B. C. Casto, J. Meyers, and J. A. DiPaolo, Enhancement of viral transformation for evaluation of the carcinogenic or mutagenic potential of inorganic metal salts, Cancer Res. 39:193 (1979).
52. Bureau of National Affairs, Inc., National Wildlife Federation seeks defense phase-out of cadmium dust, Environ. Reporter Aug. 29:703 (1975).
53. IARC Monographs, Vol. 2, IARC, Lyon, France (1972), pp. 74-99.

54. IARC Monographs, Vol. 11, IARC, Lyon, France (1976), pp. 39-74.
55. C. L. Potts, Cadmium proteinuria--The health of battery workers exposed to cadmium oxide dust, Ann. Occup. Hyg. 8:55 (1965).
56. M. D. Kipling and J. A. H. Waterhouse, Cadmium and prostatic carcinoma, Lancet 1:730 (1967).
57. R. Lemen, J. S. Lee, J. K. Wagoner, and H. P. Blejer, Cancer mortality survey of workers exposed to cadmium, Ann. N.Y. Acad. Sci. 271:273 (1976).
58. L. N. Kolonel, Association of cadmium with renal cancer, Cancer 37:1782 (1976).
59. W. R. Bruce and J. A. Heddle, The mutagenic activity of 61 agents as determined by the micronucleus, Salmonella, and sperm abnormality assays, Can. J. Genet. Cytol. 21:319 (1979).
60. A. W. Hsie, J. P. O'Neill, J. R. San Sebastian, D. B. Couch, P. A. Brimer, W. N. C. Sun, J. C. Fuscoe, N. L. Forbes, R. Machanoff, J. C. Riddle, and M. H. Hsie, Quantitative mammalian cell genetic toxicology: Study of the cytotoxicity and mutagenicity of seventy individual environmental agents related to energy technologies and three subfractions of a crude synthetic oil in the CHO/HGPRT system, in: "Application of Short-Term Bioassays in the Fractionation and Analysis of Complex Environmental Mixtures," M. D. Waters, S. Nesnow, J. L. Huisingh, S. S. Sandhu, and L. Claxton, eds., Plenum Press, New York (1978), p. 291.
61. N. Kanematsu, M. Hara, and T. Kada, Rec assay and mutagenicity studies on metal compounds, Mutat. Res. 77:109 (1980).
62. L. L. Deaven and E. W. Campbell, Factors affecting the induction of chromosomal aberrations by cadmium in Chinese hamster cells, Cytogenet. Cell Genet. 26:251 (1980).
63. D. W. R. Bleyl and H. J. Lewerenz, Dominant lethal test in the mouse with repeated oral application of cadmium chloride, Arch. Exp. Vet. Med. Leipzig 34:399 (1980).
64. N. Gilliavod and A. Leonard, Mutagenicity tests with cadmium in the mouse, Toxicology 5:43 (1975).
65. S. Sutou, K. Yamamoto, H. Sendota, and M. Sugiyama, Toxicity, fertility, teratogenicity, and dominant lethal tests in rats administered cadmium subchronically. II. Fertility, teratogenicity, and dominant lethal tests, Ecotoxicol. Environ. Safety 4:51 (1980).
66. H. A. Schroeder, A sensible look at air pollution by metals, Arch. Environ. Health 21:798 (1970).
67. A. M. Baetjer, Pulmonary carcinoma in chromate workers. I. A review of literature and report of cases, Arch. Ind. Hyg. 2:487 (1950).

68. A. M. Baetjer, Pulmomary carcinoma in chromate workers. II. Incidence on basis of hospital records, Arch. Ind. Hyg. 2:505 (1950).
69. W. Machle and F. Gregorius, Cancer of the respiratory system in the United States chromate-producing industry, Pub. Health Rep. (Washington) 63:1114 (1948).
70. P. L. Bidstrup and R. A. M. Case, Carcinoma of the lung in workmen in the bichromates-producing industry in Great Britain, Br. J. Ind. Med. 13:260 (1956).
71. M. R. Alderson, N. S. Rattan, and L. Bidstrup, Health of workmen in the chromate-producing industry in Britain, Br. J. Ind. Med. 38:117 (1981).
72. Y. Ohsaki, S. Abe, K. Kimura, Y. Tsuneta, H. Mikami, and M. Murao, Lung cancer in Japanese chromate workers, Thorax 33:372 (1978).
73. F. L. Petrilli and S. De Flora, Toxicity and mutagenicity of hexavalent chromium on Salmonella typhimurium, Appl. Environ. Microbiol. 33:805 (1977).
74. E. R. Nestmann, T. I. Matula, G. R. Douglas, K. C. Bora, and D. J. Kowbel, Detection of the mutagenic activity of lead chromate using a battery of microbial tests, Mutat. Res. 66:357 (1979).
75. S. Bonatti, M. Meini, and A. Abbondandolo, Genetic effects of potassium dichromate in Schizosaccharomyces pombe, Mutat. Res. 38:147 (1976).
76. I. Knudsen, The mammalian spot test and its use for the testing of potential carcinogenicity of welding fume particles and hexavalent chromium, Acta Pharmacol. Toxicol. 47:66 (1980).
77. G. Raffetto, S. Parodi, C. Parodi, M. De Ferrari, R. Troiano, and G. Brambilla, Direct interaction with cellular targets as the mechanism for chromium carcinogenesis, Tumori 63:503 (1977).
78. R. F. Whiting, H. F. Stich, and D. J. Koropatnick, DNA damage and DNA repair in cultured human cells exposed to chromate, Chem.-Biol. Interact. 26:267 (1979).
79. W. D. Macrae, R. F. Whiting, and H. F. Stich, Sister chromatid exchanges induced in cultured mammalian cells by chromate, Chem.-Biol. Interact. 26:281 (1979).
80. A. G. Levis and F. Majone, Cytotoxic and clastogenic effects of soluble chromium compounds on mammalian cell cultures, Br. J. Cancer 40:523 (1979).
81. M. Umeda and M. Nishimura, Inducibility of chromosomal aberrations by metal compounds in cultured mammalian cells, Mutat. Res. 67:221 (1979).
82. L. Fabry, Relationship between the induction of micronuclei in marrow cells by chromium salts and their carcinogenic properties, C.R. Soc. Biol. 174:889 (1980).

83. D. Wild, Cytogenetic effects in the mouse of 17 chemical mutagens and carcinogens evaluated by the micronucleus test, Mutat. Res. 56:319 (1978).
84. L. J. Cralley, R. G. Keenan, and J. R. Lynch, Exposure to metals in the manufacture of asbestos textile products, Am. Ind. Hyg. Assoc. J. 28:452 (1967).
85. F. W. Sunderman, Jr., A review of the carcinogenicities of nickel, chromium and arsenic compounds in man and animals, Prev. Med. 5:279 (1976).
86. R. Doll, Cancer of the lung and nose in nickel workers, Br. J. Ind. Med. 15:217 (1958).
87. R. Doll, L. G. Morgan, and F. E. Speizer, Cancers of the lung and nasal sinuses in nickel workers, Br. J. Cancer 24:623 (1970).
88. E. Pedersen, A. C. Hogetveit, and A. Anderson, Cancer of respiratory organs among workers at a nickel refinery in Norway, Int. J. Cancer 12:32 (1973).
89. J. A. Virtue, The relationship between the refining of nickel and cancer of the nasal cavity, Can. J. Otolaryng. 1:37 (1972).
90. IARC Monographs, Vol. 2, IARC, Lyon, France (1973), pp. 126-149.
91. IARC Monographs, Vol. 11, IARC, Lyon, France (1976), pp. 75-112.
92. J. E. Cox, R. Doll, W. A. Scott, and S. Smith, Mortality of nickel workers: Experience of men working with metallic nickel, Br. J. Ind. Med. 38:235 (1981).
93. E. Mastromatteo, Nickel: A review of its occupational health aspects, J. Occup. Med. 9:127 (1967).
94. F. W. Sunderman, Jr. and E. Mastromatteo, Nickel carcinogenesis, in: "Nickel," F. W. Sunderman, Jr., F. Coulston, G. L. Eichorn, J. A. Fellows, E. Mastromatteo, H. T. Reno, and M. H. Samitz, eds., National Academy of Science, Washington, DC (1975), p. 144.
95. M. H. L. Green, W. J. Muriel, and B. A. Bridges, Use of a simplified fluctuation test to detect low levels of mutagens, Mutat. Res. 38:33 (1976).
96. V. W. Buselmaier, G. Rohrborn, and P. Propping, Mutagenicity investigations with pesticides in the host-mediated assay and the dominant lethal test in mice, Biol. Zbl. 91:311 (1972).
97. M. Nishimura and M. Umeda, Induction of chromosomal aberrations in cultured mammalian cells by nickel compounds, Mutat. Res. 68:337 (1979).
98. S. H. H. Swierenga and P. K. Basrur, Effect of nickel on cultured rat embryo muscle cells, Lab. Invest. 19:663 (1968).
99. K. M. Lynch and W. A. Smith, Pulmonary asbestosis: Carcinoma of the lung in asbestos-silicosis, Am. J. Cancer 24:56 (1935).

100. S. R. Gloyne, Two cases of squamous carcinoma of the lung occurring in asbestosis, Tubercle 17:5 (1935).
101. R. Doll, Mortality from lung cancer in asbestos workers, Br. J. Ind. Med. 12:81 (1955).
102. J. C. Wagner, C. A. Sleggs, and P. Marchand, Diffuse plural mesothelioma and asbestos exposure in the North-Western Cape Province, Br. J. Ind. Med. 17:260 (1960).
103. I. J. Selikoff, J. Churg, and E. C. Hammond, Asbestos exposure and neoplasia, JAMA 188:22 (1964).
104. E. C. Hammond, I. J. Selikoff, and J. Churg, Neoplasia among insulation workers in the United States with special reference to intra-abdominal neoplasia, Ann. N.Y. Acad. Sci. 132:519 (1965).
105. M. Kleinfeld, J. Messite, and O. Kooymann, Mortality experience in a group of asbestos workers, Arch. Environ. Health 15:177 (1967).
106. M. A. Gerber, Asbestosis and neoplastic disorders of the hematopoietic system, Am. J. Clin. Pathol. 53:204 (1970).
107. IARC Monographs, Vol. 14, IARC, Lyon, France (1977), pp. 11-106.
108. I. J. Selikoff, E. C. Hammond, and J. Churg, Asbestosis exposure, smoking and neoplasia, JAMA 204:106 (1968).
109. M. Chamberlain and E. M. Tarmy, Asbestos and glass fibers in bacterial mutation tests, Mutat. Res. 43:159 (1977).
110. S. L. Huang, Amosite, chrysotile, and crocidolite asbestos are mutagenic in Chinese hamster lung cells, Mutat. Res. 68:265 (1979).
111. K. S. Lavappa, M. M. Fu, and S. S. Epstein, Cytogenetic studies on chrysotile asbestos, Environ. Res. 10:165 (1975).
112. A. Sincock and M. Seabright, Induction of chromosome changes in Chinese hamster cells by exposure to asbestos fibers, Nature 257:56 (1975).
113. S. L. Huang, D. Saggioro, H. Michelmann, and H. V. Malling, Genetic effects of crocidolite asbestos in Chinese hamster lung cells, Mutat. Res. 57:225 (1978).
114. F. Valerio, M. De Ferrari, L. Ottaggio, E. Repetto, and L. Santi, Cytogenetic effects of Rhodesian chrysotile on human lymphocytes in vitro, IARC Sci. Publ. 30:485 (1980).
115. A. M. Sincock, Preliminary studies of the in vitro cellular effects of asbestos and fine glass dusts, in: "Origins of Human Cancer," Book B, Cold Spring Harbor Laboratory, Cold Spring Harbor, NY (1977), p. 941.
116. IARC Monographs, Vol. 7, IARC, Lyon, France (1974), pp. 203-221.
117. T. J. Haley, Evaluation of the health effects of benzene inhalation, Clin. Toxicol. 11:531 (1977).
118. "The Merck Index," 8th ed., Merck and Co., Rahway, NJ (1968), p. 128.

119. P. F. Infante, R. A. Rinski, J. K. Wagoner, and R. J. Young, Leukemia in benzene workers, Lancet 2:76 (1977).
120. P. Delore and C. Borgomano, Leucemie aigue au cours de l'intoxication benzenique: Sur l'origine toxique de certains leucemies aigues et leur relations avec les anemies graves, J. Med. Lyon 9:227 (1928).
121. A. Forni and E. C. Vigliani, Chemical leukemogenesis in man, Ser. Haemat. 7:211 (1974).
122. E. C. Vigliani and A. Forni, Benzene and leukemia, Environ. Res. 11:122 (1976).
123. T. Ishimaru, H. Okada, T. Tomiyasu, T. Tsuchimoto, T. Hoshino, and M. Ichimaru, Occupational factors in the epidemiology of leukemia in Hiroshima and Nagasaki, Am. J. Epidemiol. 93:157 (1971).
124. P. H. Wolf, D. Andjelkovich, A. Smith, and H. Tyroler, A case-control study of leukemia in the U.S. rubber industry, J. Occup. Med. 23:103 (1981).
125. M. Aksoy, S. Erdem, and G. Din Col, Leukemia in shoe-workers exposed chronically to benzene, Blood 44:837 (1974).
126. M. Aksoy and S. Erdem, Follow-up study on the mortality and the development of leukemia in 44 pancytopenic patients with chronic exposure to benzene, Blood 52:285 (1978).
127. A. Forni, E. Pacifico, and A. Limonta, Chromosome studies in workers exposed to benzene or toluene or both, Arch. Environ. Health 22:373 (1971).
128. B. J. Dean, Genetic toxicology of benzene, toluene, xylenes and phenols, Mutat. Res. 47:75 (1978).
129. R. Snyder and J. J. Kocsis, Current concepts of chronic benzene toxicity, CRC Crit. Rev. Toxicol. 3:265 (1975).
130. J. A. Cotruvo, V. F. Simmon, and R. J. Spanggord, Investigation of mutagenic effects of products of ozonation reactions in water, Ann. N.Y. Acad. Sci. 298:124 (1977).
131. L. A. Schairer, J. Van't Hof, C. G. Hayes, R. M. Burton, and F. J. de Serres, Measurement of biological activity of ambient air mixtures using a mobile laboratory for in situ exposures: Preliminary results from the Tradescantia plant test system, in: "Application of Short-Term Bioassays in the Fractionation and Analysis of Complex Environmental Mixtures," M. D. Waters, S. Nesnow, J. L. Huisingh, S. S. Sandhu, and L. Claxton, eds., Plenum Press, New York (1978), p. 419.
132. P. Nylander, H. Olofsson, B. Rasmuson, and H. Svahlin, Mutagenic effects of petrol in Drosophila melanogaster. I. Effects of benzene and 1,2-dichloroethane, Mutat. Res. 57:163 (1978).
133. H. Tanooka, Development and applications of Bacillus subtilis test systems for mutagens, involving DNA repair, deficiency and suppressible auxotrophic mutations, Mutat. Res. 42:19 (1977).

134. M. Diaz, N. Fijtman, V. Carricarte, L. Braier, and J. Diez, Effect of benzene and its metabolites on SCE in human lymphocyte cultures, In Vitro 15:172 (1979).
135. A. Koizumi, Y. Dobashi, Y. Tachibana, K. Tsuda, H. Katsunuma, Cytokinetic and cytogenetic changes in cultured human leukocytes and Hela cells induced by benzene, Ind. Health 12:23 (1974)
136. P. Gerner-Smidt and U. Friedrich, The mutagenic effect of benzene, toluene and xylene studied by the SCE technique, Mutat. Res. 58:313 (1978).
137. J. Meyne and M. S. Legator, Sex-related differences in cytogenetic effects of benzene in the bone marrow of Swiss mice, Environ. Mutagen. 2:43 (1980).
138. R. R. Tice, D. L. Costa, and R. T. Drew, Cytogenetic effects of inhaled benzene in murine bone marrow: Induction of sister chromatid exchanges, chromosomal aberrations, and cellular proliferation in DBA/2 mice, Proc. Natl. Acad. Sci. U.S.A. 77:2148 (1980).
139. D. Picciano, Cytogenetic study of workers exposed to benzene, Environ. Res. 19:33 (1979).
140. M. Hite, M. Pecharo, I. Smith, and S. Thornton, The effect of benzene in the micronucleus test, Mutat. Res. 77:149 (1980).
141. J. C. Topham, Do induced sperm-head abnormalities in mice specifically identify mammalian mutagens rather than carcinogens?, Mutat. Res. 74:379 (1980).
142. B. C. Casto and G. G. Hatch, "In Vitro Study of the Nature of the Interaction Between Chemical and Viral Carcinogens" (unpublished).
143. F. Wesley, B. Rourke, and O. Darbishire, The formation of persistent toxic chlorohydrins in foodstuffs by fumigation with ethylene oxide and with propylene oxide, J. Food Sci. 30:1037 (1965).
144. "The Merck Index," 8th ed., Merck and Co., Rahway, NJ (1968), p. 435.
145. J. W. Embree, J. P. Lyon, and C. H. Hine, The mutagenic potential of ethylene oxide using the dominant-lethal assay in rats, Toxicol. Appl. Pharmacol. 40:261 (1977).
146. L. Ehrenberg and A. Gustafsson, On the mutagenic action of ethylene oxide and diepoxylbutane in barley, Hereditas 43:595 (1957).
147. L. Ehrenberg, U. Lundquist, and G. Strom, On the mutagenic action of ethyleneimine in barley, Hereditas 44:330 (1958).
148. C. Hogstedt, N. Malmqvist, and B. Wadman, Leukemia in workers exposed to ethylene oxide, JAMA 241:1132 (1979).
149. S. De Flora, Study of 106 organic and inorganic compounds in the Salmonella/microsome test, Carcinogenesis 2:283 (1981).
150. B. J. Kilbey and H. G. Kolmark, A mutagenic after-effect associated with ethylene oxide in Neurospora crassa, Mol. Gen. Genet. 101:185 (1968).

151. K. Krell, E. D. Jacobson, and K. Selby, Mutagenic effect on L5178Y mouse lymphoma cells by growth in ethylene oxide-sterilized polycarbonate flasks, In Vitro 15:326 (1979).
152. M. J. Bird, Chemical production of mutations in Drosophila: Comparison of techniques, J. Genet. 50:480 (1952).
153. R. B. Cumming and T. A. Michaud, Mutagenic effects of inhaled ethylene oxide in male mice, Environ. Mutagen. 1:166 (1979).
154. E. G. Star, Mutagenic and cytotoxic effect of ethylene oxide on human cell cultures, Zbl. Bakt. Hyg. I. Abt. Orig. B170:548 (1980).
155. V. F. Garry, J. Hozier, D. Jacobs, R. L. Wade, and D. G. Gray, Ethylene oxide: Evidence of human chromosomal effects, Environ. Mutagen. 1:375 (1979).
156. J. W. Embree and C. H. Hine, Mutagenicity of ethylene oxide, Toxicol. Appl. Pharmacol. 33:172 (1975).
157. A. M. Thiess, H. Schwegler, I. Fleig, and W. G. Stocker, Mutagenicity study of workers exposed to alkylene oxides (ethylene oxide/propylene oxide) and derivatives, J. Occup. Med. 23:343 (1981).
158. L. E. Appelgren, G. Eneroth, C. Grant, L. E. Landstrom, and K. Tenghagen, Testing of ethylene oxide for mutagenicity using the micronucleus test in mice and rats, Acta Pharmacol. Toxicol. 43:69 (1978).
159. W. M. Generoso, K. T. Cain, M. Krishna, C. W. Sheu, and R. M. Gryder, Heritable translocation and dominant-lethal mutation induction with ethylene oxide in mice, Mutat. Res. 73:133 (1980).
160. Y. Nakao and C. Auerbach, Test of a possible correlation between cross-linking and chromosome breaking abilities of chemical mutagens, Zeitschrift für Vererbungslehre 92:457 (1961).
161. W. A. F. Watson, Further evidence of an essential difference between the genetical effects of mono- and bifunctional alkylating agents, Mutat. Res. 3:455 (1966).
162. R. K. Karchmer, M. Amare, W. E. Larsem, A. G. Mallouk, and G. G. Caldwell, Alkylating agents as leukemogens in multiple myeloma, Cancer 33:1103 (1974).
163. R. F. K. De Bock and M. E. Peetermans, Leukemia after prolonged use of melphalan for non-malignant disease, Lancet 1:1208 (1977).
164. N. Einhorn, Acute leukemia after chemotherapy (melphalan), Cancer 41:444 (1978).
165. I. P. Law and J. Blom, Second malignancies in patients with multiple myeloma, Oncology 34:20 (1977).
166. R. A. Kyle, R. V. Pierre, and E. D. Bayrd, Multiple myeloma and acute leukemia associated with alkylating agents, Arch. Int. Med. 135:185 (1975).

167. IARC Monographs, Vol. 9, IARC, Lyon, France (1975), pp. 167-180.
168. W. F. Benedict, M. S. Baker, L. Haroun, E. Choi, and B. N. Ames, Mutagenicity of cancer chemotherapeutic agents in the Salmonella/microsome test, Cancer Res. 37:2209 (1977).
169. V. Minnich, M. E. Smith, D. Thompson, and S. Kornfeld, Detection of mutagenic activity in human urine using mutant strains of Salmonella typhimurium, Cancer 38:1253 (1976).
170. D. Matheson, D. Brusick, and R. Carrano, Comparison of the relative mutagenic activity for eight antineoplastic drugs in the Ames Salmonella/microsome and TK +/- mouse lymphoma assays, Drug Chem. Toxicol. 1:277 (1978).
171. O. G. Fahmy and M. J. Fahmy, Cytogenetic analysis of the action of carcinogens and tumor inhibitors in Drosophila melanogaster. V. Differential genetic response to the alkylating mutagens and X-radiation, J. Genet. 54:146 (1956).
172. D. S. Longnecker, T. J. Curphey, S. T. James, D. S. Daniel, and N. J. Jacobs, Trial of a bacterial screening system for rapid detection of mutagens and carcinogens, Cancer Res. 34:1658 (1974).
173. R. Lewensohn and U. Ringborg, Induction of unscheduled DNA synthesis in human bone marrow cells by bifunctional alkylating agents, Blood 54:1320 (1979).
174. B. Lambert, U. Ringborg, A. Lindblad, E. Harper, M. Nordenskjold, and B. Werelius, Sister-chromatid exchanges in smoking and non-smoking control subjects, patients receiving cancer chemotherapy and laboratory workers exposed to organic solvents, Mutat. Res. 64:138 (1979).
175. A. Banerjee and W. F. Benedict, Production of sister chromatid exchanges by various cancer chemotherapeutic agents, Cancer Res. 39:797 (1979).
176. W. F. Benedict, A. Banerjee, A. Gardner, and P. A. Jones, Induction of morphological transformation in mouse C3H/10T½ clone 8 cells and chromosomal damage in hamster $A(T_1)Cl$-3 cells by cancer chemotherapeutic agents, Cancer Res. 37:2202 (1977).
177. M. Nordenskjold, S. Soderhall, and P. Moldeus, Studies of DNA-strand breaks induced in human fibroblasts by chemical mutagens/carcinogens, Mutat. Res. 63:393 (1979).
178. IARC Monographs, Vol. 10, IARC, Lyon, France (1976), pp. 85-98.
179. R. O. Wallerstein, P. K. Condit, C. K. Kasper, J. W. Brown, and F. R. Morrison, State wide study of chloramphenicol therapy and fatal aplastic anemia, JAMA 208:2045 (1969).
180. P. S. Mukherji, Acute myeloblastic leukemia following chloramphenicol treatment, Br. Med. J. ii:1286 (1957).
181. H. S. Rosenkranz, B. Gutter, and W. T. Speck, Mutagenicity and DNA-modifying activity: A comparison of two microbial assays, Mutat. Res. 41:61 (1976).

182. J. Hemmerly and M. Demerec, Tests of chemicals for mutagenicity, Cancer Res. 15:69 (1955).
183. A. J. Müller, A survey on agents tested with regard to their ability to induce recessive lethals in Arabidopsis, Arabidopsis Information Service 2:22 (1965).
184. G. E. Nasrat, K. A. Ahmed, H. A. Nafei, and A. H. Abdel-Rahman, Mutagenic action of certain therapeutic drugs on Drosophila melanogaster, Zanco 3:214 (1977).
185. H. S. Rosenkranz and Z. Leifer, Determining the DNA-modifying activity of chemicals using DNA-polymerase-deficient Escherichia coli, in: "Chemical Mutagens: Principles and Methods for Their Detection," Vol. 6, F. J. de Serres and A. Hollaender, eds., Plenum Press, New York (1980), p. 109.
186. K. Goh, Chloramphenicol and chromosomal morphology, J. Med. 10:159 (1979).
187. G. K. Manna and S. Bardhan, Some aspects of chloramphenicol induced bone marrow chromosome aberrations in mice, J. Cytol. Genet. 12:10 (1977).
188. R. J. Sram, Effect of chloramphenicol and puromycin on the dominant lethals induced by TEPA in mice, Fol. Biol. 18:367 (1972).
189. R. R. Monson, L. Rosenberg, S. C. Hartz, S. Shapiro, O. P. Heinonen, and D. Slone, Diphenylhydantoin and selected congenital malformations, New England J. Med. 289:1049 (1973).
190. IARC Monographs, Vol. 13, IARC, Lyon, France (1977), pp. 201-225.
191. F. P. Li, D. R. Willard, R. Goodman, and G. Vawter, Malignant lymphoma after diphenylhydantoin (Dilantin) therapy, Cancer 36:1359 (1975).
192. J. Clemmesen and S. Hjalmgrim-Jensen, Is phenobarbital carcinogenic? A follow-up of 8078 epileptics, Ecotoxicol. Environ. Safety 1:457 (1978).
193. L. S. Goodman and A. Gilman, "The Pharmacological Basis of Therapeutics," Macmillan, New York (1975), pp. 204-208.
194. J. Alving, M. K. Jensen, and H. Meyer, Diphenylhydantoin and chromosome morphology in man and rat--A negative report, Mutat. Res. 40:173 (1976).
195. T. V. Ramaniah, S. D. Nandan, K. P. Rao, and M. S. Rao, Mutagenicity of phenytoin in the male germ cells of Swiss mice, ICRS Med. Sci. 8:853 (1980).
196. IARC Monographs, Vol. 1, IARC, Lyon, France (1972), pp. 74-79.
197. W. F. Melick, H. M. Escue, J. J. Naryka, R. A. Mezera, and E. R. Wheeler, The first reported case of human bladder tumors due to a new carcinogen--Xenylamine, J. Urol. (Baltimore) 74:760 (1955).
198. W. F. Melick, J. J. Naryka, and R. E. Kelly, Bladder cancer due to exposure to para-aminobiphenyl: A 17-year follow up, J. Urol. (Baltimore) 106:220 (1971).

199. V. F. Simmon, In vitro mutagenicity assays of chemical carcinogens and related compounds with Salmonella typhimurium, JNCI 62:893 (1979).
200. J. L. Radomski, W. L. Hearn, T. Radomski, H. Moreno, and W. E. Scott, Isolation of the glucuronic acid conjugate of N-hydroxy-4-aminobiphenyl from dog urine and its mutagenic activity, Cancer Res. 37:1757 (1977).
201. D. F. Krahn, Rat liver homogenate-mediated toxicity and induction of 6-thioguanine-resistance in V79 Chinese hamster cells by chemical carcinogens, Diss. Abstr. Int. B37:3726 (1977).
202. R. P. Bos, R. M. E. Brouns, R. Van Doorn, J. L. G. Theuws, and P. T. Henderson, The appearance of mutagens in urine of rats after the administration of benzidine and some other aromatic amines, Toxicology 16:113 (1980).
203. V. F. Simmon, H. S. Rosenkranz, E. Zeiger, and L. A. Poirier, Mutagenic activity of chemical carcinogens and related compounds in the intraperitoneal host-mediated assay, JNCI 62:911 (1979).
204. H. S. Rosenkranz and L. A. Poirier, Evaluation of the mutagenicity and DNA-modifying activity of carcinogens and noncarcinogens in microbial systems, JNCI 62:873 (1979).
205. V. F. Simmon, In vitro assays for recombinogenic activity of chemical carcinogens and related compounds with Saccharomyces cerevisiae D3, JNCI 62:901 (1979).
206. G. M. Williams, Further improvements in the hepatocyte primary culture DNA repair test for carcinogens: Detection of carcinogenic biphenyl derivatives, Cancer Lett. 4:69 (1978).
207. R. J. Trzos, G. L. Petzold, M. N. Brunden, and J. A. Swenberg, The evaluation of sixteen carcinogens in the rat using the micronucleus test, Mutat. Res. 58:79 (1978).
208. R. J. Pienta, A hamster embryo cell model system for identifying carcinogens, in: "Carcinogens: Identification and Mechanisms of Action" A. C. Griffin and C. R. Shaw, eds., Raven Press, New York (1979), p. 121.
209. J. S. Rhim, D. K. Park, E. K. Weisburger, and J. H. Weisburger, Evaluation of an in vitro assay system for carcinogens based on prior infection of rodent cells with nontransforming RNA tumor virus, JNCI 52:1167 (1974).
210. A. E. Freeman, E. K. Weisburger, J. H. Weisburger, R. G. Wolford, J. M. Maryak, and R. J. Huebner, Transformation of cell cultures as an indication of the carcinogenic potential of chemicals, JNCI 51:799 (1973).
211. Chem. Eng. News Feb. 11:12 (1974).
212. IARC Monographs, Vol. 1, IARC, Lyon, France (1972), pp. 80-86.
213. L. Rehn, Blasengeschwulste bei fuchsin-arbeitern, Arch. Klin. Chirugie 50:588 (1895).

214. R. A. M. Case, M. E. Hosker, D. B. McDonald, and J. T. Pearson, Tumors of the urinary bladder in workmen engaged in the manufacture and use of certain dyestuff intermediates in the British chemical industry. Part I. The role of aniline, benzidine, α-naphthylamine and β-naphthylamine, Br. J. Ind. Med. 11:75 (1954).
215. T. J. Haley, Benzidine revisited: A review of the literature and problems associated with the use of benzidine and its congeners, Clin. Toxicol. 8:13 (1975).
216. T. S. Scott and M. H. C. Williams, The control of industrial bladder tumors, Br. J. Ind. Med. 14:150 (1957).
217. M. R. Zavon, U. Hoegg, and U. Bingham, Benzidine exposure as a cause of bladder tumors, Arch. Environ. Health 27:1 (1973).
218. P. F. Meal, J. Cocker, H. K. Wilson, and J. M. Gilmour, Search for benzidine and its metabolites in urine of workers weighing benzidine-derived dyes, Br. J. Ind. Med. 38:191 (1981).
219. W. C. Hueper, "Occupational and Environmental Cancers of the Urinary System," Yale University Press, New Haven, CT (1969).
220. K. Tanaka, S. Marui, and T. Mii, Mutagenicity of extracts of urine from rats treated with aromatic amines, Mutat. Res. 79:173 (1980).
221. R. C. Garner, A. L. Walpole, and F. L. Rose, Testing of some benzidine analogues for microsomal activation to bacterial mutagens, Cancer Lett. 1:39 (1975).
222. M. J. Fahmy and O. G. Fahmy, Mutagenicity of hair dye components relative to the carcinogen benzidine in Drosophila melanogaster, Mutat. Res. 56:31 (1977).
223. V. F. Simmon, S. L. Eckford, and A. F. Griffin, Ozone methods and ozone chemistry of selected organics in water. 2. Mutagenic assays, in: "Proceedings of a Conference: Ozone/Chlorine Dioxide Oxidation Products of Organic Materials" (1978), p. 126.
224. C. N. Martin, A. C. McDermid, and R. C. Garner, Testing of known carcinogens and noncarcinogens for their ability to induce unscheduled DNA synthesis in HeLa cells, Cancer Res. 38:2621 (1978).
225. R. B. Painter, DNA synthesis inhibition in HeLa cells as a simple test for agents that damage human DNA, J. Environ. Pathol. Toxicol. 2:65 (1978).
226. R. Cihak, Evaluation of benzidine by the micronucleus test, Mutat. Res. 67:383 (1979).
227. R. J. Pienta, J. A. Poiley, and W. B. Lebherz, III, Morphological transformation of early passage golden Syrian hamster embryo cells derived from cryopreserved primary cultures as a reliable in vitro bioassay for identifying diverse carcinogens, Int. J. Cancer 19:642 (1977).

228. K. A. Traul and J. S. Wolff, report under Contract NO1-CP-55703, John L. Smith Memorial on Cancer, Pfizer, Inc. (1979).
229. IARC Monographs, Vol. 1, IARC, Lyon, France (1972), pp. 69-73.
230. A. von Mueller, Blasenveranderungen durch amine, erfahrungen aus dem industriegebeit basel, Z. Urol. Chir. 36:202 (1933).
231. R. A. M. Case and J. T. Pearson, Tumors of the urinary bladder in workmen engaged in the manufacture and use of certain dyestuff intermediates in the British chemical industry. Part II. Further consideration of the role of aniline and of the manufacture of auramine and magenta (fuchsin) as possible causative agents, Br. J. Ind. Med. 11:213 (1954).
232. D. E. Amacher, S. C. Paillet, G. N. Turner, V. A. Ray, and D. S. Salsburg, Point mutations at the thymidine kinase locus in L5178Y mouse lymphoma cells. II. Test validation and interpretation, Mutat. Res. 72:447 (1980).
233. T. Tsuchimoto and B. E. Matter, Activity of coded compounds in the micronucleus test, in: "Evaluation of Short-Term Tests for Carcinogenesis: Report of the International Collaborative Program," Progress in Mutation Research, Vol. 1, F. J. de Serres and J. Ashby, eds., Elsevier/North-Holland Biomedical Press, New York (1981), p. 705.
234. H. G. Treibl, Naphthalene derivatives, in: "Encyclopedia of Chemical Toxicology," 2nd ed., R. E. Kirk and D. F. Othmer, eds., Vol. 13, John Wiley and Sons, New York (1967), p. 708.
235. "The Merck Index," 8th ed., Merck and Co., Rahway, NJ (1968), p. 717.
236. W. C. Hueper, "Occupational Tumors and Allied Diseases," Thomas, Springfield, IL (1942).
237. IARC Monographs, Vol. 4, IARC, Lyon, France (1974), pp. 97-111.
238. L. J. Goldwater, A. J. Rosso, and M. Kleinfeld, Bladder tumors in a coal-tar dye plant, Arch. Environ. Health 11:814 (1965).
239. T. Sugimura, S. Sato, M. Nagao, T. Yahagi, T. Matsushima, Y. Seino, M. Takeuchi, and T. Kawachi, Overlapping of carcinogens and mutagens, in: "Fundamentals in Cancer Prevention," P. N. Magee et al., eds., University of Tokyo Press and University Park Press, Tokyo and Baltimore, MD (1976), p. 191.
240. D. Ichinotsubo, H. F. Mower, J. Setliff, and M. Mandel, The use of rec⁻ bacteria for testing of carcinogenic substances, Mutat. Res. 46:53 (1977).
241. V. W. Mayer, Mutagenic effects induced in Saccharomyces cerevisiae by breakdown products of 1-naphthylamine and 2-naphthylamine formed in an enzyme-free hydroxylation system, Mutat. Res. 15:147 (1972).
242. T. Ong and F. J. de Serres, Mutagenicity of chemical carcinogens in Neurospora crassa, Cancer Res. 32:1890 (1972).

243. V. W. Mayer, Induction of mitotic crossing over in Saccharomyces cerevisiae by breakdown products of dimethylnitrosamine, diethylnitrosamine, 1-naphthylamine and 2-naphthylamine formed by an in vitro hydroxylation system, Genetics 74:433 (1973).
244. D. F. Callen and R. M. Philpot, Cytochrome P-450 and the activation of promutagens in Saccharomyces cerevisiae, Mutat. Res. 45:309 (1977).
245. A. D. Mitchell, "Potential Prescreens for Chemical Carcinogens: Unscheduled DNA Synthesis," Task 2, Final Report under Contract NO1/CP-33394, Stanford Research Institute, Stanford, CA (1976).
246. M. F. Salamone, J. A. Heddle, and M. Katz, Mutagenic activity of 41 compounds in the in vivo micronucleus assay, in: "Evaluation of Short-Term Tests for Carcinogenesis: Report of the International Collaborative Program," Progress in Mutation Research, Vol. 1, F. J. de Serres and J. Ashby, eds., Elsevier/North-Holland Biomedical Press, New York (1981), p. 686.
247. B. Kirkhart, Micronucleus test on 21 compounds, in: "Evaluation of Short-Term Tests for Carcinogenesis: Report of the International Collaborative Program," Progress in Mutation Research, Vol. 1, F. J. de Serres and J. Ashby, eds., Elsevier/North-Holland Biomedical Press, New York (1981), p. 698.
248. A. Videbaek, Chlornaphazin (Erysan®) may induce cancer of the urinary bladder, Acta Med. Scand. 176:45 (1964).
249. N. I. Sax, "Cancer Causing Chemicals," Van Nostrand Reinhold, New York (1981).
250. T. Thiede, E. Chievitz, and B. C. Christensen, Chlornaphazine as a bladder carcinogen, Acta Med. Scand. 175:721 (1964).
251. E. Chievitz and T. Thiede, Acta Med. Scand. 172:513 (1962).
252. T. Thiede and B. C. Christensen, Bladder tumors induced by chlornaphazine, Acta Med. Scand. 185:133 (1969).
253. IARC Monographs, Vol. 4, IARC, Lyon, France (1974), pp. 119-124.
254. O. G. Fahmy and M. J. Fahmy, Gene elimination in carcinogenesis: Reinterpretation of the somatic mutation theory, Cancer Res. 30:195 (1970).
255. R. L. Wall and K. P. Clausen, Carcinoma of the urinary bladder in patients receiving cyclophosphamide, New England J. Med. 293:271 (1975).
256. IARC Monographs, Vol. 9, IARC, Lyon, France (1975), pp. 135-156.
257. A. D. Steinberg, P. H. Plotz, S. M. Wolff, V. G. Wong, S. G. Agus, and J. L. Decker, Cytotoxic drugs in treatment of nonmalignant diseases, Ann. Int. Med. 76:619 (1972).
258. J. C. Cline and R. E. McMahon, Detection of chemical mutagens: Use of concentration gradient plates in a high capacity screen, Res. Commun. Chem. Pathol. Pharmacol. 16:523 (1977).

259. V. W. Mayer, C. J. Hybner, and D. J. Brusick, Genetic effects induced in Saccharomyces cerevisiae by cyclophosphamide in vitro without liver enzyme preparations, Mutat. Res. 37:201 (1976).
260. D. Siebert and U. Simon, Genetic activity of metabolites in the ascitic fluid and in the urine of a human patient treated with cyclophosphamide, Mutat. Res. 21:257 (1973).
261. D. Siebert, A new method for testing genetically active metabolites: Urinary assay with cyclophosphamide (Endoxan, Cytoxan) and Saccharomyces cerevisiae, Mutat. Res. 17:307 (1973).
262. W. J. Suling, R. F. Struck, C. W. Woolley, and W. M. Shannon, Comparative disposition of phosphoramide mustard and other cyclophosphamide metabolites in the mouse using the Salmonella/mutagenesis assay, Cancer Treat. Rep. 62:1321 (1978).
263. A. Schubert, Host-mediated assay and urinary assay with the same mice for the detection of chemical mutagens in Saccharomyces cerevisiae, Biol. Zbl. 94:451 (1975).
264. A. A. Shapiro and L. M. Fonshtein, Study of the mutagenic action of cyclophosphamide on bacteria in host-mediated assay, Izv. Akad. Nauk SSSR, Ser. Biol. 6:371 (1979).
265. S. R. Sirianni, M. Furukawa, and C. C. Huang, Induction of 8-azaguanine- and ouabain-resistant mutants by cyclophosphamide and 1-(pyridyl-B)-3,3-dimethyltriazene in Chinese hamster cells cultured in diffusion chambers in mice, Mutat. Res. 64:259 (1979).
266. D. Clive, K. O. Johnson, J. F. S. Spector, A. G. Batson, and M. M. M. Brown, Validation and characterization of the L5178Y/TK$^{+/-}$ mouse lymphoma mutagen assay system, Mutat. Res. 59:61 (1979).
267. E. Vogel, W. R. Lee, A. Schalet, and F. Wurgler, Drosophila test system, in: "Proceedings of the Comparative Chemical Mutagen Conference" (in press).
268. R. B. Cumming and M. F. Walton, Genetic effects of cyclophosphamide in the germ cells of male mice, Genetics 68:S14 (1971).
269. R. E. Sotomayor, G. A. Sega, and R. B. Cumming, Unscheduled DNA synthesis in the germ cèlls of male mice treated in vivo with chemical mutagens requiring metabolic activation, Mutat. Res. 38:395 (1976).
270. W. F. Benedict, A. Banerjee, and N. Venkatesan, Cyclophosphamide-induced oncogenic transformation, chromosomal breakage, and sister chromatid exchange following microsomal activation, Cancer Res. 38:2922 (1978).
271. A. Korte, Comparative analysis of chromosomal aberrations and sister-chromatid exchanges in bone marrow cells of Chinese hamsters after treatment with aflatoxin B_1, patulin and cyclophosphamide, Mutat. Res. 74:164 (1980).

272. T. Ikeuchi, K. Sugimura, and M. Sasaki, Evaluation of mutagen-metabolizing capacity of cultured mammalian cells, as revealed by the induction of chromosome aberrations and sister chromatid exchanges, Jpn. J. Hum. Genet. 24:186 (1979).
273. C. C. Huang, K. McKernan, J. R. Pantano, and S. R. Sirianni, An in vitro metabolic activation assay using liver microsomes in diffusion chambers: Induction of sister chromatid exchanges and chromosome aberrations by cyclophosphamide or ifosfamide in cultured human and Chinese hamster cells, Carcinogenesis 1:37 (1980).
274. A. N. Chebotarev, L. Y. Telegin, and E. M. Derzhavets, Cytogenetic effect of cyclophosphamide in a culture of human lymphocytes after its activation in the mouse organism, Genetika 12:151 (1976).
275. I. Hansmann, Chromosome aberrations in metaphase II--Oocytes stage sensitivity in the mouse oogenesis to amethopterin and cyclophosphamide, Mutat. Res. 22:175 (1974).
276. P. Goetz, A. M. Malashenko, and N. I. Surkova, Chromosome aberrations induced by cyclophosphamide in meiotic cells of male mice, Tsitologiya i Genetika 14:29 (1980).
277. G. Rohrborn and A. Basler, Cytogenetic investigations of mammals. Comparison of the genetic activity of cytostatics in mammals, Arch. Toxicol. 38:35 (1977).
278. I. Sykora, K. Rezabek, D. Pokorna, and D. Gandalovicova, Experiences with methods testing the mutagenic and antifertility effects of the model drug cyclophosphamide, in: "Evaluation of Embryotoxic, Mutagenic, and Carcinogenic Risks of New Drugs, Proceedings of a 1976 Symposium" (1979), p. 263.
279. P. K. Datta, H. Frigger, and E. Schleiermacher, The effect of chemical mutagens on the mitotic chromosomes of the mouse in vivo, in: "Chemical Mutagenesis in Mammals and Man," F. Vogel and G. Rohrborn, eds., Springer-Verlag, Berlin and New York (1970), p. 194.
280. W. M. Generoso, K. T. Cain, S. W. Huff, and D. G. Gosslee, Inducibility by chemical mutagens of heritable translocations in male and female germ cells of mice, in: "Advances in Modern Toxicology," Vol. 5, Hemisphere Publishing Corporation, Washington, DC and London (1978), p. 109.
281. E. Vogel, Mutagenic activity of cyclophosphamide, trofosfamide, and ifosfamide in Drosophila melanogaster. Specific induction of recessive lethals in the absence of detectable chromosome breakage, Mutat. Res. 33:221 (1975).
282. T. Hirakawa, M. Tanaka, and S. Takayama, Morphological transformation of hamster embryo cells by cancer chemotherapeutic agents, Toxicol. Lett. 3:55 (1979).

283. V. C. Dunkel, R. J. Pienta, A. Sivak, and K. A. Traul, Comparative neoplastic transformation responses of Balb/3T3 cells, Syrian hamster embryo cells, and Rauscher murine leukemia virus-infected Fischer 344 rat embryo cells to chemical carcinogens, JNCI 67:1303 (1981).
284. P. M. Adams, J. D. Fabricant, and M. S. Legator, Cyclophosphamide-induced spermatogenic effects detected in the F_1 generation by behavioral testing, Science 211:80 (1981).
285. E. K. Inskeep, J. C. Herrington, and I. L. Lindahl, Effects of cyclophosphamide in rams, J. Animal Sci. 33:1022 (1971).
286. A. J. Pennisi, C. M. Grushkin, and E. Lieberman, Gonadal function in children with nephrosis treated with cyclophosphamide, Am. J. Dis. Child. 129:315 (1975).
287. J. C. Topham, Chemically-induced transmissible abnormalities in sperm-head shape, Mutat. Res. 70:109 (1980).
288. R. C. Shank, G. N. Wogan, and J. B. Gibson, Dietary aflatoxins and human liver cancer. I. Toxigenic moulds in foods and foodstuffs of tropical South-east Asia, Food Cosmetic Toxicol. 10:51 (1972).
289. R. C. Shank, G. N. Wogan, J. B. Gibson, and A. Nondasuta, Dietary aflatoxins and human liver cancer. II. Aflatoxins in market foods and foodstuffs of Thailand and Hong Kong, Food Cosmetic Toxicol. 10:61 (1972).
290. R. C. Shank, J. E. Gordon, G. N. Wogan, A. Nondasuta, and B. Subhamani, Dietary aflatoxins and human liver cancer. III. Field survey of rural Thai families for ingested aflatoxins, Food Cosmetic Toxicol. 10:71 (1972).
291. R. C. Shank, N. Bhamarapravati, J. E. Gordon, and G. N. Wogan, Dietary aflatoxins and human liver cancer. IV. Incidence of primary liver cancer in two municipal populations of Thailand, Food Cosmetic Toxicol. 10:171 (1972).
292. S. J. Van Rensburg, J. J. Van Der Watt, I. F. H. Purchase, L. Pereira Continho, and R. Markham, Primary liver cancer rate and aflatoxin intake in a high cancer area, S. Afr. Med. J. 48:2508a (1974).
293. F. G. Peers and C. A. Linsell, Dietary aflatoxins and liver cancer--A population based study in Kenya, Br. J. Cancer 27:473 (1973).
294. M. E. Alpert, M. S. R. Hutt, G. N. Wogan, and C. S. Davidson, Association between aflatoxin content of food and hepatoma frequency in Uganda, Cancer 28:253 (1971).
295. G. N. Wogan, Dietary factors and special epidemiological situations of liver cancer in Thailand and Africa, Cancer Res. 35:3499 (1975).
296. G. E. Deger, Aflatoxin--Human colon carcinogenesis?, Ann. Int. Med. 85:204 (1976).
297. T. C. Campbell and L. Stoloff, Implication of mycotoxins for human health, J. Agr. Food Chem. 22:1006 (1974).

298. T. C. Campbell, R. O. Sinnhuber, D. J. Lee, J. H. Wales, and L. Salamat, Hepatocarcinogenic material in urine specimens from humans consuming aflatoxin, JNCI 52:1647 (1974).
299. F. W. Larimer, A. A. Hardigree, D. W. Ramey, and J. L. Epler, Genetic activity of pro-mutagens in logarithmic phase cultures of *Saccharomyces cerevisiae*, Environ. Mutagen. 1:124 (1979).
300. T. Ong, Mutagenic activities of aflatoxin B_1 and G_1 in *Neurospora crassa*, Mol. Gen. Genet. 111:159 (1971).
301. D. F. Krahn and C. Heidelberger, Liver homogenate-mediated mutagenesis in Chinese hamster V79 cells by polycyclic aromatic hydrocarbons and aflatoxins, Mutat. Res. 46:27 (1977).
302. M. J. Lamb and L. J. Lilly, Induction of recessive lethals in *Drosophila melanogaster* by aflatoxin B_1, Mutat. Res. 11:430 (1971).
303. Y. Ueno and K. Kubota, DNA-attacking ability of carcinogenic mycotoxins in recombination-deficient mutant cells of *Bacillus subtilis*, Cancer Res. 36:445 (1976).
304. M. H. Kuczuk, P. M. Benson, H. Heath, and A. W. Hayes, Evaluation of the mutagenic potential of mycotoxins using *Salmonella typhimurium* and *Saccharomyces cerevisiae*, Mutat. Res. 53:11 (1978).
305. D. F. Callen, G. R. Mohn, and T. Ong, Comparison of the genetic activity of aflatoxins B_1 and G_1 in *Escherichia coli* and *Saccharomyces cerevisiae*, Mutat. Res. 45:7 (1977).
306. G. M. Williams, Detection of chemical carcinogens by unscheduled DNA synthesis in rat liver primary cell cultures, Cancer Res. 37:1845 (1977).
307. C. N. Martin, A. C. McDermid, and R. C. Garner, Measurement of 'unscheduled' DNA synthesis in HeLa cells by liquid scintillation counting after carcinogen treatment, Cancer Lett. 2:355 (1977).
308. H. F. Stich and B. A. Laishes, The response of *Xeroderma pigmentosum* cells and controls to the activated mycotoxins, aflatoxins and sterigmatocystin, Int. J. Cancer 16:266 (1975).
309. H. J. Freeman and R. H. C. San, Use of unscheduled DNA synthesis in freshly isolated human intestinal mucosal cells for carcinogen detection, Cancer Res. 40:3155 (1980).
310. L. Wheeler, M. Halula, and M. DeMeo, Comparison of prophage induction and mutagenicity in Ames tester strain TA1535 by aflatoxins and nitrosamines, Environ. Mutagen. 1:121 (1979).
311. S. Wolff and S. Takehisa, Induction of sister-chromatid exchange in mammalian cells by low concentrations of mutagenic carcinogens that require metabolic activation as well as those that do not, *in*: "Progress in Genetic Toxicology," D. Scott, B. A. Bridges, and F. H. Sobels, eds., Elsevier/North-Holland Biomedical Press, New York (1977), p. 193.

312. M. El-Zawahri, A. Moubasher, M. Morad, and I. El-Kady, Mutagenic effect of aflatoxin B_1, Ann. Nutr. Alim. 31:859 (1977).
313. Y. Nakanishi and E. L. Schneider, In vivo sister-chromatid exchange: A sensitive measure of DNA damage, Mutat. Res. 60:329 (1979).
314. A. Korte and G. Ruckert, Chromosomal analysis in bone-marrow cells of Chinese hamsters after treatment with mycotoxins, Mutat. Res. 78:41 (1980).
315. M. A. Friedman and J. Staub, Induction of micronuclei in mouse and hamster bone-marrow by chemical carcinogens, Mutat. Res. 43:255 (1977).
316. B. C. Casto, N. Janosko, and J. A. DiPaolo, Development of a focus assay model for transformation of hamster cells in vitro by chemical carcinogens, Cancer Res. 37:3508 (1977).
317. B. C. Casto, W. J. Pieczynski, N. Janosko, and J. A. DiPaolo, Significance of treatment interval and DNA repair in the enhancement of viral transformation by chemical carcinogens and mutagens, Chem.-Biol. Interact. 13:105 (1976).
318. J. A. DiPaolo, K. Takano, and N. C. Popescu, Quantitation of chemically induced neoplastic transformation of BALB/3T3 cloned cell lines, Cancer Res. 32:2686 (1972).
319. G. N. Egbunike, The effects of microdoses of aflatoxin B1 on sperm production rates, epididymal sperm abnormality, and fertility in the rat, Zentralbl. Vet. Med. A26:66 (1979).
320. IARC Monographs, Vol. 13, IARC, Lyon, France (1977), pp. 131-139.
321. G. C. Farrell, D. E. Joshua, R. F. Uren, P. J. Baird, K. W. Perkins, and H. Kronenberg, Androgen-induced hepatoma, Lancet 1:430 (1975).
322. F. L. Johnson, J. R. Feagler, K. G. Lerner, P. W. Majerus, M. Siegel, J. R. Hartmann, and E. D. Thomas, Association of androgenic-anabolic steroid therapy with development of hepatocellular carcinoma, Lancet 2:1273 (1972).
323. IARC Monographs, Vol. 7, IARC, Lyon, France (1974), pp. 291-318.
324. IARC Monographs, Vol. 19, IARC, Lyon, France (1979), pp. 377-438.
325. J. L. Creech, Jr. and M. N. Johnson, Angiosarcoma of liver in the manufacture of polyvinyl chloride, J. Occup. Med. 16:150 (1974).
326. R. Spirtas and R. Kaminski, Angiosarcoma of the liver in vinyl chloride/polyvinyl chloride workers. Update of NIOSH Register, J. Occup. Med. 20:427 (1978).
327. R. R. Monson, J. M. Peters, and M. N. Johnson, Proportional mortality among vinyl-chloride workers, Lancet 2:397 (1974).
328. W. J. Nicholson, E. C. Hammond, H. Seidman, and I. J. Selikoff, Mortality experience of a cohort of vinyl chloride-polyvinyl chloride workers, Ann. N.Y. Acad. Sci. 246:225 (1975).

329. R. J. Waxweiler, W. Stringer, J. K. Wagoner, J. Jones, H. Falk, and C. Carter, Neoplastic risk among workers exposed to vinyl chloride, Ann. N.Y. Acad. Sci. 271:40 (1976).
330. A. J. Fox and P. F. Collier, Mortality experience of workers exposed to vinyl chloride monomer in the manufacture of polyvinyl chloride in Great Britain, Br. J. Ind. Med. 34:1 (1977).
331. W. von Reinl, H. Weber, and E. Greiser, Epidemiological study on mortality of VC-exposed workers in the Federal Republic of Germany, Medichem. (Germany), September 2-8 (1977).
332. J. McCann, V. Simmon, D. Streitwieser, and B. N. Ames, Mutagenicity of chloroacetaldehyde, a possible metabolic product of 1,2-dichloroethane (ethylene dichloride), chloroethanol (ethylene chlorohydrin), vinyl chloride, and cyclophosphamide, Proc. Natl. Acad. Sci. U.S.A. 72:3190 (1975).
333. M. M. Shahin, The non-mutagenicity and -recombinogenicity of vinyl chloride in the absence of metabolic activation, Mutat. Res. 40:269 (1976).
334. N. Loprieno, R. Barale, S. Baroncelli, C. Bauer, G. Bronzetti, A. Cammellini, G. Cercignani, C. Corsi, G. Gervasi, C. Leporini, R. Nieri, A. M. Rossi, G. Stretti, and G. Turchi, Evaluation of the genetic effects induced by vinyl chloride monomer (VCM) under mammalian metabolic activation: Studies in vitro and in vivo, Mutat. Res. 40:85 (1976).
335. B. Z. Drozdowicz and P. C. Huang, Lack of mutagenicity of vinyl chloride in two strains of Neurospora crassa, Mutat. Res. 48:43 (1977).
336. I. E. Mattern and W. B. Van der Zwaan, Mutagenicity testing of urine from vinylchloride (VCM) treated rats using the Salmonella test system, Mutat. Res. 46:230 (1977).
337. F. C. Barsky, J. D. Irr, and D. F. Krahn, Mutagenicity of gases in the Chinese hamster ovary cell assay, Environ. Mutagen. 1:167 (1979).
338. C. Drevon and T. Kuroki, Mutagenicity of vinyl chloride, vinylidene chloride and chloroprene in V79 Chinese hamster cells, Mutat. Res. 67:173 (1979).
339. F. G. Verburgt and E. Vogel, Vinyl chloride mutagenesis in Drosophila melanogaster, Mutat. Res. 48:327 (1977).
340. S. Peter and G. Ungvary, Lack of mutagenic effect of vinyl chloride monomer in the mammalian spot test, Mutat. Res. 77:193 (1980).
341. J. D. Elmore, J. L. Wong, A. D. Laumbach, and U. N. Streips, Vinyl chloride mutagenicity via the metabolites chlorooxirane and chloroacetaldehyde monomer hydrate, Biochem. Biophys. Acta 442:405 (1976).
342. I. Hansteen, L. Hillestad, E. Thiis-Evensen, and S. S. Heldaas, Effects of vinyl chloride in man: A cytogenetic follow-up study, Mutat. Res. 51:271 (1978).

343. D. Anderson, C. R. Richardson, I. F. H. Purchase, H. J. Evans, and M. L. O'Riordan, Chromosomal analysis in vinyl chloride exposed workers: Comparison of the standard technique with the sister-chromatid exchange technique, Mutat. Res. 83:137 (1981).
344. A. Basler and G. Röhrborn, Vinyl-chloride: An example for evaluating mutagenic effects in mammals in vivo after exposure to inhalation, Arch. Toxicol. 45:1 (1980).
345. I. F. H. Purchase, C. R. Richardson, and D. Anderson, Chromosomal and dominant lethal effects of vinyl chloride, Lancet 2:410 (1975).
346. D. Jenssen and C. Ramel, The micronucleus test as part of a short-term mutagenicity test program for the prediction of carcinogenicity evaluated by 143 agents tested, Mutat. Res. 75:191 (1980).
347. R. D. Short, J. L. Minor, J. M. Winston, and C. Lee, A dominant lethal study in male rats after repeated exposures to vinyl chloride or vinylidene chloride, J. Toxicol. Environ. Health 3:965 (1977).
348. D. Anderson, M. C. E. Hodge, and I. F. H. Purchase, Vinyl chloride: Dominant lethal studies in male CD-1 mice, Mutat. Res. 40:359 (1976).
349. C. L. Young, "Cancer Control Monograph: Diethylstilbestrol," Project 4418, SRI International, Stanford, CA (1978).
350. A. L. Herbst, H. Ulfelder, and D. C. Poskanzer, Adenocarcinoma of the vagina. Association of maternal stilbestrol therapy with tumor appearance in young women, New England J. Med. 284:878 (1971).
351. S. J. Robboy, R. E. Scully, W. R. Welch, and A. L. Herbst, Intrauterine diethylstilbestrol exposure and its consequences, Arch. Pathol. Lab. Med. 101:1 (1977).
352. A. L. Herbst, P. Cole, T. Colton, S. J. Robboy, and R. E. Scully, Age-incidence and risk of diethylstilbestrol-related clear cell adenocarcinoma of the vagina and cervix, Am. J. Obstet. Gynecol. 128:43 (1977).
353. IARC Monographs, Vol. 21, IARC, Lyon, France (1979), pp. 173-231.
354. C. Drevon, C. Piccoli, and R. Montesano, Mutagenicity assays of estrogenic hormones in mammalian cells, Mutat. Res. 89:83 (1981).
355. H. W. Rudiger, F. Haenisch, M. Metzler, F. Oesch, and H. R. Glatt, Metabolites of diethylstilboestrol induce sister-chromatid exchange in human cultured fibroblasts, Nature 281:392 (1979).
356. S. Abe and M. Sasaki, Chromosome aberrations and sister-chromatid exchanges in Chinese hamster cells exposed to various chemicals, JNCI 58:1635 (1977).
357. J. L. Ivett and R. R. Tice, Cytogenetic effects of diethystilbestrol-diphosphate (DES-dp) in murine bone marrow, Environ. Mutagen. 1:184 (1979).

358. A. J. F. Griffiths, Neurospora and environmentally induced aneuploidy, in: "Short-Term Tests for Chemical Carcinogens," H. F. Stich and R. H. C. Sans, eds., Springer-Verlag, New York/Berlin (1981), p. 187.
359. N. P. Bishun, N. Smith, H. Eddie and D. C. Williams, Cytogenetic studies and diethylstilboestrol, Mutat. Res. 46:211 (1977).
360. N. Bishun, S. Forster, N. Valera, and D. C. Williams, The clastogenic effects of diethylstilboestrol on ascitic tumour cells in vivo, Microbiol. Lett. 13:27 (1980).
361. L. Molina, S. Rinkus, and M. S. Legator, Evaluation of the micronucleus procedure over a 2-yr period, Mutat. Res. 53:125 (1978).
362. R. J. Pienta, In vitro carcinogenesis, in: "Frederick Cancer Research Center Annual Progress Report," Vol. 11-D (1979), p. 7.
363. J. C. Topham, The detection of carcinogen-induced sperm head abnormalities in mice, Mutat. Res. 69:149 (1980).
364. A. Wyrobek, L. Gordon, and G. Watchmaker, Effect of 17 chemical agents including 6 carcinogen/noncarcinogen pairs on sperm shape abnormalities in mice, in: "Evaluation of Short-Term Tests for Carcinogenesis: Report of the International Collaborative Program," Progress in Mutation Research, Vol. 1, F. J. de Serres and J. Ashby, eds., Elsevier/North-Holland Biomedical Press, New York (1981), p. 712.
365. R. W. Andonian and R. Kessler, Transplacental exposure to diethylstibestrol in men, Urology 13:276 (1979).
366. M. Bibbo, W. B. Gill, F. Azizi, R. Blough, V. S. Fang, R. L. Rosenfeld, G. F. B. Schumacher, K. Sleeper, M. G. Sonek, and G. L. Wied, Follow-up study of male and female offspring of DES-exposed mothers, Obstet. Gynecol. 49:1 (1977).
367. "The Merck Index," 8th ed., Merck and Co., Rahway, NJ (1968), p. 410.
368. IARC Monographs, Vol. 11, IARC, Lyon, France (1976), pp. 131-139.
369. B. A. Bridges, On the detection of volatile liquid mutagens with bacteria: Experiments with dichlorvos and epichlorohydrin, Mutat. Res. 54:367 (1978).
370. D. J. Kilian, T. G. Pullin, T. H. Conner, M. S. Legator, and H. N. Edwards, Mutagenicity of epichlorohydrin in the bacterial assay system: Evaluation by direct in vitro activity and in vivo activity of urine from exposed humans and mice, Mutat. Res. 53:72 (1978).
371. K. Hemminki and K. Falck, Correlation of mutagenicity and 4-(p-nitrobenzyl)-pyridine alkylation by epoxides, Toxicol. Lett. 4:103 (1979).

372. R. E. McMahon, J. C. Cline, and C. Z. Thompson, Assay of 855 test chemicals in ten tester strains using a new modification of the Ames test for bacterial mutagens, Cancer Res. 39:682 (1979).
373. R. K. Vashishat, M. Vasudeva, and S. N. Kakar, Induction of mitotic crossing over, mitotic gene conversion and reverse mutation by epichlorohydrin in Saccharomyces cerevisiae, Indian J. Exp. Biol. 18:1337 (1980).
374. H. Heslot, A quantitative study of biochemical reversions induced in the yeast Schizosaccharomyces pombe by radiations and radiomimetic substances, Abhand der Deutschen Akademie der Wissenschaften zu Berlin Klasse fur Medizin 1:193 (1962).
375. H. E. Brockman, "Report on Epichlorohydrin (ECH) Using the ad-3 Test System (Heterocaryon-12) of Neurospora crassa," report under Contract NIH-75-0-17300, National Institutes of Health (unpublished).
376. A. D. Laumbach, S. Lee, J. Wong, and U. N. Streips, Studies on the mutagenicity of vinyl chloride metabolites and related chemicals, in: "Proceedings of the Third International Symposium on Prevention and Detection of Cancer," Vol. 1 (1977), p. 155.
377. A. D. White, In vitro induction of SCE in human lymphocytes by epichlorohydrin with and without metabolic activation, Mutat. Res. 78:171 (1980).
378. R. J. Sram, M. Cerna, and M. Kucerova, The genetic risk of epichlorohydrin as related to the occupational exposure, Biol. Zbl. 95:451 (1976).
379. M. Kucerova and Z. Polivkova, Banding technique used for the detection of chromosomal aberrations induced by radiation and alkylating agents TEPA and epichlorohydrin, Mutat. Res. 34:279 (1976).

THE SEARCH FOR BIOLOGICAL MODELS TO INVESTIGATE HUMAN CARCINOGENIC RISKS: HUMAN PATHOLOGY AND EXPERIMENTAL CARCINOGENESIS CORRELATIONS AT THE ORGAN, TISSUE, AND CELLULAR LEVEL, *IN VIVO* AND *IN VITRO*

Umberto Saffiotti

Laboratory of Experimental Pathology
Division of Cancer Cause and Prevention
National Cancer Institute
Frederick, Maryland

INTRODUCTION

The use of human cells for the assessment of risks from physical and chemical agents - the subject of the present course - is rapidly evolving in the field of carcinogenesis. Its methodology is emerging from basic advances in experimental pathology, cell biology and biochemistry. The use of human tissues and cells for the study and evaluation of human carcinogenesis is becoming a highly productive area of cancer research, although much work remains to be done toward establishing its precise role in the complex process of risk assessment. Considerable progress has been made in establishing appropriate methods and models for the study of the pathogenesis of human cancers. Partiular attention was given to models for epithelial cancers, which constitute the vast majority of human neoplasms. A variety of closely related biological systems was developed to link together the pathology observed in whole human organisms and in the corresponding whole animal models for the chemical induction of the same types of tumors, derived from the same organs and tissues. When appropriate chemically induced organ-level animal models were established, the subsequent development was devoted to organ culture models for the *in vitro* maintenance of the tissues of origin of the main types of tumors and the study of their response to carcinogens. When the organ culture models were established from experimental animal tissues, the next step was aimed at developing their human counterparts, using culture methods for the corresponding human tissues of origin. Finally, from these organ culture systems - or in parallel with them - the next stage of model development was that of systems for the culture of isolated cells from the target epithelia, both from the experimental animals and from their human counterpart. Once all these were established, linking together animal and human pathology at the organ, tissue and cellular levels, it became possible to study mechanisms of induction of neoplastic transformation in progressively linked biological systems and particularly in the isolated target cells, directly comparing animal and human cellular responses.

The advantage of embarking on such a wide-ranging effort of developing systems at these different levels is that it becomes possible to correlate the findings from biochemical and morphological mechanism studies across previously unsurmounted barriers. A firm ground is thus provided for closely related comparisons of organ, tissue and cellular responses, of in vivo and in vitro responses, and - at all levels - of animal and human pathology responses.

The methodology for investigating the experimental pathology of carcinogenesis has rapidly developed in the last 10-15 years, after relatively slow beginnings that date back to the establishment of the field in the 1930s and to its origins in the preceding two decades.

Initial studies of chemical carcinogenesis started with the use of a few simple models such as: a) skin tumor induction by topical application in rabbits and then more extensively in mice, first with tars and then with individual polycyclic aromatic hydrocarbons; b) liver tumor induction in mice and rats by feeding of azo-compounds and later of 2-acetylaminofluorene; c) subcutaneous sarcoma induction by topical injection of carcinogens in both mice and rats; and d) induction of lung adenoma in mice by systemic administration of carcinogens.*

In the 1960s and 1970s an extensive research effort was directed to the development of animal models that would mimic as closely as possible their human pathology counterpart for the induction of major forms of cancer. This development was helped by the identification of classes of carcinogens with a wide spectrum of organotropic effects such as the N-nitroso compounds. The activity spectrum of such com-

---

*A particularly comprehensive early review of the state of the art of the experimental pathology of cancer and of carcinogenesis research was provided by Pietro Rondoni in his 1945 book on cancer [1]. As the present course is held in San Miniato, Rondoni's birthplace, on the 25th anniversary of his death, I wish to dedicate this paper to the memory of this pioneer who was my teacher of general pathology and carcinogenesis at the University of Milan and first inspired my interest in this field.

Table 1. Major Chemically Induced Animal Models of Human Cancers

Epithelial	
- Epidermis	- Mammary gland
- Bronchus	- Kidney
- Larynx	- Bladder
- Esophagus	- Endometrium
- Stomach (glandular)	- Uterine cervix
- Colon and rectum	- Ovary
- Pancreas	- Prostate
- Liver	- Thyroid
- Biliary passages	- Other endocrine organs
Non-epithelial	
- Lymphomas	- Nervous system
- Leukemias	- Connective tissues

pounds [2] suggested that they would be likely to induce tumors in a variety of animal target tissues from which new pathogenetic models could be derived, more closely resembling their human counterparts.

The main types of human cancers are of epithelial origin, from such organs as the bronchus, the stomach, the colon, the rectum, the pancreas, the breast, the uterine mucosa, the bladder and the kidney. To study the induction of most of these cancers and several others, few, if any, good experimental models were available as recently as 12-15 years ago. Experimental pathology research in carcinogenesis has now successfully developed good models for most of the major forms of human cancers, that have been reproducibly induced in animals by chemical induction (Table 1). The opportunity therefore arose to investigate the pathogenesis of different types of tumors and to establish its analogy with human pathology.

DEVELOPMENT AND USE OF BIOLOGICAL MODELS FOR EPITHELIAL CARCINOGENESIS AT THE ORGAN, TISSUE, and CELLULAR LEVELS

The first example of model development I shall discuss is that of respiratory carcinogenesis models, to which I devoted a considerable portion of my efforts in terms both of direct laboratory research and of collaborative research planning and development. This topic and its relation to risk evaluation were discussed in recent reviews [3-5].

During an initial period I studied the penetration of inorganic particles in the respiratory tract by inhalation and by intratracheal instillation and their tissue distribution, uptake by macrophages and subsequent cellular responses, particularly in relation to the mechanisms of fibrogenesis in experimental pneumoconioses [6-8]. I then evisaged the role of particles as carriers of carcinogens into the respiratory tract and developed a methodology for intratracheal administration to hamsters of aqueous suspensions of a finely particulated carcinogen such as benzo[a]pyrene (B[a]P) attached to fine carrier particles of a nonfibrogenic material such as ferric oxide. High incidences of bronchogenic carcinoma were obtained and the tumor morphology was found to be closely similar to that of the analogous human tumors [9-11]. This model was then investigated to define its response to different doses of carcinogen and of carrier particles, to different schedules of exposure, and to changes in the physical characteristics of the carrier particles [12-16]. Other studies were undertaken in this initial phase of model development to investigate how the carrier particles, which were clearly not carcinogenic by themselves, produced their marked enhancement of the effect of carcinogens [9, 10, 12, 17-19]. The histogenesis and cellular pathogenesis of the carcinomas induced in the bronchial, tracheal, and laryngeal epithelium in this experimental hamster model was analyzed in comparison with human pathology at the light and electron microscopic levels [20-25]. Following the establishment of this system as a representative experimental model of human respiratory carcinogenesis, further studies were undertaken to provide an in-depth analysis of the experimental model in comparison with the human counterpart, by morphological criteria including light and electron transmission microscopy, scanning microscopy, and histochemistry. These studies elucidated the pathogenetic sequences leading from the cells of origin, through changes in their morphological differentiation, to the final establishment of various morphological types of respiratory epithelial tumors. Such studies definitively demonstrated the close qualitative similarities of the animal model [26-28] to the corresponding human disease [29-31].

Functional studies were also undertaken to investigate the pathogenetic mechanisms involved in respiratory carcinogenesis. The distribution and localization of carcinogens in the respiratory epithelium were studied by autoradiographic methods in the hamster model *in vivo* [22]. The inhibitory effect of vitamin A on epithelial squamous carcinogenesis in the respiratory tract was demonstrated with this experimental model [32] and led to the development of extensive research programs on the inhibition of carcinogenesis by related compounds (retinoids) [33-35] and on the mechanism of action of retinoids in the control of glycoprotein synthesis and cell surface properties [36-38]. Pathogenetic mechanisms at the tissue, cellular, and molecular level needed to be further investigated through coordinated studies by morphological, biochemical, and biological methods [39]. For this purpose we started to make use of organ culture techniques, removing the target tissues, i.e., the tracheobronchial mucosa, from either intact or pretreated animals and placing them in culture for maintenance and timed observations, with or without *in vitro* treatment by carcinogens and/or modifiers.

Organ culture methods were used to study the biochemical pathways of carcinogen metabolism and interaction in the target cells, the binding of carcinogens to target macromolecules, and the early morphological and biochemical responses. The advantages of such organ culture studies are many and, although obviously limited by the artificial microenvironment for the tissues, they offer a unique opportunity to characterize the pathological changes induced by carcinogens and cofactors directly in the target cells (reviewed in [3]).

The results obtained by the use of organ cultures from the target tissues of the animal models suggested that similar studies could be conducted in the corresponding organ cultures derived from human tissues. Normal human target tissues, such as bronchial mucosa, were obtained from immediate autopsies performed in cases of accidental traumatic death or from surgical material; methods for the obtainment, preparation and maintenance of human tissue explants in culture were developed. The study of the response of cultured human tissues to carcinogens became a major activity in our laboratory as a result of the work of C. C. Harris and co-workers. The extensive progress recently made in this area was described in several reviews [40-46]. These studies, initially devoted to the respiratory tract epithelium, were subsequently extended to several other human target tissues for which there were good animal model counterparts for studies in carcinogenesis (e.g., colon, esophagus, and pancreatic duct). These studies were developed by C. C. Harris and co-workers in our laboratory in collaboration with B. F. Trump and co-workers at the Department of Pathology, University of Maryland School of Medicine and with others. They included several directions of research: identification of the cellular distribution and localization of carcinogens in the human target epithelia; characterization of the pathways of metabolic activation and interaction of carcinogens in human epithelial target cells; morphological and histochemical analysis of the early stages of the human cellular response to carcinogens; and cell culture studies to characterize the properties of epithelial cells isolated from human tissue explants after carcinogen exposure. Analysis of the response to carcinogens in human target tissues and in their counterparts from animal models revealed a remarkable qualitative similarity, extending from the morphological characteristics of the cellular and tissue response to the biochemical pathways of enzymatic carcinogen activation and to the formation of the same ultimate carcinogen metabolites and the same carcinogen-DNA adducts. Much further support has thus accrued for the use of experimental animal studies as reliable qualitative indicators of the potential human response to carcinogens.

In relation to risk evaluation for human populations, the qualitative and quantitative implications of these studies, which demonstrate wide interindividual and interspecies variations, were discussed recently [4, 5]. The latest developments are addressed to the establishment of human bronchial epithelial cell lines and to their possible transformation by chemical carcinogens, presently under investigation.

The second example of model development I shall briefly discuss is that of epidermal carcinogenesis. In the human population epidermal cancer has a very high incidence but a relatively low mortality. The induction of epidermal tumors by application of carcinogens on the skin of experimental animals, especially mice, represents the earliest and one of the most extensively tested _in vivo_ models for chemical carcinogenesis. Mouse skin carcinogenesis studies _in vivo_ provided early evidence of dose-response relationships in carcinogenesis by chemicals and by ultraviolet light and provided a valuable visual record of the patterns of tumor progression [47]. The use of this model in the 1940s led to identification of the two-stage mechanism of initiation and promotion [48-50]. The model was extended by the use of systemic administration of either initiators or promoters [51]. The biological response that follows initiation differs substantially depending on whether the secondary treatment is constituted by promoting agents or by carcinogens [52-53]. An extensive literature has developed on the _in vivo_ model of mouse epidermal carcinogenesis.

The development of an _in vitro_ model, closely related to the human and animal _in vivo_ counterparts, became the object of considerable effort in our laboratory by S. H. Yuspa and co-workers. Initial establishment of culture methods for isolated epidermal cells from newborn BALB/c mice [54, 55] showed the analogy of the _in vitro_ model to its _in vivo_ counterpart and provided the opportunity for a series of studies to characterize this _in vitro_ system with respect to cellular kinetics, biochemical and histochemical markers of epithelial differentiation, metabolic competence for carcinogen activation, DNA binding of carcinogens, DNA repair characteristics, and mechanisms of neoplastic transformation of the epithelial cells in culture by tumor initiators and promoters (reviewed in [56-58]). This _in vitro_ system has been used to isolate a series of continuously growing mouse epidermal cell lines for studies of transformation mechanisms. Carcinogen-initiated cell lines, which transform when further exposed to promoting agents, may provide a unique _in vitro_ counterpart to the _in vivo_ response to tumor promoters [59-62]. A few other laboratories have worked on this system. Effective methods were recently established by Rheinwald and co-workers for the culture of human keratinocytes [63]. The mechanisms of carcinogenesis and tumor promotion and markers of epithelial differentiation are now being actively investigated in these biological models linking _in vivo_ and _in vitro_, animal and human studies.

A valuable perspective on methods for the culture of human organ explants and cells, particularly epithelial cells, and on methods for the _in vitro_ transformation of epithelial cells from differ-

Table 2. Organ Culture Models of Target Epithelial Tissues of Both Animal and Human Origin

- Epidermis	- Mammary gland
- Trachea/bronchus	- Kidney
- Lung	- Bladder
- Esophagus	- Endometrium
- Colon	- Uterine cervix
- Pancreatic duct	- Prostate

ent organs is offered by two recent books [42, 64] that review these important methodological advances.

The target epithelial tissues, for which organ culture models have been so far developed for both animal and human tissues, include an already extensive list (Table 2).

In general terms, we can now reasonably expect that the major human target tissues from which human cancers arise, as well as their counterparts from appropriate animal models, can be maintained as explant cultures in good conditions of viability, differentiation and function for a period of time sufficient to investigate their metabolic, cellular and molecular response to carcinogens.

An important methodological development concerns the selection of optimal culture conditions to extend the viability of organ cultures and to support the growth of isolated epithelial cells in culture. The selection, isolation and growth of the target epithelial cells is dependent in large part on the development of particularly suitable culture media containing appropriate additives (e.g., hormones, amino acids and proteins) that contribute to the control of cell growth in culture. A particularly important aspect of this work is the development of optimal chemically defined media, i.e., media that do not require serum additions. Serum is a variable "unknown" factor in the composition of the medium: its replacement in the medium by a carefully selected mixture of additives has opened the way towards the goal of chemically defined culture conditions as shown by the pioneering work of Gordon Sato and by several other investigators. The recent literature on culture methods for epithelial tissues and cells, particuarly of human origin [42, 64] suggests that each type of tissue or cell from different epithelial organs may have its own somewhat different optimum requirement to provide growth support for extended periods of time.

Epithelial cell cultures can be derived from the target epithelial tissues by various techniques. Cells can be derived from animal or human tissues; the latter can be obtained from biopsy,

Table 3. Development of Epithelial Cell Cultures from Target Epithelial Tissues

Sources:	Animal cells Human cells	from:	Biopsy Surgery Immediate autopsy
Cutlure methods:	Explant outgrowth Dispersed cells Isolation of cell lines		
Chemical induction of:	Metabolic activation Cytotoxicity DNA damage and repair Altered cell growth Mutation Neoplastic transformation		
→ By treatment:	*In vivo* Of organ cultures Of cell cultures		

surgery, or immediate autopsy. Epithelial cell cultures can be established from the outgrowth around organ culture explants, from suspensions of cells disaggregated from their tissues of origin, or by the selection and isolation of epithelial cell lines, which can be further cloned to select for special biological characteristics. In the epithelial cell cultures thus obtained, one can study the effects of chemical treatments by carcinogens, including pathways of metabolic activation, cytotoxicity, DNA damage and repair, chromosomal damage, altered cell growth, altered biochemical functions, mutation and neoplastic transformation. The effects of chemical carcinogens can be studied after treatment *in vivo* in the animals from which the tissues and cells are derived, after treatment *in vitro* of the organ explants from which cell cultures are derived, or after direct treatment of the target cells in cultures (Table 3).

In addition, the co-cultivation of human and animal target tissues and cells, together with cells more sensitive to certain specific effects (such as mutation) can be used to reveal the ability of the former to activate chemicals metabolically [65, 66] so that they can induce the effect detected by the latter.

The actual induction of neoplastic transformation by chemicals in epithelial cells in culture has been more difficult to achieve and to demonstrate in comparison with fibroblasts, partly because the epithelial cells lack the morphologic markers of colony transformation so typical of the fibroblast systems. Chemical induction of neoplastic transformation in human cells has proven much more difficult and time-requiring than in rodent cells. Rapid progress however is taking place in this field and it is reasonable to expect that several cell transformation models will eventually become available for different types of epithelial cells.

Chemically transformed epithelial cells in culture can be inoculated into appropriate syngeneic or immunosuppressed host animals and grow as carcinomas. This end-point of the process of carcinogenesis obtained from cells in culture can be compared with the morphologic and functional characteristics of the corresponding tumors induced from the same target cells by treatment in vivo. Mechanism studies can therefore be addressed to defining how specific and how essential a given response pathway can be for the process of carcinogenesis in a given target tissue or cell of origin, by recognizing how persistent and treatment-dependent it remains through all these levels of biological organization linking experimental models and human pathology.

RELEVANCE FOR RISK EVALUATION

How can we contribute to the issue of risk evaluation through studies on the experimental models described above? In order to evaluate a human carcinogenic risk, we need to know not only the properties of the physical or chemical exposure agents, but also the exposure conditions and the susceptibility of the hosts. Susceptibility is a comprehensive term that encompasses all the host factors that influence the penetration, distribution and retention of exogenous agents in the organism, the metabolic activation and detoxification of chemicals, their interactions with target macromolecules, DNA repair, as well as many other cellular and humoral defense mechanisms. We have to consider, therefore, both those aspects that pertain primarily to the exogenous agents and those that characterize the host response.

We want to investigate the effects of carcinogenic agents as they operate in human subjects who are obviously the goal of our prevention-oriented research; but we also want to be able to use the experimental method, for its critical investigative power and for its value in determining cause-and-effect relationships. Obvious reasons preclude experiments with carcinogens directly on living human beings, but studies on the pathology and histogenesis of cancers in human subjects can give us a clear picture of the end-points. Research approaches, such as those described above, were therefore, systematically addressed to bridging the gap between animal and human as well as in vivo and in vitro levels, developing closely related models, connected step-by-step with each other. This research made it possible to establish a large basis of reproducibility at different biological levels for pathways of carcinogen activation, carcinogen-DNA adduct formation, induction of morphological and functional changes, mutational and transformational events. When a close identity of animal and human pathogenetic pathways is demonstrated at the organ, tissue, cellular, and molecular level, such as it was for the respiratory carcinogenesis models discussed above, the results of carcinogenesis studies conducted in the animal sustems acquire a high degree of direct qualitative applicability to the human situation. Because of marked interindividual variations in the human quantitative response, however, the process of direct quantitative risk extrapolation from animals to humans becomes unreliable even in such qualitatively superimposable systems. One can however, come closer to establishing some quantitative correlations by measuring those parameters that are identified as critical for carcinogen activity pathways and that are present in all these model systems: judicious use of these measurements can suggest how to bracket the extent of the response compatible with such parameters in a population exposed to a carcinogen or category of carcinogens in a given set of conditions.

The study of the experimental pathology of carcinogenesis appears to be the safest way to safety evaluations.

REFERENCES

1. P. Rondoni, Il Cancro, Istituzioni di Patologia Generale dei Tumori, Casa Editrice Ambrosiana, Milano (1980), 860 pp.
2. H. Druckrey, R. Preussmann, S. Ivankovic, and D. Schmahl, Organotrope carcinogene wirkungen bei 65 verschiedenen N-nitrosoverbindungen an BD-Ratten, Zschr. f. Krebsforsch., 69:103 (1967).
3. U. Saffiotti and C. Harris, Carcinogenesis studies on organ cultures of animal and human respiratory tissues, in: "Carcinogens: Identification and Mechanisms of Action," A. C. Griffin and C. R. Shaw, eds., Raven Press, New York (1979), p. 65.
4. U. Saffiotti, Identification and definition of chemical carcinogens: Review of criteria and research needs, J. Toxicol. Environ. Health, 6:1029 (1980).
5. U. Saffiotti, The problem of extrapolating from observed carcinogenetic effects to estimates of risk for exposed populations, J. Toxicol. Environ. Health, 6:1309 (1980).
6. U. Saffiotti, The histogenesis of experimental silicosis. I. Methods for the histological evaluation of experimentally induced dust lesions, Med. Lavoro, 51:10 (1960).
7. U. Saffiotti, A. Tommasini Degna, and L. Mayer, The histogenesis of experimental silicosis. II. Cellular and tissue reactions in the histogenesis of pulmonary lesions, Med. Lavoro, 51:518 (1960).
8. U. Saffiotti, The histogenesis of experimental silicosis. III. Early cellular reactions and the role of necrosis, Med. Lavoro, 53:5 (1962).

9. U. Saffiotti, S. A. Borg, M. I. Grote, and D. B. Karp, Retention rates of particulate carcinogens in the lungs. Studies in an experimental model for lung cancer induction, Chicago Med. Sch. Q., 24:10 (1964).
10. U. Saffiotti, F. Cefis, L. H. Kolb, and P. Shubik, Experimental studies of the conditions of exposure to carcinogens for lung cancer induction, J. Air Pollut. Control Assoc., 15:23 (1965).
11. U. Saffiotti, F. Cefis, and L. H. Kolb, A method for the experimental induction of bronchogenic carcinoma, Cancer Res., 28:104 (1968).
12. U. Saffiotti, Experimental respiratory tract carcinogenesis and its relation to inhalation exposures, in: "Inhalation Carcinogenesis," M. G. Hanna, Jr., P. Nettesheim, and J. R. Gilbert, eds., AEC Sympsoium Series No. 18 (CONF-691001), p. 27 (1970).
13. R. Montesano, U. Saffiotti, and P. Shubik, The role of topical and systemic factors in experimental respiratory carcinogenesis, in: "Inhalation Carcinogenesis," M. G. Hanna, Jr., P. Nettesheim, and J. R. Gilbert, eds., AEC Symposium Series No. 18 (CONF-691001), p. 353 (1970).
14. U. Saffiotti, R. Montesano, A. R. Sellakumar, F. Cefis, and D. G. Kaufman, Respiratory tract carcinogenesis in hamsters induced by different numbers of administrations of benzo[a]-pyrene and ferric oxide, Cancer Res., 32:1073 (1972).
15. U. Saffiotti, R. Montesano, A. R. Sellakumar, and D. G. Kaufman, Respiratory tract carcinogenesis induced in hamsters by different dose levels of benzo[a]pyrene and ferric oxide, J. Natl. Cancer Inst., 49:1199 (1972).
16. A. R. Sellakumar, R. Montesano, U. Saffiotti, and D. G. Kaufman, Hamster respiratory carcinogenesis induced by benzo[a]pyrene and different dose levels of ferric oxide, J. Natl. Cancer Inst., 50:507 (1973).
17. M. C. Henry and D. G. Kaufman, Clearance of benzo[a]pyrene from hamster lungs after administration on coated particles, J. Natl. Cancer Inst., 51:1961 (1973).
18. M. C. Henry, C. D. Port, and D. G. Kaufman, Role of particles in respiratory carcinogenesis bioassay, in: "Experimental Lung Cancer, Carcinogenesis and Bioassays," E. Karbe and J. F. Park, eds., Springer-Verlag, New York (1974), p. 173.
19. R. L. Farrell and G. W. Davis, Effect of particulate benzo[a]-pyrene carrier on carcinogenesis in the respiratory tract of hamsters, in: "Experimental Lung Cancer, Carcinogenesis and Bioassays," E. Karbe and J. F. Pard, eds., Springer-Verlag, New York (1974), p. 186.
20. C. C. Harris, M. B. Sporn, D. G. Kaufman, J. M. Smith, M. S. Baker, and U. Saffiotti, Acute ultrastructural effects of benzo[a]pyrene and ferric oxide on the hamster tracheobronchial epithelium, Cancer Res., 31:1977 (1972).
21. C. C. Harris, M. B. Sporn, D. G. Kaufman, J. M. Smith, F. Jackson, and U. Saffiotti, Histogenesis of squamous metaplasia in the hamster tracheal epithelium caused by vitamin A deficiency of benzo[a]pyrene-ferric oxide, J. Natl. Cancer Inst., 48:743 (1972).

22. C. C. Harris, D. G. Kaufman, M. B. Sporn, H. Boren, F. Jackson, J. M. Smith, J. Pauley, P. Dedick, and U. Saffiotti, Localization of benzo[a]pyrene-^{3}H and alterations in nuclear chromatin caused by benzo[a]pyrene-ferric oxide in the hamster respiratory epithelium, Cancer Res., 33:2842 (1973).
23. C. C. Harris, D. G. Kaufman, M. B. Sporn, and U. Saffiotti, Histogenesis of squamous metaplasia and squamous cell carcinoma of the respiratory epithelium in an animal model, Cancer Chemother. Res., 4:43 (1973).
24. C. C. Harris, D. G. Kaufman, M. B. Sporn, J. M. Smith, F. Jackson, and U. Saffiotti, Ultrastructural effects of N-methylnitrosourea on the tracheobronchial epithelium of the Syrian golden hamster, Int. J. Cancer, 12:259 (1973).
25. U. Saffiotti and D. G. Kaufman, Carcinogenesis of laryngeal carcinoma, Laryngoscope, 85:454 (1975).
26. P. J. Becci, E. M. McDowell, and B. F. Trump, The respiratory epithelium. II. Hamster trachea, bronchus, and bronchioles, J. Natl. Cancer Inst., 61:551 (1978).
27. P. J. Becci, E. M. McDowell, and B. F. Trump, The respiratory epithelium. IV. Histogenesis of epidermoid metaplasia and carcinoma in situ in the hamster, J. Natl. Cancer Inst., 61:577 (1978).
28. P. J. Becci, E. M. McDowell, and B. F. Trump, The respiratory epithelium. VI. Histogenesis of lung tumors induced by benzo-[a]pyrene-ferric oxide in the hamster, J. Natl. Cancer Inst., 61:607 (1978).
29. E. M. McDowell, L. A. Barrett, F. Glavin, C. C. Harris, and B. F. Trump, The respiratory epithelium. I. Human bronchus, J. Natl. Cancer Inst., 61:539 (1978).
30. E. M. McDowell, J. S. McLaughlin, D. K. Merenyl, R. F. Kieffer, C. C. Harris, and B. F. Trump, The respiratory epithelium. V. Histogenesis of lung carcinomas in the human, J. Natl. Cancer Inst., 61:587 (1978).
31. B. F. Trump, E. M. McDowell, F. Glavin, L. A. Barrett, P. J. Becci, W. Schurch, H. E. Kaiser, and C. C. Harris, The respiratory epithelium. III. Histogenesis of epidermoid metaplasia and carcinoma in situ in the human, J. Natl. Cancer Inst., 61:563 (1978).
32. U. Saffiotti, R. Montesano, A. R. Sellakumar, and S. A. Borg, Studies on experimental lung cancer: Inhibition by vitamin A of the induction of tracheobronchial squamous metaplasia and squamous cell tumors, Cancer, 20:857 (1967).
33. M. B. Sporn, N. M. Dunlop, D. L. Newton, and J. M. Smith, Prevention of chemical carcinogenesis by vitamin A and its synthetic analogs, Fed. Proc., 35:1332 (1976).
34. M. B. Sporn and D. L. Newton, Chemoprevention of cancer with retinoids, Fed. Proc., 38:2528 (1979).
35. M. B. Sporn, D. L. Newton, A. B. Roberts, J. E. DeLarco, and G. J. Todaro, Retinoids and the suppression of the effects of polypeptide transforming factors. A new molecular approach to

chemoprevention of cancer, in: "Molecular Actions and Targets for Cancer Chemotherapeutic Agents," A. C. Sartorelli, J. R. Bertino, and J. S. Lazo, eds., Academic Press, New York, p. 541 (1981).
36. L. M. De Luca, The direct involvement of vitamin A in glycosyl transfer reactions of mammalian membranes, Vitam. Horm. (N.Y.), 35:1 (1977).
37. L. M. De Luca, S. Adamo, P. V. Bhat, W. Sasak, C. S. Silverman-Jones, I. Akalovsky, J. P. Frot-Coutaz, T. R. Fletcher, and G. J. Chader, Recent developments in studies on biological functions of vitamin A in normal and transformed tissues, Pure Appl. Chem., 51:581 (1979).
38. S. Adamo, L. M. De Luca, I. Akalovsky, and P. V. Bhat, Retinoid-induced adhesion in cultured transformed mouse fibroblasts, J. Natl. Cancer Inst., 62:1473 (1979).
39. D. G. Kaufman, M. S. Baker, C. C. Harris, J. M. Smith, H. Boren, M. B. Sporn, and U. Saffiotti, Coordinated biochemical and morphologic examination of hamster tracheal epithelium, J. Natl. Cancer Inst., 49:783 (1972).
40. C. C. Harris, V. Genta, A. Frank, D. G. Kaufman, L. Barrett, E. M. McDowell, and B. F. Trump, Carcinogenic polynuclear hydrocarbons bind to macromolecules in cultured human bronchi, Nature, 252:68 (1974).
41. C. C. Harris, H. Autrup, B. F. Trump, and G. D. Stoner, Carcinogenesis studies in human respiratory epithelium. An experimental model system, in: "Pathogenesis and Therapy of Lung Cancer," C. C. Harris, ed., Dekker, New York p. 559 (1978).
42. C. C. Harris, B. F. Trump, and G. D. Stoner, eds., Methods in Cell Biology, Vol. 21, Normal Human Tissue and Cell Culture. A. Respiratory, Cardiovascular, and Integumentary Systems. B. Endocrine, Urogenital, and Gastrointestinal Systems. Academic Press, New York (1980).
43. M. G. Valerio, E. L. Fineman, R. L. Bowman, C. D. Harris, G. D. Stoner, H. Autrup, B. F. Trump, E. M. McDowell, and R. T. Jones, Long-term survival of normal adult human tissues as xenografts in congenitally athymic nude mice, J. Natl. Cancer Inst., 66: 849 (1981).
44. C. C. Harris, R. C. Grafstrom, B. F. Trump, and H. Autrup, Differences in metabolism of chemical carcinogens in cultured human epithelial tissues, in: "Mechanisms of Chemical Carcinogenesis," C. C. Harris and P. Cerutti, eds., R. Liss, New York (in press).
45. H. Autrup, Carcinogen metabolism in human tissues and cells, Drug Metabolism Reviews, Vol. 13 (in press).
46. H. Autrup, R. C. Graftstrom, and C. C. Harris, Metabolism of chemical carcinogens by tracheobronchial tissues, in: "Organ and Species Specificity in Chemical Carcinogenesis," J. M. Rice, R. Langenbach, and S. Nesnow, eds., Plenum Press, New York (in press).

47. L. Foulds, Neoplastic Development, Vol. 1, Academic Press, London, 424 pp. (1969).
48. I. Berenblum, The cocarcinogenic action of croton resin, Cancer Res., 1:44 (1941).
49. J. C. Mottram, A developing factor in experimental blastogenesis, J. Pathol. Bacteriol., 56:181 (1944).
50. I. Berenblum and P. Shubik, A new quantitative approach to the study of the stages of chemical carcinogenesis in the mouse's skin, Br. J. Cancer, 1:383 (1947).
51. A. C. Ritchie and U. Saffiotti, Orally administered 2-acetylaminofluorene as an initiator and as a promoter in epidermal carcinogenesis in the mouse, Cancer Res., 15:84 (1955). (Erratum 15:700, 1955).
52. U. Saffiotti and P. Shubik, The effects of low concentrations of carcinogen in epidermal carcinogenesis: A comparison with promoting agents, J. Natl. Cancer Inst., 16:961 (1956).
53. U. Saffiotti and P. Shubik, Studies on promoting action in skin carcinogenesis, Natl. Cancer Inst. Monogr., 10:489 (1963).
54. S. H. Yuspa, D. L. Morgan, R. J. Walker, and R. R. Bates, The growth of fetal mouse skin in cell culture and transplantation to F_1 mice, J. Invest. Dermatol., 55:379 (1970).
55. S. H. Yuspa and C. C. Harris, Altered differentiation of mouse epidermal cells treated with retinyl acetate in vitro, Exp. Cell Res., 86:95 (1974).
56. S. H. Yuspa, H. Hennings, and U. Saffiotti, Cutaneous chemical carcinogenesis: Past, present, and future, J. Invest. Dermatol., 67:199 (1976).
57. S. H. Yuspa, Mouse epidermal cell cultures as an in vitro model for the study of chemical carcinogenesis, in: "In vitro Carcinogenesis. Guide to the Literature, Recent Advances and Laboratory Procedures," U. Saffiotti and H. Autrup, eds., Natl. Cancer Inst. Tech. Report Series No. 44, DHEW Publ. No. (NIH)78-844, p. 47 (1978).
58. N. Colburn, Chemical transformation of epidermal cell cultures, in: "In vitro Carcinogenesis. Guide to the Literature, Recent Advances and Laboratory Procedures," U. Saffiotti and H. Autrup, eds., Natl. Cancer Inst. Tech. Report Series No. 44, DHEW Publ. No. (NIH)78-844, p. 57 (1978).
59. S. H. Yuspa, U. Lichti, H. Hennings, T. Ben, E. Patterson, and T. J. Slaga, Tumor promoter stimulated proliferation in mouse epidermis in vivo and in vitro: Mediation by polyamines and inhibition by the antipromoter steroid fluocinolone acetonide, in: "Mechanisms of Tumor Promotion and Cocarcinogenesis," T. J. Slaga, A. Sivak, and R. K. Boutwell, eds., Raven Press, New York, p. 221 (1978).
60. N. H. Colburn, U. V. Vorder Bruegge, J. Bates, and S. H. Yuspa, Epidermal cell transformation in vitro, in: "Mechanisms of Tumor Promotion and Cocarcinogenesis," T. J. Slaga, A. Sivak, and R. K. Boutwell, eds., Raven Press, New York p. 257 (1978).

61. H. Hennings, S. H. Yuspa, D. Michael, and U. Lichti, Modification of epidermal cell response to 12-O-tetradecanoyl-phorbol-13-acetate by serum level, culture temperature and pH, in: "Mechanisms of Tumor Promotion and Cocarcinogenesis," T. J. Slaga, A. Sivak, and R. K. Boutwell, eds., Raven Press, New York p. 233 (1978).
62. N. H. Colburn, Tumor promotion and preneoplastic progression, in: "Carcinogenesis, Vol. 5: Modifiers of Chemical Carcinogenesis," T. J. Slaga, ed., Raven Press, New York, p. 33 (1980).
63. J. G. Rheinwald, Serial cultivation of normal human epidermal keratinocytes, in: "Methods in Cell Biology, Vol. 21A," C. C. Harris, B. F. Trump, and G. D. Stoner, eds., Academic Press, New York, p. 229 (1980).
64. L. M. Franks and C. B. Wigley, eds., Neoplastic Transformation in Differentiated Epithelial Cell Systems In Vitro, Academic Press, New York (1979).
65. I. C. Hsu, G. D. Stoner, H. Autrup, B. F. Trump, J. K. Selkirk, and C. C. Harris, Human bronchus-mediated mutagenesis of mammalian cells by carcinogenic polynuclear aromatic hydrocarbons, Proc. Natl. Acad. Sci. U.S.A., 75:2003 (1978).
66. I. C. Hsu, C. C. Harris, M. Yamaguchi, B. F. Trump, and P. W. Schafer, Induction of ouabain-resistant mutation and sister chromatid exchanges in Chinese hamster cells with chemical carcinogens mediated by human pulmonary macrophages, J. Clin. Invest., 64:1245 (1979).

THE CAUSES OF CANCER: QUANTITATIVE ESTIMATES OF AVOIDABLE RISKS OF CANCER IN THE UNITED STATES TODAY

Richard Peto

Oxford University
U.K.

My lecture spanned not only the hour allocated for it in the morning, but also the first half of the round table that afternoon, where it acted as an introduction to the round table discussion that followed. The break between the two sessions was determined only by administrative and not by scientific matters, and so in this published account, the two may be read as a unit.

The title of my lecture was the same as that of our long review article on the causes of human cancer which appeared in the June 1981 issue of the JNCI (Doll, R., Peto, R., J. Natl. Cancer Inst., 66:1191-1308). Copies of that review were made available to all the participants at this meeting, and the structure of my lecture followed that of the review article so closely that there would be little point in reproducing it at length. Instead, I shall merely summarize a few of the major points, and outline their possible implications. Although the numerical data that I shall discuss relate only to the United States, their qualitative implications, in terms of cancer prevention, probably apply equally to most developed countries.

The four main points that I addressed were, first, why it is believed that cancer is largely an avoidable disease; second, whether there is really any reliable evidence, once the major sources of bias in the available data have been avoided, for any generalized increase in U.S. cancer rates over and above that which could plausibly be attributed to tobacco; third, what is known about the quantitative importance of the currently known or suspected causes of cancer in the U.S.; and finally (as an introduction to the round table discussion) what general implications are suggested by the first three conclusions which future research directions towards the prevention of human cancer best combine practicability and promise. The first three points depend on a review of reasonably well-established scientific knowledge, and can be considered in isolation from the possibly unjustifiable speculation inherent in the final point, where my aim was to suggest a certain approach and to learn from other people's reaction to it. All of these questions are dealt with at greater depth in our JNCI review, to which interested readers are referred.

1. Avoidability of the Majority of Human Cancer

The basic evidence that human cancer is largely an avoidable disease is that whenever different populations are compared, large differences in the onset rates (among people of similar age) of many types of cancer are observed. These differences are not (except for skin cancer, and perhaps also a few types of lymphatic neoplasm) chiefly of genetic origin, for: 1) the rates of particular types of cancer among people of similar age in different countries are closely correlated with certain social characteristics (and although these correlations do not suffice to tell us what the causes of these cancers are, they do suffice to tell us that these cancers have causes); and 2) cancer rates among the descendants of migrants from one country to another often resemble the cancer rates in the new country far more closely than they resemble the cancer rates in the country from which the migrants originated.

Comparison of lung cancer rates in America with rates in those parts of the world where lung cancer is least common suggests that about 90% of U.S. lung cancer might be avoidable, a conclusion that is reinforced by comparison of national U.S. lung cancer rates with the lung cancer rates observed in prospective studies of self-described U.S. non-smokers.

Likewise, comparison of the onset rates for cancer of the large intestine in the United States with the corresponding rates in those parts of the world where cancer of the large intestine is least common suggests that about 90% of all U.S. intestinal cancer might be avoidable, a conclusion reinforced by comparison of the rates among blacks in West Africa with the tenfold higher rates among blacks in the U.S.

The same is true for cancer of the breast; although it is common in America there are several other countries (particularly Japan) where it is so much less common as to suggest that the large majority of U.S. breat cancer might be avoidable, a conclusion reinforced by study of the high onset rates observed among Japanese who have been born and brought up in the United States. When, moreover, it is remembered that a quarter of a century ago Japanese breast cancer rates were even lower than they now are, it seems likely that nearly 90% of U.S. breast cancer might be avoidable.

Cancers of the lung, breast, and large intestine are currently the commonest types of cancer in the U.S., and collectively they account for half of all U.S. cancer deaths. The foregoing arguments suggest that each is largely an avoidable disease, although only for lung cancer are means of avoidance reliably known. Similar arguments, based on comparison between different parts of the world, can be adduced for the partial avoidability of many remaining types of cancer, though the percentages of these that appear to be avoidable are not all as extreme as the figures of about 90% suggested by the data on cancers of the lung, breast, and large intestine. Indeed, for stomach cancer (which is, in many parts of the world, the commonest neoplastic cause of death) the U.S. rates are among the lowest in the world, so comparison with other countries gives no evidence as to whether a large proportion of the U.S. stomach cancer deaths could be avoided. Ascribing on the basis of geographic comparisons suitable "numbers avoidable" for each type of cancer other than cancer of the skin leads, when these estimates are added up, to the suggestion that in the U.S. today about 75-80% of internal* neoplasms might be avoidable by means that some human population happens already to have adopted. The total percentage that is avoidable must presumably be even greater than this, and for some types of cancer (e.g., stomach, where U.S. rates are continuing to halve every generation) such comparisons must underestimate the proportion that is avoidable. Conversely, however, it is uncertain whether, once the means of prevention that underlie the geographic differences have been identified, they will prove socially acceptable, for there are many aspects of the lifestyle of the impoverished that affluent people would not willingly adopt.

Nevertheless, it is already known that one-third of all U.S. cancer deaths are due to tobacco, and it seems very reasonable to hope that, of the remaining two-thirds, at least half, and possibly more, will turn out to be avoidable by practicable means, either by mechanisms corresponding to those that underlie the existing international differences or in other ways. This conclusion (that at least 70%, and perhaps more, of all cancer is avoidable) has often been expressed as that 70, 80, or 90% of cancer onsets are due to "environmental factors" (which is acceptable only if it is understood that "environmental factors" includes not only everything one absorbs but also everything one does - for example, early pregnancy is an "environmental factor" that greatly decreases the mother's subsequent risk of developing breast cancer in old age). The same

---

*Geographic comparison of skin cancer rates are not valid, as genetic determinants of skin color influence them so profoundly, but the large majority of all U.S. skin cancer onsets are known to be due to the effects of strong sunlight on white skins. Fortunately, in view of the difficulty of controlling this type of exposure, cancer of the skin is easily treated and seldom fatal.

finding has also been mistakenly interpreted to mean that 70, 80, or 90% of cancer is due to environmental pollutants; this is not acceptable and there is no good evidence that it is true.

2. Lack of Generalized Increase of Cancer among Nonsmokers

Cancer is much more talked about nowadays than in previous decades, but this is not evidence that (apart from the delayed effects of tobacco) cancer rates among people of a given age are rising. For, public awareness is determined by the extensive media coverage of the growing body of cancer research; by the increasing willingness of cancer patients and their friends to discuss the disease rather than to hush it up; by the increasing number of people who live on into old age nowadays (for cancer rates are now, and always have been, far greater among the old than among the young); and by the decrease in the toll taken by most other fatal diseases (for, as the percentage of deaths that are due to other diseases falls, so the percentage of deaths that are due to cancer will automatically rise, even if cancer onset rates do not change). For these and various other reasons, one cannot take the increasing public awareness of cancer as evidence for increasing onset rates of cancer, and more objective data must be sought.

The assessment of trends in cancer onset rates is, however, more difficult than might be imagined, because standards of medical diagnosis and record-keeping change with the passage of time. Improvements in medical care particularly affect cancer death certification rates among old people, who might previously have died of cancer with the cause of death mis-certified as being some infective or (for cancer in or of the brain) neurological disease. They have, however, less effect on the trends in cancer death certification rates among people in youth or middle age, since for the past few decades it has been so unnatural for such people to die that the nature of their terminal illnesses have been reasonably thoroughly investigated. The true trends in cancer mortality may therefore be best assessed by the age-standardized trends among people under 65 years of age. Since there has, during the past quarter century, been little improvement in curative treatment for the common cancers (despite large improvements in the treatment of certain embryomal and/or diffuse neoplasms), these trends in cancer mortality rates among people under 65 give a reasonable indication of the true trends in cancer onset rates. Indeed, these trends in mortality may be even more accurate than the superficially more attractive trends in the total incidence (fatal plus nonfatal) of "cancer." For, the definition of what constitutes "cancer" may be evolving, with increasing numbers of lumps that are histologically "cancer" but biologically benign being sought, discovered, excised, and counted among the "cancer" statistics (even if, left alone, many such lumps would never have caused any serious trouble in that patient's remaining normal lifespan). Thus, of the various imperfect sources of data that are currently available to assess trends in cancer onset rates, the most reliable appears to be the study of the trends in age-standardized cancer death certification rates among people aged under 65 years (using, of course, population estimates that have been corrected for the variable degree of undercount that occurs in the U.S. census).

When this is done, there is clear evidence of a generalized increase, in both sexes, in cancers of the mouth, throat and respiratory tract (chiefly lung cancer, of course). This increase is, however, no larger than could plausibly be explained by the delayed effects of changes in U.S. smoking habits earlier this century, diluted by the effects of the more recent decreases in tar yields per cigarette. This is not to say that no environmental changes other than those in tobacco usage affect the trends in lung cancer (indeed, we know that some other effects are involved, the increasing effects of asbestos being one example), but it is to say that the trends in lung cancer do not of themselves offer any evidence for the recent emergence of any other large causes. Moreover, it is encouraging to note that among U.S. males aged under 50 lung cancer mortality is decreasing, due presumably in part to the decreasing yields of noxious chemicals per cigarette.

However, apart from these increases in mortality from cancers of those sites (mouth, throat, and respiratory tract) that are strongly affected by tobacco, there is no evidence of any generalized increase in U.S. cancer rates. A few sites are increasing (e.g., melanoma, and certain lymphomas), a few are decreasing (stomach, cervix, and, interestingly, bladder), many are roughly constant and no generalized increase is evident in non-respiratory cancer mortality among Americans aged under 65 years. This suggests that many of the important determinants (apart from tobacco) of U.S. cancer onset rates must be things that have characterized the U.S. lifestyle throughout much of this century. This is an extraordinarily strict, and hence useful, constraint on speculation (and it is not one which particularly implicates the sort of environmental pollutants that "risk estimation" is commonly concerned with).

What Do We Know Quantitatively about the Causes of U.S. Cancer?

Briefly, the only cause which is both large and reliably known is tobacco. In 1978 tobacco accounted for about 30% of all U.S. cancer deaths. This figure will rise to 33% by the mid-1980's and unless substantial changes in U.S. cigarette consumption or composition take place fairly quickly it will continue to rise steadily throughout this century (as may the probably even greater number of tobacco-induced deaths from non-neoplastic diseases).

The above-mentioned comparisons of the onset rates of various types of cancer in different parts of the world do, however, strongly suggest that some other large causes of cancer still await discovery in the U.S., and various quite plausible suggestions have been made about the possibility of a really large role for certain dietary, hormonal, or infective factors. But, although some of these suggestions may eventually be proved correct, at present definitive proof is still lacking.

Many other factors have been reliably shown to affect human cancer risks (alcohol, 3% of all U.S. cancer deaths; asbestos, 1-2%; sunlight, 1-2%; background radiation, 1-2%; effects of sexual activity on cancer of the uterine cervix, 1%; medical use of x-rays, 1/2%; other medical procedures, 1/2%; and so on), but none seem to cause a large percentage of the national total.

In short, apart from tobacco, all causes of cancer are <u>either</u> small <u>or</u> uncertain, although some large cause(s) probably still lie buried, awaiting discovery among some long-established aspect(s) of the American lifestyle. Partly by default of any particularly plausible alternative suggestions, and partly for more positive reasons (for review, see Section 5.3 of Doll and Peto, 1981, JNCI, 66:1191-1308), I suspect that dietary factors will prove the most fruitful category of agents among which to seek these important causes. But, the dietary factors that at present appear most plausible are perhaps not those that involve either ingestion or endogenous synthesis of traces of powerful carcinogens, but rather factors which affect the natural history of partially altered cells, affecting the probability that such cells will evolve into the seeds of neoplastic clones.

Implications for Future Research

If this view of the main determinants of current U.S. cancer rates is accepted, it certainly suggests that we have been paying too little attention to the relevance of nutritional factors to human cancer risks. However, whether or not the current effects of chemical carcinogens other than in tobacco smoke is at present small, this does not imply that the future effects of current chemical exposures will be small. So, it does not follow that we should greatly reduce our research into the likely effects of various pollutants of the workplace, of food, of air, or of water, although our continuing colossal ignorance about the causes of human cancer should make us extremely sceptical about any program of research which purports to offer, now or in the next few years, any method of direct estimation of absolute human cancer risks from any laboratory studies. A more realistic, though perhaps less saleable, aim of laboratory research might be to help regulators decide which dozen out of a hundred different pesticides to ban or to restrict, or to help committees on the safety of medicines to decide which few among the many alternative medicaments for some particular condition (e.g., avoidance of sunburn) to restrict. Laboratory research has helped and can continue to help agencies to frame prudent restrictions even in the absence of any direct estimate of human hazard. But (fortunately, in view of its shaky scientific basis) "risk assessment" is not a necessary part of the proper use of laboratory toxicology. It would be marvellous if human risk assessment for toxic chemicals could be reliably achieved from laboratory studies, but at present it cannot, nor do I expect it to be able to be achievable this century.

In Section 4.2 of our JNCI review we discussed certain ways in which the heuristic use that is already being made of laboratory data for priority setting rather than for risk estimation might be somewhat refined, and I shall conclude by drawing your attention to the excellent monograph that was published last year by the International Agency for Research on Cancer (IARC monographs, Supplement 2 (1980): Long-term and short-term screening assays for carcinogens: a critical appraisal). In this monograph, after a careful review of current knowledge, it was concluded that useful quantitative predictions of the carcinogenic potency of chemicals based on short-term laboratory tests were not possible even for <u>rodent</u> carcinogenicity, despite the fact that experiments with rodents have provided us with hundreds of reasonably reliable measurements of the carcinogenic effects of various chemicals. How much less reliable must predictions of <u>human</u> carcinogenicity be, where we have virtually no reliable quantitative measurements of the carcinogenic effects of chronic exposures to particular chemicals with which to calibrate our potency estimates? Also, there is no sound basis for expecting that rodent and human hazards will be approximately similar: they may be, but humans have had to evolve some extraordinarily effective biochemical strategies to allow most of us to escape cancer in a body a thousand times the size of a mouse for a lifespan thirty times longer than that of a mouse. These biochemical differences between mice and men are, of necessity, of enormous quantitative relevance to cancer risks, and they completely undermine the scientific basis for expecting (without direct evident) approximate similarity of absolute risks in mice and men exposed to particular chemicals.

ROUND TABLE: REASONS FOR DISTRUSTING HUMAN RISK ASSESSMENT BASED SOLELY ON *IN VITRO* OR ANIMAL TEST RESULTS

Leader: Richard Peto

Oxford University
U.K.

PETO

I apologize for having exploited my position as leader of what should have been a round table discussion deliberately to monopolize the first half of it, but you've had nearly two weeks to discuss what causes cancer in cells, and I wanted two hours to discuss what causes it in people.* Could I now invite comments not so much on the epidemiological perspective, which is probably more or less correct, but on my much less soundly based belief that risk assessment, by which I mean the estimation of *absolute* human risks from the results of laboratory studies, is not scientifically justifiable now or in the foreseeable future?

SETLOW

I would want to think about that carefully before I made any comment.

PETO

You've had two weeks in a meeting on human risk assessment. You must have some opinions as to whether it's a good idea or not.

---

*The lectures actually given comprised not the abbreviated text published here, but rather an extended account of much of what was in our JNCI review, to which interested readers are referred for the detailed arguments for any suggestions that, stated in isolation, may seem unconvincing.

SETLOW

Sure: I think it's a good idea.

PETO

By that you mean human risk assessment, trying to make some estimate of absolute cancer risks for humans based on laboratory studies?

SETLOW

Yes. We heard this morning from Dr. Osterman-Golkar some suggestions as to how to make internal dosimetric measurements in people for particular classes of carcinogens, such as the alkylating agents, and I think it will be possible to go from cellular studies to animal studies, knowing, for example, the number of adducts per unit of molecular weight of DNA, and make some estimate of human risk. I think this is perfectly possible. Unfortunately, we don't necessarily know everything about what to measure and, for a number of chemicals, we are still completely in the dark as to what to measure, but nevertheless, for a few of them, I believe we do know what to study. Therefore, even though they may be errors of factors of 10 or even more, I think it is useful to attempt to get some estimates of these numbers. If no-one tries, you'll never get an answer to your question.

PETO

But how is this to be calibrated against human risk? I would be very happy with tenfold errors; they would be fine, but how do you expect to get as close as tenfold errors in the foreseeable future? What measurements of human risk will you use to calibrate these laboratory findings?

SETLOW

I think we have estimates, or could get estimates, in the case of rodents, as to the risk of certain cancers; let's say the probability of getting cancer for a certain number of DNA adducts, and if we knew something about the lifetime of such adducts in rodents and in humans, I would say that the first extrapolation would be to assume that you have similar risks in the two instances. The extrapolation, however, would be based on a DNA-damage level and not on a measure of milligrams per kilo. I want to bypass all the activation, detoxification, etc., and use some estimate of the actual extent of damage in what we believe at the moment to be one of the target molecules. Of course, the unknown in all this is that all that we are measuring, when we measure effects on DNA, is what we believe to be the degree of cellular initiation, and the subsequent steps in carcinogenesis, about which we unfortunately know comparatively little, could amount to modulating factors which are overwhelming, such as 100 or a 1000. I'm just a believer that research will eventually enable us to determine something about these modulating factors. Nevertheless, if I found that in mice a certain level of adducts gave rise to a probability of 1% of cancer induction and that in humans we were observing a similar level of DNA adducts, I would be worried.

LEGATOR

I think that any time we put out an absolute number in this general area, we are probably going to be wrong. I suspect the best we can do is look at a number of different systems, knowing that we can make quantitative comparisons within each system of one chemical with another. However, the second we move up the order of biological complexity, a number derived from a simpler system is going to be totally wrong, perhaps by several orders of magnitude. Therefore, what I think we should do is what you suggested, and that is to set rough categories but go no further than that, and within each category to estimate a measure of concern. This proposal has already been made in the area of animal carcinogenicity by Bob Squire of Johns Hopkins.

PETO

I would tend to agree with that, of course. Dr. Setlow seems undisturbed really by the great difference between the human and the rodent lifespan and by the need for there to be real biochemical mechanisms behind those differences. I don't see how, with factors of thousands or millions floating around, you can start talking about risk assessment. This troubles me, really.

SETLOW

Sure, you're worried about the extrapolation from mice to people, and I'm worried about such an extrapolation, but I just sort of have faith that we are going to find out something about what determines the differences in the lifespans of mice and of people. We already know a number of differences between mice and people. Whether these are going to be the important ones there is no way of my saying at the moment. I just have confidence that things that are bad for mice are going to be bad for people, and it's going to be a question of developing, with certain chemicals that we know about, some sort of rules for extrapolation, even though the extrapolation may be over a factor of ten to the ninth.

PETO

The trouble is, I can't really foresee anything, at least within the next decade, being anywhere near a scientifically respectable basis for such an extrapolation. And the other thing that worries me about all this is that concentration on these chemicals, because we can measure them, may divert attention from what are at present the important determinants of human cancer. For example, I think that the concentration on a variety of chemicals has already diverted legislative attention away from tobacco, to the very considerable detriment of the national health. My fear is that this emphasis on the categories of chemicals which turn out to be active in rodent systems may be diverting attention from the really important factors which are at present the determinants of the big international differences between human cancer rates that already exist.

SETLOW

I couldn't agree more with what you are saying. Nevertheless, I think that there are experimental ways of approaching an extrapolation from rodent tissues to human tissues, and one of these ways has to do with the induction of neoplastic transformation in cells in culture, rodent versus human. It's well known that it is more difficult, experimentally at least, to transform human cells in culture. The reasons for that difference are not known, but nevertheless we will get some estimate of what the magnitude of that difference is, which is another extrapolation factor that in the next few years probably may become a rather firm number.

PETO

I should throw this discussion much more open. Who else wishes to contribute to this question, or perhaps to the more general question of, if we want to prevent cancer, what should the ways that we adopt include? We are devoting so much of our resources in cancer prevention to the investigation of mechanisms, the investigation of chemicals, etc., and so little to investigation of the reasons for the differences that currently exist between the different populations in the world today, although I suppose that is really out of the main line of the present workshop.

SAFFIOTTI

Some of the major items that were discussed at this course in the past ten days or so have dealt with the development of a large number of new research methods, many of which are addressed to defining conditions under which the effects of a variety of agents, chemicals, radiation, can be studied directly in human tissues and cells. This is not irrelevant, I think, to the point that you yourself are making, that it is important to be able to study differences in different populations. Many of us are experimentalists and I think we believe that the experimental method offers a lot in probing real, relevant mechanisms, not just to investigate an academic problem of what fancy mechanisms may occur. Studies of mechanisms can really be very useful to help identify cause-and-effect relationships. If we do not have more sophisticated methods to analyze differences between different human groups that have different responses to certain environmental, genetic, nutritional, and other changes, we will continue to argue without solid data. I think that what is encouraging to me in this field is that, as this course has shown, there are many stimulating new approaches to trying to, gradually and obviously with a lot of work, fill in the gaps of our knowledge as to how we might compare what happens to the Japanese in Hawaii and with what happens to them in Japan and in the U.S., to study what happens to the stomach mucosa in these people in different conditions, and all these other questions. Now, let me go on from there. I agree with the point, and I've expressed it before, that it is extremely difficult, and in many cases impossible, to arrive at reliable "risk estimates" from many of these environmental exposures, as far as human cancer risk is concerned. I have been at the same time emphasizing the importance of not ignoring qualitative risk assessment, again in the sense of trying to study interactions, early changes, model mechanisms, etc. There is again a growing awareness of similarities and some areas where differences are beginning to appear that allow us a much more discriminating insight into what to take as a good model for human carcinogenesis and what perhaps to take with a great deal of caution. In response to your point about priorities, are we almost doing ourselves a disservice by studying so many problems when there is one overwhelming problem, such as tobacoo, that should take all our energies? My reaction to that is that we do not really waste our time studying a variety of problems. The problem of tobacco is indeed well posed. A lot of the consequences for public health are consequences that are no longer in need of basic biological research in that area, so these are now political, economic, or sociological problems. I think that we as biologists cannot do much more to convince people that tobacco is indeed a carcinogenic factor. By this same token, one of the major points I made at the beginning of the course in discussing the framework of "risk assessment" is to give more importance than, for instance, even you are giving in the context of your own present ranges of risk estimates to overlap. We have discussed this on other occasions. This was one of the major points for which the famous, or infamous, report by people from several government agencies was written (Bridbord et al., 1978; reproduced as appendix to Banbury Report No. 9, Cold Spring Harbor Publications, New York), which was to draw the attention of people involved in this risk assessment to the fact that there were widely overlapping factors. Now the more I have been thinking about this problem since those days, the more I am convinced that we should not settle down for a relatively small overlap; I think in your range estimates (in Doll and Peto, JNCI 66, Table 20) even the higher ranges you give have only about a one-and-a-half cycle of overlap. I would anticipate many, many layers of overlap, genetic, nutritional and a number of other components including exposure to a variety of agents for which the causative role is more difficult to pin down.

PETO

Yes, when the causes of cancer are understood, then they'll probably add up to well over 100%; we discussed this in Section 4.4 of our JNCI review.

SAFFIOTTI

Then you will have many hundred percent. The advantage of recognizing that is that you don't have to worry about taking away something from one factor when you discover more about the role of others, because they all overlap. If you do find that there are indeed many more overlaps, I think you simply have more chance to intervene. You have given some examples of interactions that have already been demonstrated, tobacoo, alcohol, asbestos, radiation; there may well be many more. That doesn't mean that tobacco is not so important, but it means that there are other ways to intervene that may be useful in certain areas and have in fact been very useful already in certain areas in prevention.

PETO

The one point I would like to comment on in what you said is that you feel that there is a possibility, a likelihood, that laboratory investigations will develop good models for human carcinogenesis. I am much less hopeful about this for various reasons, one of which is that I have not seen yet good evidence as to which are the causative agents, the important causative agents, in tobacco smoke. There are substances there, it's been studied for 25 years and nobody can really say which are the important initiating agents and which are the important late-stage agents in tobacco smoke; although we do know that both are there and that they are probably qualitatively different. The failure to find it out even when you actually know where to look is not terribly encouraging.

Another thing is that we are still at a stage of ignorance where John Cairns (Nature 289, 353) is arguing that one particular category of translocational DNA lesion is important and other people say, no, it's point lesions. You can't even agree what category of DNA lesions is important. You don't know the important processes whereby, for example, early reproductive history affects breast cancer. I don't know where there are good models for the important processes of human carcinogenesis and even if they exist I don't know how we would recognize them.

I feel I'd like to plead in this context for a "black blox" approach, where you just say, look, the one thing I do know is that I am ignorant, and I am going to study the human body like a black box. I'm just going to find out what seems to correlate with the incidence of cancer in humans. If you have that philosophy, then one of your research directions (not to the exclusion of laboratory research) might be, for example, to store a few hundred thousand blood samples from apparently healthy people, store them for years and then find out who gets cancer and who doesn't; and then to go back to your stored blood samples and find out what in the stored blood sample - if anything - might have discriminated between those likely to get cancer and those not. Wherever this has been done, it has yielded results, but they have never been the results that the people setting up the blood samples were after. It has always yielded results that were completely out of line with what was expected. I fell that there is a need in this area for not only a laboratory approach but also a complete "black box" approach based on recognized ignorance. Does anybody want to make a final comment?

BOREK

I agree that the complexity of the animal system is really horrendous. That is the reason we have gone to the cellular systems where we study cell transformation. You can raise many doubts about cellular systems, and ask whether they include the actual mechanisms of what measure of transformation is the most appropriate end-point. The conversion of cells into having the potential for growth in agar may not be sufficient, because you really have to show that such cells are tumorigenic, and then you run into other problems. However, you can study *in vitro* the interaction among different agents, and synergism is of exceptional importance. I think one of the problems in whole-animal systems has been in recognizing and defining agents which interact to enhance carcinogenesis. And there I think the *in vitro* systems are very useful.

PETO

I'm sorry, I really have not at any point been trying to say the *in vitro* systems are not useful. I merely fear that there is an insufficient effort to step back from all this research and look at what is actually happening to human beings. I'm really not trying to discourage *in vitro* research, *in vivo* research, or whatever; I'm just trying to argue that sometimes it may be useful to treat the whole human much more as a "black box" than we have been doing up till now. I think perhaps, as it's now half past five, I'd better declare this discussion closed. Thank you very much indeed for your tolerance of my exploitation of it.

ROUND TABLE: QUANTITATIVE RELATIONSHIPS, IF ANY, BETWEEN HUMAN AND ANIMAL CARCINOGENESIS: BIOLOGICAL ASPECTS

Leader: J. D. Jansen

SIRM B.V., Group Toxicology
P. O. Box 162
2501 AN The Hague
Netherlands

JANSEN

I see that I am the first discussion leader who is not an expert and therefore I would like to introduce the discussion on Risk Assessment for carcinogenicity in general terms.

Life is a hazardous activity because there is an (almost) certainty for any newborn baby that eventually he or she will die. In Western countries, cancer is the cause of death for roughly 25% of the general population, so I put the risk of cancer to 1/4. This means that it is a great risk for everybody.

Although this risk applies to the general population, it does not apply equally to parts of the population, e.g., it did not apply to one particular group of distillers of B-naphthylamine who all developed bladder cancer. Although this is an extreme example, it does illustrate that occupational cancer can be a great risk also, and therefore is of the greatest importance in its own right even if it disappears as a noticeable risk after dilution over the general population. However, during this discussion, I would like to concentrate on population risk. Is our primary aim indeed to bring down cancer as a percentage of total deaths? For this purpose, the fate of Seventh Day Adventists in contracting colon cancer may be illustrative (Fig. 1).

Apparently, the Seventh Day Adventists are "spared" the fate of colon cancer appreciably longer than the normal population. However, at the end, the percentage of Seventh Day Adventists dying of colon cancer is slightly higher than the percentage of the American popu-

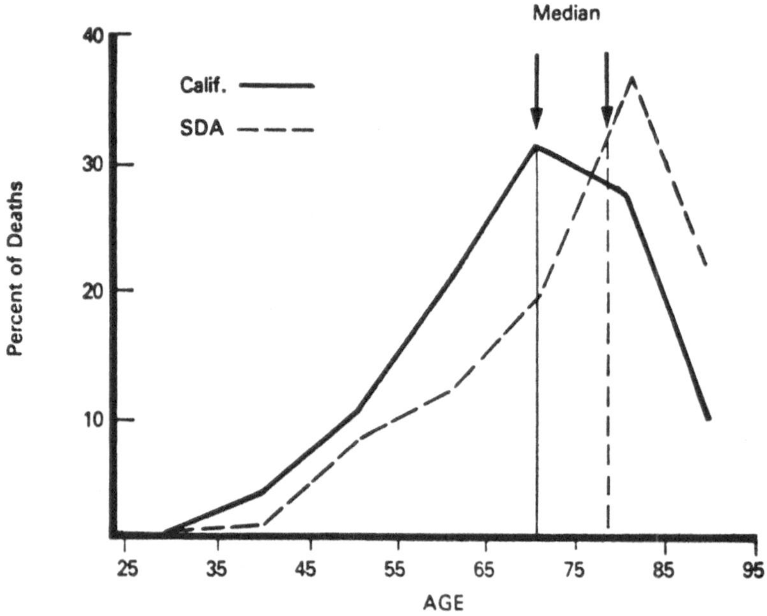

Fig. 1. From R. L. Philips, Cancer among Seventh Day Adventists, in: Cancer and the Environment, Demopoulos, Mehlman, eds., Pathotox Publishers, Inc., 1980.

lation. So perhaps a more practical primary aim should be to postpone cancer rather than to eradicate it (Table 1).

In order to start the dicussion, I have projected some, deliberately provocative, statements on what we do not know. Being provocative means that I feel myself, like a tightrope walker: I believe that my statements are not too far from true at the actual state of the art. However, they deliberately show one side only of the picture and therefore they are intended to give an unbalanced perspective. I hope that the discussion will yield the balance to this perspective. The reason for stressing our areas of ignorance is to arrive at a better sense of direction of future research - because many present areas of ignorance are not eternal and can be covered by presently available research techniques.

The provocative statements are the following: 1) Risk assessment of one single chemical is because of the added problems of metabolism a larger problem than the entire effort on risk assessment of ionizing radiation. 2) Risk assessment of a chemical on the basis of one test only, even if that is a NCI cancer study, is impossible. 3) DNA-alkylation as a simple test for the presence or absence of carcinogenic activity is now untenable. 4) Mutagenic

Table 1. Proportionate Mortality for California SDAs and all California Residents Age 35 and Over by Cause of Death, Both Sexes, 1958-1965

Cause of death	Percent of total deaths SDAs %	Calif. %
Disease of the heart	40.8	41.4
Coronary heart disease	30.1	32.3
Other heart disease	10.7	9.2
Malignant neoplasms	17.8	17.9
Colon-rectal cancer	2.9	2.5
Other malignant neoplasms	13.9	15.4
Cerebral vascular disease	12.9	12.0
Accidents and violence	4.8	6.2
Influenza and pneumonia	3.1	2.9
Diabetes	1.2	1.3
Arteriosclerosis	7.4	6.4
Cirrhosis	0.4	2.5

tests as simple tests for carcinogenicity are untenable. 5) There is no known relation between mutagenic tests and genetic disease. 6) There is no known human mutagen, not even radiation. 7) However, there are known human carcinogens.

I want to mention one more consideration on population cancer: in the USA and many other countries, stomach cancer incidence has rapidly diminished and cigarette induced lung cancer has rapidly increased. As a total age-adjusted cancer incidence is (almost) constant. This means that society has done something extremely well - without any scientific background or understanding - and something very bad (cigarette smoking), again with little scientific understanding of why this is so bad.

Dr. Saffiotti has shown a slide on a total number of chemicals known, total number of animal carcinogens known, ending with the few known human carcinogens.

In order to put these data in perspective, I construct now a slide on your daily food - roughly 1.5 kg/day. I am sure that anybody with a good chromatograph can identify, say, 100,000 chemicals in each single tomato or potato - although nobody yet has tried. I am equally sure that he could recognize at least 100 animal carcinogens in 1.5 kg of food. So that in this sense we are indeed living in a sea of carcinogens and moreover, in a sea of inhibitors and promotors.

The subject of the discussion is hoped to be: what direction should we go in science and society in order to achieve the goal of substantially lowering the cancer incidence which we all see around us? After some private discussions, I made a few rules for the discussion:

1) No experimental details. 2) No discussion of occupational cancer - this may sound strange but we want to discuss population cancer, we have not discussed occupational cancer during this course and we could easily spend the entire Round Table on occupational cancer only. 3) No discussion of laws or regulations - again, we could spend our entire time on that subject alone.

May I now invite comments?

SETLOW

I do not wish to comment in detail on the rules and guidelines you have put up except to point out one. The world of physical science has advanced a great deal by constructing theories because, for example, you cannot test every instance of an object falling toward the surface of the earth. And just as in physical science we also have rules in biological science and we have heard some of these rules today. The biological rules that govern replication, transcription, translation hold for all biological systems we know of. So it should be possible, if there is any regularity in biology, to find out something about lower systems and to extrapolate to higher systems. The fundamental laws of biology as applied to mice also apply to man.

JANSEN

I completely agree with you; the statements were not put up to show how bad we are but as a point of departure to see how we should go from here. In this context, I would like to emphasize that at no time have we had so many exquisitely sensitive tests and methods available and that some of the newest methodology enables us to go down to DNA and individual differences in DNA. I am certain that these powerful tools will lead to great discoveries, in mutagenesis, carcinogenesis or whatever entirely unsuspected direction. So these methods are fully justified in their own right. But I would like to discuss how we should go from this excellent scientific base into the direction we all want to go, i.e., a diminishing risk of cancer for the entire population in the face of so many possible hazards. How to pick out the real ones? And where should we look for them?

LEGATOR

We make a definite error by making absolute statements where data is lacking and inferring because of lack of data that there is no effect. In reality we do not have information to draw any conclusions. You say there is a not known relation between mutagenic agents and genetic diseases in the population. The real question is do we have the tools or the methods to determine if a chemical can indeed induce genetic disease. I would suggest that at the present state of knowledge we do not have the information to conclude that there may not be an effect.

I would suggest that information on increase in spontaneous abortions among wives whose partners were exposed to halothane may give us cause for concern, this is analogous to the dominant lethal effect in animals. Now in the area of chemical carcinogens we know that there are 12 known human carcinogens and about 4000 carcinogens that are known to be active in animals. Of the 4000 animal carcinogens how many have been studied in man? To conclude what percentage of these 4000 animal carcinogens are active in man is impossible without the epidemiological data that we cannot obtain. Among those 4000 chemicals I think it is probably safe to assume that a significant number of them are carcinogenic in man. Looking at the 12 known human carcinogens all of them could have been picked up in animal studies with the possible exception of trivalent arsenic. Therefore we can already say that the animal model has proved to be a fairly good qualitative indicator for human carcinogens. I do not however believe that the quantitative extrapolation from animals to man is meaningful.

My bottom line is: a) if we don't have evidence for something it doesn't mean that it doesn't occur, b) we probably can't wait for epidemiological data, and c) we have systems that will detect at least qualitatively chemicals that are potentially hazardous to man.

JANSEN

I agree with what you say, except in your reference to epidemiology coming too late. If you discuss public policy on the introduction of new chemicals, I fully agree that epidemiology cannot help. However, I feel that the importance of epidemiology, as a science, is vastly underrated.

Much of this discussion is intended to be an introduction to the talk of Dr. Peto. I have mentioned the decreasing incidence of stomach cancer in order to indicate that it is possible to do something about it - if only we knew how we did it. Epidemiology does not come too late for the cancer which has always been with us and for exposures which have existed for several decades. I completely agree that the fact that we know only about 12 human carcinogens does not mean that there are no more. For instance, I find it hard to believe that some nitrosamines would not be carcinogenic in humans sufficiently exposed. However, I feel it is still questionable whether nitrosamines actually cause an important number of cancer cases in man at the levels now encountered in the environment. This is still a question of very important research. During that research, we have to keep in mind what Dr. Setlow said, i.e., that there is unity of biologic behavior and there are problems which can much better be studied in bacteria or mice than in man. However, there are also major species differences and therefore to my mind human experience is still the ultimate arbiter of the validity of our test systems.

The availability of cancer registries has directly led to the discovery of the two major cancer hazards in man, i.e., cigarette smoking and our daily diet. Americans may not realize that in most European countries, with the exception of the UK and Scandinavia, a rigid separation is made between the registry of the personal mortality data and the purely statistical registry of causes of death. It is therefore not unexpected that good epidemiological studies in Europe are almost entirely confined to the UK and the Scandinavian countries. I am sure that having good registries also in countries such as Holland, Germany, and France would immensely enrich and speed up the discovery of factors of major importance for the cancer incidence.

I feel equally strongly that we should have registries of genetic disease if we want to break the now existing barrier between mutagenic tests and genetic disease, even if the difficulties in starting them are obviously scientifically and practically greater. If epidemiology is not fostered, then after 20 years of testing we would still be as wise or unwise as we are now. That is why I feel that especially the institutional and legal ways to promote epidemiology have been sadly neglected and even thwarted by the otherwise quite legitimate drive for the safeguarding of privacy.

WATERS

I would like to ask you, Dr. Jansen, to clarify your third point that mutagenesis tests as simple tests for carcinogenic activity are untenable.

JANSEN

Fortunately, I have underlined simple. I think I can argue it scientifically that there are too many carcinogens which have no or hardly any mutagenic activity.

WATERS

Are you thinking primarily of the human carcinogens?

JANSEN

Also, some of the human carcinogens, yes. Further there are now a number of mutagens which are not carcinogenic, for instance, quercetin. I do not say that there is no relation between mutagenesis and carcinogenesis. Certainly at this stage there is no scientifically definable causal relation between the two. Personally, I feel that there are too many tests which indicate that there may be a hazard: that we know already without testing. However, I do not know of tests which will pick up the future asbestos or benzenes and that is what is required.

WATERS

Would you not say that the results which have been discussed at this meeting on, for example, AF-2 the Japanese food additive or the results that have been obtained in short-term tests on "tris" which causes us to re-examine our position in terms of carcinogenic potential represent examples of the utility of these mutagenesis test systems?

JANSEN

AF-2 is a perfect example of the difference between reasonable public policy and scientific facts. Although I do not know all the data, I feel that the public policy of the Japanese was probably very wise. However, good public policy does not make AF-2 a human carcinogen which would be a scientific fact.

WATERS

I don't quite understand your position because apparently it was believed that the tests were positive, the action was taken to remove these chemicals. Do you not believe the results of the test or did Sugimura feel that the results were a convincing lead for public policy?

JANSEN

They are two completely different questions. There is the question whether AF-2 has indeed been an actual hazard in Japan. This is important of course but there is no way of finding that out. In the presence of the information they had I would feel it irresponsible public policy if they had not taken it off the market. That doesn't mean that they have proven a scientific fact. That is a completely different question.

WATERS

I agree with your conclusion. What concerns me is that there seems to be implicit in these arguments, the feeling that we have to wait to see the effect in man before we can feel comfortable that we have identified the problem. And I think that is an unfortunate position if that is true.

JANSEN

In setting public policy you cannot wait until all the scientific understanding has been achieved - you would hardly need public policy if that was the case. Personally, as a citizen, I would hope sincerely that the regulators would not wait until everything is fully understood. However, equally, public policy should not act on the basis of clearly insufficient evidence or on the basis of entirely unvalidated scientific concepts: if we really do not know - why act? Public policy is something quite different from scientific discovery: I have previously discussed aflatoxin. I feel it is a valid scientific speculation that aflatoxin may be only a weak carcinogen in humans (although Dr. Cerutti in his latest work may well have disproved that speculation). At the same time, I very strongly feel that the regulators have followed the only sensible and wise strategy to deal with the problem in the Western countries and as a citizen, I would have felt disturbed if they had ignored the problem and ignored the very persuasive facts. However, again, that excellent policy does not prove that aflatoxin is a potent human carcinogen. I still feel that proof has not yet been obtained. To us in developed countries, such a discussion is merely an academic exercise. To underdeveloped countries the ultimate scientific answer may be a vital matter.

SAFFIOTTI

There are several points I would like to comment on. One of the difficulties in this area is to try and look at the state of our knowledge without excessive generalizations.

I think that some of the statements that you have put on the board, I am sure intentionally, as provocative statements, would be more appropriate if tuned down to be less drastic, because in several of these areas we do have extensive information from experimental studies that have gone part of the way in clarifying some of these problems. To say there is no known relation between mutagenic and carcinogenic activity is too drastic a statement. In the relation between mutagenic tests and genetic disease there is a lot of research that has qualified areas of knowledge and distinguished what we know and what we don't know. Certainly there are areas in which we still don't know many aspects and that prevents the entire picture from being clarified. One point is "let's be careful with drastic statements that can be misinterpreted," as you yourself pointed out. That doesn't mean we don't know anything: we know a lot, so let's try to qualify that point.

Some of the problems I wanted to bring up concern the first part of your talk where you referred to the epidemiologic situation and pointed out that death risks involve a risk of 100%, and cancer death risks about 25%. You deal here with total population studies and some of the examples you have given are very important pertinent aspects of such total population trends, for example, the downward trend of stomach cancer and the upward trend for lung cancer in several countries.

I have been often concerned whether we are not obscuring some more specific trends as they may develop in more select population groups which are better defined biologically than those obtained by taking a whole large mixed population, such as the entire population of the USA, with over 200 millions, which includes all kinds of ethnic backgrounds and all kinds of climatic, nutritional, geographic, occupational and cultural differences, and lumped together. The fact that, with the exception of two types, the overall cancer incidence appears somewhat steady may in fact represent an averaging out of a lot of differences. If you look into specific subgroups by sex, by age, by geographic area, or by many other factors, you do find a number of cancer types whose incidences go up or go down in different ways. In fact, in some cases, you have very marked trends one way or another.

So I am more and more skeptical as to the value of using studies on very heterogeneous large populations for the purposes of understanding what is going on in carcinogenesis. On the stomach cancer story, allow me a personal speculation. It is true that this is a major form of cancer that has gone down and that we don't know how to explain this finding; but suppose that it were a more general trend for other cancer types, and that we were doing a lot of things right: it may be that many other cancers would equally have gone down had we not continuously introduced other factors that were in fact themselves carcinogenic and which counteracted these downward trends to make their incidence stay up. Why is not cancer of the colon going down as much as cancer of the stomach? Maybe it would have gone down as much, had we not created more and more cancers of the colon by introducing more carcinogenic factors, e.g., new chemicals in the environment. We don't know that this is so, but we can't generalize, from the very broad overviews given by mixed population studies, directly to a pathogenetic hypothesis.

JANSEN

I fully agree with your comments on the pitfalls of dealing with large populations only and of considering overall cancer incidence instead of incidence of cancer of specific sites. I also fully agree that population incidence is of no interest to the workers who could possibly be exposed to a very substantial cancer hazard in their - relatively small - manufacturing plant. Therefore, these have to be looked at and studied separately. However, only on the basis of a well designed cancer registry, will all this become possible. On the incidence of colon cancer, I might mention an alternative hypothesis which is more easily testable: if regulatory authorities (quite rightly at the time) had not kept the amount of antioxidants in food to technologically necessary levels, it could be that colon cancer might have decreased as much as stomach cancer incidence.

LEGATOR

I would like to turn to point 3. "Our mutagenic tests are not very reliable in terms of tests for carcinogenic activity." I believe that under that point you suggested that there are many mutagens that are not carcinogens and frankly I cannot think of many. The example that you gave was a quercetin which is the work of Sugimura, as I recall indicate a highly active compound in the Ames test. Very little other studies were done in animal systems and then it was found to be non carcinogenic. I would suggest that this would be possibly an analogous case to benzene where all of the in vitro studies are uniformally negative but where we have very good animal data in terms of the cytogenetic endpoint. The fallacy here is to equate mutagenicity with the bacterial test. I could construct 65 to 100 chemicals and say there is no correlation between carcinogenicity and mutagenicity but that was based on a simple in vitro test. Those same compounds when tested by additional tests specifically in animals would be positive. Again I think that the mutagenic tests have served us well when we look at the totality of activity in many tests and do not dwell on any single test.

JANSEN

I agree and I fully agree with the remarks of John Ashby on the predictive power of validated mutagenic tests for the carcinogenicity of, e.g., new aromatic amines. I agree that mutagenic tests are or can be a very important facet in a much wider research program. I feel that the real significance of Cairn's recent publication is that he is able to suggest that entirely different compounds may be responsible for cancer in man than those identified by mutagenic tests without immediate and cogent contradiction: the facts are simply not there. We simply do not yet understand the real importance of DNA-alkylation: it may be very important outside carcinogenesis. Certainly, whenever definite proof of its importance in carcinogenesis was tried (admittedly not yet frequently) it has failed. This makes it impossible to regard DNA-alkylation as either sufficient or necessary for initiation of cancer.

SETLOW

If I could make my point of view clear. I agree with your call for better epidemiology, but epidemiology has two faces to it. One is the enumeration of human disease. That enumeration by itself is useless unless one has a comparable enumeration of the environmental circumstances or what I would call the dose that gives rise to that human condition. Our difficulties in most circumstances are that we may be able to measure human disease but we have no idea as to the dose that gives rise to it.

I give two examples from my own experience. One is the relation between human cancer and ionizing radiation. Unfortunately the major data relating these two come from an accident - the dropping primarily of a bomb. The doses involved are in question even more so in present than in past times and the doses that are known are distributed over populations. Moreover, the observations of cancer arising from ionizing radiation are usually confined to high doses - doses that we would not normally anticipate receiving in the chemical world except from a gross accident. So we may never be going to get an answer perhaps from epidemiology, and as a matter of fact a recent NCR report (FREIR) has said that epidemiological studies on ionizing radiation exposure are probably useless unless the doses are very high, and we may not have such cases to study.

The second example has to do with the increased incidence of malignant melanoma especially among Scandinavian populations, especially Norway, indicating that melanoma incidence is increasing at the rate of about 7% per year over the past 20 years. But no one has any idea as to the cause, the dose that gives rise to this epidemic of malignant melanomas. There are many hypotheses. The favorite is that they spend more time going to southern Spain to take their vacation and so get more sunlight. But that is only a hypothesis. What I am trying to emphasize is that this is an important disease and it is important to enumerate it, but we have no idea as to the dose. We have only half of the dose-response relation - the response but no dose. We don't even know that malignant melanoma arises from exposure to sunlight. Part of the reason for this gap in our knowledge is the fact that there is no good animal model for light induced melanoma.

Let me make other comments on your list just so that you will see my point of view. You say the assessment of one single chemical requires more work than the entire effort of radiation. I think that is an exaggeration. A fantastic amount of work has gone on with radiation and part of the problems in dealing with it is that we know very little about the products that are formed, whereas with chemical agents we have a good way of determining something about the products, primarily by immunological procedures for determining concentrations of products in DNA. I suspect that alkylation, even though there may be complications to its measurement, will yield answers long before radiation, at a minute fraction of the money spent on radiation.

Mutagenic tests as tests for carcinogenic activity imply the hypothesis that damage to DNA may be initiating events in carcinogenesis. That is not meant to imply that there are not many other steps in the carcinogenic process. What one is really looking at when you look at mutagenic compounds is compounds that have the ability to react with DNA. Compounds that react with DNA are by their very nature bad. There is no question about it. They change the base sequence, they change replication, they change the transcription. The question is how bad are they? That really gets to be a public policy question that I don't wish to get into but there is no question that agents that react with DNA are bad. I, for one, would not willingly swallow compounds that have been shown to be strong mutagens or carcinogens in any animal or bacterial test systems.

BOREK

I would just like to amplify Dr. Setlow's point of view on the radiation aspect. I think it is wrong to take it as a simple agent. Although the effects of radiation do not require metabolism such as you have with chemicals, there exist a variety of complexities related to different latency periods depending on the target tissue and sometimes age. For example, a young thyroid is much more sensitive to ionizing radiation than aged thyroid. Thus there are many aspects which one has to consider when evaluating the effects of radiation, some of them similar to those monitored for chemicals.

JANSEN

I agree with all the differences of carcinogenic activity of radiation in relation to, e.g., age, rate of exposure, etc. However, I suspect that the same may apply to chemicals as soon as we start investigating such differences. But chemicals are not usually investigated in that way.

Regarding Dr. Setlow's comments, I agree. Epidemiologic investigations are no panacea to solve all our problems in the absence of further experimental research and testing. However, currently, I see a great gap between the grossly unexploited epidemiologic research and experimental research and I do believe that a close cooperation between these aspects would yield great dividends. After Dr. Setlow's citing of the difficulties of interpreting epidemiologic research, I will cite an example of neglected opportunities: the Netherlands happen to have more precise nutritional data over a longer period than any other country. However, due to the absence of a scientific cancer registry this wealth of nutritional information cannot be correlated with cancer incidence data.

KOTTARIDIS

I would like to make a statement and also like to ask a question. A few years ago it was found that some particular hair dyes were mutagenic. Of course there was no proof or it wasn't proven that these compounds were carcinogenic. In this case would it be justified to let these products circulate among millions of women and men in this case because men dye their hair occasionally, or would we consider it better public policy to withdraw these compounds from the market or to remove these compounds from some of the dyes as it was the case?

JANSEN

Personally, I do not know too much about the data on hair dyes. Certainly, to obtain relevant toxicological evaluation must be difficult. I thought there were several discrepancies between mutagenic test results on some of the hair dyes and the results of carcinogenic tests. I gather that several components have been changed for non-mutagenic components and some animal carcinogens deleted from the formulae: that seems successful public policy to me and a reasonable satisfactory sense of direction for the industry. I understand that there is no epidemiologic indication of a real hazard but that epidemiology is inherently difficult to do in this area. However, the intense publicity, scaring women unnecessarily and the attempts in some countries to ban some components on the basis of one microbiological mutagenic test only seems to me exaggerated and wrong.

LEWIS

The way in which you have worded many of your statements has very conveniently put us into the position of being absolutely correct about any of our tests. Now I will use the example of DNA alkylation, because I work in that area. Your statement requires, if I wish to thoroughly answer it, for me to prove DNA alkylation to be the absolute test and indicator of all time. I would like to turn the tables on you and have you convince me beyond any doubt that DNA alkylation has nothing to do with carcinogenesis. This would put you in the same position that many of us find ourselves in responding to these types of worded statements.

JANSEN

Thank you very much, I fully agree with you. Yet, I feel that my outspoken bias is as useful for finding out the limits of our knowledge as the more customary bias.

PARODI

I have the impression that perhaps there is a way of looking at the relationship by mutagenicity for instance in the Ames test, and carcinogenicity, from a quantitative point of view. We could find a way of measuring carcinogenic potency in animals; it is perfectly true that there are many many problems, but at least we can try. We can start, as many people have started (for instance, Meselson and Russell), taking in consideration the animals bearing at least one tumor and, on the bases of the multistep progression of the tumors, use some formula, to give an index of carcinogenic potency. We can try to compare these carcinogenic potencies in the animals with the potencies in the mutagenicity test. There are many pitfalls in this way of proceeding but, at least, it is an operational way. Not only do I think that this is pretty much possible, but I think also that there are already preliminary results on groups of 50-60 compounds where mutagenic potency in the Ames test was compared with carcinogenic potency. Unfortunately, from what I am aware of in these cases, in terms of the correlation coefficient r and in terms of regression line between the two logs of the potencies, the correlation was relatively poor. r was around 0.4 and 90% confidence limits were so large that practically they were including a large range of carcinogenic potencies. Let's say a range of 40,000 times. In conclusion, we have probably the means of studying the quantitative relationship between mutagenicity in the Ames test and carcinogenic potency, even if I think it is true that the first results suggest that the correlation is relatively poor.

SAFFIOTTI

I would like to follow up, as I usually do when I hear the word "potency," with some comments. "Potency" is basically a very difficult, for me almost impossible, concept to use practically, because potency obviously is intended as a measure of an interaction of the chemical with a biological target: therefore it varies with the variation in the biological target. Depending on a variety of biological targets, you can attribute almost any "potency" to a given chemical depending on what biological measurement you choose. Particularly for carcinogenicity, which is dependent on so many factors besides the chemical itself to express the neoplastic response, you can have very high and very low levels of activity for the same chemical just by varying the host system, whether it is an animal or a cellular system in vitro. So all the attempts that were made, starting with Meselson and Russell and continued by Ames's group, to establish direct correlations between response in a test system and a theoretical "potency" level, I think are really destined to prove that the hypothesis is untenable, because the problem is too complex to be simply reduced to a single numerical correlation. If some day we could narrow it down to a very precise measurement of the critical molecular interactions (that we still don't know how to define), then perhaps we will have a different and more specific set of data to relate.

At the present time, I think that we must specify what is the carcinogenic activity in what system, by what route, with what co-factors, with what nutritional state, what sexual, hormonal, environmental modifiers that can be brought in and could give you data so different that they would overlap widely the different orders of magnitude that are used in the classification of "potencies." Some people are now suggesting an order of magnitude classification of carcinogens and even that might be a very dangerous thing to do unless one defines it much more narrowly within certain biological systems and within certain methodological confines. The more you narrow the biological system that is used for these comparisons the more the internal comparisons are valuable. It becomes more difficult to extrapolate between two entirely different systems such as to a human population.

LEGATOR

We know with chemicals, as you stated, we can certainly spend many life times determining the specific mode of action. In the case of aflatoxin where the initial adduct is not the important one, indeed the important adduct may be transitory. One could come to all sorts of erroneous conclusions with very fine basic studies. I suspect that what we really need is operational tests that will tell us if we have activity in terms of final expression of the mutagenic activity. With most of the chemical carcinogens we really don't know the exact molecular action, we really don't know the basic mechanism of action. For instance, one can look at a compound like halothane and it doesn't make much difference if this compound is operating in a conventional way, causing mutations or if it is causing any chromosome aberrations by affecting spindle mechanism. The result as to different mechanisms may be the same. I think one of the most important questions is what kind of information must we generate and at what level to draw meaningful conclusions. I am afraid that if we wait to know exactly the mode of action for all our chemicals, we will do absolutely nothing. The trick is to determine the minimum amount of information that we have to generate from our various tests to take action.

JANSEN

I fully support Dr. Saffiotti with his remarks on potency: I do not know all the data but experimentally I doubt whether B-naphthylamine or smoking can be regarded as potent carcinogens. Nevertheless, the former was possibly the most devasting occupational health hazard and the latter, possibly after diet, the most important single cause of cancer.

Therefore, I have also great difficulties in relating experimental potency to human hazard which is the aim of all our work.

SAFFIOTTI

I would like to add on to this dicussion to emphasize how in many cases the kinds of correlations we can best make are qualitative correlations. They involve comparability of certain mechanisms of action, of certain measurable effects, of the pattern of response (e.g., in tissues and cells of animal test species versus the human, or even in isolated cell systems of different origin). Qualitative correlations can tell us that we seem to be within the same type of response, that we are not too far different. I think that in the case of many of the major types of carcinogens we now have a reasonable extensive data basis that shows how certain biological systems are fairly closely related to others and ultimately to the human, in terms of metabolic pathways, in terms of enzyme induction, in terms of intracellular localization of carcinogens and in terms of pathogenetic response in animal and human tissues. I think that there are now many good models that show how you can actually induce this main progressive sequence of events that leads a normal tissue to become neoplastic under the effect of a given chemical exposure in different biological systems. For the problem of risk assessment, I think it is important that we emphasize how useful it can be to do more research at all these levels. It certainly takes time and effort and resources to do this research. But let's think of the lengthy controversies and administrative and legal procedures that have often been required for decisions on environmental control, in the absence of good qualitative data: they have required enormous expenditures of money and manpower that could have been spent by our society to obtain better data in research that would have solved the problems at hand more readily and more logically.

One of the difficulties I have found is that a lot of people tend to equate the concept of risk assessment with that of quantitative numerical risk assessment, i.e., they want to come down to a number. We should try and build up an awareness of the fact that there is a qualitative component to risk assessment and that can be the most reliable basis we have at the present time. I think we can go further by trying to understand better the comparability at the biological level than by trying to pin down specific numbers. I think this understanding has underlined many of our discussions. I mentioned some of these points at the beginning of the meeting, but Dr. Setlow and some of the other participants were not here yet, and this is why I repeat some of these concepts, perhaps to stimulate their discussion of these points. I think we should emphasize that risk assessment in some cases, whether it is for chemicals or for physical agents, could be just qualitative and not quantitative in precise terms.

JANSEN

I was thinking that I should have added more statements: a) We do risk assessment daily and we are not too bad in this game. However, such assessment is always based on a number of quite different considerations which ultimately all go back to human experience. b) Consequently, formalized risk assessment based on a fixed line of thought seems entirely impossible but wise risk assessment is not necessarily impossible - unfortunately, that cannot be described in regulations and formalized test procedures. Further, it must be stated that perfect legislation is not possible and is not even a practical goal. However, the important consideration is whether it steers society in a desirable direction and whether there is a mechanism to check whether single decisions were bad or not. Legislation as well as science should be able to profit from its own mistakes!

PARODI

I agree that it is impossible to establish a correlation between the carcinogenicity in humans and carcinogenicity in animals because the epidemiological studies present tremendouse problems with the question of the dose. However, I think it can at least be explored if, when we compare short-term tests and carcinogenicity in animals, we have only qualitative correlations, such that saccharin and aflatoxin B_1 are the same thing or, if we have a more quantitative relationship. I think that this can at least be explored. It is quite possible that we come out with the answer that the correlation is so poor, at least at the present stage, that we cannot distinguish between saccharin and aflatoxin B_1, but at least we can explore how the things are from a quantitative point of view.

GOULD

I agree with Dr. Saffiotti that it is not going to be easy to put a potency value on everything. However, if we take the case of radiation, we know that qualitatively it is a risk. If we are unwilling to estimate a potency value then it becomes impossible to balance the risks and benefits of radiation in formulating public policy. The same would occur with any environmental contaminant that we do not generate a potency value for. A second point is that potency should not be a simple value but should also take the shape of the dose-response curve into account. This will better let us extrapolate our experimental data to man.

LEGATOR

I think we have examples of where we have formulated public policy without relying on specific numbers. Let me give you examples. In the case of aflatoxin obviously to work towards a zero tolerance since it is a potent carcinogen. However, we accept a certain amount because if we go below specific levels we will do away with the corn crop. This is an example of where the biological information and any quantitative extrapolation is not a factor in determining permissible levels. We are tolerating aflatoxin because the consequence of not tolerating it would be far worse. Another example would be vinyl chloride. It is impossible to know if 5 parts is much safer than 1 part per million. The decision on the permissible level in the workplace was based on technological considerations, i.e., on how low we could go without eliminating V.C. I would contend that in the majority of cases we take the biological information, possibly pay some attention to potency, but the actual amount we allow is usually a social, economic and even engineering decision. Biology plays a less important role than we think in terms of actual permissible exposure. There are other factors that usually play a principal role in this kind of decision.

MONTI BRAGADIN

Do we believe that each human cancer is caused by something, chemicl or radiation, or do you suppose that strictly "spontaneous" cancers exist, which are the result of the way the human body is organized? Furthermore, do you believe that such a question is relevant to this discussion or not?

JANSEN

I fear that your question is so important that you could fill an entire symposium trying to give approximate answers. May I give one example of the difficulties: the effect of early menarche on breast cancer incidence is well established epidemiologically. Early menarche is again dependent on the quantity and composition of food which again influences hormone production. Now, what do we call "cause" or "secondary cause?" Except for some occupational cancers and some cancers caused by drugs it is semantically difficult to assign one single cause, although sometimes you can assign a main cause.

SAFFIOTTI

I would like to comment on this point which is a very important one because in the evaluation of risk assessment, which is our main subject of concern at this meeting, we tend to relate risk evaluations to individual factors and I think there is a general agreement that we have concurrent causative factors of a different type. A good example of this point was given when Dr. Kraemer showed data on xeroderma pigmentosum patients that had been shielded from sunlight. The area of the skin which was shielded did not produce tumors. A photograph of the young XP man, who is now about 20 years old who has so far been thoroughly shielded, showed he is completely tumor free. In such a case we can say that skin cancer is a genetically determined by a physical external agent, ultraviolet light. They are both true statements. There are probably other factors we don't know yet how to define with certainty, e.g., nutrition. What is the causative factor? It is the combination of all these factors. When we talk about risk, the point I made on the first day, in emphasizing the overlapping causative factors, is that probably no single factor could be given even near a 100% causative burden, because there would always be room for some of these others. As for the discussion about spontaneous versus induced cancer, I always remember the comment made by Dr. Hueper, who was the pioneer in the field of environmental cancer at the National Cancer Institute, about "spontaneous" cancer: he would always say: "That is the wrong term, we should say cryptogenetic!"

JANSEN

I fell that it is the basis of scientific progress to try to establish causal relationships. You may well establish several causal factors. You may also find modifying factors. I do not know how well we will succeed with cancer, but I fell that Doll and Peto have convincingly shown that we have come a long way already, not yet in finding single causes of cancer but in grossly defining the main causes of cancer. I do hope that this gross understanding will also be reflected in the direction of experimental research because it is the combination and critical interaction of epidemiologic and experimental results from which the most important progress may be expected to come.

ROUND TABLE: QUALITATIVE AND QUANTITATIVE PROBLEMS IN THE EXTRAPOLATION OF RISK TO HUMANS FROM ANIMAL DATA

Leader: U. Saffiotti

Lab. of Exper. Path.,Div. of Cancer Cause and Prevention

National Cancer Institute, Frederick, Maryland

SAFFIOTTI

The task of this round table is to address qualitative and quantitative problems in the extrapolation of risk to humans from animal data. The emphasis is therefore on the extrapolation from animal studies to human risk as distinct from the extrapolation from human cells to human populations; but I believe that we will probably be able to discuss the whole area to some extent. The round table will be followed by some specific presentations and maybe we will have some time at the end for a general discussion. I would like to ask the participants to feel free to address questions to the speakers of the day on any problems that we did not have time to discuss after the individual presentations.

I would like to start with some brief general comments on the problems of risk extrapolation, especially as they concern the extrapolation from animal data to the human. We have tried, this morning, to put the accent on the rapid development of human tissue studies which are beginning to fill the gap between animal and human situations, but in many cases we don't have quite enough data from such studies to interpret them in terms of risk assessment. Therefore, we still have to make some judgements on the basis of correlations between data obtained strictly in animal systems and risk estimates in human populations.

This problem has been extensively debated in Europe and in North America and to some extent also in other countries, and several groups have worked to construct at least some conceptual approach to these various aspects. For example it took a long time to identify clearly the distinction between quantitative and qualitative risk assessment procedures, although they really belong to obviously related, but different, spheres of concerns. The qualitative aspects are, in a sense, easier to deal with in terms of relating the findings in one area of toxicology to the corresponding risk assessment, but they may still be difficult when they cover a broad range of complex biological phenomena. The quantitative aspects, on the other hand, may be deceptively easy from a methodological point of view. If we were to choose among a restricted number of mathematical models and make our calculations on this basis alone, the problem would appear simpler, but it becomes really very difficult if we try to go beyond these simple calculations to attempt a real assessment of the intrinsic risk involved in very different and complex biological situations. I would like to refer to a report prepared by the Risk Assessment Working Group of the Interagency Regulatory Liaison Group (IRLG). This is a governmental interagency group that has worked intensively in the last few years to develop common sound bases for the criteria to be used in scientific evaluations of carcinogens by the regulatory agencies in the U.S. This report, entitled "Scientific basis for identification for potential carcinogens and estimation of risks"(JNCI 63:241, 1979), has represented an attempt to analyze all these different aspects.

I would like briefly to refer to its last part, which deals with the problem of quantitative extrapolations (or at least attempts at quantitative extrapolations) based on data from an animal system or from a particular epidemiological study in a limited population, which then need to be extrapolated to a large or to a different human population, for example the population of a whole country or a whole geographical area. If we go from the animal models to the human population, the differences are obvious to all of us, but even if we take epidemiological data on a particular type of population (e.g. an occupational group) and want to extrapolate them to the general population, we must consider the different characteristics of the two populations. A workers' population examined for exposure to a given agent is often a population of relatively healthy and relatively young people in comparison with the general population that includes older people, diseased people, pregnant women, newborns, infants and children.

In order to consider these different approaches, needed for risk evaluation, the IRLG Working Group identified the following five steps as necessary components of the process of quantitative risk assessment.

1) Definition and quantification of exposures. If we are concerned about the effect of a given exposure in the population, we have to make sure that we know how to define precisely, in qualitative and quantitative terms, what the exposure is like, and this is often not easy. Even as we relate to the analysis of exposure and not to the biological effects, we need quantitation to define

the exposure. For ionizing radiation and some other physical factors there are at least certain common methods for measuring exposure, but for chemical exposures to a variety of agents we are dependent on analytical chemistry methods of very different reliability. When it comes to estimating environmental exposures to mixtures of chemicals (e.g. combustion products), the problem of determining the conditions of exposure involves a complex set of chemical and physical parameters.

2) Characterization of the exposed populations in quantitative terms. This process requires an attempt to determine the size of the population, the period and mode of exposure and the characteristics of the population, in terms of age, sex, and many other factors. This characterization is important because we may have to correlate data obtained in one type of population with the effects estimated in a different kind of population.

3) Characterization of the chemical and physical properties of the substances and their chemical reactivity in relation to exposure. This step can be very difficult especially in the case of mixtures, but even in the presence of single compounds one has to be concerned with such properties as metabolic and environmental changes, and particularly with the precise characterization of purity of industrial chemicals (controversial cases have arisen when materials were tested in commercial preparations that contained sometimes high levels of impurities). The first three steps are therefore devoted to defining the situation; i.e. quantifying the exposure, characterizing the population and characterizing the chemical and physical agents.

4) Prudent quantitative mathematical extrapolation of the responses from observed to estimated exposure ranges within the observed biological system. In order to correlate effects observed at high doses with effects predicted at low levels of exposure some guidance is needed as to how to project the effect of a low level exposure from data obtained at a higher level: this step involves the selection of mathematical models for such an extrapolation, within the same biological system. From data in animal tests, a mathematical model can predict the effect that would be detected at a much lower level of exposure in the same animal system. It does not tell us what will happen to other animal species or humans. The estimate, calculated on the basis of a somewhat educated guess in the selection of a mathematical model, gives us an indication of the expected response to low level exposures in the original biological system.

5) Qualification of the estimated risk for the population in light of identifiable biologic and toxicologic differences that may be present in the exposed human population. This last step considers all the available knowledge about the differences between observed

and projected biological systems. This process is still very difficult. Only in some cases we can rely on pretty good existing human observations to project our estimates to very similar populations, for example in two closely similar occupational exposure groups.

In many occupational situations fortunately the greatly increased awareness of these problems has led industry as well as governments, unions and other interested parties, to implement preventive measures; the populations that are exposed now to some of the qualitative risks that were identified by retrospective studies to have been very hazardous 20 or 30 years ago, have now a much lower hazard because the exposure is much lower and the people are much more protected. But that does not mean that the risk is entirely wiped out, if some exposure persists. Obviously we are striving to come closer to a realistic predictive approach.

Let's open the discussion on all these points and have your comments on the evaluation of the models that have been discussed, particularly the cellular transformation models that Dr Borek has discussed, and the models that I have alluded to in both human and animal experimental pathology in vivo and in vitro, while giving serious consideration to the problems brought to your attention by Dr Jansen, of correlating different types of toxicology for risk assessment.

LEGATOR

I was very interested in the various models you mentioned of explants from organ sites. It occurs to me that when one does that in culture, it is for one or two reasons. Either you expect something unique about the cells you are culturing depending upon their tissue or origin, such as metabolism of the specific chemical, or there is a non-metabolic characteristic of the tissue carried over in the culture that alters the ability to detect organ or site specific carcinogens. If I recall your slide correctly, the bronchial epithelial cell in every case picked up every single agent that was tested regardless of site specificity. As an example, the hepatotoxin, aflatoxin, was active on the bronchus. I fail to see the advantage of using bronchial epithelia unless you can demonstrate that they can selectively detect carcinogens that cannot be detected by cell lines.

SAFFIOTTI

The question really is, is there any specificity to these interactions and the answer is that basically we don't know yet, we haven't got enough data in this area. I want to make clear that most of this work is not my personal work, but was done by Dr C.C. Harris and his group in my laboratory in the last few years in collaboration with several other research groups, particularly Dr B.F.Trump's at the University of Maryland. I am getting into it from a different angle at this present time, and let me mention that one of the angles that interest me particularly is the study of multiple exposures to different carcinogens at the same time, which is common to all of us in real life and about which we know very little. One of the possible problems here is that there may be indeed a great deal of common susceptibility of many different tissues to a large range of carcinogens. It may indeed be the case that, if you have a sufficient amount of policyclic hydrocarbons and aflatoxin and aromatic amines circulating in your blood stream, many tissues will be affected by them. The question is: under what conditions will these tissues manifest some toxic effect? I was impressed by one of the first experiments of my cancer research career (Ritchie, A.C. and Saffiotti, U., Cancer Res. 15:84-88, 1955), which studied the effect of 2-acetylaminofluorene (AAF) in mice, that are highly susceptible to this carcinogen by feeding, responding with tumors at a variety of sites but not with tumors of the skin. AAF is not a skin carcinogen under any conditions when tested by itself. We were interested at that time in combinations of factors for 2-stage skin carcinogenesis. That experiment showed that in mice that had received AAF by feeding the skin was initiated and when further exposed to the promoting agent croton oil (applied only to the skin) it developed a significant number of tumors. Conversely, if the skin had been previously treated with a topical carcinogen as initiator, i.e. DMBA, that skin would respond significantly to the subsequent systemic action of the carcinogen AAF that otherwise we would not know to be active in the skin. We may have a variety of carcinogens, none of which could be picked up as being primarily responsible for inducing a significant incidence of tumors in a given tissue; but these carcinogens reach that tissue and are biologically reactive with critical target molecules. Such interactions may increase the background sensitivity in that tissue and contribute to a complex effect. Now, how can we use human tissues in this area? It is a field that is now developing and we will have to see what patterns come out of these studies.

Aflatoxin seems to be a particularly good example in that it binds significantly to the colon epithelium, especially if the level of aflatoxin-DNA adducts is considered. Adrienne Rogers and Paul Newberne some years ago showed that in some conditions, namely in vitamin A deficient animals, aflatoxin produced colon carcinoma, a target effect that was not otherwise revealed. There are some anecdotal human case reports that suggest that aflatoxin may be involved in tumor induction at sites other than the liver. I am simply throwing this up for discussion as I am not convinced that we should rule out the role of a widespread carcinogenic contaminant such as aflatoxin in the pathogenesis of cancers as common as colon cancer. We would not pick it up epidemiologically unless it had a very strong role. The target effect of carcinogens is still an open question. A lot more work is needed to see whether a battery of different cells would indeed eventually pick up specific patterns of response.

LEGATOR

I quite agree, but maybe it is too early to tell; but I would suggest from the non-specificity that we have seen to date, that a wide spectrum of carcinogens regardless of their target site, can be detected by cell culture or cell lines that are derived from non-selected organs. On the basis of existing data I see little advantage to using explants or primary cell cultures from specific organs.

SAFFIOTTI

By the way, to follow up on your comment, we are by no means saying that the DNA binding, or even the specific adduct formation, is a direct measure of carcinogenicity: it may well not be one, because of the other interplaying factors. Let me add some more data on the aflatoxin story. Dr Jansen mentioned this morning the fact that mice have been reported as being not sensitive to carcinogenicity by aflatoxin except in the study in which newborn mice were treated. This is on the basis of three strains that were tested as adult by Dr Wogan at MIT. The newborn study was done in a different strain yet, so we don't really know for sure that we can say all mice are resistant to aflatoxin. In cell transformation models we have interesting data. Dr Heidelberger and others have tested aflatoxin in 10T½ cells that derive from the C3H strain, which seems to be negative in vivo, and found it negative in the transformation assay. Dr Cortesi and I have tested aflatoxin in the BALB 3T3 clone A31-1-1 cells that I mentioned this morning and we found aflatoxin to be quite active as a transforming agent in those cells. I am now planning an in vivo study on the BALB/c mouse: there is a possibility that if its cells are transformed by the aflatoxin maybe the whole animal will also respond to it. If it does, it would then provide a very good in vivo model to compare resistant and susceptible strains. If it doesn't, it would still be very interesting to compare why some of its cells are highly responsive to aflatoxin when the whole animal is not. This study therefore will provide us with a set of comparisons to try to clear up some of these problems of species specificity. But this kind of fine tuning will have to go on for quite a while to pin down all these problems of specificity.

GOULD

Since we are trying to screen chemicals that will transform cells of specific organs we have to develop specific assays. These assays should screen for functional endpoints. Screening for macromolecular adducts, even relevant ones, may be misleading since only a small subpopulation of cells in an organ is a target for transformation. Thus if we screen the whole organ for adducts, adducts in target cells may not be apparent because of "noise" from other cell types.

SAFFIOTTI

That is a very good point. I wonder if Dr Borek has any comment on this problem of specificity and transformation.

BOREK

What kind of specificity? Specificity of the carcinogen, or specificity of the cells?

SAFFIOTTI

Specificity of the interaction.

BOREK

When studying interaction we have to be concerned with the kind of tissue we are working. Tissues vary in their response to a particular carcinogen at a particular dose level. As Mike pointed out, we might be deriving in culture different types of epithelial cells from the various organs we were working with. One should therefore define the question more precisely, namely how specific is transformation in a particular cell type? Can one extrapolate from one cell type to another? The answer is that we do not know with epithelial cell systems. In the case of fibroblasts one can use fibroblasts from various tissues and among them there exists more of a homogeneity, as compared to the epithelial cells. I personally am concerned with working with more than one species, with diploid as well as heteroploid cells, primary cultures as well as cell lines. The data are quantitatively different but qualitatively results are similar to some degree. The cell types are diploid hamster embryo cells and the mouse 10T½ fibroblast system. Expression time of transformation differs in these two cell types. With the hamster embryo cells it is 8 days whilst with the 10T½ system 6 weeks are required to see a transformed focus. There are some additional complications with these two systems, which I am not sure there is the time to go into. The basic point is that the 10T½ cells, similar to the 3T3, can not be considered as based on normal cells, because they are heteroploid. Thus in some ways one can consider them "pre-initiated cells". The processes of carcinogenesis in these cells may take on a different time scale, but the ultimate result of transformation seems to be the same in both systems. If one wants to extrapolate these experiments to epithelial cells one must be absolutely sure that one is working with a differentiated epithelial cell. Namely that the cultured cells carry in vitro the characteristics which they possess in vivo. Once the cells are in culture, at least in cell culture but not in organ culture as Dr Saffiotti indicated, they lose their differentiated quality with time in vitro. Of course we are limited by our knowledge of the optimal conditions for preserving these differentiated qualities and until we elucidate these we cannot be sure we are working with the cell type with which we started. This is therefore one difficulty with transformation of epithelial cells. A second difficulty is the question of quantitation. Quantitation of transformation at early stages is what we need for dose-response relationships related to risk estimates. In the fibroblasts we have an early assay. We are of course aware that values are not in absolute terms. However, the availability of a large body of data from many experiments and good statistical evaluation (which I shall show on Thursday) makes it possible to get a good idea of the dose-response relationship. Epithelial cells present a problem. For example, with liver, a system with which I am familiar, in order to get transformation one has to maintain the carcinogen in contact with the cells for two months, and one can evaluate the transformed nature of the cells by growth in agar and in the animal. During 2 months in culture many things can happen. Consequently, in this system we cannot get the actual quantitation at the early stage of the target cell-carcinogen interaction. Thus one ideally should work with many cell types and with many carcinogens in order to establish some kind of generalization.

WATERS

I just wanted to make an additional comment about organ specificity. It doesn't pertain to the transformation systems, where it has not worked, but involves the co-cultivation methods that Dr Saffiotti referred to this morning. The original work was done by Huberman and Sachs and employed Syrian hamster embryo "metabolizer" cells co-cultivated with V79 "indicator" cells. Further work by Dr Robert Langenbach in our laboratory has involved co-cultivation of primary liver, bladder and lung cells with V79 cells. He has been able to show that these primary cells retain some of their organ specificity. I think that this approach using mutagenesis as the endpoint and using primary cells for organ specific metabolism may be advantageous for certain classes of compounds that are not effectively evaluated in other short term tests. Hydrazines and certain nitrosomines, for example, respond very well in the co-cultivation system. I would not advocate its use in routine screening at this time, but rather for mechanistic studies or for detection purposes when you know the class of compounds you are dealing with.

JANIAUD

I just want to say some words about the tentative comparison of the human system and the animal system and that is the safrole story. You know that safrole, which is a simple molecule, is carcinogenic in mice and rats but negative in the Ames system. We studied it with rat liver epithelial cell culture and we compared metabolism in the rat liver culture and in the animals. We also compared the metabolism obtained when we tried the Ames system with microsomes and we could not demonstrate the safrole to be mutagenic with either strain of salmonella. We measured the metabolites and we first found that there was not enough of the product we had analyzed either in vivo in the rat or in vitro. We modified the procedure a little bit and learned why safrole was not mutagenic in the Ames system, and that was because safrole oxide (which is for us the active form of safrole) was alkylating the proteins of the microsomes and the cytochromes were killed in a sort of suicide process. The physiological effect on the liver is first the formation of oxide then alkylation of cytochrome P450; in the animal afterwards there is the other class of cytochromes which is quite the same cytochrome activating polycyclic hydrocarbons or P448. In relation to the human situation, safrole is a widely used product as a food additive, a flavouring agent and also as a natural product present in a lot of things. A study was made by giving to some volunteers ^{14}C-safrole and in this study no mutagenic compound was detected in the urine of the volunteers and no metabolite of safrole was found. But when we took human epithelial cells, of which I would speak later, we found a rather interesting system, i.e. a moderate level of the activating enzyme, which is the monoxigenase, and a low level of the detoxification enzyme which is the epoxide hydrolase. The situation for this tissue is that if safrole comes from the circulation some oxide is made and this oxide is not detoxified. It is a low level of enzymes as compared to rat liver in vivo, but the fact is that because of an unbalance between activating and detoxifying pathways, there is a risk. That is one thing. The second thing is, we have looked at the animal liver situation of the enzymes since we know all the metabolic chart for this simple molecule. We have 51 different metabolites of which six oxides and these oxides have different activities as mutagenic agents when synthesized and added to bacteria or other systems. When we compared 12 different strains of mice available in France, we found 1-30 variations in the level of the different enzymes. I think that if we have no idea of the pharmacokinetics of products and the metabolic abilities of different tissues, we cannot exactly compare different systems. Then the question of transformed cells. We have compared the metabolism in a continuous line from breast cancer, MCF7, and we have found a completely different pattern in the enzymatic pathway. That means that some enzymes are 100 times more inducible than in the primary culture or replicative culture. So I think it is a good reason to try to work with the epithelial cells.

GOULD

I have a question about using the MCF7 cell line. You were comparing this cell line to normal breast primary cells. I think the actual comparison is not tumor versus normal in this case but a cell line versus primary cells. It is known that cell lines lose various differentiated traits. Thus I think if you are going to try to compare transformed cells to normal primary tissue you should use primary malignant tissue instead of a cell line.

SAFFIOTTI

I would like to add a note to the safrole story. We have studied safrole together with several other compounds in mutagenicity tests in the Ames system in the course of a study on combined effects of different carcinogens. We have confirmed the finding that it is negative as a mutagen in the TA 100 and the TA 98 strains of the Ames test in Salmonella with rat liver S9. However, we found to our surprise that it is a good synergist with several other carcinogens, namely benzo/a/pyrene, benzidine and aflatoxin B_1, enhancing considerably the mutagenic response to these other agents when tested in combination. So it is interesting to speculate that an agent that is not detected as a mutagen and that has, as Dr Janiaud has reported, this particular metabolism, can be picked up as having some particular effect in the Ames test if it is tested in combination with other carcinogens, as we did, while in straight tests by itself it would not have been picked up. In those combination tests a particular biological effect was picked up and it is interesting to hear of the metabolic studies on this material because they could eventually help in explaining these interactions.

JANSEN

I would like to discuss one additional consideration as to the role of management in avoiding cancer, i.e. normal technological development. In oil refineries scrotal cancer had disappeared by the time it was realized there was such a problem. The reason was the entirely independent technological development of solvent extraction of paraffin wax instead of filtering in filter-presses, thus eliminating a source of heavy exposures. This development took place without any interference by toxicologists (who were very rare at that period). Technological development does not automatically solve toxicological problems as illustrated by the nickel refinery in the U.K., studied by Richard Doll. This refinery had largely solved the occupational problem of lung cancer before they knew they had the problem. However, when an even more modern plant using the same process was built in Norway, occupational lung cancer was unwittingly re-introduced. The blame must lie with cancer research: the actual culprit has still not been identified and in the absence of such identification, occupational cancer problems are equally unwittingly introduced as abolished. So cancer researchers have their own role to play as well as management which can hardly be expected to react efficiently to vague exhortations, even if completely willing to solve defined problems.

SAFFIOTTI

I want to make sure that I wasn't misunderstood on that issue. I was in fact pointing to the role that industrial technology development can have in preventing further exposures or in cutting down the risk considerably. Obviously part of the problem of risk assessment will be that of applying these criteria to the evaluation of alternative technologies. It is often difficult to determine whether a technological change can indeed be deemed to be a considerable improvement from the risk point of view, and we need to exert our skills in predicting hazards in that direction too. There is a potential danger of having a technology which solves a problem and creates another or that removes the exposure to a certain type of product and creates another. We have seen many situations in industry that have been in fact cleaned up by better technology and that is a very encouraging situation. I wonder if there are any other specific questions related to the presentations made earlier in the day?

KOTTARIDIS

I would like to comment on this specificity that we are just discussing this afternoon. I think we may run into a risk if we really say that we have got a system and that it is working and we will just try it and if a compound is carcinogenic we would pick it up or not. If we just think a little bit what happened in Japan a few years ago with the compound AF180 which was added as a preservative to food. This compound was checked for two years or so, in an animal model, I don't recall correctly, I think rats, and it was found that this compound was not carcinogenic or mutagenic so it was used for a number of years; then new tests came along and showed this compound was mutagenic, so they went back and tested it again in the same animal model and it was indeed found that this compound was highly carcinogenic, so it was immediately taken off the market. Now what happened here? There is a system that was tested before and then tested again and it was found to be affected the second time. I mentioned that just to stress the point that we run into a risk if we rely on an epithelial cell system to check a particular compound. Maybe this is a risk that we are taking, and we should really try to assess the risk of a compound in as many different ways as we can.

SAFFIOTTI

This is an important problem: we had some comments yesterday on the need to address a battery of test systems. Dr Legator had discussed that point, and I hope that the development of the human cell model systems will help in providing a variety of components to a battery, all of which can gradually be used for studies of toxicological problems so that we are not bound to a single model or one or two models with all their limitations, however good the models may be, but really try and cover a spectrum of biological systems.

LEGATOR

This discussion may be appropriately concluded by the statement made by a pioneer toxicologist, Dr Brodie, at the National Institutes of Health. When he was asked the question, 'Is rat like a man?', his answer was: 'What man?'. I think that in this statement there is a world of wisdom. We vary tremendously as a species and a segment or sub-group of our population can mimic almost any response we see in experimental animals.

ROUND TABLE: RISKS FROM AMBIENT CHEMICALS AND RADIATIONS

Leader: M.D. Waters

Genetic Toxicology Div., Health Effects Research Lab.

U.S. EPA, Research Triangle Park, NC 27711

WATERS

This morning we heard three very excellent, and yet distinctly different, presentations. With the permission of Drs Saffiotti, Legator and Arlett, I would like to reiterate several of the major points of their presentations and to raise a question to each of them. Then perhaps we can hear from each of them to offer them an opportunity to clarify or expand on any of the points that they made in their presentations. I'd like to suggest that we then open the floor to general discussion following each of their brief presentations regarding this morning's discussion.

Dr Saffiotti emphasized the differences between terminal and self-replicating toxic phenomena relating carcinogenesis and mutagenesis to the latter category. He mentioned the problem of identifying carcinogens in the ambient environment and estimating their number. He showed that the number of agents to which man is actually exposed, for which there is good evidence of carcinogenic potential, is actually rather small such it does seem realistically feasable to deal with the problems using available bioassay technology. He raised concern over the ability of investigators to determine the relative 'potency' of chemicals based upon short-term test results, and he suggested that single numerical estimates of cancer risk should be avoided. He went on to discuss the thesis that cancer is a multi-factorial process with multiple causative factors as distinct from a one cause-one cancer process. With either view, however, it appears that there is a fair degree of uncertainty as to the range of involvement of the various causative agents. Specifically he mentioned that we don't know the impact of physical agents - a topic for this conference.

I'd like to ask Dr Saffiotti: How might we avoid single numerical estimates of cancer risk? Or, in other words, in accord with the topic of our round table, how should we go about estimating the individual contribution of risk from ambient chemicals and radiations in the environment? While I give Dr Saffiotti an opportunity to consider this question, I'd like to reintroduce the other two presentations.

Dr Legator described two major objectives in the field of chemical mutagenises, a qualitative objective and a quantitative objective. He expressed concern about 1) heritable genetic effects in man, 2) our ability to quantitatively estimate mutagenic risk, and 3) our capability to predict other toxicological properties of chemicals, particularly their potential of inducing cancer. This latter concern relates to the use of short-term, especially microbial, in vitro tests. He felt that mammalian cells in culture would be useful since at least they possessed the genetic machinery necessary to relate results obtained in these systems to results obtained in intact animal systems. He stated that risks should be based upon final phenotypic expression and not, I take it, on indicators of primary damage.

A question for Dr Legator is: 'What approach do you recommend to obtain mutagenesis data from whole animal systems? Which systems and at what cost in terms of time and resources? Please keep in mind our concern for ambient chemicals and radiation'.

Dr Arlett spoke about the use of human cells in risk assessment. He described some of the genetic details of the Lesch-Nyhan syndrome, xeroderma pigmentosum and ataxia-telangiectasia genetic disease states, as well as polyposis coli and Huntington's chorea. He spoke specifically of the differing relative sensitivities of skin fibroblasts obtained from these genetic variant individuals to radiations both gamma and UV, and to the chemicals, 8-methoxypsoralen and 1,8-dinitropyrene. He emphasized the importance of concentration, as well as time, in the process of risk estimation and he was generally positive on the issue of risk assessment, provided that the impreciseness of the estimates were recognized. My question for Dr Arlett is 'Do we have any estimate of how variable human beings are?'

SAFFIOTTI

The questions Dr Waters addressed to me are obviously difficult ones. I should try to clarify my thoughts in this area. Dr Waters has referred to my very brief comment on the problem of potency estimates and I would like to restate here that the reason I don't like to use the word potency as applied to a particular chemical is that we deal with data generated by the interaction of a chemical or physical agent with a biological target system; therefore each interaction has a component from the agent and a component from the host. The data do not derive solely from the agent itself. In simple terms, there is no 'potency' as a property of the chemical in the bottle. The effect of the chemical is measured in a given biological system, and if the biological system changes, the level of effect may very well change. For these reasons I am against the common use of the term 'potency' and I replace it with the term 'observed levels of effect'. This term deals with a much more concrete concept, i.e. that of effects that obviously have been observed in a particular system, and not with an abstract generalization.

Risk estimation is really an exercise in comparative toxicology, or comparative pathology, since it is an attempt to correlate observations of effects made in a particular biological system with predictions of effects in other biological systems, such as an exposed human population.

Dr Waters asked me the following question: if we try to avoid risk estimates by single numerical indexes, how do we estimate the role of different contributing factors? This is a crucial issue for the topic of our symposium. I think that we should first determine whether a quantitative type of risk evaluation is indeed possible from the kind of data we have in a given situation. If it isn't - i.e. if we do not have sufficient data to correlate conditions of exposure, species, tissue and other differences in one system to the other system - then no manner of theoretical formulations will replace this lack of knowledge and we should recognize that we don't know how to express a precise reliable estimate in numerical terms. We have heard the argument that in order to issue certain regulations one needs to have numerical risk estimates. It is true that a regulator cannot afford to regulate without such numbers or is it perhaps more true that a regulator could not afford to regulate on the basis of unreliable or fictitious numbers? This dilemma has been well identified by the Committee on Prototype Explicit Analyses of Pesticides (1980).

My answer to the problem of how to estimate risk if we cannot use reliable numbers to recognize that there are degrees of estimates and that in some cases the risk can be estimated only qualitatively and not quantitatively. Certain types of effects are quite constant throughout various biological models, various species, various human and animal tissues and cells. When many studies are all concurrent in a certain direction they may bring to a reasonable scientific conclusion that a type of effect could be confidently extrapolated to a human population. In other cases, there may be marked qualitative differences among individuals or amoung groups: for example, required metabolic pathways may be present in one system and absent in another and under those conditions we may not be able to extrapolate even qualitatively.

The use of an extrapolation approach which is unreliable by definition can be worse than recognizing that we don't know how to do it. In such cases, one extreme approach to regulation is to ignore the problem, even if it allows potentially a serious risk of toxic effects to go uncontrolled. The other extreme approach is to eliminate the problem by eliminating the exposure altogether, even for low level exposures. These decisions are embodied in certain types of legislation; in the US the area food additives legislation in the so-called Delaney clause that if an agent has been found to cause cancer in animals by ingestion or by methods adequate for the evaluation of food additives it should not be added to food. It takes action by the Congress itself to overrule that law, as it has done in the case of saccharin. In all other segments, the US regulation of carcinogens is less rigid. One alternative that has been proposed is to recognize our uncertainties and to move towards the categorisation of carcinogens as major hazards, not so major hazards, and lower levels of hazards by comparison with reference standards. There are still many difficulties in this approach and we need much more research in this general area.

GOULD

In regard to your talk this morning about the multifactorial models of carcinogenesis - I think you won't find much general disagreement. However, for example when you take a look at the risks associated with radiation where we have a reasonable idea of the quantitative risks associated with this singular agent. How does that blend within your concept of multifactorial design?

SAFFIOTTI

My view of the problem of dealing with one well quantified component, while others are not quantifiable, is that we should take into account the contribution of the quantified components but we should not forget the existence and interplay of the others. Even with radiation, where exposures can be quantitatively comparable in different biological systems, and there is no interference from metabolic activation pathways, there remains the problem of translating the measures of exposure in terms of measures of basic molecular effects which are dependent on a variety of host factors. Then there is the problem common to all types of carcinogens of translating the measurement of the triggering event at the molecular level into their expression as neoplastic or genetic changes. I have the impression that, because there is this large body of data on risk measure by radiation, if has often been forgotten that radiation itself is usually a component of a larger etiologic picture. Uranium mining exposure to radiation and tobacco smoke show marked synergism for lung cancer. I think this is not an isolated case, but it is probably an example of synergism by a variety of chemical exposures. In addition to several other exposure factors, there will be genetical, nutritional, hormonal, sexual and other differences to account for. I haven't seen any method for translating the interaction of many different factors into mathematical terms.

LEGATOR

I agree in principle that we are better off without numbers for risk estimate if the numbers are meaningless. Other strategies such as categorization of response is a better approach. The question I have for Dr Saffiotti is that since we have had years of experience using various mathematical models to derive risk estimates for human populations from animal studies and since these models are conservative, do you, Dr Saffiotti, believe that we have been ill served by using these mathematical models and deriving a precise number or, if indeed, we have been fairly well protected because of the conservative nature of the models we have been using?

SAFFIOTTI

Some of the mathematical extrapolation models, after they have been applied and studied and in a number of systems, have turned out to be much less conservative than they were claimed to be when they first came out. The Mantel Bryan model was proposed largely as a conservative estimate and it is now considered to be much less conservative than the linear extrapolation model. The linear extrapolation model was considered to be a conservative one in the sense of not underestimating the risk, but now I understand that it has been found that in certain circumstances actual data suggest that it may underestimate the risk at low doses because there can be a shoulder above the extrapolation line in certain situations. The problem is: how conservative can we trust the model to be? Are there situations in which it can result in an underestimate? There was a second part to your question.

LEGATOR

In those few chemicals where we have some epidemiological data such as aflatoxin, if we look back upon the predicted value of the models in the light of our human experience, how accurate have they been?

SAFFIOTTI

Another problem is how far down in the dose response scale can one extend the use of these mathematical models. If data are observed at a certain level and you want to extrapolate them somewhat further down but not much further down, then there is no great divergence among several of the mathematical models. But if you want to extrapolate a long way down below the observed levels, different mathematical models give you highly divergent extrapolation levels. My main concern here is again that we should maintain the use of these mathematical models for extrapolation from high dose to low dose strictly to the biological systems from which the data were derived, because they are really not intended to handle intrinsic biological differences. In a recent paper Anderson, Hoel and Kaplan (Toxicol. Appl. Pharmacol., 55:154, 1980) attempted to develop a somewhat more complex mathematical formulation to allow for the additional variable of differences in pharmaco-kinetics. I do not know how well this more complicated formulation can cope with the complexities of pharmaco-kinetic phenomena, and besides there will always remain several other biological differences among systems. However, it is encouraging that highly qualified bio-statisticians have tried to cope with this problem.

LEGATOR

It would seem to me that one of the major problems in using mathematical models for extrapolation can be illustrated with vinyl chloride. When one uses mathematical models for extrapolation we are usually assuming the same target organ in animals and in man. With vinyl chloride, if we assume angiosarcoma and later find that central nervous system tumors may be the most important effect, our extrapolation from mathematical models is quite misleading.

For some time our group has asked the question of how many tests can we run concurrently in the same animal experiment. Assuming that most of the chemicals we are interested in, human exposure is usually sub-acute or chronic, over a period of days or weeks, we can therefore administer our chemical to animals. The administrating of the chemical by multiple injections we have eliminated the need for specific timing that may be a requisite for specific tests. The question is: how many tests can we conduct in a single animal experiment? The rational of this approach, multiple endpoints could ne detected from a single experiment, thus saving both time and money. We call this approach the 'combined testing protocol'.

What can we do with one animal experiment? We can do cytogenetics, including micronucleus test and metaphase analysis, we can look at spermatagonia to see if we have an effect on germinal cells, and we can look at body fluids, usually the urine, using various tester strains or even a mammalian cell culture to see if we detect genetically active compounds. This assay can be improved substantially by correlating the urine after treatment. If we have some prior information about the chemical we include determining the alkylation of haemoglobin, we can possibly do a repair study, as well as the host-mediated assay. At the present time we do approximately six discreet tests on the same animal experiment. In addition to saving money and time, it allows us to interrelate one test with another under the same treatment conditions. There are some problems with this procedure because you are looking at multiple endpoints, it requires that you have a cytogeneticist, microbial geneticist and capable animal handling personnel. All the tests are short-term, that is, you can complete your tests within a matter of weeks or a month depending on duration of your initial treatment. As in all animal tests, we are deficient in assays to detect gene mutations and we are relying on tests which detect ongoing processes rather than final toxicological outcomes. If at all possible, pharmaco-kinetic studies should be carried out with mutation studies. Knowledge about the distribution and absorption of the chemical can assist in the design of the 'combined testing protocol'. It's hard to give you an exact cost estimate for this approach. Using three concentrations of the chemical and depending how long we treat our animals, the cost would be several thousand dollars per compound. We can complete the work in a matter of a month.

SAFFIOTTI

I'd like to ask a question to Dr Legator. We have been interested in recent years in the problem of combined effects of different carcinogens and mutagens. We have seen in the Ames test a series of agents that have marked mutual synergistic interactions and others that are mutually inhibitory. The question then arises how to evaluate concurrent exposures to mixtures of agents which may produce an interactive effect. In the Ames test we have found that a group of polycyclic aromatic hydrocarbons are all mutually inhibitory. This observation may be important in the evaluation of mixtures, such as Diesel fuels and various combustion products: for example, if this kind of inhibition does not take place in a chronic long-term exposure as we have it in people, then the Ames test of the mixture may underestimate the risk. Conversely, we found examples of synergism of different carcinogens, which may give us a clue to potential effects that may be higher than one would predict from the level of activity of individual components tested separately. Have you found any examples of such interactions in your cytogenetic studies and with the other tests you mentioned?

LEGATOR

A modification of the mutation response has frequently been seen with induced animals, i.e. methyl cholenthrene induced animals, for instance, I presented the benzene data: the methyl cholenthrene induced animals show about a ten-fold increase in chromosome aberration after benzene treatment. A metabolite is produced through a methyl cholenthrene induced enzyme. With other chemicals you can show the opposite effect, enzymatic detoxification. There is also information by the Oak Ridge group and others where antioxidants decrease chemical induction of mutagenesis. I'm sure there are many other examples where in animal tests you can alter the mutagenic activity by what you add either prior to or at the time of chemical administration. The advantage of mutagenicity studies over carcinogenicity studies is that we are dealing with short-term responses and complex interactions can be tested more conveniently.

WATERS

An additional thought in Dr Saffiotti's question was 'do you believe that there is a substantial difficulty in assessing the biological activity of components of complex mixtures using animal approach as opposed to a microbial approach?'

SAFFIOTTI

There is a distinct possibility that some effects might be masked.

ARLETT

The question is: 'Do we have any ideas or data on human variability? As a result of working for several years with human cell cultures we are starting to accumulate data and are beginning to get a feel for human variability at the cellular level. I have put in a few slides which might help to illustrate this, while we cannot yet give a real answer to the question, there exist some data which might help.

The first slide shows us the response of cells to the lethal action of UV light. We believe that there is little variation in cellular response to UV amongst normal individuals. The sensitivity of normal cells can be contrasted with that of excision defective xeroderma pigmentosum (XP) cell strains which are clearly hypersensitive. The excision component XP variants may show some limited hypersensitivity but many are normal in their response. A second syndrome with cellular hypersensitivity to UV is Cockayne syndrome. While there is no direct evidence for a repair defect in this syndrome the failure of these cells to reinitiate DNA synthesis as demonstrated by my colleague Dr Alan Lehmann is strong circumstantial evidence for such a defect. With respect to ionizing radiation we see immediately that there is considerable variability in response to the lethal effects amongst different normal individuals. The fact that we cannot demonstrate a biopsy effect suggests that these differences are real and may have important implications at many levels. For example at the level of radiotherapy, it may well be that unrecognized radioresistant individuals will bear more radioresistant tumors and possibly be given insufficient radiotherapy doses.

Turning to variability with regard to mutation we now have available after some five years' work three classes of information, spontaneous and induced mutation frequencies to 6-thioguanine resistance following treatment with UV or gamma irradiation. With spontaneous mutation we have accumulated data on 27 different cell strains amongst which are 5 from clinically normal individuals. One of these cell strains, 1BR, is our reference normal and we have a considerable body of data on these cells giving a spontaneous mutation frequency of $3.8\pm0.9\times10^{-6}$ which we regard as being very accurate. A proper estimate of spontaneous mutation would utilize the Luria-Delbruck fluctuation test and generate mutation rates, but this is impracticable except in very special circumstances. Such a test was performed recently by Trosko (Proc. Natl. Acad. Sci., USA, 78:3133-3137, 1981) on Bloom's syndrome cells and claims for enhanced spontaneous mutation rates have now been made. We have not yet examined spontaneous mutation in Bloom's syndrome but have to report that cells from cancer prone syndromes such as xeroderma pigmentosum, basal cell naevus syndrome and retinoblastoma all appear to have essentially normal spontaneous mutation frequencies. The absence of an intrinsically elevated mutation frequency in the cancer prone syndrome implies that the increased cancer seen in the individual is likely to be a consequence of damage to DNA.

For UV-induced mutation we have data on cell strains from four normal individuals and from a further five who, while not clinically normal, show no hypersensitivity. The data from these nine individuals is relatively uniform and gives us a feel for UV-induced mutation frequencies. Similar data for ten individuals for gamma irradiation again shows little variation. Thus our information on UV and gamma-induced mutation is consistent with limited variation in response amongst normal individuals. Clearly more will have to be examined and the response to chemicals similarly evaluated. Preliminary data with 4NQO indicated a considerable difference in lethal response amongst normal fibroblast cell strains. It is not known whether this is a consequence of differences in repair capacity or metabolism between the strains.

WATERS

Is some of the variability that you see possibly due either to the age of the donor or the age of the culture? That is, the number of passage levels.

ARLETT

I don't think we have enough data to answer that in relation to mutation, but in terms of cell killing, I guess we have. Most of our experiments are cell killing experiments. We have been able to take that data and look at it in terms of passage number and cloning efficiency and I am convinced in fact that there is no passage or cloning efficiency effect on cell killing.

KRAEMER

I would like to make a cautionary comment and point out some of the difficulties we have found in making correlations between X-ray survival curves and predicting the patient's clinical response. We can consider survival curves like Colin was showing for three different diseases, all three having cancer. Ataxia telangiectasia, hereditary retinoblastoma and a particular patient that we came across, a 16 year old boy with dermatomyositis and a basal cell carcinoma of the eye-lid (Smith, P.J., Patterson, M.C., Kraemer, K.H., Lancet i:216, 1981). All three types of fibroblast strains had X-ray hypersensitivity in terms of survival, but the ataxia telangiectasia strains are more sensitive than the others. The ataxia telangiectasia patients in general, if they have developed tumors previously and are treated with radiation therapy, get a tremendous over-reaction to standard doses of radiation. This would be in accord to their greatly increased sensitivity to X-ray, in terms of these survival curves. Now fibroblasts from hereditary retinoblastoma patients do not have that great sensitivity. In fact, some of the cases are absolutely normal, others have a slight sensitivity. Retinoblastoma patients develop this tumor of the eye and are treated with radiation. Standard doses of radiation result in normal responses. However, in a long-term analysis, these patients are more prone to develop osteosarcomas in their radiated areas than elsewhere. The patient with juvenile dermatomyositis and carcinoma of the eye-lid was actually treated with radiation for the basal cell carcinoma. He had a normal response to the therapy. Very much earlier in his life he had received superficial X-radiation for his skin rash. We do not know if in this particular individual the radiation might have induced the cancer with a long latent period. We do know that even though his cells show a moderate hypersensitivity to radiation, the acute effect of radiation was a normal response in him and in the retinoblastoma patients. Only where the cells are extremely hypersensitive you see any early effects. Thus it may be hard to see any clinical effects in the short-term where we find only minor differences in survival curves.

ARLETT

My point was that a possible consequence of variability in survival amongst normal individuals would be that some might be receiving insufficient radiation in therapy regimes. I would accept your caution in supposing that we might extrapolate from survival curves to individuals. We must be even more cautious with respect to extrapolation of the mutation data since we are still limited to the HGPRT system for practical mutation studies.

GOULD

The X-ray survival curves you present don't seem to have shoulders on them. Do you feel this represents the in vivo condition or do you think it's an artifact of the culture system you are using?

ARLETT

That is a very difficult question. As far as I am aware very small or not measurable shoulders are the usual result of ionizing radiation survival curve experiments with human fibroblasts. A system where a shoulder is seen is in very late passage foetal fibroblast cultures as was shown by Cox at Harwell (Cox and Masson, Int. J. Radiat. Biol. 26:193-196, 1974). I would suggest that shoulderless survival curves are probably characteristic of stem-line cells and may reflect a true in vivo situation for this particular cell type.

GOULD

Well, as you say, if it's related to radiotherapy patients, we know that these patients do have recovery between fractions which would indicate a shoulder. Again, it may not be the same cell type, but if this is true when you go to work with mutation or transformation in vitro are you possibly ignoring a major repair phenomenon, that may exist in vivo and therefore give us false risk estimates for transformation and mutation because of lack of repair.

ARLETT

I can put a shoulder on our survival curves by doing two things either separately or together. If we liquid hold cells (or stop the cells cycling), recovery of potentially lethal damage occurs putting a shoulder on the survival curve. If one reduces the dose rate down to 0.1-0.01 rad per minute you can also get a large shoulder. I think what is happening is that the liquid held cells have gone into a G_o phase typical of most non-cycling cells in the body.

We have yet to do these liquid holding experiments with mutation in our laboratory, but V. Maher has already shown the capacity for a repair process to eliminate UV-induced mutants under such conditions (Maher et al., Mutation Res. 62:311-323, 1979). I agree that unless we achieve more realistic in vivo like conditions which may be represented by both clycling or non-cycling cells then we may both over- or under-estimate induced transformation or mutation frequencies.

GOULD

In the 'potentially lethal dose' experiments would you expect to see any individual variation which you don't see in the normal exponential growth such as for survival and mutagenesis following UV radiation?

ARLETT

Not enough individuals have been looked at to give an answer to that question, but I anticipate that we may reveal hidden variability.

CERUTTI

I have two comments. One is a word of caution. Equating increased sensitivity automatically to repair deficiency is dangerous. The second thing is that while passage in our hands is not really related to cloning efficiency and sensitivity, cell cycle differences can be a factor determining sensitivity. It's clear for instance for Bloom syndrome that cells have a tendency to skip rounds of replication. They are not dead, they just wait a little while before resumption of division. This non-dividing cell portion may be more sensitive than the cycling portion. Such phenomena may contribute to interindividual differences in sensitivity.

ARLETT

We have very little information on cell cycle kinetics in our system. I guess part of the problem is we don't live long enough to do that component of the experiment and I would very much accept your comment about ascribing a repair at the drop of a survival curve. I imagine you will be making some further points about this later in the week. One has other ways in which the cells may appear sensitive. One can have different targets and one can have the ability to take off the damage by the involvement of clastogenic agents.

CERUTTI

It seems to me also relating shoulders in survival curves to repair is equally dangerous. A shoulder does not necessarily reflect a repair process which is saturable and the absence of the shoulder by no means excludes repair processes.

BOREK

The fact that liquid holding wipes out transformation is interesting because liquid holding also wipes out transformation *in vitro*. I wonder if you could comment a little more about this, specifically on the fact that you add a shoulder to the survival curve by liquid holding. Is the shoulder modified by the length of time of liquid holding?

ARLETT

I can only speak really of our own experiments which have not yet reached the stage of mutation. We have been concerned with looking at cell survival and chromosome aberrations and showing recovery for these endpoints. All we have done is achieve conditions which absolutely stop cells cycling. We put cells up in culture and change the medium to ½ percent foetal calf serum, after a period of 24 hrs, we perform our experiment 5 days later and allow a further 24 hrs for recovery and then the cells are returned to standard culture conditions. This has absolutely no effect on the cloning efficiency of the cells.

ROUND TABLE: HUMAN AND OTHER MAMMALIAN CELLS: THEIR ROLE IN RISK ASSESSMENT

Leader: C. Borek

Radiation Research Laboratory and Dept. of Pathology

Columbia University, New York, NY 10032

BOREK

In recent years it has become increasingly clear that environmental factors including diet play a significant role in determining cancer rates. These factors are a composite of what people do, or what is done to them and are superimposed on the genetic makeup which may in part play a role as a risk determinant. Some of these risk factors may be available but as we have clearly seen in various talks this week the difficulty lies in characterizing them and in identifying agents which may interact in an additive or synergistic manner, thus potentiating their hazardous effects.

Chemicals are present in abundance and may vary in their mode of action and in their effect on specific target tissues. Radiation while being a weaker carcinogen compared to some chemicals at an equitoxic level is the most universal and the most accurately measurable oncogenic agent. Latency and specific target tissue and its age are important factors in determining radiation carcinogenesis. Recently public concern has focussed on the biological hazards of the low levels of radiation at the dose levels of 1 rad, and less, the kind of exposure to which one may be subjected from medical diagnostic procedures or from sources of nuclear energy which are increasing in number in our environment. Low dose levels are of concern both with physical and chemical agents for we are ignorant of the actual determining primary processes which serve in initiation. At low dose one cannot discount the possibility that "potentially transformable" lesions may be initiated and will predispose the human cells to neoplastic transformation following further exposure to the same or other environmental factors; such factors would serve as promotors and could act concurrently or at a later stage and allow full expression of the lesion in the initiated cells. When evaluating all oncogenic agents we are faced with a conundrum; in the chain of events initiated by these agents we are still unable to establish what is the primary event and what is secondary. Epidemiology and animal studies are limited in the establishment of risk at low doses and low dose rates, the kinds of exposure we are faced with constantly. Thus we turn to cell culture where we are able to assay several million cells, instead of thousands of animals. However, being in vitro systems we must realize that factors associated with man such as genetics, age, sex and various environments cannot be fully represented.

Several points have come out of the discussion today. First, as we have seen, even in animal cell studies it is of crucial importance to test one potential carcinogenic agent in cells of different species as well as in primary and long term cultures for at least two obvious reasons. a) The agent may appear as positive in one system but not in others. b) Because we do not know which animal cell model reflects most closely the human situation. Another point to be borne in mind is the fact that we must distinguish between mutagenesis and carcinogenesis. A recent paper from Barett's lab evaluating diethylstilbestrol (DES) in hamster embryo cells indicated that within the same cell system DES was carcinogenic but not mutagenic. Thus for optimal studies we seek systems in which we can study both types of toxicity, mutagenesis and carcinogenicity at the same time to evaluate both types of risk. Another problem to consider is whether animal epithelial cell systems are ready for quantitative evaluation or carcinogenesis. In transformation studies the required time of exposure of epithelial cells to a chemical carcinogen will be up to 4 weeks. Many undefined events may take place during this long period.

After evaluating the usefulness of animal fibroblasts versus epithelial cell we must evaluate animal cells versus human cells. As Dr Saffiotti pointed out, human epithelial cell systems are not yet ready for quantitative assays. Within the human cell spectrum currently available for quantitative in vitro studies of mutagenesis we have lymphocytes and fibroblasts and for carcinogenic studies we have fibroblasts and efforts to use epithelial cells. While transformation studies with human cells are still at early stages, they are of crucial importance. Besides being an end in itself for evaluating risk in the appropriate system, we hopefully will be able to evaluate how they differ from or are similar to animal cells. Such information would render our animal studies more meaningful. Thus, how ready are human cells for these various studies on mutagenesis and carcinogenesis? Can we use them to identify cancer-prone individuals? How do we deal with suitable controls, who is a normal reference point? These are questions which we should tackle in this discussion.

Dr Schleiffer-Strauss, would you like to amplify your talk today and tell us what is the future of your particular assay and what are the limitations?

SCHLEIFFER-STRAUSS

I think I can extend what I have already said and clarify. There are several possibilities for further characterizing the TG-resistant peripheral blood lymphocytes (Pbls) which we have been enumerating from humans and animals. I mentioned that we find very high variant frequencies in renal transplant recipients, especially where there exists significant graft-host antigenic disparity and consequently a stimulation of lymphocyte proliferation. As a result of in vivo selection in favor of the TG^R variants, we are able to observe amplified numbers of these resisting cells which can be removed from the body easily in large numbers for comparison with Lesch-Nyhan cells. There is obviously a problem with this system in that we have not yet determined what percentage of TG^R Pbls are Lesch-Nyhan-type mutants and what percentage are phenotypic pretenders. One interesting experiment I didn't describe this morning subjected TG-resistant lymphocytes taken from patients who have been treated with mutagens during anti-cancer chemotherapy, from purine analogue immunosuppressed transplant patients and from Lesch-Nyhan heterozygotes to HAT medium (containing amethopterin) which, as I said, blocks the de novo pathway for DNA synthesis. In this case, cells truly lacking purine salvage pathway activity are inhibited and fail to become autographically labelled. As it happens certain percentage of TG^R-HAT^R cells exist. Robert De Mars called fibroblasts from LN hemizygotes having this characteristic, type 2 cells. We find that 98% of TG^R Pbls from LN heterozygotes were, in fact, completely inhibited. The transplant recipients evaluated often develop very high variant frequencies, as high as 10^{-2} in some cases. About 70% of these lymphocytes are indeed killed by methatrexate in the Strauss-Albertini test. About 85% of TG^R Pbls from mutagen exposed individuals were HAT sensitive. Results from normal individuals show that most, but not all, of these TG^R Pbls are killed by the addition of methatrexate. An interesting possibility in the problem of characterizing lymphocytes emerges in the transplant recipient. I use these people extensively because at times some of them possess many TG^R Pbls which we can study. As you know, the assay consumes the test cell and we cannot have a further look at it after the test. To overcome this problem, in one sense, I took some blood from transplant recipients and normal people and separated them as I have shown. These cells were cultured and transformed with Epstein-Barr virus to produce long term B-lymphocyte lines. These experiments were successful in all cases. In addition, I also, in each case, attempted to culture cells in the presence of TG at $3x10^{-4}$M. Only one line grew under these conditions. The original cells had come from a transplant recipient on the verge of rejection containing high numbers of TG^R Pbls. The culture grew for 2 months until it was lost to infection. There is no question that these cells were selected in vitro and grew very well. Dick Albertini has also carried out the experiment we discussed before, but rather than transforming the lymphocytes with E-B virus, he used T-cell growth factor. T-cell growth factor is specific for T-cells and can produce long term lines which can be cloned. Albertini was able to produce a line of T-cells from a transplant recipient with a high TG^R variant frequency. This opens up another possibility, a modification of this method which would allow us to re-examine events in vivo, using an in vitro culture system, carefully controlled, with knowledge of the starting numbers of variant cells. In this system we can find out by enzyme assays and other means whether these cells are mutants and what they represent as markers of damage to DNA and health in human beings at risk.

BOREK

Could you just enumerate what are the advantages or the limitations of your method in the terms of risk estimate?

SCHLEIFFER-STRAUSS

I think the primary advantages are, or will be, when this system is characterized to give sufficient confidence, that it can be utilized to monitor in vivo, in a longitudinal fashion, events in individual human beings. I should think that until modifications including automation of the method are effected, it will be best used in targeted individuals, perhaps individuals at special risk because of exposure or susceptibility. It can be used quite well in animals and the results are very similar to those we have seen in humans. Therefore, as I said this morning, it should be possible to extrapolate back and forth as may be required. In the animals of course we also can look for a further endpoint and carcinogenicity may be correlated with somatic cell mutation, this is a most intriguing and desirable possibility.

BOREK

Dr Arlett, you mentioned at some point that your assays have a good potential in picking out victims of various genetic diseases.

ARLETT

Your question anticipates my talk tomorrow on our attempts to detect heterozygotes for repair defective/cancer-prone genetic diseases. I would like to delay my response until tomorrow but use this opportunity to move the discussion on to other areas.

The frist of these is concerned with population surveys: Gary Strauss's method presents us with the potential of using human blood to measure mutational damage at the population level. It still remains, however, to prove that he is actually looking at mutants. It would seem to me that this also brings into focus the core topic of this meeting which is our ability to assess risk in man. The Strauss methodology allows us to go directly to human populations and could mean that we need not bother with cells in culture. I realize, however, that this is not practicable at the moment.

If we simply wish to know whether a compound is genotoxic or not then the bacterial tests will suffice. If we require to know if a compound is genotoxic in human beings then there is no question in my mind that we should go directly to human cells for the answer. A nice example of where animal cells might mislead us is with 1-8 dinitropyrene which is a very effective mutagen for mouse LS178Y cells but negative for human cells. It is still not clear which human cell type is the most useful for measuring genotoxicity and we are, in our laboratory, attempting to set up a comparison of fibroblasts and lymphoblastoid cell lines for this purpose.

An area which I should also like us to consider is the importance of chronic effects. Most of the model mutagenesis experiments utilize short treatment times such as a two hour treatment with ethyl methanesulphonate. In nature, on the other hand, we are more likely to receive chronic exposure at low dose rates. Not only do we have a problem here relating to measuring extremely low doses but there is still the unresolved possibility that adaptive responses might exist, viz. a continuous, chronic, low dose treatment with alkylating agents might even be good for you.

To be more specific about adaptive responses, these have been demonstrated very clearly by John Cairns and his co-workers who showed that continuous non-toxic treatment of bacteria by MNNG or MNU protect the cells against the lethal and mutagenic effects of these same chemicals and many other alkylating agents. Attempts are in hand in many laboratories to extend these observations to mammalian cells and Leona Samson has recently produced some very convincing evidence that such effects can also be seen in cultured Chinese hamster cells. She has also shown an effect on sister chromatid exchanges in human fibroblasts and we have produced preliminary data that indicate an adaptive response for lethal responses in human cells.

CERUTTI

It should be mentioned that a considerable amount of work is being carried out at the IARC of the effect of pretreatment with low doses of carcinogens on the tumorigenicity of a second major dose.

KOTTARIDIS

I would like to ask Dr Strauss: were there leukemia patients included among your group of cancer patients? That is one question.

And I imagine you know why I ask this question. And the second question is, if I understood correctly, you work your system with a mixed lymphocyte population, am I right? Now I wonder if you fractionate your lymphocytes, or have you intended to do it and can you speculate what is going to happen? Is there any particular lymphocyte that is reacting or acting in your system?

SCHLEIFFER-STRAUSS

We did test people suffering from hematological malignancies including various leukemias. We eliminated them from our general considerations because in some cases the test cell is directly involved in the disease process. We did, however, consider that this might represent a situation in which tremendous proliferation of lymphocytes results in the production of mutants which with the appropriate selective and regulatory mechanisms may be required for normal immune functions. That is a highly speculative issue which needs a lot of work. The leukemia patients we did study (and have not yet reported) were acute lymphocytic leukemia, pediatric patients. These were children who as you know are receiving chemotherapeutic modalities for their tumors which are often successful. The protocols we studied included treatment with TG followed by methatrexate. The clinical oncologists using this treatment didn't seem to realize exactly why this sequential combination approach might be effective. It seems that these two agents were components of a very large combination of agents studied over a period of time which were found to be the effective. When we studied these children we discovered that if the individuals were given TG without methatrexate they developed very high TG^R Pbls frequencies, When these treatments with TG were followed by methatrexate the number of TG^R lymphocytes fell to normal and this probably accounts for the therapeutic effect.

As for your second question: we didn't attempt to fractionate our lymphocyte populations. We mainly stimulated T-cells when we used PHA. The monocytes aren't apt to participate. We compared other mitogens including pokeweed mitogen which mainly acts to stimulate B-cells and we found no difference in variant frequencies from one individual at a given time. I don't think the source of the mitogenic stimulation is of great consequence in this test as we apply it. I think mixed lymphocyte reactions would also produce this sort of effect in our system.

BOREK

Dr Waters, I wonder if you could comment on the point that in all the battery of elegant tests you have shown us, there is little concern with the use of human cells. Is that deliberate? Is it because of cost? or time? or for any other reason?

WATERS

No, I don't think that there is a bias against the use of human cells. Certainly not. I think it is largely a matter of the state of development of these bioassay systems. I might point out that the bioassays selected for review under the Gene-Tox Program were chosen in part on the basis of the numbers of chemicals that had been evaluated in each of them. Since there are relatively few scientists that are working with human cell systems in DNA repair and mutagenesis bioassays and even fewer individuals involved in transformation bioassay systems, there obviously will be only a limited data base available from these systems for some time. However, that is not to say that there should be any discouragement, just the opposite, in my opinion. Those of us who have worked in the field of cell culture have long awaited the capability to routinely cultivate human cells, especially human epithelial cells. Now that techniques are available for cultivating cells in the absence of serum or in low serum and there are special factors for growth and differentiation, these factors will permit the more effective research with human cells in culture. Certainly there should be more encouragement of this sort of work. I think that this encouragement is present within the regulatory agencies, such as the one that I represent. Our own laboratory has a major investment in intramural human cell research. In the area of metabolic activation, we are combining human cells with other types of indicator cells such as the V79 Chinese hamster lung cells, and in mutagenesis studies we are employing human foreskin fibroblasts to study forward mutation of the HGPRT locus. We are being encouraged to do this work and, certainly, I think that the regulatory agencies look forward to the time when information obtained using such systems is more readily available. I think that this information will be very useful.

BOREK

Dr Saffiotti, can you estimate within what period of time in the future will the human epithelial systems be available for quantitative transformation studies?

Also I would like to have your comment on the uses of human fibroblasts for chemical transformation. The frequency of radiation induced transformation in human cells seems to be lower than with rodent cells. Thus low doses studies are going to be very difficult. I wondered if you and Dr Legator could comment whether in chemical transformation of human fibroblasts and epithelial cells a similar situation may take place.

SAFFIOTTI

My speculation in this area, which of course we don't know for sure, is that there will be several aspects in which fairly rapid progress will occur in the development of model systems. If we take as a frame of reference the time that was needed to define transformation systems in rodent cells and to make them generally available, I think that it may be reasonable to expect that in the next decade we will have a reasonable basis to use some human cell models as established transformation models. There are, however, certain inherent drawbacks and complications, such as the limited lifespan of human cells in culture. Decisions will eventually have to be made on the choice of systems, for example whether one should try to develop human cell lines comparable to the mouse 3T3 or 10T½ cell lines, which are not normal cells but considerably anenplaid cells, already selected to be halfway towards transformation. In spite of these limitations, the mouse cell line transformation systems have proven to be very useful. There is a possibility that human cell lines will be developed that would become the counterpart to those. I am not personally familiar with the development of the human embryo cell systems you have mentioned, and I don't know how much to expect from it. For any human cell system based on primary or secondary cultures, the high individual variability of human subjects will be a much more serious problem than with the animal counterparts. If we take cells from different individuals we expect marked variability and therefore it will be difficult to standardize any such method for bioassays and quantitative studies. You were asking about human fibroblasts usage in chemical transformation.

BOREK

Do you think the assay is good enough to show quantitatively risk assessment of these agents?

SAFFIOTTI

No, I don't think that we are anywhere close enough to having sufficiently standardized systems to generate a large enough data base to use for risk assessment. The human cell systems that have been developed so far are useful in helping to appreciate their qualitative correlations, in the terms of qualitative risk assessment. When we see the same metabolic pathways, the same cell lesions, the same sequences of cellular events, the same patterns of cellular control mechanisms, in the rodent systems and in their human counterpart, then we feel more confident that the rodent systems are good models of the human cells. On the other hand, we may be able to pick up differences, which I expect will eventually be demonstrated for certain types of chemical or physical agents in relation to certain types of responses in human cells. We will indeed find in what respects human cells are not exactly like mouse cells or rat cells. It's very difficult to venture any guess in that area, but I think that there are good chances that many of these problems will be sorted out in the next decade. We shall then know better how to evaluate what is reliable and what is not in a cell model and for what purpose is a model good. As to the question whether we will move more towards developing human fibroblast cell line systems comparable to rodent systems or move more towards the epithelial systems - as a spectrum of target issue systems to study different parameters - I don't know the answer, but I hope that we will be able to do both.

BOREK

The transformability of both hamster embryo and human embryo cells by radiation decreases with progressive passage of the cells in vitro. We showed this with hamster cell exposed to X-ray in 1966. Recently, Dr Sutherland has found this to be the case with human cells initiated by UV and we are finding the same for human embryo cells exposed to X-rays. These facts introduce an important limiting factor in terms of using primary cultures for risk estimates because the more you passage the cells the less transformation you are going to get. Thus your idea of developing human "cell lines" might be a very good solution.

TAYLOR

Just before you questioned Dr Saffiotti you implied that human fibroblasts generally could be transformed by ionizing radiation. Is this the case?

BOREK

Yes. My work has been with ionizing radiation, with X-rays.

TAYLOR

But it is generally not the case that human fibroblasts can be transformed by X-rays, you are referring to particular lines. Is that correct?

BOREK

I am referring to particular experiments. The whole area of cell transformation is very young.

TAYLOR

I just thought it was unfair to generalize on all human fibroblasts, that is all.

BOREK

My generalization on transformability decreasing with cell passage is on the basis of my work and Dr Sutherland's in indicating that embryonic fibroblasts become less transformable with progressive passage in culture. This may be a limiting factor for long term experiments if late passages are to be used. This is what I wanted to point out.

GOULD

I would just like to address a general question to Dr Saffiotti, Dr Waters, Dr Arlett. In general we have been talking about cell systems whether they be human or rodent and concentrating on genotoxicity assays. Is it possible that most of our cells have already been initiated? Maybe we should be directing these assays more towards trying to identify promoting agents. There doesn't seem to be much work in this area. It has been demonstrated that promotors do work in culture but are we not ignoring this in much of our environmental screening efforts in cell culture systems?

WATERS

Since you mentioned the EPA, I suppose I should respond to the question. Certainly, there is no lack of concern over promoting agents. The agency is interested in in vitro and in vivo techniques for detection of promotors and has actively supported research to develop such techniques. At the present time, however, we don't have well standardized short-term assays for promotors. The best established method employs the original mouse skin model, and this procedure is time consuming. We are concerned about the phenomenon of promotion and believe that the development of short-term assays to detect promotors should be encouraged.

ARLETT

Since my name was associated with the collective question, I will respond. First of all since Jim Trosko first published the observation on the modulation of mutation in Chinese hamster cells with TPA, Madam C. Lasne from Chouroulinkov's lab was visiting us and tried to check those observations with mouse lymphoma cells. We were totally unable to modulate mutation using three different mutagens and a couple of endpoints with TPA. Has anybody else here followed up Trosko's subsequent publication that the modulation was really via metabolic co-operation? You could use a metabolic co-operation experiment, put on your suspect promotor and either wipe out or have no effect on metabolic corporation. This would function as a cellular test for promoting activity.

GOULD

In the light of this, the original work actually was originated by Lankas. He has worked with the ouabain system. At the densities he was working with there wasn't much cross-feeding. Thus it would be hard to explain these results with promotors based on the modification of cross-feeding.

ARLETT

Well, the specific point is that with ouabain we can avoid the complication of metabolic corporation altogether. My comment was that Jim Trosko went on to use metabolic co-operation as a test for promoting agents and I'm just asking as a collective question whether there is anybody here who has followed it up and whether it has come to anything?

CERUTTI

Carrano and collaborators at San Francisco have re-investigated the mutagens and no-mutagens effect of TPA in several types of cells. In general, TPA was inactive in contrast to earlier results by Trosko and collaborators. I'll show tomorrow that TPA indeed is a very weak inducer of SCE, but a strong clastogenic agent. This property might potentially be useful for the testing of promotors.

ARLETT

I am aware of two studies which say the original Trosko results couldn't be repeated. My question was, does anybody know whether his series of experiments on TPA and promotors on metabolic co-operation have been repeated and whether it is a usable system? It seems to me, since we happen to be talking about promotors, that Trosko has a very exciting system and I am not sure if anybody is following it up.

CERUTTI

It depends entirely on the cell type, some cells have it and others don't.

BOREK

It has been persued by a group in Australia, Murry's group. My early work in the field, in 1969, using electrophysiological intercellular communication indicated that cell communication varied with cell type. This is possibly the case with the modifying effect by promotors.

ARLETT

Since we are supposed to be teaching, I will use this opportunity to give a brief description of the mechanics of metabolic cooperation. What we are talking about here is the transmission of gene product or information from one cell to another through gaps between cells. If a cell is of the HGPRT- phenotype and it touches a cell which is HGPRT+, it can be modified into an HPPRT+ by the transfer of gene product from the plus to the minus cell. This then makes the cell phenotypically normal and sensitive to 6-thioguanine. Cell to cell contact is necessary for the effect to occur. Now it seems almost certain that the same sort of cell system can be used to transfer information relating to thymidine kinase activity as well. What Trosko showed is that if he mixed the two cell types together and then added 6-thioguanine to the system which would normally kill the HGPRT+ cells, the metabolic co-operation capacity could be removed by promoting agents. His idea was to use the metabolic co-operation experiment to establish the existence of promoting activity.

BOREK

I think that potentially it sounds like a marvellous idea. Dr Legator, do you have any comments?

LEGATOR

I have just examined a review article of Jim's and as far as I can tell it hasn't been expanded over his original paper as far as new experimental data is concerned.

BOREK

Returning to the original question by Dr Gould, we must realize that the distinction between initiators and promotors is very fine. Every initiator at the right dose in the right target tissue is a complete carcinogen, namely it will act as an initiator and a promotor. Thus one of the uses of in vitro systems is to assess the action of initiators and promotors. In culture one can expose the cells to the oncogenic agent at low doses in which one cannot observe transformation above spontaneous level. However, once the initiated cells are exposed to a promotor, they will express transformation suggesting that cells which did not appear to be initiated are now promoted to full expression following the treatment, indicating that initiation did take place.

KOTTARIDIS

The work with Epstein bar virus has shown that TPA has been used to initiate or to enhance the expression of the virus. Although it has been used in different concentrations, high, low, medium doses and in different cells still nobody is able to make this virus go into any other cell except the B lymphocytes and the only observation here is on this particular cell, so what is a promotor? Really if EBV regularly infects B-cell and you observe by using TPA a somewhat better expression of this virus, there is not too much that anybody can do actually. If this TPA would work let's say on fibroblasts infected with EBV or on some other cell then we could really be able to speak seriously about TPA as a promotor. In this case, I don't know how anybody can take this as a promotor if it just enhances one or two-fold the expression of the virus in cells.

BOREK

Perhaps Dr Lambert has some comments on the question of promotion in human cells.

LAMBERT

Yes, thank you Dr Borek. We are now actually engaged in studies using TPA and benzo pyrene looking at excision, gene amplification and the expression of integrated viral sequences in human cells but as yet are unable to differentiate between intitiating events and a promotional event.

BOREK

I would like to ask Dr Jansen if he has any comments in this area on the use of human cells in risk estimates. I know you will be giving us a comprehensive talk, your own talk, but would you like to comment in the context of this discussion?

JANSEN

I am extremely encouraged that it is now possible to use human cells because this is a great step forward. We have to wait and see how to incorporate this development into a wider research program to see what their contribution is going to be. I would like to make one further comment. Several people have remarked that human cells are far less sensitive than cells of rats, mice and hamsters. I wouldn't be surprised if one or two chemicals would be found where the opposite would be the case and they might be the chemicals which could pose a real human health risk. But I think it is very dangerous to generalize before we have a far greater data base than now.

BOREK

Dr Perry, would you like to comment on your experience using human cells versus animal cells for assessing compounds which produce various chromosomal changes as the endpoint such as sister chromatid exchanges?

PERRY

In general I use Chinese hamster cells in preference to human cells because we have them growing in the lab the whole time and we have them well characterized. I think we discovered some time ago that Chinese hamster cells in general are quite a lot more sensitive than human cells. We were somewhat worried some years ago that if we did start using human cells we would have to try several individuals because of the variation between people. That did worry us for some time and right now whenever we do experiments testing chemicals we usually test these chemicals over a range of individuals to see if there is any difference in response. In general, taking for example a population of non-smokers there is very little difference from one individual to another.

BOREK

Do you find variations between cells from different sources?

Do you find a similar chromosomal alteration if you take peripheral blood cells as compared to skin fibroblasts? Do you have similar patterns of SCE in response to particular carcinogens?

PERRY

I am sure there is a difference although in fact I have not done these experiments. I think it was Beek and Obe who investigated chromosomes in fibroblasts and lymphocytes and other types of cells. In fact, there was a considerable difference in sensitivity but that doesn't really surprise me because there is a big difference in, for example, cell cycle time between the two types of cells and that will make a difference to the SCE response.

BOREK

Then what is the choice cell? If we want to use human cells for risk estimates should we suggest using lymphocytes and fibroblasts? Which type do we rely on?

PERRY

Well, I don't think I am really prepared to give a definite answer on that. As far as I am concerned you just use every type of cell you can get your hands on. We are not really at the stage of making a black and white answer yet. We just need a lot more data on this.

BOREK

Dr Kraemer would you have any comments on the uses of human cells in these risk estimates using cells from individuals afflicted with diseases you have been dealing with?

KRAEMER

I have been working with human lymphoblastoid cell lines that have been transformed with EB virus. We will be talking more about that in a couple of days. These cells may be the mammalian cell answer to bacteria in that they grow to high numbers in suspension culture and they are fairly easy to handle. Unfortunately, instead of doubling in 20 minutes the bacteria their doubling time is closer to 20 hours but that is the way it is with mammalian cells. There is a lot of technology being developed at present to work with lymphoblastoid cells. It may even be possible to automate analysis of cell survival and mutability. One advantage over fibroblasts and that is that you can get a large number of cells for biochemical work in a short period of time. Since the cells are transformed, we must always be cautious in ascribing properties to the original human that may be related to the process.

ROMMAELERE

Actually we are looking at mutagenesis in a rather indirect way: indeed, we are measuring viral mutagenesis and we test whether certain cell treatments modify the ability of the cells to mutagenize an infecting virus. We performed those studies both with rodent and human cells. So far we couldn't detect any significant difference, neither kinetic nor quantitative, with respect to viral mutagenesis.

BOREK

That is interesting. It is one of the important things to establish, namely the differences and similarities that exist when comparing human with animal cells.

SAFFIOTTI

Since I have been talking primarily in support of the use of human cells, I want to relate some opposing arguments too. Some years ago at a symposium on developments in research pathology, the exciting developments in the methods for the study of carcinogenesis in human cells have been discussed. An authoritative dissenting view was voiced by Arthur Kornberg, the Nobel laureate molecular biologist and biochemist, who warned against the use of experimental models based on human cells since they are so poorly defined in molecular terms. He advocated the use of simple and well defined biological systems, such as certain bacterial, viral or phage systems. We explained that we were talking of a different type and level of research approach, and that we were interested in studying the pathology of human tissues and cells. After a long discussion I guess that he accepted that we may need to use human cells to study the diseases of human cells, as long as we were not really trying to elucidate basic molecular mechanisms in a poorly defined biological system, such as human cells, just because they were human and therefore apparently "relevant". It is an important argument, and a sobering note, that one should not use human cells just to be able to say that one is doing research relevant to human disease - if one is really interested in studying basic molecular mechanisms that need to be studied in better befined biological systems. We should not force the use of human cells for the purpose of studying mechanisms that can be learnt better in simpler and better defined systems. If we are interested as experimental pathologists in the study of human disease and in relating the non-human models to human disease, then at some point we should eventually undertake careful studies of human tissues and cells and of human diseases, but remembering how difficult it is to control these studies critically.

CIARROCCHI

The different sensitivity between rodent and human cells brings to my mind a paper authored by Ruth Ben-Ishai. She said in that paper that rodent cells, as soon as you start to culture them, lose part of their ability to repair DNA damages. We don't see this change in repair ability in human cells.

CERUTTI

If I can refer to some of our own work. In 1974 we did some studies on repair capacity as a function of passage with WI38 fibroblasts (the Hayflick system). Extracts from cells at about passage 40 precipitously lost their capacity to repair gamma ray type damage, i.e. several passages before they stop dividing and die. The question was, of course, whether the loss of repair capacity is the cause of death or vice versa. Similar experiments with skin explants (fibroblasts) from young and old people again suggest a diminution of repair capacity in the older individuals. I think you should talk to Dick Setlow when he is here, he has much more experience in this area which is open to a lot of criticism.

YAROSH

When I was in Dick Setlow's lab we attempted to follow up the initial observation of Ben-Ishai that rodent cells lost the ability for excision repair during passage or aging. Our approach was to say that if they lost the ability of excision repair it might be because they lost the ability to incise DNA that had been UV irradiated. Our approach was to permeabilize rodent cells and introduce an endonuclease which recognized UV irradiated DNA from micrococcus luteus. The results of these experiments were that the endonuclease got into the cells and nicked the DNA, but the rodent cells were still unable to excise the dimers. If the cells lost the ability to excise dimers during passage or during the aging process, the loss was more than just shutting off the incision of dimers, but included the complete loss of all the steps of excision repair even if the DNA had been incised. So I think that there is certainly a lot more research to be done before we can say that aging shuts off the excision repair processes in rodent cells.

ROUND TABLE: MEASUREMENTS OF DNA REPAIR ACTIVITY IN HUMAN CELLS

Leader: P.A. Cerutti

Dept. of Carcinogenesis, Swiss Institute for Experimental

Cancer Research, Epalinges s/Lausanne, Switzerland

CERUTTI

First we'd like to discuss questions which are directly relevant to the lectures of this morning, very shortly, only burning questions are being accepted. Then I'd like to ask 5 speakers to give the short presentations for which they have signed up and which are relevant to the topic of the round table discussion for this afternoon. In the third part I'd like to discuss with you the possible role of DNA repair for interindividual differences in cancer susceptibility. Maybe we can come up with some recommendations of what system could be used to explore this question. For the fourth topic, it has been suggested that we discuss radical mechanisms which might be involved in human carcinogenesis.

Short questions relating directly to the lectures of this morning:

LEWIS

I was interested in the role of the active oxygen in the diseased states in which most of the tumors seem to come from the immunocompetent cells. The role of the active oxygen, especially hydrogen peroxide, in the killing of intracellular bacteria is well known. It also may be a very important mechanism in macrophage mediated cytolysis of tumor cells. Could it not possibly be in some of these diseases, and I understand that these people frequently die from infection, that just by encountering of bacteria, they are continually and chornically damaging the DNA of their immunocompetent cells. These mechanisms you described could be easily tested or has this been tested already?

CERUTTI

This is a very interesting comment. The word I liked best in your comment is 'chronic'. I think the chronic exposure which is typical for inflammation and some of the rheumatoid diseases I mentioned this morning could well play a role in tumor promotion and progression and possibly even in initiation.

ARLETT

Phil Lawley and his collaborators have been looking at immunodeficiency diseases over the last few years. For information, they are fairly convinced now that a large number of these patients are defective in O_6-methyl-guanine excision. While we have been at some pains to try and play down the cry 'repair' here comes 'repair' throwing itself out at another level.

CERUTTI

Something which I find particularly striking in the chromosome breakage disorders: so many apparently unrelated abnormalities have been discovered on the molecular level. This is hard to explain on the basis of a single gene mutation. Some mechanism of the type mentioned by Dr Lewis could be involved. For example a deficiency in detoxification of active oxygen species may result in chronic macromolecular damage. This could result in partial enzyme deficiencies rather than total lack of a function.

KRAEMER

As you have been pointing out the damage may be ubiquitous but the diseases are well defined. The clinical characteristics fall into certain categories, for instance we talk glibly about xeroderma pigmentosum patients having neurological abnormalities (and so do ataxia teangiectasia patients) but the specificity of the type of abnormality is much different in the two of them. We are really at a loss to explain this specificity particularly in view of a general mechanism of damage.

CERUTTI

I totally agree. I would like to stress we are not proposing that the abnormality in oxygen metabolism which apparently exists in these diseases represents the primary genetic defect in these diseases. It may be a secondary expression of the pathology in these diseases, however.

LEWIS

The tissue specificity of the reaction to injury, may be very different for neural tissue, but back to the immune system, these tumors do seem to be specific. I don't mean to offer the solution, but merely put forth a hypothesis. The technology exists to test it.

KRAEMER

Now, I'll be talking about unscheduled synthesis. This is one of the measurements of repair and involves irradiating cells and then adding tritiated thymidine. If repair is going properly the dimer will be removed. A patch will be created and if there is tritiated thymidine in the medium it will be incorporated into DNA. Auto-radiography can assess the amount of thymidine incorporated. This is performed by using a photographic emulsion and then analyzing the amount of repair on a single cell basis. Unirradiated cells in S phase will be very black indicating that they can incorporate tritiated thymidine. In other cells nuclei contain only few grains. The S phase is the 'scheduled' phase of synthesis and if the cells are repairing, there would be incorporation in the 'unscheduled' phase. The unscheduled DNA synthesis may be quantitated by actually counting the number of grains over each nucleus. The following result is obtained when this type of procedure is carried out with cells from a patient with xeroderma pigmentosum. Again we see S phase cells that are heavily labelled, showing that the cells can incorporate tritiated thymidine (in S phase) but the other nuclei do not have any grains, indicating a much reduced rate of unscheduled DNA synthesis in XP patients as compared to the normal.

We can also measure this type of repair in circulating peripheral blood lymphocytes. This is a very rapid test, which can be applied to the diagnosis of XP and also for doing studies of DNA repair. The lymphocytes are treated with UV and, in this case, hydroxyuria is added to reduce the very low residual rate of DNA synthesis. Normal lymphocytes but not XP lymphocytes have an increase in this type of repair synthesis after UV. We have obtained evidence suggesting that there may be no absolute block of repair in XP. Rather repair may be slower. This has been evident when we pulsed with thymidine for successive periods of time. By 6-9 hrs the normal lymphocytes had ceased doing any measurable repair, but the XP cells continued. Again by 9-12 hrs, the normal was 0 and the XP had 174 counts. We kept this up for two days. The total amount of repair in the normal was 851 and in the XP was 899. Therefore, for peripheral blood lymphocytes the total amount of repair was the same in the normals and XP, but the rate was much slower in the XP. We use this type of information when we test patients to see if they have XP. (Robbins et al., Ann. Intern. Med. 80, 221-248, 1974).

CERUTTI

A comment to completeness of repair: R. Setlow and collaborators have shown that pothodimer excision in xeroderma cells may merely occur at a strongly reduced rate. In our own work with 313 mm irradiation a similar result has been obtained. It now follows a short contribution by Dr Lewis. He pointed out to me that he observed a discrepancy between the kinetics of product removal measured by fluorescence technology and unscheduled DNA synthesis. Measuring unscheduled DNA synthesis may be simple but it doesn't give you the whole truth.

LEWIS

When we are doing the experiments with SDMH (1.2-dimethyl hydrazine) we measured the disappearance of O6-methylguanine (O^6MG) while the animals were continuously drinking the carcinogen for 28 days. This means they were continuously alkylating their DNA. In the hepatocytes, O^6MG was rapidly removed reaching almost the limit of detection by 3 days. However, concurrently we were quantifying unscheduled DNA synthesis. This was very high at the beginning of the experiment but by 28 days there was no measurable unscheduled synthesis. This was occurring at a time when (after 28 days of exposure) the hepatocytes were repairing O^6MG as fast as it was formed. It appears that unscheduled synthesis may not be the main mechanism by which O6-methylguanine is repaired. It is interesting that after 28 days of exposure to SDMH there was no unscheduled DNA synthesis in hepatocytes which are thought to have the ability to invoke specific mechanisms for DNA repair. Is there an initial general response and an induced specific response?

CERUTTI

Looking at DNA repair and replication may also not give a complete answer about the metabolism of damaged DNA. Chemical carcinogens may have other effects which indeed may be more relevant to carcinogenesis than the processes we have been mostly discussing now.

I'd like to mention that Sarah Lavi has described phenomena on induction and amplification of SV40 sequences in rodent cells upon treatment with carcinogens. She has also demonstrated that the DNA which has been amplified could then be used to transfect and transform carcinogen induced rodent cells in Cooper-Weinberg type experiments.

While the methodologies used in this type of experiment seem very sophisticated and laborious, there is no reason that later they could be standardized and simplified and that they could be made amenable to carcinogen testing.

BOREK

I think one should be very cautious in extrapolating from studies *in vitro* on gene amplification to *in vivo* situation, e.g. acquisition of cell resistance to the chemotherapeutic agent methotraxate is correlated *in vitro* with gene amplification but it is so far strictly an *in vitro* phenomenon.

CERUTTI

The somatic mutation hypothesis of cancer is very old but far from being proved. All I'm saying is that those tests may be as justifiable or unjustifiable as mutagenesis tests etc. which are presently in use.

LAMBERT

I would like to make two brief comments. The first is that we are interested in trying the transfection experiments with the extracts from our excision experiments to see whether indeed we can induce morphological transformation.

The second point is that we are interested in establishing a dose-response relationship for this excision phenomenon and in comparing this with standard assays of point mutation and transformation as a way to compare these various biological endpoints and perhaps to improve our understanding of this possible molecular mechanism of carcinogenesis.

CERUTTI

The bext presentation will be by Dr Yarosh. The topic of his short presentation is: incision of carcinogen treated DNA by extracts of human cells.

YAROSH

I would like to describe a new assay for the incision of carcinogen damaged DNA. The basis of the assay begins with supercoiled plasmid. Two different preparations are used. One labelled with tritium, and one labelled with (14C). These plasmids can essentially be of any type but the ones I've selected contain a gene which can be selected, the glactokinase gene, from *E. coli*. The treated plasmid is treated with a DNA damaging agent. This can be of any type either UV light or radiation or any sort of chemical mutagen. The second plasmid is held as a control, the (14C). The two plasmids are then mixed and always treated together. Any difference between the treated tritium plasmid and the (14C) plasmid represents something which is specific to the DNA lesion. The plasmids are mixed together and then treated with an extract of human cells. I prepared the extract by sonication, although any method for preparing cell extracts can be employed. There is an activity in human cell extracts which incises the DNA. It will incise at the site of a lesion and supercoiled DNA which contains an incision is relaxed. The control plasmid which does not contain a lesion is not incised by the human extract and retains it's supercoiled structure. The plasmids are loaded onto a column and this column contains acridine dye bound to bisacrylamide. Acridine is a dye. It is a planer molecule and it intercalates into DNA and for energetic reasons it prefers to interact with supercoiled

DNA. The DNA is loaded on the top of the column and eluted with a salt solution. The DNA which has been nicked and relaxed doesn't interact much with the acridine and flows through very fast or elutes at a lower salt concentration. The supercoiled DNA interacts with acridine dye and is retained on the column. The material which comes out early is relaxed DNA which has been nicked and the material which elutes later is supercoiled and it has not been nicked. By comparing the amount which comes out relaxed in the treated versus the amount which comes out relaxed in the control one can determine the incision activity. The log of the percentage of supercoiled plasmid at the end of the assay divided by the percentage of supercoiled plasmid at the beginning gives the total number of breaks per plasmid. This is assuming a Poisson distribution of breaks.

There are two factors which have to be subtracted from this equation. One is non-specific nuclease breaks and the second factor is breaks directly produced by the carcinogen treatment. UV doesn't cause a great deal of breaks directly and this second number is small. For other carcinogens such as alkylating agents this number might be a little bit larger. Let us examine a sample profile. The untreated plasmid elutes at the latter stages of the elution profile. If you irradiate the plasmid with UV very few breaks are produced and it continues to elute late. If you irradiate the plasmid with 100 jouls per meter squared which introduces quite a few dimers and then treat with the _M. luteus_ endonuclease which recognizes dimers and makes incisions most of the DNA elutes early. DNA has been irradiated with a small dose, 5 jouls per meter squared and treated with the _M. luteus_ endonuclease which nicks the dimers.

Here we see two populations, the group of plasmids which contained a dimer and were nicked and the group of plasmids which did not contain a dimer and which were not nicked. This technique is very accurate. I have plotted the number of breaks per plasmid versus jouls per meter squared. Between 0 and 1 break per plasmid there is a very good linear relationship. The technique is accurate for these very small doses of UV and very low levels of nicks which are ordinarily very difficult to measure. This data can be used to show endonuclease activity against UV irradiated DNA. Plasmid DNA labelled with tritium has been irradiated by 40 jouls per meter squared and the 14C-labelled plasmid has been left unirradiated. These have been treated with an extract from a human tumor cell which is completely normal in UV repair. The irradiated plasmid has been nicked and most of the DNA elutes in the region of relaxed DNA. The unirradiated plasmid remains mostly supercoiled. The number of breaks which are introduced in 14C-DNA represents the non-specific breaks from the nuclease activity.

We have examined normal human fibroblasts, tumor cells and lymphoblastoid cells and have measured breaks produced in the DNA. The dose of irradiation that was used was 40 jouls per meter squared which introduced about 1 or 2 dimers per plasmid. If the extract is heated at 70° for an hour you can inactivate its nicking activity. We have taken a number of different cell lines with normal UV sensitivity and we have measured in extracts the ability to nick plasmid DNA. HH4 is a normal lymphoblastoid cell line which has been transformed by Epstein-Barr virus. It has normal UV sensitivity and at two different protein concentrations we measured nicking. Here we are looking at two of the diseases which have been discussed, xeroderma pigmentosum and Cockayne's syndrome.

The point was made that the problem with xeroderma pigmentosum is not necessarily the complete absence of incision but a very slow nature. We have measured endonuclease activity in xeroderma pigmentosum cells and these cells have been measured by Dr Kraemer to be hypersensitive to UV light. Nevertheless one can detect in these cells endonuclease activity. Cockayne's syndrome cells are hypersensitive to UV light although as Dr Arlett has mentioned, there is no evidence of a defect in UV repair. We have measured endonuclease activity against UV irradiated DNA in these cells. Dr Lewis mentioned that it is possible that when alkylating agents produce O6-methylguanine it may be repaired in a mechanism which doesn't involve incision. We have data which support this point. Here we are using methylnitrosourea-treated DNA. It has been treated with 100 mmolar and it creates a whole spectrum of lesions including N7 methylguanine and O6-methylguanine. We have characterized in our laboratory a series of cell lines some of which we call Mer+ and some of which we call Mer-. The Mer+ cells are able to remove O6-methylguanine, the Mer- cells are not able to repair O6-methylguanine. Normal fibroblasts are able to nick MNU-treated DNA. This DNA has about three methyl adducts per plasmid so we are nicking up to a third of the methyl groups on the DNA. Normal cells are able to nick and a series of tumor cells that can remove O6-methylguanine also nick MNU-treated DNA. However, cells which are unable to repair O6-methylguanine nevertheless are still able to nick MNU-treated DNA.

The conclusion in both these instances are that we may find cells which fail to repair certain lesions, but when we look at the first step, that is the ability to recognize an incise DNA, these cells may contain endonuclease activity. As a final comment I'd like to encourage the use of this technique. It is a very rapid and easy technique. One can complete the elution, clean the column and reuse it in a matter of an hour. By washing one column while using another one can do a whole series of these assays in a day so it is a very quick and, as I hope you have seen, a very sensitive technique for measuring the incision step. It may also be useful in determining whether human cells can recognize carcinogens. You can use a chemical of an unknown nature and determine whether human cells have the ability to recognize the lesions. If they don't have the ability to recognize the lesions perhaps we will be at risk that some lesion will persist in DNA because of our inability to repair it.

CERUTTI

Since you advertised the procedure, do you make the conditions available to the audience? There is a law in commerce that if a product is publicized it also has to be sold. It also should be mentioned that Dr Thielmann (Heidelberg) has used similar technology using PM2 bacteriophage DNA. In this system he was apparently able to distinguish normal and xeroderma pigmentosum extracts in that the latter were incision defective, in contrast to earlier work by Mortelmans et al.

I would now like to discuss with you the possible role of DNA repair in determining individual susceptibility to carcinogen exposure. The fact that repair deficiencies have not been demonstrated with certainty in the chromosome breakage disorders does not exclude the possibility that DNA repair may represent an important step in carcinogenesis and may contribute to inter-individual differences in susceptibility. Cancer susceptibility in xeroderma pigmentosum patients remains to be a very impressive *in vivo* example.

LAMBERT

I just want to make a general comment about the utility of using repair as a screening method. From the evolutionary and human population genetics perspective it certainly does make sense to believe that there could be some genetic heterogeneity in repair response since a biochemical pathway such as this must have been subject to some selective pressure during human evolution. But at the same time geneticists would argue that there may also be environmental variability underlying the observed distribution of spontaneous mutation rates in man. Here I refer to Jim Neil's work, who has compared mutation rates in traditional versus urban societies, and seems to be able to explain the observed differences on the basis of endogenous mutagens in the environment. In other words, those people who live in traditional societies seem to have a higher background mutation rate, but also seem to be eating foods which may contain mutagens. So, the observed difference in spontaneous mutation in his study population does not seem to have a direct correlation with genetic variability in repair, a fact which strikes me as possibly reducing the overall utility of using repair as an assay in large scale population screening for susceptibility to cancer, although it obviously doesn't rule out the utility of using repair in studying specific genetic isolates, or for tracing the incidence of heterozygous carriers of the recessive repair disorders like xeroderma.

CERUTTI

I don't think we have time to go into this, but I would not dare to eliminate the possibility of a contribution of repair capacity to differences in individual cancer susceptibility.

GOULD

I just want to comment on patients we see in high risk clinics for cancer, many risks that are based on family history. These people have specific risks for certain organs. For example, high risk for breast cancer, high risk for colon cancer. Thus even if we don't find any major differences of repair by looking at peripheral blood lymphocytes or fibroblasts that doesn't eliminate the possibility that there are going to be repair differences, if you look at the target organ for specific susceptibility. In other words, you may have to look at breast cells or colon cells. We find this sort of organ specific susceptibility in rats. Strains of rats may have a high susceptibility for chemically induced breast cancer but no differences for liver cancers. Thus we should concentrate more effort on target cells as opposed to non-target cells such as lymphocytes and fibroblasts.

CERUTTI

I think there is some supporting evidence to this point from Rufus Days' laboratory. Is there anybody who would like to comment to this?

YAROSH

The reasoning is really quite simple. We have seen that germ line mutations can arise which can inactivate DNA repair mechanisms resulting in cancer and that is XP. There can be somatic mutations which arise in someone's body during development which results in a clone of cells within the body which are DNA repair defective. That clone of cells within the body may be more likely to be transformed by agents in the environment and the supporting evidence is to simply survey tumors. We use an assay using a damaged virus to measure the ability of tumor cells to support the virus. The results are that about 20% of human tumor cells are deficient in the repair of the damaged virus and these are the cells I referred to as being defective in repair of O6-methylguanine. Cells can undergo somatic mutation, these somatic mutations may be in DNA repair mechanism, and result in a cluster of cells which are hypersensitive and may represent cells susceptible to transformation.

KRAEMER

The model that has been used is the xeroderma model. In XP all of the cells that have been examined in a given patient have shown an equal defect in DNA repair. These include the ones we have mentioned previously, in the dermal fibroblasts and the lymphocytes or lymphoblastoid cells. In addition epidermal cells, ocular cells, liver cells, muscle cells and epithelial cells all have been checked and found to show the defect (Kraemer, K.H. Xeroderma Pigmentosum, In Demis, Dobson, McGuire, Clinical Dermatology, 1980, Harper & Row, unit 19-7). This has been the model for genetic susceptibility to cancer, whereas the one that Dan Yarosh was talking about may be a non-genetic mechanism involving a somatic mutation.

The test I showed before using the lymphocytes to detect deficient UV repair has not been able to pick up small differences in repair. The XP patients that we have looked at had large differences where the residual rate of repair was from 0-50% of normal. If it is greater than that we will have difficulty to determine it. Actually you can't even pick out all the xeroderma patients with that test in that the xeroderma variants would be normal. One way we have tried to amplify the sensitivity was to look at an early time and also at a late time where we can see the reversal of it. Now if you use PHA-stimulated cells this would increase the repair but would also increase the background and might give you a problem. An alternative method that may be suitable to discriminate between the scheduled synthesis and the repair synthesis is that of the BND cellulose that Strauss and Scudiero had used. This has been able to pick up differences and may be suitable for examining lymphocytes on a large scale.

CERUTTI

I think that leads us to the next point, i.e. what are the technologies which could be used to test the hypothesis that DNA repair represents an important step in the carcinogenesis process. Immunological methods may become particularly important since they promise to be highly sensitive, rapid, cheap and are amenable to cytological studies. I would like to ask Dr Rommelaere, who has been involved in preparing antibodies against DNA lesions and has used immunological techniques in studies of DNA repair, to address some comments to this point.

ROMMELAERE

I would like to emphasize the potentiality of immunological methods in measuring the induction and removal of lesions. I think that those methods could be standardized and used to screen human cells for their repair capacity. About six years ago Jan Cornelis in our Department, prepared antisera directed against UV-irradiated DNA, these antisera apparently recognize UV-induced pyrimidine dimers. Several laboratories are involved in the preparation of antisera directed against other types of radiation- or chemically induced lesions.

Most importantly, the technique of monoclonal antibodies production is being used by a few groups, including Cerutti's and Lohman's, in order to improve the specificity of these preparations. I think that availability of such antibodies provides a unique probe for measuring lesions in treated cells and for determining their removal. Indeed, lesions can be quantitated either in vitro by radio immunoassay or in situ by the autoradiographic measurement of the cell-binding of radio-labelled antibodies. Both types of methods are convenient, rapid and very sensitive. The radio-immunoassay, in particular, allows one to measure the induction of a small number of lesions which would not be detected by classical fractionation procedures. We used the in situ immunolabelling technique to study the time-course of the removal of pyrimidine dimers in different types of cells. To that purpose, cells were fixed at different times following irradiation and were incubated with radio-labelled antibodies directed against dimers. The amount of antibodies which bound to the cells was quantitated by autoradiography and provided a measurement of the number of lesions. Since individual cells are scored, this in situ procedure can be applied to a heterogeneous culture, as far as the different cell types can be differentiated microscopically. Moreover, the resolution of the in situ immunolabelling technique makes it possible to localize damage within cells exposed to a narrow beam of radiation. If the cultures are fixed immediately after irradiation, the binding of the antibodies is indeed restricted to the area of the cells which has been hit by the beam.

BOREK

I would just like to point out the possibilities of human in vitro cell transformation. In recent ongoing studies in collaboration with Allan Andrews we have been evaluating the oncogenic effect of UVB on XP and Bloom's syndrome cells. We find that the XP cells require shorter treatment time than the Bloom cells to achieve an equal result in terms of morphological transformation and growth in agar. Thus, human cell transformation in vitro, with reproducible reliable endpoints could be useful in determining directly the susceptibility of the human cells from various individuals to the action of various carcinogens.

CERUTTI

This is clearly important and could be a topic for a future conference.

I'd like to give you some food for thought for the evening. The last topic to be discussed was 'the involvement of radical mechanisms in cancer initiation and promotion'. I'd like to ask Dr Jansen to express a few words in this regard.

JANSEN

I am a bit hesitant because I am trying to formulate a theory which an organic chemist is trying to develop in our group. His language and expertise is too difficult for me and I may well misrepresent important parts of his 'theory'. He is first an organic chemist in polymer chemistry but is not a toxicologist and he was struck by the fact that if you write up the equation of DNA alkylation by polynuclear aromatic compounds you must, by force, end up with an electron liberated at the same time. This electron should be added to the pool of active oxygen species which you described so beautifully this morning in your slide. Indeed excessive production of active oxygen without enough oxygen dismutase would be one of the most devastating things which could happen to the cell.

He was also struck by the fact that if he looked over the alkylation data with the eyes of an organic chemist that the yield in terms of organic chemistry of these alkylation products was extremely low indeed. Now his suggestion was, and I hope that I am giving it in a not too bad fashion, that what is happening in transformation is actually the excessive production of active oxygen and he came back to the theory of Walpole who published about 1960 about cross-linking at a time that one did not know about DNA yet so he could not formulate his theory in terms of cross-linking of DNA, although he defined the necessary distances. But this colleague of mine made some calculations and saw that the singlet oxygen (or some other active oxygen) was excellently suited in dimensions to the cross-linking of DNA and to the dimensions proposed by Walpole as early as 1960. Now if it is true that a carcinogen is really a compound which produces an excess of singlet oxygen in the cell then DNA alkylation would be the side reaction only and active oxygen the real initiator. I wonder whether you have any comments on this theory which would fit the situation depicted in your slide.

ROUND TABLE: RISK ASSESSMENT FOR LOW-DOSE AND LOW-DOSE-RATE RADIATION

Leader: Richard Burton Setlow

Brookhaven National Laboratory

Upton, Long Island, New York 11973

SETLOW

I doubt if we will come up with an answer for this assessment, but I am sure a number of you have something to say on the subject. Let me introduce it by pointing out that there have been several US National Research Council studies on the subject of assessment of risk from ionizing radiation. One is called BEIR III (the Biological Effects of Ionizing Radiation). It created a great deal of controversy because it represented the average view of the committee and had two dissents. One said the report was too conservative and the other said just the opposite. So perhaps it was a good average after all. A second report which has recently appeared is called FREIR (Federal Research Efforts in Ionizing Radiation). This report was wise and made no attempt to assess the risk from ionizing radiation but indicated the kinds of research that might be useful in reaching conclusions about the quantitative effects of ionizing radiation.

Ionizing radiation is more complicated than many chemicals and it is also more complicated than UV radiation. Let me outline some of the terms that may appear in the discussion. One is LET (linear energy transfer), the special rate at which radiation distributes energy. Most people agree that for high linear energy transfers, such as from alpha particles or neutrons, the biological effects of high LET radiation are to a large extent a linear function of dose. Having said that I need say no more because a linear function has no threshold and if we knew the effect at a high dose we can interpolate and find the effect at a low dose. The problem of major uncertainty is the low LET effects arising from X-rays and gamma rays. These effects are complicated by split doses and dose rates. Most experiments are carried out at high dose rates. In the real world, except for cataclysmic events, we have low doses. The problem is how to extrapolate from one to another. The National Research Council's report reached a golden mean and described the low dose rate effects as being a composite of linear and quadratic terms. This was the point of controversy. I want to illustrate some of this controversy by a Figure based on some of the NRC calculations.

It represents calculations made to describe human data obtained with doses in the range of 100-150 rads. They represent the average mortality from leukemia or bone cancer per 10,000 males as a function of dose. The experimental points if they existed at all, would lie in the high dose range, 100-150 rads. Three curves are drawn, linear (L), quadratic (Q), linear quadratic (LQ). They are theoretical curves from BEIR III drawn through the experimental data at high doses which fit these data. Also indicated is the dose - 0.1 rad/yr - that one receives from average radiation background. The experimental problem we face is to distinguish between these three curves. The consensus of opinion is that it is impossible to distinguish between them because we cannot do the appropriate experiments on people. We can't get enough people so as to decrease the

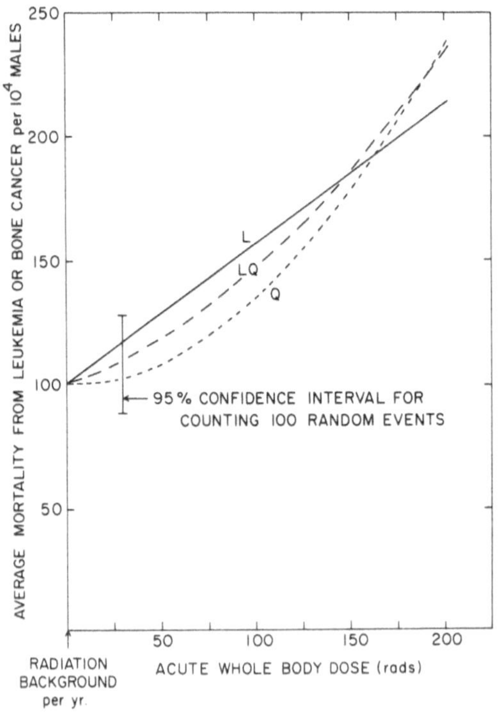

confidence interval for counting random events at low doses. This Figure illustrates the fact that many of our data have the complication of a background rate and we are always trying to observe an effect above the background. If the background rate is 1% and we wish to distinguish one curve from another we need large numbers of people. We obviously need more than 10,000 males, we probably need more than 100,000 males. So the conclusions were 1) we should use the linear quadratic curve because theory - not human data - says that is better, and 2) because of the experimental and statistical uncertainties one should not attempt to do epidemiological experiments below 30 rads. Any experiments carried out below such doses have tremendous experimental uncertainty and measure variances in populations or techniques rather than a dose response curve. To distinguish between the various curves in the Figure you can adopt an optimistic or a pessimistic attitude. The optimistic attitude is that there isn't a tremendous difference between the three curves. The pessimistic attitude is that if one subtracted backgound then there is a big difference between them. From my point of view the important question to answer is what are the effects of radiation compared to the effects of no radiation? We have to work with what we know from basic biology. For low LET radiation, using theories of microdosimetry, we have good evidence that two events - nature unknown - are often needed to get a biological effect. The two events may arise from one ionizing ray or by a cooperative effect from two rays. The effects of cancer induction in animals of low dose rates are usually less than at high dose rates. This is not true for high LET radiation. We really don't know how to extrapolate to very low dose rates except to know that there are split-dose effects and low dose rate effects.

PETO

There is always bound to be some uncertainty as to what the exact effects are at very low doses. This is, as you say, virtually inescapable, although if you observe linearity in some higher dose range then it becomes very plausible biologically to extrapolate that linear dose-response relationship that you have observed in a high dose range on down to doses where the effect is not measurable. But, if you haven't observed linearity in the high dose range, then there is always going to be real uncertainty as to the true shape of the dose-response relationship in the low dose range. Despite this, however, certain theoretical considerations suggest that it would be prudent, but not ludicrously prudent, to assume linearity as you go on down to low doses. I summarized these theoretical considerations in a short paper in the February 1978 issue of Environmental Health Perspectives, where references to various more detailed papers may be found.

The first of them is that, no matter what class of mathematical models you fit, if you assume there is some sort of background of cellular damage on which the damage from radiation is superimposed then quite general arguments suggest that the upper confidence limits for the effect at low doses will be linear. For example, you have described the fit of linear and/or quadratic models to radiation dose-response data. Now, suppose you assume any mixture of linear and quadratic and assume an unknown background effect and thenfiddle around with the statistics a bit to work out what your upper confidence limit for the effects of low doses will be, you will always find that the upper confidence limit derived from any set of experimental data will be approximately proportional to dose at low doses. So, although your lower confidence limit may indicate a negligible risk, especially if you assume rather implausible mathematical model, always, no matter what mathematical model you assume, your upper confidence limit tells you that the true effect could well be linear at low doses.

It thus seems as though you are never going to get proof of non linearity at low doses. Moreover, linearity is biologically quite plausible, so I think one should assume linearity, with no threshold, in interpreting such data and in setting human risk standards even though this conclusion cannot be strictly verified until one knows far more than at present about radiation biology and carcinogenesis.

SETLOW

I think you are much more pessimistic than I am. I would hope that some of us might be able to determine more and obtain good experimental data indicating, for example, that the linear quadratic was the appropriate function even though one couldn't distinguish between the curves by human data.

PETO

Yes, but if it is linear quadratic then as soon as you get down to low doses the linear term predominates and the quadratic term becomes negligible, so you have linearity at low doses again.

SETLOW

But that is a different linear function than the one you are describing.

PETO

Over the years a variety of statistical models have been proposed for dose response relationships. If in any of these models you assume that some background of biologically equivalent damage is possible (which is an assumption so plausible that one could hardly exclude it) then this has the surprising result that no matter what mathematical family you assume you finish up with the upper confidence limit for the radiation effect being linear. This holds irrespective of what class of mathematical functions you assume - linear, quadratic, linear quadratic, probit, log normal, or anything else you like. No matter what mathematical class of dose/response relationships you assumed, if you merely admit that some biologically equivalent background cannot be excluded by mathematical hypothesis then it follows that your upper confidence limit would be proportional to dose at low doses. That doesn't prove that no threshold exists, and it doesn't prove that the true effect at low doses is not much lower than linear, but it does mean that no experimental data that you can adduce (other than some kind of complete biological understanding which gives you theoretical predictions) can ever exclude linearity at low doses. It also implies that, at low doses, the appropriate constant of proportionality is not very strongly dependent on the choice of model. It may vary by perhaps a factor or two but it is unlikely to vary by an order of magnitude. So, for practical purposes I think one should always, in interpreting such data, assume linearity because it is quite plausible biologically, and it cannot be excluded on any valid mathematical grounds (because it is invalid just to slip in a mathematical assumption that no biologically equivalent background could possibly exist). In a sense I think this bypasses, at least to within a factor of two or so, the question of whether the committee should assume that the true relationship is linear or whether it is linear with a bit of quadratic.

SETLOW

I don't think you can disprove the linear hypothesis, but I think the factor of two is not at all definite for many systems nor do I think there is any good biological reason for feeling that the background rate of leukemia arises from similar kinds of changes as does leukemia from ionizing radiation.

JANSEN

I fully agree with Peto's mathematical argument which I think is inescapable, but I have a semantic problem. Everybody, especially in genetics, is always saying that 'we have learned so much from radiation'. As far as I can see we have learned how to scare the outside world without intending to do so. I am quite prepared to accept your use of the word 'risk', but if we do that as a scientific community we have also to explain that if we are moving house from London to Edinburgh this too is a 'risk' because of the increase in background radiation. I do not think that anybody, not even a radiation-biologist, will consider this 'risk' in the midst of all the other risks he is taking anyway (e.g. by making the move by car). I feel that if we say both things at the same time, then we really remove all practical significance from the unquantitated word risk and we really only say life is risky which everybody knows already. Could somebody give me some guidance on this question because I think we are really misinforming the outside world. The word 'risk' as it is used by outsiders is quite different from what mathematical theory or scientists are proposing.

SETLOW

I am not an authority on the subject but we are just talking about probabilities when we speak about risks for developing a particular disease. The numbers may be incorrect and they may be upper confidence limits but nevertheless they are numbers. It is the outside world that worries when we say something about such numbers and this worry is a question of communication between us and the outside world.

PETO

Rather in support of what Dr Jansen was saying I would like to quote something from the NY Times Business Section of April 12 this year. They had a full page spread on the Reynold's Tobacco Co., which apparently has just enjoyed a record year with a further 2% increase in US cigarette sales. In explaining why all wise New Yorkers should put their money into Reynold's the Business Section had a quotation from the chairman who had been asked why 'the cancer problem' was no longer hitting cigarette sales as much as it had in earlier years. The chairman replied that 'so many other things have been linked to cancer' that the public are beginning to take 'a more objective (sic!) view of the health issue'. Basically, he was just saying that the enormous effects of cigarettes have been diluted in people's minds by the media coverage of innumerable other minor risks. So, we really do need to be very careful in communicating.

SETLOW

The problem with risk is that people don't appreciate its quantitative significance.

PETO

Yes: the difference between a risk of one in ten, one in a thousand and one in a million is not really understood.

SETLOW

This is a question of education.

JANSEN

Could I make one more comment on it. I think to use the same word 'risk', for risks which are quite obviously entirely different is already making our communications very difficult. I don't know an easy answer but I wonder what the real meaning is of a low risk. At these low doses, we are down risks which are far below the very normal risks of life. Is there not any way in which we can convey that in a scientific manner? As you have said already, Dr Setlow, experimentation at these very low dose levels yields such small numbers of tumors that it is simply not worthwhile. I am dramatising what you said, but in effect that was what you were saying.

Now I think by that you have implicitly removed nearly all biological significance from the effects of these very low doses. Although I am deliberately exaggerating, I don't think I am exaggerating very much.

PETO

The question of how to communicate low dose risks is not directly relevant to Dr Setlow's original question of what those low dose risks actually are. You are putting the question of how to sell ideas before the question of what ideas to sell.

BOREK

Before we determine the risk we have to know what is the potential of a particular carcinogen in producing certain events. One of the approaches has been, in recent years, to use animal cells in culture, the endpoints being survival and cell transformation. Of course we realise the fact that these are *in vitro* studies but at least we evaluate at a cellular level the interaction of the agent, e.g. radiation with particular cells and determine both the potential of the particular radiation in producing toxicity as well as in modifying cells to become transformed. I will limit my comments to ionizing radiation with which we have been working. *In vitro* systems are useful for the study of mechanisms underlying transformation as well as for evaluating dose response relationships at very low doses. We have been using two types of fibroblasts, one is hamster embryo cells and the other is mouse IOT ½ fibroblasts which are an established line. If you look at the dose response relationship for transformation, you will see there is a dose related response for transformation, the endpoint being morphological transformation for both cell types. However, if you look more carefully you will see that the relationship for both cell types at the lower dose levels is much more complicated.

The *in vitro* systems have provided us with unexpected information on protracted radiation. At low doses splitting the dose into two fractions, with an interval of 5 hrs, enhances transformation by 70%, whilst at higher doses by splitting the dose you get a decreased transformation rate. So this is one of the ways to look at the effectiveness of radiation at low doses. Another question of protracted radiation which can be addressed by these systems is the question of dose rate. In our lab we find that at low dose rate we have enhanced transformation. These data are in contrast to those of Elkind who suggests that at low dose rate you have decreased transformation. But the methods of using these cells are not the same. These two pieces of data were obtained in different ways. In Elkind's lab the cells are exposed to radiation and then they are cloned out into single cells whilst in our lab you irradiate, in many dishes, the cells which have already attached, and then allow them to grow into colonies some of which are transformed. The possibility that there is a difference here lies in the fact that if you expose the cells first and then trypsinize them you may perturb the cell cycle and transformability depends on position in the cycle. In IOT ½ cells the expression of transformation after trypsinization is related to the time after exposure at which the cells have been trypsinized. If you start with single cells which have been plated and have already established their efficiency you do not have this problem.

Our knowledge of the effectiveness of very low doses and of different radiations can also be derived from these systems. We have studied transformation with doses as low as 0.3 rad of X-rays and 0.1 rad neutron. If we compare the transformability of X-rays and gamma rays which are another low LET radiation, we find that X-rays are more efficient in transforming than are the gamma rays at the very low dose level. The RBE of the gamma rays compared to the X-rays is about 0.5 at low doses. So this is one answer to the possibility of studying the effects of radiation at low doses and since we now can transform human cells we aim to carry out with them the same studies we have done with rodent cells.

SETLOW

Do you believe that these data indicate that low dose rates are liable to be more harmful than high dose rates?

BOREK

In these systems yes. These are animal cells and an *in vitro* system but still we have an endpoint which has been proven to be associated with a state of malignancy of the cells.

SETLOW

On the other hand to the best of my knowledge there aren't any animal data that say this sort of thing.

BOREK

The animal data don't go to such low doses.

SETLOW

My only worries about these results are that there are no explanations for the discontinuities in dose response relations.

BOREK

I agree. One of the deficiencies of the *in vitro* system is the fact that we dissociate the cells and a variety of cells which have been intact and non-dividing, and have been in tissue specific arrangement, are now allowed to proliferate in a very free and fancy way. Thus they can express something which they have not been able to do before and of course there is the possibility that establishing the cells in culture is a kind of 'initiation', a possibility which one can't prove or disprove.

SETLOW

This gets us to a point that Dr Peto was making - that there may be other effects, that result in a background, that add on to a particular system.

BOREK

I think it is a very valid point since the work we have done in utero shows that we have about a ten-fold less transformation by inducing transplacentally and assaying in vitro compared to in vitro studies. The data suggest that there may really be in vivo cell communication or some repair mechanisms which are transmitted from one cell to another which is a saviour to us I suppose.

GOULD

My first comment is a specific one. The split dose transformation data presented seem to be based on a 5 hour interval between doses. Will it apply to other intervals or is it unique?

My second comment is general. Today we are talking now about radiation and yesterday we talked about chemicals. When we discussed chemicals yesterday Dr Legator and Dr Saffiotti were very unwilling to associate any quantitative value of potency with chemicals. Today when we are talking about 'how many angels can dance on the head of a pin' with regard to radiation we no longer talk of not using potency. When one goes out into the community and talks about chemical risks or radiation risks the radiation people are really at a disadvantage because we talk about potency and the general public sees that radiation at a very low dose can be harmful maybe one in a million or maybe one in every ten million and labels this as a 'risk', but with chemicals that do not have potency values this is not done. I am therefore asking Dr Saffiotti and Dr Legator if we should be consistent with chemicals and radiation and if so are we just wasting our time debating the effects of low level radiation. Should we just go with the minimum amount of radiation that is possible as one does with chemicals.

LEGATOR

We have spent an awful lot of time speaking about a concept that can neither be proved nor disproved. I recall the AEC select committee when we went through the same exact kind of deliberation and came to the conclusion of our inability to determine effects of low level radiation without spending an inordinate amount of money, which might result in inconclusive findings. Risk should be viewed as a continuum, there is no cut-off point, there is no absolute line. For radiation we may derive accurate figures, but not for chemicals.

SETLOW

This morning Dr Osterman-Golkar alluded to the concept of rad equivalent for chemicals that she will speak about later. There was a scheme proposed to relate chemicals to radiation in terms of rad equivalents.

LEGATOR

When we looked at Dr Osterman-Golkar's beautiful data we should also keep in mind that in relating chemicals in terms of rad equivalence we may be comparing quite dissimilar processes. Given the differences in mechanism of action and dose response curves it may be a little misleading to relate chemicals to rad equivalents even though rad equivalents may mean something to us conceptually.

SAFFIOTTI

In relating individual exposures to various chemicals to the model of the radiation equivalent we should not lose sight of the fact that we are dealing with a potentially large number of chemicals that are detected by a variety of different analytical techniques as opposed to radiation that can often be reduced to a single measurement. For chemicals, in most cases, we don't have any information on what combination of events might take place to modify the response when multiple concurrent exposures occur. We would have to compare not just split doses of two or three fractions of the same agent but potentially dozens or hundreds of exposures by a variety of different agents, all of which may act on the same target cells, possibly by different mechanisms including genetic toxicology mechanisms and epigenetic cellular regulatory mechanisms. In the world of low level chemical risk estimates, there is still much ignorance in terms of ultimate mechanisms although a lot of progress has been made in elucidating different metabolic requirements and pathways, and different cellular interaction. The estimation of effects well below the observed levels requires a margin of uncertainty even greater than in the radiation models. I am concerned that some people might take the concept of 'radiation equivalence' too literally and use it to estimate chemical exposures as if they were radiation exposures, implying the same biological effects, when chemical effects on the same target cells may be much more complicated.

GOULD

When we were comparing chemical carcinogens we employed equivalent survival doses. If we take a look at radiation on an equivalent basis, i.e. equivalent survival, radiation really turns out to be a fairly moderate carcinogen and mutagen. In the light of this if we employ the 'rad equivalent' and also employ the same controls on chemicals as we currently use for radiation, we may wind up having to give up many of our major agricultural and industrial processes.

SETLOW

I don't think we should get into a real discussion of rad equivalent at this session except to note that if the concept is to be a useful one the proportionality has to be independent of dose or of concentration.

PUGH

I would like to comment briefly on the dose response data which Dr Borek showed. She showed us some curves with steps in them and talked about the difficulty this would give in extrapolating low dose effects downwards and that is certainly one way of looking at it. I think that, for me a dose effect relationship is only valid if one can be certain that the agent producing the effect is acting in exactly the same way on exactly the same target up and down the whole dose response range investigated. I would like to suggest to Dr Borek that her stepped curves could be interpreted in rather a different way from the one which she offered. That is, to suggest that the steps indicate points in a dose response relationship where either the agents starts to act in a different or additional way perhaps on a different or additional set of targets. Perhaps you would like to comment on that as a feasible explanation.

BOREK

I think you are perfectly right, there is so little we know about the mechanisms of how ionizing radiation acts. We have seen that our work indicates that free radicals may be involved in the process of transformation as well as in cell killing. If you treat the cells with free radical scavengers along with the radiation or even along with the radiation and the tumor promoter TPA you are able to greatly inhibit the effect of both radiation and its promotional effect by the tumor promoter. Thus one cannot really discuss what you say, I think more work is required. I wonder if Dr Setlow has any more comments?

SETLOW

I have two comments. One is to correct the record, there are enzymes that can act on DNA damaged by ionizing radiation. A number of groups have reported their existence and used such activities as probes for radiation damage. What is not kown is the precise molecular nature of the substrate for these enzymes. The second is a point you alluded to. Even though we speak about ionizing radiation it is important to remember that the effects of ionizing radiation arise not only from the direct effect of the ionizations on cellular material but also by indirect effects by activated solute molecules. That latter subject gets us into chemical carcinogenesis.

PETO

What comes out of all this, and what always comes out when you look at a lot of complicated experimental results in relation to all this, is that no conceivable set of experimental results is going to make it particularly implausible that at low doses a linear dose response relationship should obtain. It is always going to remain biologically quite plausible that linearity should obtain at lowish doses. None of the epidemiological data are going to be sensitive enough to exclude it - in fact, they fit it really remarkably well. So, linearity is quite plausible, it is moderately suggested by the epidemiological data, and, in conclusion, you are unlikely to be wrong by more than a factor of about 2 if you just take your epidemiological data and draw a straight line down to zero risk at zero dose. You are not going to be wrong by orders of magnitude, at least for epidemiological studies of low, chronic radiation exposure. I wouldn't maintain this as confidently for the results of epidemiological studies of the effects of high acute exposures because it could be that those high exposures not only transformed but also killed off the stem cells, i.e. the very cells which are relevant. But, for chronic exposure, I think that we know roughly where we are: we know roughly what chronic high dose exposure does and linear extrapolation down from this seems to me to be extremely satisfactory.

What really makes me shudder is the idea of what would we do if we did not have the human data. Just imagine the range of reasonable uncertainty that would exist if all we had to go on for our human risk assessment was the results from these laboratory studies of animals, cultured cells and so on. We could never guess what radiation was going to do to human beings.

SETLOW

But I hope you are not implying that we need some chemical accidents to obtain data on humans.

PETO

Actually there is virtually no chemical for which we have any reliable quantitative estimates of the human effects of chronic exposure. The only things where we have got really good dose response relationships are alcohol, which seems not to be a carcinogen in almost any animal system (although it can be mutagenic in yeast), and tobacco smoke, where we have no idea which of the vast array of chemicals in tobacco smoke are important carcingens and which are the unimportant carcinogens. In addition, one can get some idea of the effects of chronic exposure to aflatoxin from the studies in Africa. There is thus not a single chemical for which we have good dose response data, unfortunately. Maybe if there were we could start to approach the question of whether, quantitatively, humans are generally a thousand times more sensitive than animals, a thousand times less sensitive than animals, or roughly the same as animals. All we can really do with a set of a few hundred chemicals (e.g. a large collection of pesticides) is to use particular laboratory tests to help rank them in order of likely hazard, as a guide to which to restrict which is, unfortunately, not calibrated with respect to human risk. Possible ways of doing this are discussed in Section 4.2 of our recent JNCI review article (J. Natl. Cancer Inst. 1981, 66, 1191-1308). In radiation by contrast it seems to me that we have more or less got the answer as to roughly how hazardous it really is for people. And laboratory experiments on radiation are probably not going to add materially the information that epidemiology has provided and is providing. The one further thing that we do need, however, is to follow the irradiated populations that have only been followed for 25 years on to 50 years. It could be that when we do this we shall find that the absolute effects continue to escalate. For example, perhaps women who were irradiated at the age of ten in Hiroshima will at the age of 70 have a very large absolute excess of breast cancer. But, we will learn whether or not this is so only by continuing to observe people.

LEGATOR

Not to be outdone by the radiation biologist I must admit that at least we made an attempt to determine a threshold for AAF, the bladder carcinogen. The National Centre for Toxicological Research has as their major initial effort to see if AAF given to rodents, using a large number of animals would show a no-effect level. The results indicated that for bladder cancer there could conceivably be a threshold, however an unexpected finding was hepatomas that occurred at all doses.

RINDI

I am now referring to what may be a possibility of adding points to the dose-effect curve at low dose levels. If I understand well one of the several difficulties on performing experiments at low doses is that when you say low doses you mean of the order of or even less than the natural background. Could it be of any interest to have a laboratory to perform experiments where the background is of the order of one tenth - one 50th of the natural background? We are planning to build for a physics experiment (measuring the half-life of the proton), a lab under the Gran Sasso mountain which is some 2500 meters underground where the cosmic ray background will be of the order of one 10th - one 50th of the natural cosmic background; by using particular materials we can reduce also the other part of the natural background. I was wondering if such a lab can be any use for biological experiments.

SETLOW

The general answer to the question is 'no' because of the difficulty of measuring biological effects at these low doses. It makes no difference which dose response curves you extrapolate through the point representing background radiation per year (0.1 rad). If you extrapolate tenfold closer to the origin you are still at the origin. On that basis I predict no one will take you up on your offer of laboratory space. If they did they must have some reason other than extrapolation in the back of their minds.

Investigations have been made on small human populations living at natural backgrounds much higher than average. They have shown no significant increases. Reducing background below the average will not get you that much closer to zero on a linear scale.

ROUND TABLE: DIFFERENCE IN CANCER SUSCEPTIBILITY AMONG INDIVIDUALS AND WHAT DETERMINES THE DIFFERENCES

Leader: A.M.R. Taylor

Department of Cancer Studies, The Medical School

Birmingham, U.K.

TAYLOR

'Difference in cancer susceptibility among individuals and what determines the differences' I am going to try and say something about this particular topic.

Cancer is many diseases and cannot be treated as a single entity and it seems not unreasonable to suggest that in all types of cancer it will be possible to group patients into those showing a strong genetic component for that particular cancer and those showing a weaker component. Now an example of a strong genetic influence is given by basal cell naevus syndrome, which I think Colin Arlett has mentioned and probably several other people, where the patients develop basal cell carcinomas in large numbers and at an earlier age than the rest of the population. At the other end of the extreme we would expect instances where an environmental influence was so strong, in determining the cancer, that any variation in the genetic susceptibility or influence would be totally swamped and of little consequence.

Cancer cells can show many properties which suggest that there has been an alteration in either the structure or the regulation of the genetic material. Let me just mention structural genetic change for a moment. This can be suggested by one or two different pieces of evidence. Firstly there are the chromosomal changes seen in cancer cells and perhaps along the same line is the variation in the nuclei of histological sections of tumors. Thirdly, the fact is that carcinogenic agents are often also mutagenic, that is they are known to interact with the genetic material. All these might suggest that structural changes in the DNA are important. But equally well, there is evidence that change in the regulation of the genome is important and this can be suggested by the observation of ectopic hormone production in some tumors or the appearance of embryonic antigens or antigens associated with immature cells. Examples of embryonic antigens, of course, are carcinoembryonic antigen (CEA) and α-foetoprotein (AFP). Acute lymphocytic leukemia cells are associated with antigens of immature precursor cells. Thirdly, further evidence for changes in regulation in the genome come from some work involving transplantation or tumor nuclei into enucleated ova, which can result in a normal fully differentiated adult animal. This implies that normal regulatory procedures are retained. This evidence all points to a genetic change in the cell which leads to malignancy whether this be structurally determined or regulatory. Now there is controversy surrounding the evidence I have quoted and for example as far as structural changes are concerned in the chromosomes of tumor cells it is not clear which comes first; whether there is an aberration in the chromosomes of the cell which then forms the clinical tumor or whether the tumor is formed first and by selection chromosome abnormalities arise.

If we believe that the host genome does influence malignant change then how in broad terms could this occur? This is the difficult question which is posed by the topic. Well, I have divided this into two parts: the host genome may control the probability with which the initiating event occurs. And I think Peter Cerutti has touched on this problem already. A good example of this is xeroderma pigmentosum, where there is an inability to repair pyrimidine dimers following exposure to UV light, and we have heard a lot about this. This only occurs when patients are of course exposed to sunlight. Patients not exposed to sunlight do not get skin tumors. The host genome controls the likelihood of that first initial event occuring. Susceptibility to cancer may also occur by loss of host control over potentially malignant focus. And here I am really talking about the control of progression to the clinically recognizable tumor. Genetically determined features of host metabolism, of hormone balance of the immune status and so on, will control progression and perhaps a change in these is necessary for progression. In genetically determined conditions where there is an abnormality in one of these features this could be associated with increased incidence of cancer. A good example, I think here of susceptibility to cancer by loss of host control is polyposis coli. In patients with this disorder there is a predisposition to form many colonic polyps. Now there is a probability in any of us, if we have a colonic polyp, that the polyp will become malignant. But in these patients the numbers of polyps are so huge that the probability of developing a malignancy is so much greater. An example of hormonal involvement might be in Klinefelter's syndrome and Dr Jansen this morning touched on chromosomal disorders. Klinefelter's syndrome patients are 47 XXY males. There is an increased predisposition to breast cancer so perhaps hormonal influence is important there. Now there are many other ways of categorizing what determines cancer susceptibility. One can for example class several disorders into immune deficiency disorders, Wiskott-Aldrich syndrome, agammaglobulinaemia and so on. And each of these seems to have its own spectrum of tumors. Many of the immunodeficiency disorders have tumors of the lymphoreticular system but they should not be lumped together. For example in ataxia telangiectasia the tumors are quite specifically of the lymphocytes, lymphomas and also T-cell leukemias. We could contrast this with Wiskott-Aldrich syndrome for example, which again has leukemias but in this case they are mainly myeloid leukemias. So there are important differences. And of course there are other disorders without immune defects and one can class virtually all of them in this group, albinism, xeroderma pigmentosum, polyposis coli and a host of others. Thirdly, the chromosomally determined disorders which again Dr Jansen spoke about this morning; Down's syndrome which has a very greatly increased incidence of lymphoblastic leukemia, Klinefelter's syndrome which I have already mentioned, gonadal dysgenesis. These latter are 46XY females where there is a clear association with gonadal tumors. There is a fourth category where there is an inheritance of the tumor susceptibility alone and a good example of this is retinoblastoma. This is inherited as autosomal dominant gene and the tumor seems to be the only manifestation of this gene apart from some evidence suggesting an increased susceptibility to osteosarcoma of the long bones. So it is quite clear therefore that in some cases we know why there is cancer susceptibility in some individuals in the terms that I have mentioned. In others there may be more than one feature, for example in ataxia telangiectasia, which could be important in the development of malignancy and this was argued over a little the other day when we were talking about the putative DNA repair defect in ataxia versus the immune deficiency. In other disorders like the chromosome disorders the relationship of the extra chromosome for example to the malignancy is quite unclear.

CERUTTI

I think you are right in every sentence you said.

ARLETT

What I have to say needs to be illustrated on the board. It could be regarded as not quite being appropriate to the title, but since I am leaving tomorrow morning I will need to take this opportunity to ask 'Can we use human cells to measure risks?' and to be more precise can we take advantage of the fact that we have some human cells that are particularly sensitive to some DNA damaging agents. I will quote you the example we usually use in our undergraduate teaching. We give the students a set of cell strains and access to ionizing radiation and UV and we ask them to tell us what the cell strains are. Now it is perfectly possible to turn that experiment on its head and to give them an XP and an A-T and some others as I shall illustrate in a moment and then give them the equivalent of liquid X-rays or liquid UV and ask them to tell us what it is with the prior knowledge that XP cells are sensitive to UV-like compounds and A-T is sensitive to ionizing radiation and to some radio-mimetic compounds. I think this is actually very central to the stated topic of this course'can we use human cells in this way'. I am trying to argue the case that we can and I would submit that if we can get undergraduates to do it in an albeit very simple experiment or set of experiments, then it should be perfectly possible to extend them in a more scientific manner.

We are able to produce a table of hypersensitivities by a variety of different human cell strains against a set of DNA damaging agents as shown in the table:

Cell strain	UV	γ	MMC	MMS	EMS	ENU
XP	++	N	N	N	N	N
A-T	N	++	N	N	N	N
FA	N	+	++	N	N	N
11961	+	N	N	N	++	++
46BR	+	+	+	++	++	N

XP = xeroderma pigmentosum, A-T = ataxia-telangiectasia, FA = Fanconi's anaemia, 11961 = sunsensitive individual (probably Cockayne syndrome), 46BR = unknown syndrome. N = normal sensitivity, ++ = hypersensitive, + = slightly hypersensitive, UV = ultra-violet light (254 nm), γ = gamma radiation, MMC = mitomycin C, MMS = methyl methanesulphonate, EMS = ethyl methanesulphonate, ENU = ethyl nitrosourea.

This data is by no means exclusive because we are always extending it by adding more cell strains or more DNA damaging agents. What should be clear here is that we are in a position to detect, γ, UV, cross-linking agents, ethylating agents or methylating agents by the use of specific cell strains.

I think it is an example which is central to the subject of the meeting. Human cells can be used to detect damage and therefore I submit that they can be used to detect risk. I think that is a substantial enough short statement.

LEGATOR

I agree the information that one can generate is extremely useful. A more important question though is can that same kind of information with diverse agents be determined as accurately with less energy and less time by using other systems? Perhaps we can accomplish our goal much easier in non human cells or even in microbial systems. In most cases we are faced with looking at materials whose mode of action is unclear or unknown. Given the fact that we have unknown materials to look at, we need a number of systems covering various genetic lesions, and the use of human cells may be a secondary consideration.

CERUTTI

I really don't see what you are getting at Colin with this. I think there is ample evidence that cytotoxicity is not directly related to tumorigenicity and transforming potency. We already have a problem studying mutagenesis as an endpoint which is also not necessarily related to the carcinogenic process.

ARLETT

What I have talked about is my example of the use of human cells for the assessment of risk from physical and chemical agents. It is a specific example where we have a potential in human cells. They are human equivalents of the Ames' tester strains. This is perhaps a very pretentious way of putting it. Would you be happier if instead of cytotoxicity we either had transformation or mutation as the endpoint? Would you like to think it was more meaningful? It is our ambition that we will ultimately be able to score these endpoints as easily as we can presently measure cell survival.

JANSEN

I completely agree with Dr Cerutti. What you are describing is to catalogue the kind of effects the substance can have. That is the kind of thing which we can ask the organic chemist to do and he can tell us right away whether it could be a cross-linking agent, even frequently whether the Ames' test will be positive, whether it will be an alkylating agent or a methylating agent etc. The only trouble is, as referred to by Dr Cerutti, that this qualitative cataloguing does not help us. We know that any substance is poisonous; even water is a poison. It is precisely the business of the experimental toxicologist to find out at which level of exposure symptoms arise and which ones. In comparing his data with mutagenic data he may find that cytotoxic effects will kill the cell well before any mutagenic effect would occur. Your scheme would be very nice as a catalogue of some of the possibilities of mutagenic effects, but your scheme would not teach us whether mutagenic effects occur at a time that the cell is already dead for other reasons or before transformation takes place or after transformation takes place. So therefore I don't think that your scheme will really add to what you called risk estimation. It will help with cataloguing the possibilities.

KRAEMER

Part of the problem in the past with using the mammalian cells has been the difficulty with working with fibroblasts which in general have a limited life-span, are difficult to subculture and are hard to grow to large numbers of cells for biochemical studies. Human lymphoblastoid lines may be another source of material that is much easier to work with. Technology is advancing and it may be much easier to make some of these determinations. The utility of a test depends on whether you can pick up things that you would not have been able to pick up elsewhere and that is just an empirical question. We will need some data to find out but I don't think we have it yet.

ARLETT

I think the concept I am evolving in my mind and putting forward to you is the possibility that there may be a tremendous range of repair or sensitivities in man and that we might have to put a very large figure in our estimates of risk. Our data suggests to me differential repair in different individuals for particular DNA damaging agents and that in fact we may have enormous variation not only between but within agents.

LEWIS

This is a plea for basic science. I have just been involved in a very successful attempt to design a battery of tests to detect women who would have thrombo-embolic problems from taking oral contraceptives. It was successful because the clotting systems and controls were already worked out and therefore the ability to detect weaknesses or lack of response was possible. I think one of the problems we have here is that we all want to run home and use human cells and we don't know what we want to measure. What are the lesions? I would suggest if you want to measure repair, measure repair; the technology is available.

CERUTTI

A point which is ignored in your box scheme: each agent produces a whole spectrum of lesions each of which may be processed with a different efficiency and possibly by a different repair pathway. A good example is the repair of O6-methylguanine relative to N^3-methyl-adenine lesions. I think that if you want to study repair, it is particularly informative if the removal of individual lesions is followed.

ARLETT

Obviously Peter you are absolutely right, the existence of the hypersensitive cell strains may make it possible for us to investigate specific lesions. Thus it is of considerable interest to discover why cell strain 46BR is hypersensitive to EMS but not ENU. This is again an example where a human cell strain may be particularly useful.

WATERS

This may be a bit unfair but I would simply like to point out that one of the reasons that the Ames' test was so successful was that it was provided with exogenous metabolic activation and in the discussion thus far I think we are leaving out that point. I would like to make a plea that while we are pursuing various repair deficiencies and proficiencies in human fibroblasts in culture, we might keep in mind a need for exogenous metabolic activation.

ARLETT

It is easy to say 'no problem at all' we can just sprinkle some microsomes into the systems if we wish, but that doesn't happen to be the way we are working with the system at the moment.

LEGATOR

I think perhaps when we talk about risk we are considering all forms of DNA damage and its final phenotypic expression. We may want to consider systems that will allow us to measure as many different genetic events as possible. You can do it in two ways, you can have a system with a number of different endpoints or you can have a number of different systems giving you different endpoints. Very few chemicals behave in a completely predictable manner. It is important to measure as many multiple points as we can either in the same system or using different biological systems. For instance one could use a CHO cell where you can evaluate point mutations, repair, transformation, etc. I think that is the kind of information we should be looking for.

Mike Waters says if we are talking about risk assessment then there is no way that we can neglect the entire metabolism of an intact animal. I think there is just no way around that. One final point I would hesitate to say that an organic chemist can identify with any degree of accuracy the kind of activity one would anticipate at a molecular basis. I think that is beyond our capabilities at the present time.

JANSEN

I just want to react on that last part. If you ask an organic chemist how a compound is going to behave in the body, an animal or human body, he will make enormous mistakes. If you ask him whether it can act as a cross-linking agent or a methylating agent or an ethylating agent he can tell you right away. You don't need a human cell for that and the organic chemist can be as accurate. However, if you ask the organic chemist what will be the predominant action in the cell, which metabolites will be formed and at which relative speed to each other then the difficulties are coming in. But not in the classification of chemicals and not in the prediction of how they will react. To find that out we need the living animal body but not isolated cells.

TAYLOR

Would anyone like to say something on a slightly different topic?

GOULD

If we know that a certain individual is susceptible to a type of cancer, say colon cancer or breast cancer because of their family history, how do we assess their risk to environmental contaminants? For example let us consider breast cancer. We know we don't want to do mammography on the general population at age 35 but the question is what to do with high risk individuals around age 35. The question is if these individuals are also susceptible to X-ray radiation then we may gain nothing and shouldn't do mammography. Are high risk individuals to 'spontaneous cancers' also high risk individuals for induceable cancers? Is there any way we can investigate this using cell types?

ARLETT

I have a response. I showed earlier in the meeting data where we had estimates of spontaneous mutation frequencies from individuals of normal and cancer-prone syndromes. Now if we accept that the assays of mutation are some measure of cancer-proneness and I suspect that that could be debated quite effectively, then there was no evidence of any enhanced spontaneous mutation frequency. But the 'take home' message as far as I am concerned is that the increased cancer in the individuals was a consequence of damage. I do think that cancer-prone individuals are at risk from environmental agents. Have I answered your question or not?

GOULD

There are obviously cells that may be prone to UV mutagenesis but may not be any more susceptible to X-ray radiation. If we could get some type of understanding about what environmental agents individuals with a genetic susceptible to various organ specific disease are also sensitive to, we may better be able to assess their risks. Is there any work in that type of an area?

ARLETT

I think we should take Mac Paterson's hard-luck families and find out if they have any susceptibility to this array of DNA damaging agents. If they don't we are no further ahead, if they do we are substantially further ahead. However, I would tend to believe that if there is any truth in the claims that XP heterozygotes have enhanced cancer susceptibility then it is a direct response to UV light and not to other things.

TAYLOR

I am going to ask Dr Kraemer if he would like to say something.

KRAEMER

We have been talking about using cells from people to get estimates of risk from certain agents but it may be possible to use the people themselves. I would like to suggest a study of xeroderma pigmentosum. The patients are sensitive to ultra violet as we have seen before and their cells in the laboratory are also sensitive to a number of known mutagens and carcinogens. If XP patients are exposed to UV they get skin cancer. We are supposedly living in a cesspool of environmental mutagens. If XP patients have the susceptibility we have been talking about in all of their cells and not just their skin cells one may study the types of cancers they get. You would expect they might get cancer other than in the skin. This susceptibility to environmental mutagens is significant in terms of oncogenesis. We are beginning a study of this question by looking through the literature. I am still evaluating the data and I do not have the denominator but this is what we have been able to find in terms of tumors of patients with xeroderma pigmentosum other than in the skin.

Table I. Primary internal neoplasms in xeroderma pigmentosum

Anatomic Site	Age (years)	Number reported
Oral cavity	3 - 18	17
Brain	14,15,21	3
Leukemia	3, 32	2
Breast	38	1
Lung	62	1
Uterus	51	1
Testis	12	1
Eye (uveal tract)	33	1
Peritoneum (metastatic)	27	1

Since XP patients have a known susceptibility we don't really have to worry in asking whether this model can be adapted to the human because these are humans already. When considering ultraviolet radiation the XP patients get similar tumors to people who do not have xeroderma. For example, farmers and sailors who receive a tremendous amount of UV exposure. The xeroderma patients get their tumors much earlier in life. This table shows what I have found so far and I can't say for any of these whether there is a significant increase yet, just that these neoplasms have occurred. Oral cavity tumors were found in 19 patients and these were relatively young, 3-18 years old. There are two firm reports and one possible report of a primary brain tumor. Two reports of XP patients with leukemia, a 38 year old woman with a breast cancer, a 62 year old man with lung cancer, a uterine cancer, a 51 year old and a 12 year old with a testicular cancer. There is a very unusual case of a 33 year old Japanese woman with xeroderma pigmentosum who developed a malignant melanoma in an ultraviolet shielded portion of the eye. Thus this is not a UV-induced lesion. The very first patient described by Kaposi with xeroderma pigmentosum in an article published in 1874 was said to have died of the cancer of the peritoneum. Now at this point we don't have an autopsy and we don't know if this was metastatic from a skin tumor but it might possibly have been a non-cutaneous neoplasm. In this regard I think studies in xeroderma pigmentosum and some other disorders may be quite useful. In the USA we are attempting to set up a prospective registry of xeroderma pigmentosum. I am doing this in collaboration with Dr Alan Andrews at Columbia University, James German at the New York Blood Center and Clark Lambert. If anyone has any information about xeroderma pigmentosum patients in the USA, I would certainly appreciate getting it. I am aware of another XP registry in Japan run by Dr H. Takebe of Kyoto.

ARLETT

It is really absolutely essential to establish whether XP's have a higher frequency of tumors in sites other than the skin and the only way this can be established is on the basis of prospective studies. In Britain we are fortunate in having a somewhat more accessible computer system that deals with Health Service records. XP patients and A-T patients and their families are being tagged so that we should get information prospectively about what is happening in these families.

KRAEMER

The question at the next stage would be that if in fact there is an increase in oral cavity neoplasms in these patients, why? They are not really walking around with their tongues out and their mouths open to the sun all the time. Maybe it is an environmental mutagen or carcinogen that is causing it. What would it be? Possibly pyrolysis products, nitrosamines or flavenoids. These patients are too young to be smoking but maybe they are eating a lot of barbecued fish or something. This type of study raises interesting questions as to what the environmental exposure might be.

TAYLOR

You said that Dr Takebe in Japan was doing the same thing. Does he know whether these tumors occur with the same frequency in his patients?

KRAEMER

Dr Takebe has performed studies of the DNA repair deficiencies of more than 180 XP patients. He is just beginning to gather this clinical information.

LEGATOR

If we assume that a significant number of individuals who have genetic handicaps have a higher degree of susceptibility to cancer generally, and if we assume that this may even occur in heterozygote condition, then should there be some effort to screen out those individuals, and eliminate these individuals from working sites with chemicals some of which may be carcinogens.

KRAEMER

I think you have stated the problem accurately. The diseases which we have been talking about are very rare but they are also autosomal recessive. That means that the heterozygous carriers are much more common. Do the heterozygotes have increased susceptibility to these agents in terms of acute or chronic toxicity or in terms of developing cancer? Unfortunately the only studies to date are retrospective epidemiologic studies without definitive identification of the heterozygote. I think that until we can have a test to say whether a person is heterozygous for ataxia tangiectasia or xeroderma pigmentosum we cannot rely on this type of retrospective study. My view of the role of the retrospective study is to suggest the prospect of one. Once we have a test for the heterozygotes, which at present we don't have, then we can test individuals and see. A problem we have come across as we have been screening unusual individuals for one reason or another is that when we find small changes in the survival tests it is very hard to assess the significance of these.

CERUTTI

I think the real issue is whether repair plays a central role in carcinogenesis in the general population. I look at these diseases more as models, as mutants available for biological investigation. Of course, the goal to protect these rare individuals is valid at the same time.

KRAEMER

One of the reasons for establishing the xeroderma pigmentosum registry is our vast ignorance of many of the basic epidemiologic questions. How many XP patients are there? How long do they live? I have made estimates of 1-4 per million in the USA so that would be somewhere between a few hundred and a thousand. I may be shown to be wrong soon. The only way you can tell if a person is a heterozygote at present is if they have an affected child.

ROUND TABLE: CALIBRATION AND MONITORING OF HUMAN POPULATION: BIOLOGICAL ASPECTS, HEMOGLOBIN ALKYLATION AND RADIATION EQUIVALENT APPROACH

Leaders: M.S. Legator and S. Osterman-Golkar*

Preventive Medicine Department, University of Texas Medical Branch, Galveston, Texas. *Radiobiology Department Wallenberg Laboratory, University of Stockholm, Sweden

LEGATOR

Concerning the alkylation of macromolecule procedure presented by Dr Osterman-Golkar, one can be impressed with its versatility and our ability to quantitate the response. I was interested in asking Dr Golkar her views as to the present status of the method, where it can be applied and her future projecting for the procedure. So I'd like to turn the microphone over to Dr Golkar and have her tell us about her inner thoughts about the alkylation of the macromolecule method.

OSTERMAN-GOLKAR

I want to say a few words about how the hemoglobin dosimetry method could be used. It could be used as an endpoint in animal studies to demonstrate pathways of activation of chemicals to electriphilic compounds. At the Wallenberg Laboratory we are currently studying the metabolism of 1,2-dichloroethane in the mouse. After treatment of animals with the radiolabelled compound it was possible to demonstrate activation by glutathion to a reactive halfmustard and oxidation to chloroacetaldehyde by determining reaction products with hemoglobin of these reactive intermediates. Generally it is easier to determine reaction products of proteins than products of DNA. It is difficult to obtain DNA in quantity and reaction products may be removed from the nucleic acid by normal repair processes.

In contrast to measurements of a chemical or its metabolites in urine or in expired air monitoring by means of hemoglobin alkylation gives a measure of the dose of a reactive compound. Long term animal experiments for genetic toxicity are generally carried out at unrealistically high concentrations of chemicals and there may be a non-linear relationship between exposure dose and in vivo dose. It is therefore recommended that binding studies are introduced as a component of the testing protocol. This would also provide a basis for interspecies comparisons.

A dosimetry in man by determination of hemoglobin alkylation could be used for the control of the hygienic standard in work environments. The method is specific to the causative agent and may therefore give a valuable endpoint in epidemiological studies.

LEGATOR

I know that yesterday when Dr Osterman-Golkar presented her work there were a few questions and I wonder if anybody has anything they want to bring up about this procedure at this time. One of the important features of this procedure is that if we look at the hemoglobin (alkylation of histidine) we record an effect that occurred within the last 63 days (half life of hemoglobin) so you have the opportunity to show a result that could have occurred a month or two prior to the analysis. I suspect, in terms of risk estimates even though we may not be dealing with DNA we are taking into account one of the major characteristics of a large group of know genotoxic agents, where quantitation can be performed. It is not a routine procedure, however, and one should have carried out in vitro studies to identify most likely products.

JANSEN

You may be interested to hear about our own experience with the method of Ehrenberg and Osterman-Golkar. We consider this currently the only available method for the medical supervision of workers which may be more sensitive than the measurement of the incidence of chromosome aberrations.

In practical terms, there are two major disadvantages: 1. Exquisitely sensitive analytical techniques have to be developed for each single chemical under investigation. We have applied the method which had already been developed on ethylene oxide but even so and despite full cooperation by Ehrenberg and Osterman-Golkar, method development in our own laboratory was a major exercise in itself. 2. The method is a major step forward in dosimetry in animals and man. It still leaves the unavoidable problem of quantitative extrapolation from animals to man.

In our own situation there was no difference in alkylation of hemoglobin between EO-exposed workers and controls. However, we found distinctly more background-alkylation than Ehrenberg and this apparent difference remains to be resolved (some background-alkylation is theoretically unavoidable because of EO-formation in the course of normal biochemical processes).

However, even though it is good to know that your own workers seem well protected because you do not find a discernible increase in hemoglobin alkylation, I do not know how to interpret findings of a definite increase - you do not analyze a hazard, you measure an alkylation which has some, but not determined relation with DNA-alkylation in different organs which in turn is related in a not determined way to the possibility of a carcinogenic effect.

LEGATOR

Is there anybdoy here, at this late date in the conference, who feels strongly that based on any of the systems we have heard or been through that we can come up with any risk estimates in man? Is there a defender here for any of the systems we heard because we just heard Dr Jansen say this comes closer than anything he knows of and so the question I would pose: is there anybody who would suggest a better quantitative estimate in man than say the alkylation procedure?

SETLOW

This morning you were speaking about chromosomal changes and chromosomal changes were just described as one measure. Is that a bad measure? I know little about it but is it a measure that could be compared to ionizing radiation because chromosomal changes as a result of ionizing radiation dose have been well calibrated. If you could make that calibration imperfect as it would be, you could say certain individuals have been exposed to chemical doses that make chromosome changes the equivalent of so many rads. What is wrong with that proposition?

LEGATOR

If we look at specific chemicals such as actinomicin D, there is a specific affinity for centromeric regions. If we look at a chemical such as halothane which affects the spindle mechanism, we are detecting effects at the cytogenetic level and they are not comparable to the non-specific effects you see with radiation. Therefore to talk about rad equivalence for chemicals may be misleading.

SETLOW

I agree. Do chemicals exist that don't have these extreme aberrant effects? Do they produce chromosomal aberrations of a more conventional type? Chromatid aberrations, deletions and so on?

LEGATOR

Even if we assumed that they don't have these specifications which we know some of them do have, we have no assurance that the dose response curve is the same. Since we are comparing agents with dissimilar curves quantitatively, we are in trouble as to dose response. I suspect we are going to find a great deal of dissimilarity between chemical and chemical radiation.

SETLOW

I was not advocating a rad equivalent. Don't misunderstand me, I am saying could you say to someone that you have been exposed to a chemical that changes your chromosomes by the equivalent of 10 rads. That is very different from saying a rad equivalent. I don't mean to imply a proportionality.

LEGATOR

I think conceptially it certainly would mean more.

JANSEN

Dr Perry is the real expert but in his absence I will try to do my best.

I understand that radiation affects DNA directly whereas most or many chemicals only act after metabolism and only during replication. Hence on theoretical grounds you would expect the relation chemicals-chromosome aberrations to be fundamentally different from the relation radiation-chromosome aberrations. This is also found in practice but we have experience with very few chemicals so that it is too early to generalize for all chemicals. (Benzene may be an exception to most chemicals).

WATERS

May I show three slides? I don't want, at this point in the discussion, to offer any solutions, but I'd simply like to offer an approach that I have considered, that I think possibly could help us with the problem of risk assessment. This slide (Fig.1) represents the parallelogram approach which was described a few years ago by

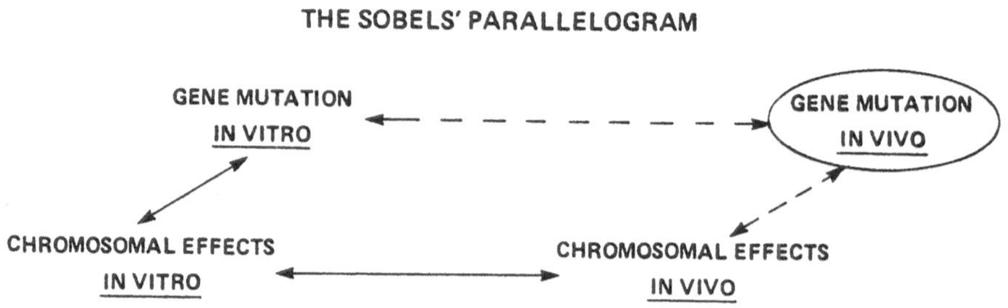

Figure 1

Dr Fritz Sobels. It is an approach that could be applied to many different parameters. Here the concern is with gene mutation in vivo. The thought is that if you understand the dose-response relationship for gene mutation in vitro and chromosomal effects in vitro and if you also understand the dose-response relationship for chromosomal effects in vitro and chromosomal effects in vivo then you can make some prediction about the dose-response relationships between gene mutation in vitro and gene mutation in vivo, or chromosomal effects in vivo and gene mutation in vivo. So you are projecting the dotted lines to obtain information about gene mutation in vivo.

The next slide (Fig. 2) takes a similar sort of approach focusing on gene mutation in germ cells in humans as the unknown parameter. This was an approach developed by Dr Heinrich Malling and again the endpoint of concern is mutation. But let me go on to the third slide (Fig. 3) where we expand the parallelogram to the consideration of multiple parameters. Many of these parameters have been described by Dr Legator earlier in the session. I would like to suggest that, if we were to take an integrated approach such as this one, using lymphocytes, fibroblasts, perhaps even sperm in vivo, that it might be possible to develop better correlative information for use in quantitative risk estimation. Using chemotherapeutic agents wherein we have a known exposure and can calculate half-lives in various compartments, and can determine alkylation and so forth, we should be able to relate quantitatively dose and effect for multiple parameters. This slide focuses, as you see,

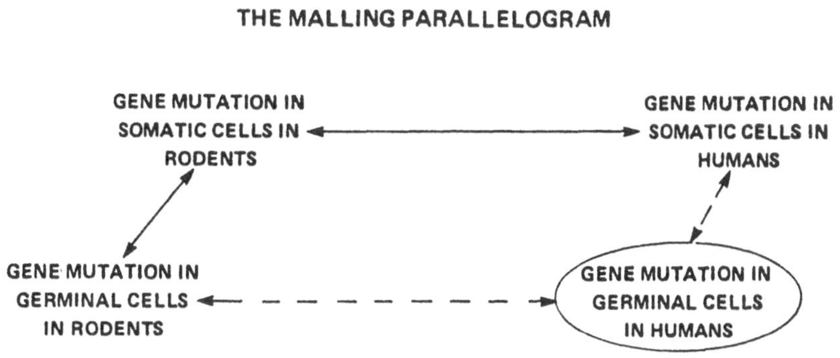

Figure 2

APPLICATION OF HUMAN GENETIC BIOASSAYS
IN HEALTH HAZARD EVALUATION

[SYSTEMS INVOLVING IN VITRO OR IN VIVO EXPOSURE WITH IN VITRO ANALYSIS]

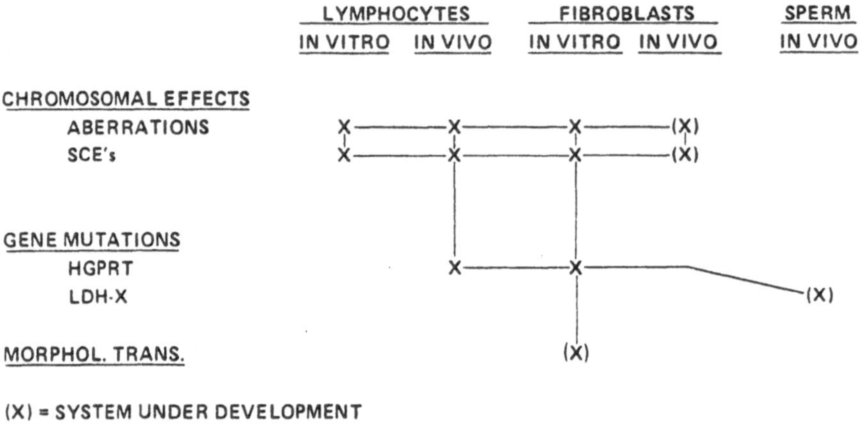

Figure 3

on the use of human materials; but I would suggest that not only in vitro and in vivo responses in the human materials be examined, but also the relationship between these responses in the human situation and the corresponding effects in experimental systems. Since we have people who are being exposed to chemotherapeutic agents at prescribed doses it seems reasonable to apply these methods to the human subjects and then to try to relate the observations to the experimental animal and in vitro systems where a wider range of doses can be employed and more precise dose-response curves can be generated. Such an approach should help us to understand the dose-response relationships among these three types of systems.

JANSEN

I agree and I do believe it is possible to calibrate systems. However, most attempts have been made for industrial populations and these have scientifically speaking an enormous disadvantage: as soon as exposure is known to be excessive in terms of a chemical or analytical criterion, exposures are reduced and the "experiment" is ruined. This does not automatically apply to a small company but the scientific disadvantage remains because the same considerations which make it less possible for a small company to be fully aware of all hazards, make it also unlikely that they have the detailed medical, administrative and industrial hygiene information available which is needed for a scientific study. So, the industrial situation is inherently adverse to this kind of scientific research. The scientific situation with regard to patients treated with chemotherapeutics is intrinsically more profitable for carrying out the scientific research indicated by you because precise information on dosing and precise epidemiologic follow-up is possible, at least in theory.

LEGATOR

I suggest all this is great and I am entirely for the Sobel's parallelogram, but I would also suggest that we have, for the last several years, been looking at the same alkylating agents over and over again in various systems and I must admit that I get a little bit restless when somebody proposes that we go back and look at the alkylating agents and see whether those in vitro, in vivo studies correlate with effects in cancer patients. I would just suggest that we have a adequate body of information in human subjects and we have already been able to demonstrate by these techniques that they can detect active chemicals. What is needed is more human studies. We should not neglect animal systems, but also evaluate high risk populations by available techniques. In limited studies, these non-invasive procedures that can be used with human subjects have already demonstrated their value.

ABBONDANDOLO

There is another Sobels parallelogram where the four corners are DNA alkylation in vitro, DNA alkylation in vivo, mutation in vitro and mutation in vivo. In this scheme, in vitro means in vitro cell cultures or any other simple laboratory system and in vivo means mammals.

The idea is that molecular dosimetry data can be used to extrapolate the most inaccessible information from the three other data which are relatively easy to obtain experimentally. It is recognized that molecular dosimetry data are not more difficult to obtain in vivo than in vitro while mutation studies are incomparably more laborious in animals than in cellular systems.

I wanted to stress again the idea that this approach may turn out to be both feasible and appropriate for the problem of risk estimates.

JANSEN

I would like to take issue with Dr Legator if he feels that we have come a long way with test systems. Personally, I feel that most compounds 'picked up' by the numerous test systems now available will in fact not produce any mutagenic or cancer hazard in man under the conditions of use. However, a few may actually be really hazardous. The problem is that we do not know how to pick out the future equivalents of asbestos, benzene and β-naphtylamine. I maintain that we do not have satisfactory tests for doing that and the problem is: how can we develop such tests in the future. Mere adding of yet another test system does not help but further study of human experience is necessary for understanding the real significance of test systems.

LEGATOR

Let me just give you an illustration of exactly what I mean as to completed epidemiological studies. Dr Myra Karstadt, Mount Sinai Hospital, did an interesting survey. She picked 76 IARC animal carcinogens. These are materials that are in commerce now, most of them are industrial products. She sent a letter to the manufacturer of each one of these 76 products and asked the following question: 'Can you tell me of any human data that you have gathered or that you know of?'These are chemicals known to be carcinogenic in animals and are in commerce. Of the 76 requests, the manufacturers responded in all cases if I remember correctly. It turns out that of the total of 76 animal carcinogens, only eight had been looked at in human studies. No reference was made as to the quality of the studies carried out with the eight chemicals. I would suggest that given the fact that there are known animal carcinogens in commerce, we could identify exposed populations and utilize our short term procedures to determine potential adverse effects. We could also identify chemicals which, on the basis of structure or preliminary information, we might suspect to be a problem. These procedures could also be used as part of an industrial medical surveillance program. Dow Chemical employed these techniques for over ten years.

WATERS

May I clarify the position I was trying to take? It certainly is not to argue against the utility of the human monitoring method. However, I don't think it is really feasible to argue that we can do the necessary dosimetry for very many compounds in the human situation. We will have to do that kind of work in vitro and in experimental animals. Therefore, the point I am trying to make is, for those situations where we do have known exposures, where we can get careful dosimetry in man, let's make us of those, and then use the animal models and the in vitro models to gain the additional information that we will need to evaluate other compounds. It seems to me that by combining the human monitoring and the laboratory approaches we will learn a lot more about the problem.

PUGH

One issue which has come up several times in the course of the meeting and which intrigues me as a pharmacologist is the constant concern about the need to establish dose-response relationships and the desirability of achieving parallelism between compounds in different test systems and so on. Dr Legator mentioned this morning that as a criterion for his proposed test system (this is the one in which substances would be categorized into a, b, c, as substances of different levels of concern) that only if a dose-response relationship was apparent would a substance be considered as something of concern. I don't see why it is that you need to see a dose-response relationship before something can be considered as a substance of concern. Perhaps you could explain that for me?

LEGATOR

I am absolutely convinced that the best we can do is to determine categories of concern rather than use risk analysis to determine a specific number. In the area of carcinogenesis, where there is a great deal more experience with risk estimate, than in the field of mutation research, the numbers arrived at are sc soft as to be meaningless. The best we can hope for from animal studies is the qualitative identification of a mutagen, and the establishment of categories of potency.

WATERS

It seems to me we will be taking a step back if we decide that we should not do as much as possible towards quantitative risk assessment. We can use the information in many different ways in terms of public policy, but I think what we are talking about here is the science of risk assessment.

LEGATOR

I take just the opposite stand Dr Waters, I'll tell you why. If we come up with a meaningless figure in using the information from cancer bioassays, it isn't scientific and we are doing it only for political reasons. I come up exactly the reverse conclusions of what you have stated.

JANSEN

I support Dr Waters and I do feel that we can make real progress in scientific risk estimation if we would really try. There are now so many systems and approaches available that I feel that it is quantitative human information which is mostly lacking for such an effort. It is a slow and difficult process but I feel it can be done and should be done. Sobel's parallelogram has been discussed by several people around this table and his approach in some form or another seems inescapable.

I agree with Dr Waters that more attention to this approach (which is costly, will involve several laboratories and disciplines and will take much time, especially for collecting necessary epidemiologic data) is far more profitable in terms of real scientific understanding than mere extension of yet more test systems. More screening tests merely means more compounds which could possibly be hazardous: yet we know already that there is possibly a risk even before we start testing at all. The problem is how to arrive at a test which will reliably predict the conditions of use which are really hazardous.

For the development of such a test, Sobel's approach seems the only way of progress.

LEGATOR

Let me ask you a question, Dr Jansen. Do you have any confidence in the numbers that we generate from the Brian Mantell or any mathematical model when we extrapolate from rodents to man with a specific carcinogen; do you have any confidence in that number?

JANSEN

I think I have more confidence in the astrologists in the papers!

LEGATOR

That is not the question. We generate numbers, by use of mathematical models with carcinogens in a field where we have had a great deal more experience than in the field of mutagenicity. What do these numbers mean? We estimate the risk of vinyl chloride for inducing argiosarcoma and find that this may not be the most important tumor induced by vinyl chloride. Depending on selected mathematical model, the results with saccharin can vary as much as 100,000 fold. Given the state of the art, we are no better in the field of mutation research when it comes to risk estimate.

JANSEN

We have been talking at length about Flagyl this morning where a great number of people are exposed for a short time period. During this whole meeting, except for Peto's talk, we have not discussed the fact that people normally have an enormous amount of mutagens in their food and that is probably connected with colon cancer. Not much work is going on in this field because we do not know the precise factors involved. However, with Flagyl we look at a defined chemical compound used on a defined population. I would submit it would be more useful to do epidemiology research on this defined population rather than extend the number of mutagenicity tests on this compound. We want to obtain informations which are useful for risk estimate.

LEGATOR

Epidemiology will always be of limited use in identifying chronic hazards. Animals will be our essential data base. As to risk assessment, I am convinced categorization is the best we can do in determining the extent of the hazard.

SAFFIOTTI

I think we are polarizing this discussion a bit too much, and we should be looking ahead to what could be developed in the future. If I understood the discussion correctly, on one end of the discussion is the question of whether we should use or try to use quantitative measurements of risk and on the other end is the suggestion that we should not bother to do that and rely on other types of indicators. I think you both would agree that at the present time, in many situations, we do not have these quantitative measurements in a reliable and practical fashion.

The question is: can we eventually move, through our research, towards a situation in which we can really fill quite a few of these gaps? We still have many gaps, but we are beginning at least to identify them as gaps that are not completly our of reach of our research. These points have come out throughout the meeting as gaps that, when filled, would give us a basis for being much more comfortable about estimates of risk extrapolated through the various corners of our parallelograms.

My view in this respect is that there is a need for systematic research at all levels, from tissues to cells to molecular mechanisms, with risk evaluation as a kind of ultimate goal in mind, so that we can actually begin to fill many of these gaps with data. Many of these data can already be obtained, for example, from work done directly on human cell targets, as you have illustrated, and on several other human cell systems that have been discussed at this course and will eventually become a basis for work on risk evaluation. What I am now concerned about is what happens in the meantime.

In the history of environmental policies there have been controversies based on the two opposite sides with a lot of intermediate levels of action. One policy was not to worry about any product for which we do not now have overwhelming evidence of human damage: this was the old traditional policy derived from the toxicology of acute effects, which implies that once you see people actually developing toxic effects you can then cut down the dose and the effects will eventually go away and so you learn to reduce the exposures. Now obviously this policy has become obsolete once the long-term delayed effects have become a matter of concern. The opposite extreme position, that has been taken in some cases is that of requiring to eliminate entirely from the environment anything that has any endpoint in genetic toxicology and induces any harmful effect. Both extremes are, in my view, practically and in many cases scientificially unnecessary. In cases where we have reasonably solid evidence of a type of damage which, at the present stage of knowledge, is considered likely to occur also in human beings, the question is whether we can base our actions on certain presumptions. For example, Dr Jansen the other day has expressed his view that most compounds will not produce carcinogenic effects at low levels. We don't really know that this is the case, what we know is that we can't detect the effects below certain levels, since there is always a problem of detectability; but the effects may add up with those of many other compounds and participate in the causation of a damaging effect. So this is where the answer to these problems becomes a matter of policy.

Some policy discussions can become excessively polarized, but I think that, ultimatly, as investigators in the field we can offer a solid voice of hope to both sides by identifying how to get a lot more data in a coordinated fashion to provide specific answers to these questions. I would say that quantitative risk assessment at the present time, especially for genetic endpoints in the human and for cancer in the human, is practically so difficult or so elusive that it is not reliable, but it should not be eliminated from our attention and in fact it could become an ultimate goal for a lot of our research so that we will be able to narrow the gap progressively. Would that be a conciliatory statement?

LEGATOR

Exactly! We go with the best we have and hope to improve our ability to quantify the data but we have to make decisions in the meantime with meaningful data.

WATERS

I would just like to make it clear, if I may, that what I offered was simply an approach to the systematic collection of information. It is not to be taken as the way to do risk estimation. I think we need to develop better scientific information in laboratory studies and in human clinical and field studies before we will be in a very good position to do quantitative risk estimation.

LEGATOR

And again this is not to say that we should not be doing exact quantitation within a specific system in ranking chemicals on the basis of well conducted experiments that is not the point. The point is when we make that jump from animals to man we have problems and therefore we have to use the 'weight of evidence' instead of any specific figure.

I suspect we had better stop at this point and turn the meeting over to Dr Saffiotti who has been making all sorts of notes!

SUMMING UP OF THE MEETING

SAFFIOTTI

I have been asked to chair the last session of our Round Tables as a concluding Round Table. I hope we will have some stimulating final thoughts from the participants on the many different types of findings that have been presented and on the points that have been raised for discussion in the last two weeks. We considered, with our organizer Dr Castellani, the possibility of having a more formal final session, but concluded that it would be better just to have a brief summary here and some final discussion, and I was asked to give you some concluding remarks.

I have been trying to keep notes throughout the meeting. While I confirmed the depth of my ignorance, at the same time I felt encouraged by the opportunity to learn many facts that were new to me or else were not as clear as they are now after having been thoroughly presented. I think that we saw considerable advances that are fundamental to our understanding of those biological relationships that relate to the possibility of evaluating risk from physical and chemical agents more accurately and more precisely. Even allowing for a large proportion of my feeling of ignorance to come from my own personal deficiencies, I think we are all aware of major areas in which ignorance is still pervading the whole field of methodologies for risk assessment. It is a relatively young field and it has a long way to go. Of course I am referring primarily to the general field of toxicology applied to long-term delayed effects, particularly genetic effects and cancer induction effects. There are certain aspects of long-term risks from physical and chemical agents that we have barely touched upon during this meeting and I presume that they will become more amenable to direct study in the future, particularly immunotoxic effects, neurotoxic effects, and behavioral effects. We have given a relatively limited attention during this course to the problem of teratologic effects that are in many ways more closely related to mutagenic and carcinogenic effects. The latter two categories of effects have concentrated our attention most of the time.

A particularly positive result of the course, I think, is that it showed that a lot of good work is being done and the field is moving forward fairly rapidly in several different directions. These different directions begin to have bridges that connect them, so that one can go from one model system to another, from one type of biological or biochemical determination to another, building up more links. These links appear more complex than the four corners of a parallelogram, and almost become a cobweb, a net of interrelations that will perhaps eventually give us a map to guide us through this difficult field.

During the meeting we have heard these problems analyzed at different levels of biological organization, including molecular level events, cellular level events and tissue and organism level events. I have had a particular interest in my research career in the correlation of the different levels of biological organization for carcinogenesis studies, and I am interested to look at mechanisms with methods that could be as comparable as possible at all these levels so that we can learn how to correlate molecular events to the cells, and the cells to the tissues, and the tissues to the organs in which they are contained and ultimately to the response of the whole individual across species barriers, sex differences and variations in individual and environmental conditions.

We had a good demonstration at this meeting of the rapid progress in the methods for neoplastic cell transformation by physical and chemicals agents, because we now have a variety of these systems, extending to the human, where one can study the process of transformation of a normal (or in some cases abnormal but non-neoplastic) cell population to a clearly neoplastic cell population that can be perpetuated and give rise to tumors in appropriate hosts. So we are beginning to narrow down the biological model systems to managable proportions that can be well controlled and reproduced and we know that the critical effect is occurring somewhere in a much smaller black box than we knew when we were studying whole animals or whole human beings.

Dr Borek gave us an excellent introduction to the general characteristics of transformation models and criteria. These systems have been discussed throughout the meeting, pointing to the need for defining our criteria for measuring effects such as transformation by biological parameters such as growth in soft agar and tumorigenicity of the transformed cells. A large area of consensus has developed on how to use these parameters and different laboratories are able to exchange their data in a fairly homogeneous way.

An exciting new aspect of neoplastic cell transformation studies by chemical and physical agents is the appearance of methods for the transformation of human cells directly exposed in culture to these agents: Dr Sutherland has given us an impressive report on her studies on transformation of human embryo cells. I think it is not an excessively optimistic hope, that with the refinement of cell culture conditions one can move towards an increasing number of model systems that will include eventually epithelial cells and a variety of differentiated cells representing the tissues of origin of many of the tumor types that we want to correlate with in vitro transformation models. The advantage of this approach, as I have pointed out in my talks, is that one can go back to the problem of risk correlations so that carcinogen metabolism and several cellular parameters that can be studied in the human tissues can be correlated to the final event of transformation.

DNA repair has taken a central position in this area of studies perhaps for two reasons: because elegant methodologies have been developed to measure it quantitatively and to interpret the molecular events that underlie the phenomenon, and because it is so suggestive as the central event in the control of the initial lesion of neoplastic transformation. It has been pointed out, however, that there are alternative pathways that could be considered in the mechanisms of carcinogenesis and there are certainly certain types of carcinogens, that were also considered in this course, that do not seem to go through a genotoxic pathway and yet may be important carcinogens nonetheless. There is still some confusion about the proper definitions for these different types of carcinogenic events, including in vitro models for them.

An area which has been discussed at the meeting, but perhaps not in great detail, is that of the correlations between carcinogens and co-factors, particularly promoting agents. Some tests were discussed here which are particularly addressed to the study of promoting agents. I think we should remember that modifying factors can act through a variety of pathways and that the agents that have been more strictly called by the name of promoting agents may be only a relatively narrow category of this more general area of modifiers or enhancers of carcinogenesis. Some of the work which has been done with the phorbol esters has been taken to represent almost a prototype model for a portion of the cancer process as a whole. About this comparability, I have serious reservations. A point that remains to be clarified further, and on which I am planning to do some work in the laboratory, is a more specific comparison of the effects of promoting agents (when they follow a carcinogen in the classical two-stage model), with the effects of other agents (including other carcinogens) which may follow an initiating carcinogen.

Some studies I did with Dr Shubik many years ago, looking at skin carcinogenesis, did point out the very striking differences between the quality of the biological response induced by initiation followed by croton oil promotion, in comparison with the same initiation followed by repeated exposures to small amounts of carcinogens. The promoting agent induced a high proportion of benign tumors, many of which regressed and had practically only a marginal influence on the induction of carcinomas, while the effect of a carcinogen followed by additional low doses of carcinogen leads to fewer benign tumors, none that regress, and a lot of carcinomas. A similar type of response one can see in some other systems that have now been identified as good models for two-stage induction, such as rat liver where some of the promoting treatments produce liver cell nodules of which a proportion will regress, while many of the classical carcinogens given repeatedly or in combination give rise primarily to liver cell carcinomas directly.

These differences suggest underlying differences in mechanisms that are now beginning to be demonstrated. In terms of evaluation of potential risks for humans, I think that one should be very careful in using the terms of promotion or promotors as being relevant to the human and comparable to the effects of those few promotors that have actually been studied so far in animal systems, partly because those promotors that have been studied in the animal systems have given us endpoints that are really different from the ones we are looking for in the study of the human carcinogenic process. By comparing these processes we will eventually be able to make a better judgement of the similarities and differences of the two phenomena.

The problem of mutational effects received considerable attention at this course. The important point has been made from the start that although induced mutation rates in the human are still unknown, methods have become available to measure mutation frequencies in human cells, using selected systems. Obviously they are like small points in a large map, but they are beginning to provide precise measurements. One point that concerns the risk evaluation of these events, is that we seem to have indirect, preliminary or soft indications that several of the agents so far studied produced mutation rates in human cells that are relatively very low. One may eventually come to the conclusion that exposure to certain agents produces a very low mutation rate in humans. Now, what does that mean in terms of population risks?

It seems to me that for practical purposes a tendency to look at the effect of mutagenic agents one by one tends to mask to some extent the evaluation of their cumulative effects. If we have a low mutation rate from agent 1 and we have a low mutation rate from agent 2 and a low mutation rate from agent n, and we put them all together, we may end up with a cumulative mutation rate which is well within the realistic boundaries of serious health problems and may be responsible for patterns of genetic damage and disease in the population. The fact that each contributor is acting at a low level does not eliminate our concern if we are taking into account the multiplicity of factors, even if we are unable at the present time to estimate risk values directly for their possible mutual interactions. We have seen some interactions experimentally, in mutagenesis as well as in carcinogenesis experiments, both in terms of inhibition and in terms of synergism. One doesn't really know what is the final total sum resulting from these individual interactions of components. These factors suggest a note of caution in our trying to draw conclusions in terms of risk assessment for humans.

Another aspect that is becoming more and more evident from different types of studies is the interindividual variation in the human in response to specific challenges. Dr Arlett has reported mutation frequencies in human fibroblasts with 4-nitroquinoline-1-oxide showing two orders of magnitude in variation from individual to individual. That is the same range of two orders of magnitude that was found by Curtis Harris's group in our laboratory in studies on the DNA binding of a variety of carcinogens in different types of human tissues. Similar results were obtained in other laboratories, for example by Montesano's group at Lyon on human liver cells. There seems to be therefore at least a two orders of magnitude spread in the interindividual response of human tissues to genotoxic agents. Most of these studies were done with human cells or tissues derived from groups of human beings that were not selected for being homogeneous but also did not really include extremes of susceptibility. They were usually adult hospital patients or adult 'normal' trauma victims, and they do not seem to include the type of susceptibility to certain types of damage that may be present at very early ages in life or in extreme cases equivalent to xeroderma pigmentosum. If this sort of 'median' sample of human tissue in adults gives us two orders of magnitude of variation, the real variation existing among the more extreme cases may well be of another order or magnitude, extending the total variation to three orders of magnitude. If we look at the spread of the levels of effect found in a variety of biological test systems for different carcinogens and mutagens we see that this spread is as high as 6 orders of magnitude. But the compounds that represent the extremes of this spread are very few and the bulk of the chemicals seems to fall within a range of about 4 orders of magnitude of levels of effect (i.e. 'potency', as it is often inappropriately called). Now if 3 out of these 4 orders of magnitude of variation are already superimposed to the spread of individual variations, I find it very questionable to estimate the location of a chemical in this range of levels of effects on the scanty basis of data from one or two or even a few experimental systems, as if these were a good quantitative index of the response in people, when in fact the variation among individuals in the human population may almost completely overlap the variation in the experimental level of effect of the chemical in the activity scale. These caveats I think we should keep in mind, before accepting optimistically direct quantitative risk extrapolations. These concerns, however, should certainly not prevent us from working to fill more of the gaps in our quantitative model studies, because we need to have a more cohesive and complete picture.

There is no time to review all the specific methods that were presented. Many exciting biological systems were presented which make use of a variety of cell systems, particularly of human cells: each of them promises to be valuable to collect more data to establish a better basis for biological risk evaluations. I am hoping that meetings like this one will lead to more parameters being looked at in the same system by different investigators and to more systems being used by an investigator for comparative evaluations of the same factors. I hope it will encourage those investigators who have good biological systems in their laboratories to share them with others who have special techniques for looking at different types of events comparatively, so that we can obtain more data in wider matrices.

Biological variation due to metabolic differences came up time and again in our discussions. Each biological system can be characterized for its ability to offer metabolic activation or detoxification pathways to any of the chemical agents that we are dealing with. We need to define our biological systems, as much as possible, in terms of metabolic capability: I think it is very important to do so for those new bioloigical systems that are being entered into the general matrix of models. Some good examples of such approaches were presented here.

Dosimetry is another important issue that was discussed in different situations. It includes dosimetry of exposure to the whole organisms, and dosimetry of exposure to the target cells and tissues. The problem includes variations of dosimetry within the same total dose, e.g. splitting the dose, or fractionating the dose by chronic exposure to low doses versus exposure to relatively few large doses or single doses. The consequent multiplication of possible experimental designs in any given system is a problem that faces all of us, when we go back to our laboratories, with their limitations of resources and time, after having our interest stimulated by many new topics. We can't stop everything else every time we run into a new interesting biological model to study all the possible permutations suggested by these types of research. I still favor giving more emphasis than is currently being given, for example in the USA, to some careful planning of research to select an appropriate range of studies to encompass such general needs as defining and quantitating biological models in more details. This process of model definition may seem somewhat repetitious and less original than trying to discover another new molecular mechanism, but it is a necessary investment if new basic molecular biology advances need to be eventually related to pathological events and validated for the evaluation of human pathology. Funding agencies in various countries have recently taken different attitudes to this problem. Some of the European countries have developed specifically targeted programs in which priorities are given largely on the basis of decisions made by advisors and experts in the framework of a general priority plan. This approach has been prominent in the USA from the mid-1960s to the mid-1970s, but in the last 6 or 7 years the emphasis has been switched very strongly in the opposite direction, by supporting primarily independent projects in basic research by independent investigators, with a strong premium on new and original ideas. This approach provides a very important safeguard of basic research, no doubt. I am saying, however, that we should not lose sight of the need to support the development, definition and validation of the advances that the original inventive ideas have generated, since such support provides a more solid foundation to our knowledge. In our field, this consolidation work is needed for defining and characterizing new models and mechanisms, so that we would know exactly where they stand, especially as reference systems that are being used for public health evaluations. It seems to me that a lot of time, money and effort are spent in arguing about the possible extrapolation from one system to another - sometimes in cumbersome administrative or legal procedures - when a lot more could be gained by supporting systematic research needed for the definition and documentation of the critical biological interactions that need to be interpreted.

We have generally agreed, I think, that the best estimates of total human risk attributions come from the comparative analysis of several different biological systems. Any single system is difficult to use as a sole base for extrapolation: therefore the concept of batteries of tests has become more and more prominent, as Dr Legator and Dr Waters have particularly stressed. I have contributed to some of these efforts in the past, particularly in the area of animal carcinogenesis studies and in the development of some of the short-term approaches. But I think that we need a balanced view of the concept of batteries of test systems. There is a danger in taking a battery of a fairly large number of systems, including cumbersome ones like the animal test systems for long-term studies, and just pouring chemicals in and getting data poured out. Sometimes great difficulties are encountered in having them analyzed well enough to make critical sense. It is however necessary that a certain part of the total research effort in different countries be devoted to filling the present gap in the comparability of a variety of biological model systems, under fairly standardized conditions of treatment, by exposure to batteries of chemicals that are applied throughout a series of biological systems. Work in this direction is now being done, more and more systematically, not only in the USA but also in Canada, in Japan and in several European countries. The IARC has had a valuable role as a coordinating agency for some of these studies, and so have several national governments. The scientific community cannot deal at the individual level with the resources and responsibilities required by these large efforts, which are dependent on science planning at the national and international level. Balanced planning is vital, so that one does not block out essential resources for basic research in universities and research institutions to do routine testing. However, I think that resources designed for the purpose of testing are most effective when they are operated in proximity and close contact with the competence and the critical judgement of basic scientists, who are best qualified to monitor that test efforts are conducted in a qualitatively critical way and who can examine the problems that inevitably will arise and that may lead to difficulties of interpretation unless they are carefully and critically evaluated. Private industry has emerged, especially in the last 10-15 years, as a major contributor to this field: in several countries it has not only the necessary economic resources but excellent modern facilities and expertise to undertake some of the larger scale studies. Without going into a discussion of the complex issue of the relationships of industry research with government-supported research and university research, it is important to stress the need for communication, openness of information and availability of results. The openness of discussion meetings, such as this one, can help in this direction. After an initial tense period, during which in some countries adversarial relationships have clouded the discussion of several public health related research issues, my personal impression is that there is now more willingness to co-operate towards scientific solutions to the problems. One still needs to be very careful that sectorial interests, on any side, do not mask the objectivity and the quality of the results, but there is a need in our society for a great deal of co-operation from any sector that is willing to contribute.

Acceptability of risk is the last point I wanted to comment on. It is the issue that is ultimately going to decide whether our attempts to risk assessment have any weight in our society. Dr Cerutti commented on this point saying that the social acceptability of a risk may be very different from the economic acceptability of that risk. The problem of risk acceptability is characterized by the traditional questions: 'Benefit to whom and risk to whom?'; 'Who is paying for risk to a given sector or society?'; 'Can the risks be controlled by individuals or by society?'; 'What is the value of investments made on certain products, in relation to the cost of doing certain toxicity tests on those products?'.

I would like to add a third prospective to the distinction of social acceptability of risk versus economic acceptability: I would like to add scientific acceptability, in the sense that if we fail to provide scientific acceptability and credibility of our risk assessment, no economic or social pressure will eventually stand up to a critical review of the scientific evidence, which may end up embarrassing those who have pushed through a risk assessment that is not scientifically valid.

All our discussions contributed to giving us an increased awareness of the problems and the progress that has been made towards a scientifically acceptable approach to risk assessment and risk evaluation. I am convinced at the present time that a lot of our risk assessments have to be more qualitative than quantitative. I think that quantitative risk assessment is still a useful goal to move towards, although in many circumstances it is very difficult to reach.

Now we have time for a general discussion. As suggested by our course director, I would like to invite comments on the general issues: what are the trends, what are the positive and negative aspects that we have got out of this meeting?

LEGATOR

I think after your eloquent summation I have nothing else to add except to make one final plea, and that is to realize that in the field of genetic toxicology, we have almost as many procedures in man as in animals. We need to move forward and detect hazardous chemicals in high risk populations by these relevant techniques.

PUGH

As another outsider to this particular field I could identify what for me is the positive gain from this meeting. Curiously, it is also a negative one in that it is the realization of quite how far away we are from an ability to make any accurate assessment of the risk to man from chemical substances. There is attached to that a considerable sense of disappointment because we are now in a position where legislation in the USA and in the EEC requires a safety assessment of all new chemical compounds. To be beneficial to man, any assessment will also require interpretation and, possibly, that most frightening step of all, the taking of positive action! I think that while we scientists would be justified in saying that we are not yet able to make meaningful comments and therefore we should make no comment at all, to do so is to put us into the ivory tower that the general public is already convinced we live in. This might be a pertinent moment to make a comment of thanks to the course organizers who have allowed us to spend a fortnight in this beautiful ivory tower! In conclusion then I simply have to sound a word of warning, or possibly a note of despair for those of us likely to be called upon to participate in some way in our various national programs for the safety evaluation of chemical compounds.

KOTTARIDIS

Of course I consider myself as an outsider in this field because I am not directly involved in chemical or physical carcinogenesis. I am working with viruses but we heard from several speakers about the use of viral probes or viruses to estimate some risk and now that makes me feel a little bit closer to the subject. I think that the methodology for risk assessment has come long ways. We heard some very good papers and some good presentations and I am almost positive that we have some tools in our hands, now, that we can utilize. Rather than waiting or trying to find out if the 70,000 chemicals that human beings are exposed to are carcinogenic or mutagenic or anything else, I think present methodology can offer us the tools to concentrate on a few of them, and just see what these compounds are doing to human beings. Basic scientists, however, should not really stop in trying to find new methods or improve the existent methodology for future assessments. Another important aspect which should be considered is that there should be a better collaboration among countries or among laboratories and it should be extended to countries with which at this moment I don't think this collaboration exists at all. I must say once again that I feel confident that this assessment of human risk from chemicals, if I may be optimistic, is going to be much better understood in the next 5-10 years.

LAMBERT

Just a couple of comments. The first concerns what I think has been an emerging scientific trend here, concerning the possibility of studying molecular mechanisms of carcinogenesis. I think the work of a number of individuals, some of whom have not actually been here but whose work has been frequently alluded to, deserves mention. The first is John Cairns who is now at the Harvard School of Public Health, who has written some intriguing words on the possibility of transposition as a molecular mechanism: we are now finding it possible to study this mechanism directly. The second is the study of chromatin: again this is a molecular phenomenon, something one can study directly at the nucleotide level and for which there is now beginning to emerge interesting observations concerning the role of gene expression in carcinogenesis. The third is the work of William Hazeltine, concerning the use of defined nucleotide sequences to study the DNA damage in mutation directly at the DNA level: his work has begun to reveal some intriguing new classes of DNA damage. So I think generally there is the possibility of building up a much more specific and resolved profile of DNA damage in mutation and to gain some interesting insights into molecular mechanisms of carcinogenesis by focusing our studies at the molecular level and utilizing some of the newly developed techniques from genetic engineering. That is the first point.

The second point, as I think Richard Peto had tried to impress on us, is the important role of epidemiology. This immediately falls outside of the limitation of the conference on the use of human cells for risk assessment, but I think it is intrinsically an important aspect to risk assessment. It may make experimentalists a bit uneasy since it deals with different phenomena, but none the less I think that the insights which emerge from genetic epidemiological studies should be closely followed by experimentalists.

The third point is much more philosophical and it concerns the nature of risk which I believe is to deal with uncertainty, a word which I have not heard used very frequently here. I would just like to suggest that since scientists are ultimately held accountable to those who fund them with public money, it is incumbent on scientists to stress what they do not know and not to feel guilty about it, simply to admit that uncertainty will continue for the foreseeable future in many of these questions.

Ultimately I think the use of information of the sort which is generated by scientists such as ourselves is subject to a political evaluation. I am sure everyone agrees that probabilistic statements are important. I would simply try to push that a bit further and to say that it may be acceptable to admit that there is a tremendous amount of uncertainty in what we know and to let it stand at that at any one particular moment in time in our dealings with regulators or with legislative or with judicial bodies.

WATERS

Just in response to Dr Pugh, I think that EPA will continue to regulate, it will continue to exercise its legislative responsibilities. I think that all the regulatory agencies will do their jobs more efficiently by making use of the best scientific information that is available. So I would suggest that the best thing we can do as scientists is to offer that information when it is requested.

JANIAUD

I think this course was very helpful for a lot of people. First I think this course has shown we need more dosimetry and it is possible to know the exposures of the cells of man, but then I think there is another point which needs some emphasis, i.e. comparative studies of metabolism and pharmaco-kinetics. I am a member of a commission of the Ministry of Health which gives advice of the possibility to introduce drugs on the market. Most of the questions that are asked in this commission are: when you have information on tests with rats or mice, you have chronic toxicology and you have genetic toxicology, what can we derive as extrapolation to man? In my own experience and in that of people I know working in France, we have found that by comparing patterns of active metabolites in several systems, man is not so different from mice or rats if we consider the tremendous level of differences we can find between different strains of mice and rats for example. This point has to be made here again because some very harmful carcinogens like DMBA, given to some strains of rats don't produce any tumor and with other strains you get 100% of tumors. The level of magnitude we find with cell culture, when we compare human cell culture with the tissues, it is not so different from the animal situation. But another thing is to have the right information for the metabolic pathways, and I think it is still a difficult problem.

I know we do not have all the parameters, but I think it is still possible to give an advice when things are done correctly and when, for example, industries cooperate. In France, in this permanent commission, for each product there are reporters and these reporters are taken from among the scientists who have some experience of mutagenicity testing and carcinogenicity testing, and these people give advice; when there is any problem, the people from industry are called to come and we discuss and every time that the people from industry are cooperative, then we came to an agreement. Another issue is that there is a commission which is supposed to survey all the problems caused by drugs in the population and which is called pharmaco-vigilance commission. Generally this commission is set at work by a scientific report and not at all by information coming from hospitals or doctors, except for some cases of acute toxicology, but generally the basis for this commission to say that a drug could cause a problem comes from scientific evidence with any systems we can have in our laboratories. So I think cooperation is needed, and so I think this conference has been very helpful.

SAFFIOTTI

I wish to express our great debt of gratitude to Dr Castellani for having organized this meeting so effectively and so pleasantly. Dr Setlow shares our gratitude for co-chairing the program committee. I would like to suggest that we put it in the final record of our session that we express our thanks and our gratitude to Dr Castellani and Dr Setlow; to Mrs Castellani for her untiring efforts in the editorial office and for her gracious role as hostess to all participants; to Alberto Castellani for his help; to Miss Tessa Capponi for the assistance and help she so kindly gave to all participants; to all the staff that has been extremely helpful and efficient; and, last but not least, to the Cassa di Risparmio di San Miniato for the very gracious hospitality in this convent of 'I Cappuccini'. Thank you once again from all of us.

RELAXATION OF SUPERCOILED DNA BY DNA MODIFYING AGENTS:

DETECTION BY GEL ELECTROPHORESIS

G. Ciarrocchi, M. Ciomei, and M. A. Pedrini

Istituto di Genetica Biochimica
ed Evoluzionistica

del C.N.R., vis S. Epifanio 14
Pavia, Italy 27100

Figure 1 shows the electrophoretic pattern of different forms of the same circular DNA on agarose gel. In the left lane, the upper band represents the relaxed form (RFII) and the lower band the naturally negatively supercoiled form (RFI) of a plasmid DNA. The RFI band contains different topoisomers that can not be resolved by this technique. The right lane shows the electrophoretic pattern of supercoiled DNA that has been partially relaxed by the action of the topoisomerase I of Micrococcus luteus (an ω-like protein, Kung and Wang, 1977). A pattern of bands is formed from DNA molecules differing by ± 1 linking number and by ∓ 1 supertwisting of the axis of the helix. The reciprocal relationship between twisting of the strands of the double helix and supertwisting of the axis of the helix may be expressed in the quantitative form through the relationship:

$$L = T + W$$

where L, the linking number, is the number of times one DNA strand goes around the other; T is the twist of one strand about the other; W is the writhing number and describes the twisting of the axis of the helix upon itself (Crick, 1976).

Relaxation of naturally supercoiled DNA is generally mediated by interruption of the sugar-phosphate backbone continuity. This event can be catalyzed by enzymes (endonucleases, topoisomerases) or can be a direct consequence of the action of agents like x-rays or γ-rays. In the case of endonucleases or radiations, one single nick will destroy all the topological properties of the circular molecule.

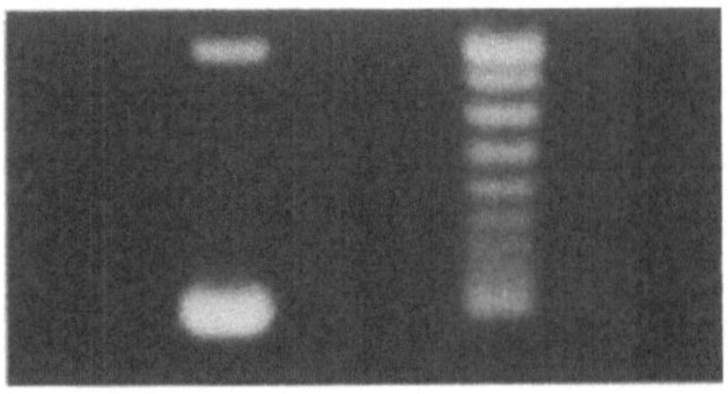

Fig. 1. Electrophoretic pattern of different forms of pAT 153 plasmid DNA.

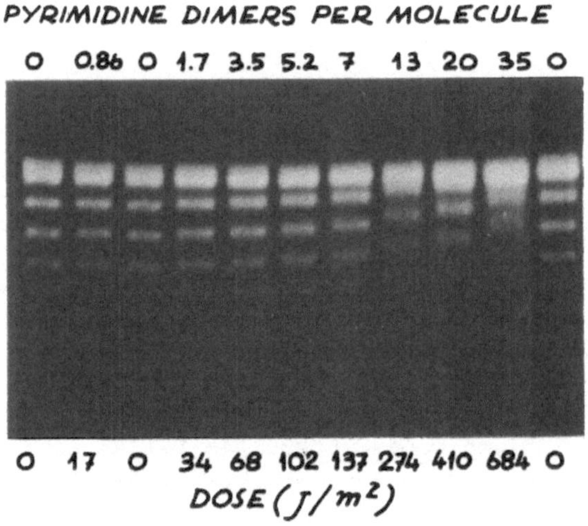

Fig. 2. Effect of UV irradiation on the electrophoretic mobility of partially relaxed pAT 153 plasmid DNA.

In the case of topoisomerases, since they nick and close the phosphodiester bond, the relaxation will take place in a stepwise manner. In addition, relaxation can occur without nicking supercoiled DNA. Intercalating agents, like ethidium bromide, or damaging agents belonging to the class which introduces bulky adducts into DNA, like psoralene (Yoakum and Cole, 1978) or benzopyrene (Gamper et al., 1980) can completely relax RFI DNA. Relaxation of supercoiled DNA can be followed by gel electrophoresis (Fig. 1), by electron microscopy or by velocity sedimentation-dye titration (Denhart and Kato, 1973).

We have decided to investigate the phenomenon of relaxation by gel electrophoresis in view of a possible application in the search of agents that damage DNA.

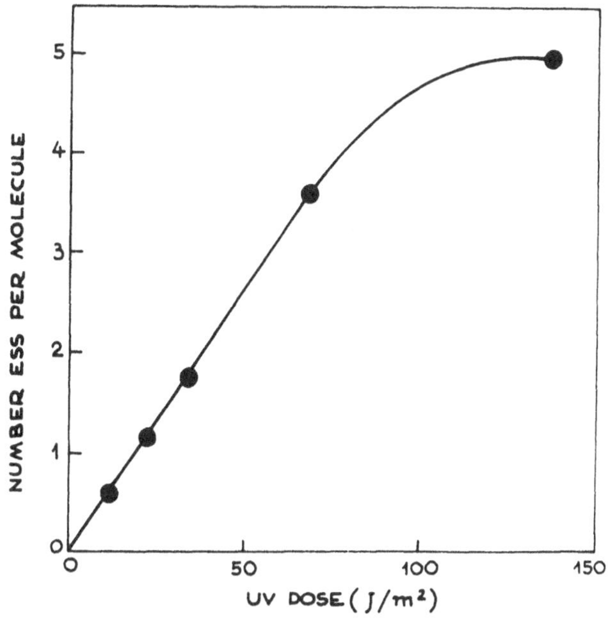

Fig. 3. Titration curve of pyrimidine dimer content in pAT 153 RFI DNA at different UV doses.

For our studies we have chosen as substrate a plasmid DNA, the pAT 153 of 3691 bp (Twigg and Sherratt, 1980). This small plasmid was chosen since treatment with topoisomerase I produces a limited number of single topoisomers which can be easily and quickly separated on agarose gel.

Figure 2 shows the effect of the presence of pyrimidine dimers on the electrophoretic mobility of DNA. Partially relaxed DNA was irradiated with 254 nm light and samples were loaded on a 0.75% agarose gel. After staining with ethidium bromide they were photographed. Peak positions were determined from negatives on a gel scanner. It has been possible in this way to measure the shift in the electrophoretic mobility produced by a single pyrimidine dimer per molecule. Furthermore, since our method uses low doses, we have also nearly eliminated the additional effects due to minor products which are known to be produced by UV irradiation at the high doses required to measure hydrodynamic changes of supercoiled RFI DNA. At these low doses we could accurately match the reduction in mobility and the pyrimidine dimer content of our substrates within the same experiment.

Pyrimidine dimer titration was obtained by the combination of a nicking assay and an enzymatic assay (Paterson, 1978). It is based

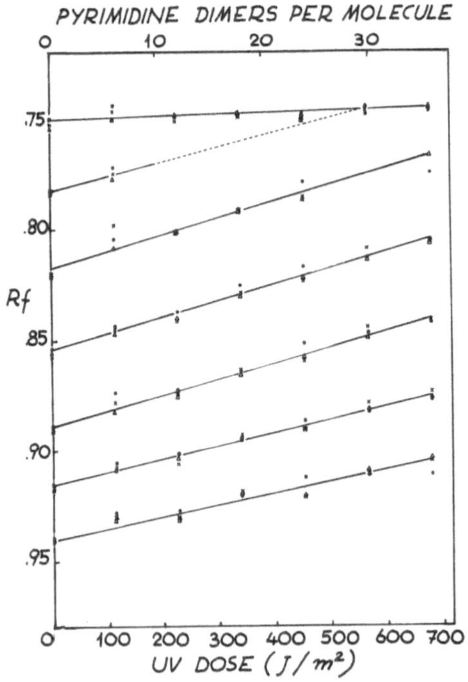

Fig. 4. Regression lines of the reduction in mobility for each topoisomer band of pAT 153 at increasing pyrimidine dimer content.

on the measurement of the conversion of the RFI to RFII on agarose gel after treatment of the UV irradiated pAT 153 with saturating amount of the dimer specific endonuclease from M. luteus (Haseltine et al., 1980). The assay shows a linear relationship with UV dose up to four pyrimidine dimers (or single strand breaks/molecule, Fig. 3).

The mobility of single topoisomers decreases with the UV dose. The reduction in mobility is observable in all visible bands and it is independent of topoisomerase I treatment which in fact can be used indifferently either before or after DNA irradiation.

Because of the topological constraint imposed on irradiated covalently closed circular DNA, the reduction of mobility on agarose gel is due to a decrease in the number of negative superhelical turns. Based on the UV dose required to reduce the mobility of each topoisomer band by one superhelical turn, we can estimate how many pyrimidine dimers are needed in order to shift the migration position of a topoisomer with linking number L_n to the position of the unirradiated band of L_{n+1}. For this purpose we ran an appropriate dose

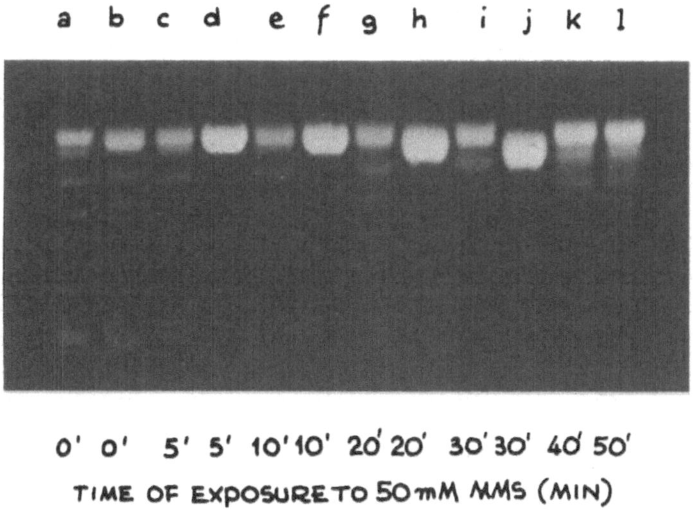

Fig. 5. Effect of alkylation on DNA electrophoretic mobility

curve with selected doses and in triplicate. After scanning of gel photographs, we measured the R_f of each band considering the RFI band as the front. From this data a regression line was calculated for each visible band (Fig. 4). Based on all regression lines, we could then determine the average dose at which one band would reduce its mobility by one linking number. This dose corresponds to 25.2 ± 0.4 pyrimidine dimers. From this number we have estimated an unwinding angle per pyrimidine dimer of -14.3° ± 0.2 (360°/25.2). This value is almost twice the 8° value expected by x-ray diffraction of thymidine dimers in solution (Camerman and Camerman, 1968), but not too far from 11.9° indirectly determined by velocity sedimentation-ethidium bromide titration (Denhart and Kato, 1973). We did not observe a differential unwinding as a function of superhelical density for all the visible topoisomers.

We have also tested a chemical agent (MMS) known to introduce a minor adduct into DNA, the methyl group. This alkyating agent is known to produce as major products N^3-MeA and N^7-MeG plus O^6-MeG as minor product. Partially relaxed DNA was allowed to react *in vitro* with 50 mM MMS for different times in the presence of potassium phosphaate buffer pH 7. As can be seen in Fig. 5 treatment of partially relaxed DNA with MMS leads to a reduction in the electrophoretic mobility of all topoisomers, as previously observed for UV treatment (Fig. 5, lane b: UV irradiated control, 5 pyrimidine dimers/molecule). In the conditions of treatment used, we observe a linear relationship between time of exposure and shift in electrophoretic mobility. However, since multiple products are generated by MMS treatment, it is not possible to calculate the unwinding angle for a single product. In addition, modified bases are unstable and are lost by the DNA molecule. Each lost base corresponds to an apurinic site (AP site). These AP sites could be eventually titrated by saturating treatment with AP endonuclease of M. luteus (Fig. 5, lanes d, f, h, j).

Therefore, we have shown that also a very small adduct like a methyl group can significantly modify the electrophoretic mobility of DNA topoisomers. We would like to propose the partially relaxed circular DNA as a very sensitive substrate for the screening of chemicals which modify the parameters of supercoiled DNA.

Since several cellular functions, such as replication, recombination, and transcription depend on the degree of supertwisting, we think that modifications of the parameters that define supercoiled DNA might influence the susceptibility of DNA to repair. We also believe that this technique could eventually be applied for detecting DNA modifications in human cells.

REFERENCES

Camerman, A., and Camerman, A., Science, 160:1451-1452 (1968).
Crick, F. H. C., Proc. Natl. Acad. Sci. U.S.A., 73:2639-2643 (1976).
Denhart, D. T., and Kato, A. C., J. Mol. Biol., 77:479-494 (1973).
Gamper, H. B., Straub, K., Calvin, M., and Bartholomew, J. C., Proc. Natl. Acad. Sci. U.S.A., 77:2000-2004 (1980).
Haseltine, W. A., Gordon, L. K., Lindan, C. P., Grafstrom, R. H., Shaper, N. L., and Grossman, L., Nature, 285:634-641 (1980).
Kung, V. T., and Wang, J. C., Biol. Chem., 252:5398-5402 (1977).
Paterson, M. C., Adv. Radiat. Biol., 7:1-56 (1978).
Twigg, A. J., and Sherratt, D., Nature, 283:216-218 (1980).
Yoakum, G. H., and Cole, R. S., Biochem. Biophys. Acta, 521:529-546 (1978).

THE MER PHENOTYPE: HUMAN TUMOR CELL STRAINS DEFECTIVE IN REPAIR OF ALKYLATION DAMAGE

Daniel B. Yarosh*, Michael R. Mattern*, Dominic A. Scudiero+ and Rufus S. Day, III*

*Nucleic Acids Section, Laboratory of Molecular Carcinogenesis, CIP, DCCP, NCI, NIH, Bethesda, Maryland 20205 and +Chemical Carcinogenesis Program, Frederick Cancer Research Center, Frederick, Maryland 21701

The integrity of DNA is vitally important to cellular function and a wide variety of organisms possess repair mechanisms to preserve DNA structure and its faithful replication. Much of our understanding of human DNA repair comes from the study of xeroderma pigmentosum (XP). Patients with this disease show sun sensitivity and a high incidence of skin cancer among their symptoms [for review see 1,2]. XP is inherited in a Mendelian fashion and cells from many tissues of XP patients show hypersensitivity to UV, suggesting that a germ line mutation is responsible for the disease. In addition to cellular hypersensitivity, XP cells are deficient in support of growth of UV-irradiated SV40, herpes simplex virus and and adenovirus[3,4,5]. XP cells grown in culture fail to remove UV-induced pyrimidine dimers from their DNA while normal cells do[6]. UV-irradiated XP cells have been permeabilized and supplied with exogenous endonucleases which incise UV-irradiated DNA, whereupon dimers were excised and cellular hypersensitivity was reduced[7,8]. These data suggest that in XP a germ line mutation results in inactivation of excision repair of pyrimdine dimers throughout the body and the persistence of high levels of pyrimidine dimers in epidermal DNA leads to oncogenic transformation.

Somatic cell mutations might also arise which inactivate DNA repair mechanisms. This would result in a clone of somatic cells hypersensitive to DNA damaging agents and more likely to undergo malignant transformation. Tumors may develop composed of cells defective in DNA repair. Thirty-nine human tumor cell strains and 22 normal skin fibroblast cell lines have been tested for their their ability to support the growth of adenovirus treated with

N-methyl-N'-nitro-N'nitrosoguanidine (MNNG) [for review see 9].Nine of the tumor cell strains but none of the fibroblast lines showed a defect in support of growth of MNNG-treated adenovirus. These nine strains were also defective in support of growth of adenovirus treated with methylnitrosourea (MNU), ethylnitrosourea (ENU) and a variety of alkyl-nitrosoguanidines[10,11]. This defect has been designated the mer$^-$ phenotype (methylation repair) and is interpreted to reflect a defect in the repair of alkylation damage to DNA.

Mer$^-$ cells show cellular hypersensitivity to MNNG compared to mer$^+$ cells[10,11,12]. However, there is no difference between mer$^+$ and mer$^-$ cells in cellular sensitivity to UV [11,12] or in the ability to support the growth of UV-irradiated or MMS-treated adenovirus[10,11,13]. There are some ambiguities in the mer phenotype. Two lung carcinoma strains, A549 and A2182, are phenotypicaly mer$^+$ by the adenovirus growth assay but show cellular hypersensitivity to MNNG compared to other mer$^+$ strains (unpublished observations). A kidney carcinoma strain, A498, was converted from mer$^+$ to mer$^-$ phenotype in the adenovirus growth assay by pretreatment of the cells with MNNG[11]. Four normal fibroblast lines are mer$^+$ while SV40 transformed derivatives of these lines are mer$^-$ in the adenovirus growth assay and show cellular hypersensitivity to MNNG[12].

Mer$^-$ cells differ from mer$^+$ cells by other criteria. Mer$^-$ strains give rise to detectible levels of sister-chromatid-exchanges at a much lower concentration of MNNG than do mer$^+$ cells, although there is heterogeneity in response among mer$^+$ strains[12]. Semi-conservative DNA synthesis after MNNG treatment is decreased in mer$^-$ cells relative to mer$^+$ cells immediately after treatment and at 24 hrs after treatment.

Mer$^-$ cells may be defective in removal of alkylation damage from DNA. After MNNG treatment the amount of O^6-methylguanine (O^6-meG) relative to N^7-methylguanine (N^7-meG) in the DNA of mer$^+$ cells is about three-fold less than found in mer$^-$ cells (perhaps reflecting active removal during MNNG treatment) and 20 hr after treatment the ratio of O^6-meG/N^7-meG delcines for mer$^+$ cells while increasing slightly for mer$^-$ cells[12]. Mer$^-$ cells sustain higher interstrand crosslinking levels following treatment with 1-(2-chloroethyl)-1-nitrosourea (CNU) than do mer$^+$ cells[14]. These crosslinks may occur because mer$^-$ cells fail to remove the CNU monoadduct and thus have a higher concentration of monoadducts available for conversion to the diadduct or crosslink.

Mer$^-$ cells do not appear to be defective in recognition and incision of alkylated DNA. Both mer$^+$ and mer$^-$ cell extracts contain endonuclease activity which incises MNU-treated *E. coli* plasmid DNA (Yarosh and Day, submitted for publication). Upon treatment with MNNG, mer$^+$ and mer$^-$ cells undergo a rapid relaxation of nucleoid DNA, as judged by sedimentation in 15-30% neutral sucrose gradients

(Mattern, Paone and Day, submitted for publication). This relaxation may reflect in vivo incision of DNA by damage-specific endonucleases. The failure of mer^- cells to remove O^6-meG may not be related to excision repair. The level of DNA glycosylase acting on O^6-alkylguanine is very low in human lymphoblasts[15]. E. coli[16] and mouse liver cells[17] contain a transmethylase activity which removes methyl adducts from guanidine in DNA without incision and transfers them to an acceptor protein. The mer defect may be related to this transmethylase activity.

After alkylation damage, DNA structure and repair replication differ in mer^+ and mer^- cells. Within 2 to 4 hrs after removal of MNNG from the media, DNA in mer^+ cells was relaxed or unwound and then was restored to the control form which sedimented rapidly in neutral sucrose (Mattern, Paone and Day, submitted for publication). In contrast, nucleoid DNA of mer^- cells remained slowly sedimenting even after 48 hrs of incubation. The delayed recovery of mer^- nucleoid DNA was MNNG-specific, since after UV irradiation all cell lines underwent relaxation within the first hour and regenerated rapidly-sedimenting nucleoids within 4 to 6 hrs (Mattern, Paone and Day, submitted for publication). Two measures of repair replication in mer^+ and mer^- cells have been used. In the BND-cellulose technique, ^3H-thymidine incorporated in the presence of hydroxyurea after MNNG treatment is measured. Double-stranded DNA (into which incorporation of label reflects DNA synthesis in response to MNNG treatment) is separated from single-stranded DNA (into which incorporation of label reflects mainly semi-conservative DNA synthesis) by benzoylated naphthoylated DEAE cellulose (BND-cellulose) chromatography[18]. Mer^- strains incorporated more label into double-stranded DNA than mer^+ strains following MNNG treatment[10]. The two mer^+ lung carcinoma strains (A549 and A2182) which showed cellular hypersensitivity to MNNG compared to other mer^+ strains also showed showed more incorporation of label than other mer^+ strains (unpublished observations). In the the bromodeoxyuridine (BUDR) photolysis assay, BUDR incorporated in the presence of hydroxyurea after MNNG treatment increases the photosensitivity of pre-labeled parental DNA to 313 nm radiation[19]. The amount of BUDR incorporated into parental DNA is reflected in the rate of breaks introduced into labeled DNA by 313 nm radiation as measured by alkaline sucrose gradients. Two mer^- strains incorporated only half the level of BUDR that two mer^+ strains did (unpublished observations). The two mer^+ strains, however, were A549 and A2182, which showed cellular hypersensitivity to MNNG. Conclusions from the BUDR photolysis technique must await the testing of more $mer+$ and mer^- strains.

SUMMARY

Some human tumors appear to contain cells defective in the repair of alkylation damage. These mer^- cells may arise from a variety of tissues. They show cellular hypersensitivity to alkylating agents and are defective in the support of the growth of alkylated adenovirus. The molecular defect has not been identified, although <u>mer</u>$^-$ cells fail to remove alkylation adducts. There is no evidence that <u>mer</u>$^-$ cells are defective in recognition and incision of alkylated DNA, but they differ from <u>mer</u>$^+$ in subsequent steps involving repair replication and restoration of nucleoid structure. The identification of the <u>mer</u> phenotype may become useful in chemotherapy of human malignancies and in the understanding of the processes leading to oncogenic transformation.

REFERENCES

1. Kraemer, K. (1980) Clinical Derm. 4:1-33.
2. Cleaver, J.E. and D. Bootsma (1975) Ann. Rev. Genet. 9:19-38.
3. Aaronson, S.A. and C.D. Lytle (1970) Nature 228:359-361.
4. Lytle, C.D., S.A. Aaronson and E. Harvey (1972) Intl. J. Rad. Biol. 22:159-165.
5. Day, R.S. III (1974) Photochem. Photobiol. 19:9-13.
6. Setlow, R.B., J.D. Regan and J. German (1969) Proc. Natl. Acad. Sci. (USA) 64:1035-1039.
7. Tanaka, K., H. Hayakawa, M. Sekiguchi and Y. Okada (1977) Proc. Natl. Acad. Sci. (USA) 74:2958-2962.
8. Tanaka, K., M. Sekiguchi and Y. Okada (1975) Proc. Natl. Acad. Sci. (USA) 72:4071-4075.
9. Day, R.S. III, C.H.J. Ziolkowski, D.A. Scudiero, S.A. Meyer and M.R. Mattern (1980) <u>in</u> "Genetic and Environmental Factors in Experimental and Human Cancer" H.V. Gelboin et al. eds. Japan Sci. Soc. Press, Tokyo, pp247-257.
10. Day, R.S. III, C.H.J. Ziolkowski, D.A. Scudiero, S.A. Meyer and M.R. Mattern (1980) Carcinogenesis 1:21-32.
11. Day, R.S. III and C.H.J. Ziolkowski (1981) Carcinogenesis 2:213-218.
12. Day, R.S. III, C.H.J. Ziolkowski, D.A. Scudiero, S.A. Meyer, A.S. Lubiniecki, A.J. Girardi, S.M. Galloway and G.D. Bynum (1980) Nature 288:724-727.
13. Day, R.S. III and C.H.J. Ziolkowski (1979) Nature 279:797-799.
14. Erickson, L.C., G. Laurent, N.A. Sharkey and K.W. Kohn (1980) Nature 288:727-729.
15. Singer, B. and T.P. Brent (1981) Proc. Natl. Acad. Sci. (USA) 78:856-860.
16. Olsson, M. and T. Lindahl (1980) J. Biol. Chem. 255:10569-10571.
17. Bogden, J.M., A. Eastman and E. Bresnick (1981) Nucleic Acids Res. 9:3089-3103.
18. Scudiero, D.A., E. Henderson, A. Norin and B. Strauss (1975) Mut. Res. 29:473-488.
19. Setlow, R.B. and J.D. Regan (1981) <u>in</u> "Techniques in DNA Repair--A Handbook" E.C. Friedberg and P.C. Hanawalt eds., Marcel Dekker, Inc. N.Y. pp307-318.

GROWTH-DEPENDENT AND AGE-RELATED CHANGES IN THE FREE AMINO ACID POOL OF HUMAN DIPLOID FIBROBLASTS

Yula Sambuy and Alan H. Bittles

Department of Human Biology, Chelsea College

Manresa Road, LONDON SW3 6LX U.K.

Free aminoacids are intermediates in protein catabolism. The size and composition of the intra-cellular pool is therefore in general determined by a balance between input, for example, from protein catabolism, uptake from the extra-cellular medium and *de novo* synthesis of non-essential aminoacids and removal, for incorporation into proteins, synthesis of other compounds (including the non-essential aminoacids) and degradation for energy production (1).

It has been known for sometime that cells have the ability to accumulate aminoacids within their intra-cellular pool, by the operation of specific transport systems (2). Recent evidence suggests that the regulation of these transport systems is effected via a complex interaction of feed-back mechanisms involving both the intra-cellular and extra-cellular aminoacid concentrations (3,4,5). It therefore seems probable that the internal aminoacid pool plays an important role in the control of protein metabolism and cellular proliferation, although it has also been suggested that the aminoacids selected for protein synthesis may be directly incorporated from the extra-cellular medium (6).

Human diploid fibroblasts have a fixed and reproducible lifespan in culture (7) that is inversely related to the age of the donor from whom the cells were obtained (8,9). These observations have led to the use of cultured cells as a model for the study of the mechanisms of cellular ageing *in vitro*. Several age-related changes have been observed in human diploid fibroblasts including altered enzymes (10,11,12), changes in morphology (13), in ultrastructure (14) and in surface properties (15) as well as altered growth characteristics (16,17). Whether they result from an accumulation of errors (18,19) or represent the expression of a genetic programme similar to that operating during growth and differentiation (20,21,22) is still a matter of controversy.

The purpose of the present study was to investigate the composition of the free aminoacid pool of human diploid fibroblasts throughout their lifespan in culture and to determine the relative roles of growth rate and of ageing in the maintenance of the system.

METHODS AND MATERIALS

A human diploid embryonic fibroblast cell line, BCL-D1, was grown in Minimum Essential Medium, Glasgow modification (G-MEM) supplemented with 2.0 mM L-Glutamine, 10% Fetal Calf Serum (FCS) and 1% antibiotic solution containing 10,000 U ml^{-1} Penicillin and 10,000 $\mu g\ ml^{-1}$ Streptomycin. All cell culture materials were supplied by Gibco Europe Ltd.,England. The growth medium was changed every three days unless otherwise stated. The cells were grown in 175 cm^2 plastic flasks at 37°C in an atmosphere of 5% CO_2 in air. When the cells reached confluence (usually after 3 to 7 days), they were subcultured by a brief treatment with 0.5 g ml^{-1} EDTA in Phosphate buffered saline, Ca^{2+}-free and Mg^{2+}-free (PBS"A") and transferred to new flasks in fresh growth medium. The age of the culture was expressed as the number of cumulative Cell Population Doublings (CPD) the culture had undergone, and was calculated from the average number of cell divisions required to reach confluence, using a 1:2 or 1:3 split at each subcultivation. Following this routine, the lifespan of the cell line was 55 ± 10 CPD.

The cells were routinely tested for evidence of mycoplasma contamination by the fluorescent DNA stain method developed by Chen (23). Karyotypic analysis of the line at different CPD levels showed that the cells maintained their diploid configuration up to the latest stages of their lifespan in culture.

For the analysis of the intra-cellular free aminoacid pool the medium was poured off and the cell monolayer was washed three times with PBS"A" at 37°C, the cells were gently scraped off the growth surface with a silicon policeman and collected in 0.03M Na-phosphate buffer, pH 6.8 at 4°C. The cells were lysed using 3 x 10 seconds bursts of maximum amplitude sonication at 0°C and the cellular debris removed by centrifugation at 12,000g for 25 min at 4°C. The clear supernatant was deproteinized with crystalline sulphosalicylic acid (5 mg ml^{-1}) for 10 min and the protein precipitate removed by centrifugation at 3,000g for 25 min at 4°C.

The analysis of the aminoacids was carried out on an automatic aminoacid analyser (The Locarte Co.,England). The sequential elution of the aminoacids from the ion-exchange resin was achieved with a series of four lithium citrate buffers of increasing pH (from pH 2.78 to pH 9.0) during an 8 hours run, the aminoacids being detected by the ninhydrin reaction.

RESULTS

Before considering the results obtained, it is important to recognize that the term aminoacid pool may, in fact, describe a multi-compartmentalized system (24,25). For this reason, it is essential that highly standardized and reproducible preparative procedures be followed consistently, so that the intra-cellular aminoacid content is always measured under comparable experimental conditions (26).

(i) Growth-related changes in the free aminoacid pool.

The effects of cell growth on the composition of the intra-cellular free aminoacid pool were investigated in parallel sets of cultures at days 1,2,3,4 and 7 from seeding, without medium changes. Since the total protein content per cell has been reported to change both during the growth cycle (27) and during the lifespan in culture (28,29), each aminoacid was expressed as a proportion of the total aminoacid content of the appropriate culture.

The results of this investigation on cell cultures at CPD26 ("young") and CPD48 ("old") are reproduced in Table 1.

Table 1

A. Cultures at CPD 26 ("young")

Aminoacid	Days 1	2	3	4	7
TAU	.0104	.0208	.0439	.0765	.0972
ASP	.0551	.0426	.0406	.0271	.0182
THR	.0860	.0966	.0995	.1048	.1137
SER	.0055	.0032	.0039	.0045	.0039
GLU	.3353	.3249	.3219	.2755	.2319
GLN	.3032	.2724	.1870.	.1590	.1292
PRO	.0165	.0231	.0632	.0668	.0691
GLY	.0180	.0223	.0342	.0544	.0700
ALA	.0312	.0517	.0764	.0932	.1301
VAL	.0257	.0256	.0251	.0275	.0252
MET	.0168	.0163	.0129	.0133	.0124
ILE	.0272	.0255	.0215	.0223	.0203
LEU	.0250	.0269	.0216	.0231	.0217
TYR	.0188	.0209	.0198	.0223	.0230
PHE	.0185	.0201	.0201	.0219	.0231
LYS	.0067	.0072	.0085	.0076	.0110

B. Cultures at CPD 48 ("old")

Aminoacid	Days 1	2	3	4	7
TAU	.0095	.0140	.0370	.0517	.0571
ASP	.0455	.0459	.0406	.0379	.0139
THR	.1039	.1078	.1141	.1158	.1252
SER	.0112	.0079	.0057	.0064	.0042
GLU	.3109	.3000	.2866	.2555	.2045
GLN	.2962	.2654	.1890	.1629	.1196
PRO	.0372	.0511	.0873	.0987	.1362
GLY	.0199	.0214	.0296	.0394	.0304
ALA	.0487	.0593	.0820	.1035	.1382
VAL	.0216	.0222	.0208	.0194	.0139
MET	.0138	.0131	.0127	.0121	.0213
ILE	.0216	.0222	.0206	.0194	.0139
LEU	.0205	.0211	.0197	.0203	.0203
TYR	.0192	.0199	.0194	.0197	.0128
PHE	.0166	.0189	.0184	.0180	.0316
LYS	.0076	.0101	.0164	.0172	.0353

Although the actual levels of each aminoacid in the two sets of cultures may be different at any one time, the pattern of change over the first four days were comparable for both cellular ages. Differences at day 7 probably represented the result both of the depletion of medium constituents and of the different numbers of cells present in the two cultures at confluence. Valine, methionine, isoleucine, tyrosine and phenylalanine did not change markedly between days 1 and 4 in either of the cultures. Lysine on the other hand, while remaining constant from days 1 to 7 in young cultures, showed a gradual increase in the old cultures. The aminoacids that increased proportionately between days 1 and 4 include taurine, proline, alanine and, to a lesser extent, glycine and threonine. Glutamine, glutamate and aspartate decreased in both sets of cultures from days 1 to 7.

(ii) Changes in the free aminoacid pool associated with cellular ageing

To assess the changes in the intra-cellular free aminoacid pool during the lifespan of the cells in culture, thirty cultures at different CPD levels were analysed 48 hours after seeding and the results pooled into three age-groups at CPD 20 to 26, CPD 28 to 39 and CPD 41 to 56. A one-way analysis of variance (30) was applied to determine whether the differences within each group were significantly different from those between groups. In order to carry out the one-way analysis of variance, the proportion of each aminoacid to the total aminoacid content of the culture was transformed into:

$$\text{arcsin}\sqrt{\frac{\text{aminoacid}}{\text{total aminoacids}}}$$

This variance stabilizing transformation (31) was required in order to meet the assumption of homogeneous variance which underlies the analysis of variance.

For those aminoacids that showed a significant difference between age-groups a Fisher's Least Significant Difference Test (LSD) was applied to determine the pattern of change between the age-groups (30). A summary of the pairwise comparison of the means of the age-groups for those aminoacids showing significant differences is presented in Table 2.

Table 2

		Significance $p < 0.05$	Significance $p < 0.01$
INCREASE			
Glutamine	$M_1 < M_2$		*
	$M_2 < M_3$	*	
Methionine	$M_1 < M_2$		*
	$M_1 < M_3$		*
DECREASE			
Taurine	$M_1 > M_2$		*
	$M_2 > M_3$	*	
Proline	$M_1 > M_2$		*
	$M_1 > M_3$		*
Alanine	$M_1 > M_2$		*
	$M_1 > M_3$		*
Glycine	$M_1 > M_2$		*
	$M_1 > \frac{M_2 + M_3}{2}$		*
Phenylalanine	$M_1 > M_3$		*
	$M_2 > M_3$		*
Tyrosine	$M_1 > M_3$		*
	$M_2 > M_3$		*
Leucine	$M_1 > M_3$	*	
	$M_2 > M_3$		*
Isoleucine	$M_1 > M_3$		*
	$M_2 > M_3$		*
Valine	$M_1 > M_3$		*
	$M_2 > M_3$		*
Threonine	$M_1 > \frac{M_2 + M_3}{2}$	*	
	$M_2 > M_3$		*

Age-related changes in the intra-cellular free aminoacid pool. Multiple comparison between the means (M) of the three age-groups.

M_1 CPD 20 - 26 M_2 CPD 28 - 39 M_3 CPD 41 - 56

DISCUSSION

As human diploid fibroblasts progress through their lifespan in culture there is an increase both in the duration of the cell cycle(16) and in the proportion of cells that lose the ability to divide (17). Furthermore, older cells exhibit density-dependent inhibition of growth at a lower cell concentration than younger cells (16); for this reason, when comparing cultures at different stages of the lifespan it is extremely difficult to standardize cell numbers, degree of confluence and growth state. In order to assess the significance of the effects of ageing on the free aminoacid pool, it is therefore essential first to consider the changes occurring during the growth of the cells.

As can be seen in Table 1, while a number of aminoacids remain relatively constant in the first four days of growth, others increase or decrease considerably over the same period of time. Since the composition of the intra-cellular pool represents the balance between a number of metabolic reactions, it is difficult to assess the real significance of these changes. Nevertheless, since the intra-cellular changes did not directly reflect the changes occurring in the medium over the same period of time (unpublished results), it is reasonable to assume that they may be caused by factors other than the extra-cellular concentration. Such factors may be related to changes in cell population density and growth state.

Although it was reported that growth rate did not affect the size and composition of the intra-cellular aminoacid pool of both normal and transformed human cells (32), more recent reports have shown that both the activity of the aminoacid transport systems and consequently the composition of the intra-cellular pool, change as the cells progress from rapid growth in sparse cultures to density-dependent growth arrest in confluent cultures (33,34,35,36). Our results agree in general with the latter reports although the findings are not directly comparable because of the use of different cell lines, different experimental procedures and handling of the data.

Since cell numbers and growth rate are the factors least easily controlled when comparing young and old cultures, they are likely to give rise to some spurious age-effects. For example, in the case of aminoacids such as glycine, alanine, proline, taurine and threonine which increased markedly in proportion during the growth of the cells, the observed decline in older cultures (Table 2) may be due to lower cell numbers or to some growth-related effect rather than to a real ageing effect. The opposite situation was observed with glutamine which decreased during growth and increased with age. Since glutamine is, with glucose, the major energy source for human diploid fibroblasts (37), it seems reasonable to assume that older, less metabolically active cells may maintain higher levels of this aminoacid than rapidly growing, younger cells because of their lower energy requirements. On the other hand, among the aminoacids that did not change during the growth of the cells, the decrease exhibited by valine, isoleucine, leucine, tyrosine, phenylalanine and the increase of methionine in old cultures as compared with young ones are likely to represent real ageing effects. It is interesting to note that all of this group are essential aminoacids in cultured human cells (32), they are all neutral and are all transported by the L-system (4) which is characterized by a broad reactivity towards aminoacids with branches or rings on the side chain (3).

In considering the possible role of the intra-cellular aminoacid pool in the regulation of protein metabolism, it is not overly important whether the precursors of protein synthesis are selected from the existing intra-cellular pool or are taken up directly from from the extra-cellular medium. The control exerted on the aminoacid transport system by both the intra-cellular and extra-cellular aminoacid concentrations (3) ensures at least an indirect regulatory role for the intra-cellular pool and hence any age-related changes will be of significance in protein metabolism.

Whether the observed age-related changes in the composition of the intra-cellular pool are part of a programmed series of events leading to senescence, or result from the breakdown of cellular control mechanisms due to the accumulation of errors at the level of protein synthesis cannot be determined on the basis of the results presented. However, if the intra-cellular pool proves to occupy a central position in the control of cell proliferation, then changes in its composition could well be associated with the loss of proliferative capacity which characterizes cellular ageing.

REFERENCES

1. Munro,H.N. (1970) In "Mammalian Protein Metabolism" vol.4 H.N. Munro ed. pp.299-386 Academic Press N.Y.
2. Christensen, H.N. (1964) In "Mammalian Protein Metabolism" vol 1. H.N. Munro ed. pp,105-124 Academic Press N.Y.
3. Guidotti, G.C., Borghetti,A.F., Gazzola, G.C. (1978) Biochim. Biophys. Acta 515,329-366.
4. Gazzola, G.C., Dall'Asta,V., Guidotti, G.C. (1980) J.Biol. Chem. 255, 929-936.
5. Gazzola, G.C., Dall'Asta, V., Guidotti, G.C. (1981) J.Biol. Chem. 256, 3191-3198.
6. Robertson,J.H., Wheatley, D.N. (1979) Biochem. J. 178, 699- 709.
7. Hayflick, L., Moorhead, P.S. (1961) Exp.Cell Res. 25, 585-621
8. Martin, G.M., Sprague, C.A., Epstein,E.J., (1970) Lab. Invest. 23, 86-92.
9. Schneider, E.L., Mitsui, Y. (1976) Proc. Natl. Acad. Sci. USA 73, 3584-3588.
10. Cristofalo, V.J., Parris, N., Kritchewsky, D. (1967) J. Cell Physiol. 69, 263-272.
11. Wang, K.M., Rose, N.R., Bartholomew, E.A., Balzen, M., Berde, K., Foldvary,M. (1970) Exp. Cell Res. 61, 357-364.
12. Holliday, R., Tarrant, G.M. (1972) Nature 238, 26-30.
13. Wolosewick, J.J., Porter, R.K. (1977) Am.J. Anat. 149, 197-225
14. Lipetz, J., Cristofalo, V.J. (1972) J. Ultrastruct. Res. 39, 43-56.
15. Aizawa, J., Mitsui,Y., Kurimototo, F., Matsuoka, K. (1980) Mech. Ageing Dev. 13, 297-306.
16. Macieira-Coelho, A., Ponten, A.J., Philipson, L. (1966) Exp. Cell Res. 42, 673-684.
17. Cristofalo, V.J., Sharf, B.B. (1973) Exp. Cell Res. 76, 419-427.
18. Orgel, L.E. (1973) Nature 243, 441-445.
19. Orgel, L.E. (1963) Proc. Natl. Acad. Sci. USA 49, 517-521.
20. Martin, G.M., Sprague, C.A., Norwood, T.H., Pendergrass,W.R. (1974) Am. J. Pathol. 74, 137-154.
21. Cristofalo, V.J. (1977) In "Senescence: Dominant or Recessive in Somatic Cell Crosses?" W.W. Nichols D.G. Murphy eds. pp.13-21. Plenum Press N.Y.
22. Bell, E., Marek, L.F., Levinstone, D.S., Merrill,C., Sher, S.,

Young, I.T., Eden, M. (1978) Science 202, 1158-1163.

23. Chen, T.R. (1977) Exp. Cell Res. 104, 255-262.
24. Airhart, J., Vidrich, A., Khairallah, E.A. (1974) Biochem. J. 140, 539-548.
25. Ward, W.F., Mortimer, G.E. (1978) J. Biol. Chem. 253, 3581-3587.
26. Melancon, S.B., Tayco, J., Nadler, H.L. (1972) Proc. Soc. Exp. Biol. Med. 141, 391-395.
27. Braun, R. (1978) Nature 273, 594.
28. Cristofalo, V.J., Howard, B.V., Kritchewsky, D. (1970) In "Organic, Biological and Medicinal Chemistry" V. Gallo L. Santamarra eds. Vol. 2 pp.95-150 N.Holland, Amsterdam.
29. Schneider, E.L., Shorr, S.S. (1975) Cell 6, 179-184.
30. Roscoe, J.T. (1975) In "Fundamental Research Statistics for the Behavioural Sciences" Holt Rinehardt and Winson. N.Y.
31. Kendall, M., Stuart, A. (1976) In "The Advanced Theory of Statistics" vol 3. p.117. Griffin, London.
32. Piez, K.A., Eagle, H. (1958) J. Biol. Chem. 231, 533-545.
33. Griffiths, J.B. (1972) J. Cell Sci. 10, 515-524.
34. Birckbichler, P.J., Whittle, W.L., Dell'Orco, R.T. (1975) Proc. Soc. Exp. Biol. Med. 149, 530-533.
35. Robinson, J.H. (1976) J. Cell Physiol. 89, 101-110.
36. Oxender, D.L., Lee, M., Cecchini, G. (1977) J. Biol. Chem. 252, 2680-2683.
37. Sumbilla, C.M., Zielke, C.L., Reed, W.D., Ozand, P.T., Zielke, H.R. (1981) Biochim. Biophys. Acta 675, 301-304.

DNA FRAGMENTATION AND SISTER CHROMATID EXCHANGES INDUCED BY COMMERCIAL AURAMINE O, PURIFIED AURAMINE, AND MICHLER'S KETONE

D. Vecchio, M. Pala, P. Russo, L. Ottaggio,
A. Albini, S. Parodi,* and L. Santi*

Istituto Scientifico per lo Studio e la Cura
dei Tumori
Istituto Nazionale per la Ricerca
sul Cancro, Genoa

INTRODUCTION

In IARC monograph No. 1 (IARC monograph, 1972) Auramine O is reported to be widely used in industry. An high increase in bladder tumors in workers engaged in the manufacture of Auramine was reported (Case and Pearson, 1954). A recent study (Report of a IARC Working Group, 1980) evaluated the data on human and experimental animal carcinogenesis. Auramine was classified in group 2, probably carcinogenetic for humans, subgroup B, lower degree of evidence.

Auramine O was reported to be carcinogenetic in rats and mice (Bonser et al., 1956; Williams and Bonser, 1962).

It was negative in the Ames test (McCann et al., 1975; Rosenkranz et al., 1976; Rosenkranz and Poirier, 1979; Simon, 1979a) and in the sporulation system of <u>B. subtilis</u> (MacGregor and Sacks, 1976), but was positive in inducing selective toxicity in <u>E. coli</u> DNA polymerase 1-deficient (pol A^-) strains (Rosenkranz et al., 1976; Rosenkranz and Poirier, 1979), and in the assay for recombinogenetic activity with <u>S. cerevisiae D3</u> (Simmon, 1979b; Simmon et al., 1979). In this report we have examined commercial and purified Auramine O for its capability to induce DNA damage, as evaluated with the alkaline elution technique, in different tissues of rats and mice <u>in vivo</u>. A human cell line grown <u>in vitro</u> was also examined for its sensitivity

*Department of Oncology, Genoa University, Italy.

to Auramine O. The capability of commercial and purified Auramine O to induce SCE increase in bone marrow cells after treatment *in vivo* was also investigated. We have also investigated the capability of inducing DNA fragmentation and SCE increment of the Michler's ketone, which is one of the major impurities of our commercial Auramine O. The Michler's ketone is hepatocarcinogenic in rats and mice (NCI bioassay, 1979).

METHODS

DNA Damage in Vivo/Alkaline Elution Assay

The *in vivo* assay for DNA damage was performed using Sprague-Dawley male albino rats and Swiss male mice (CD Charles River), aged 2 to 3 months. The products examined were suspended in 0.9% NaCl with 1% carboxymethylcellulose as suspending agent and were administered by i.p. route in 0.01 ml of vehicle/g b.w. Controls were injected with the same amount of the same vehicle. At different times after treatment rats and mice were killed by cervical dislocation and exsanguinated.

The alkaline elution was essentially performed according to Kohn et al. (1976) as previously described (Parodi et al., 1978) with minor modification. Eluted DNA and filter were assayed for DNA content by a modification of the microfluorimetric technique of Kissane and Robbins (1958), as previously described (Parodi et al., 1978). The average elution rate constant is given by the following formula:

$$K = \frac{-\ln \text{ (fraction of DNA retained on filter)}}{V}$$

Here K is the average elution rate constant (ml^{-1}) of DNA and V is the eluted volume in ml. As a first approximation K is directly proportional to the number of single strand breaks. Moreover, the above formula reflects the assumption of first-order kinetics for DNA elution, always as a first approximation (Kohn et al., 1976).

DNA Damage in Vitro/Alkaline Elution Assay

The human cell line HuF_{22} (human foreskin fibroblasts) (obtained from Dr. O. E. Varnier, Institute of Microbiology, University of Genoa) was also studied for DNA damage. Dimethylsulfoxide was the solvent for Auramine O and was present during treatment of cells at a final concentration of 1%. Cells were incubated with or without Auramine O (3×10^{-4} M) at a density of 1 to 2 $\times 10^{6}$ cells/ml in 5 ml of culture medium at 37°C and 5% CO_2 for 2 h. At the end of the incubation period, the medium containing Auramine O was removed and cells were resuspended in cold Merchant's solution. All the following steps were performed according to the alkaline elution method (Parodi et al., 1978).

Induction of SCEs in Bone Marrow Cells

The method used for SCE evaluation was essentially that of Allen et al. (1977). Mice were treated with the products examined with a single i.p. injection. The number of metaphases examined per animal varied from 10 to 20: when better spread and well contrasted, more metaphases were examined in a given sample.

Determination of LD_{50}

The 7-day lethal dose (LD_{50}), not available in the literature, was determined in male Sprague-Dawley rats according to the method of Weil (1952).

Quality Control and Purification of Auramine O and Michler's Ketone

Auramine O was purified by extraction with $CHCl_3$, dehydration of solution, filtration, and reprecipitation by partial evaporation of solvent.

The purified product was analyzed for infrared and NMR spectra. The spectra were found to correspond to spectra in the literature (The Aldrich Library of IR spectra, 1975; The Aldrich Library of NMR spectra, 1974). This purified Auramine O was used by preference for the evaluation of purity of commercial Auramine O.

The purified Auramine O in $CHCl_3$ has two absorbance maxima in UV-visible spectroscopy, $\lambda_1 max = 430$ nm ($\log \varepsilon = 4.65$) and $\lambda_2 max = 372$ nm ($\log \varepsilon = 4.33$). At these wavelengths equimolar concentrations of commercial Auramine O (at different concentrations) always showed an absorbance equal to 65% of the purified product. This suggests that the commercial product contains about 65% of Auramine O. Purified Auramine is stable for at least one month under anhydrous conditions.

Thin-layer chromatography of the commercial product (eluent chloroform) showed eight contaminant spots. One of these spots is predominant over the other seven. It is reported in the literature that Auramine O hydrolyzes easily to Michler's ketone and NH_4Cl (Holmes and Darling, 1924).

Michler's ketone was prepared by heating the commercial Auramine O in H_2O + 1% HCl, separating by filtration, and recrystallizing. The identity of Michler's ketone was confirmed by comparing the UV and infrared spectra of our compound with the spectra reported in the literature (The Aldrich Library of IR Spectra, 1975; CRC Handbook of Chemistry and Physics, 1979).

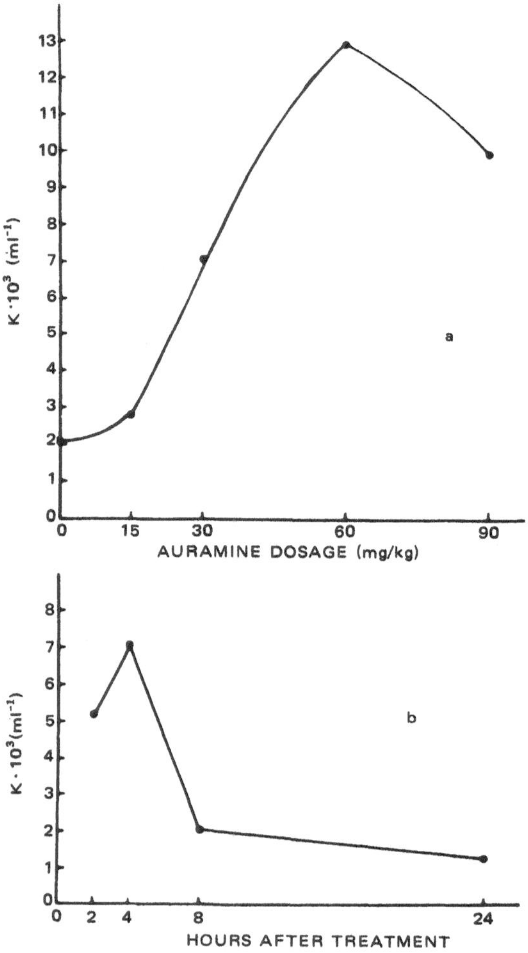

Fig. 1. a) Dependence of the elution rate constant (K) on Auramine O dosage (DNA from liver of Sprague-Dawley male rats, killed 4 h after i.p. treatment). b) Dependence of K on the time interval after treatment (Auramine O dosage 30 mg/kg i.p., same tissue, same animals). Each point represents the median value of 6-8 experiments.

The Michler's ketone was examined by thin-layer chromatography (eluent $CHCl_3$). The major spot is accompanied by a tenuous spot, suggesting the presence of a small amount of impurity in the Michler's ketone. The major spot of Michler's ketone has the same Rf as the spot of the major impurity present in commercial Auramine O.

Table 1. DNA Fragmentation Induced by Commercial Auramine O in Different Tissues and the Human Cell Line HuF_{22} after Different Treatment Schedules

Dosage and time after treatment mg/kg	hours	No. of exp.	Median $K \times 10^2$	I-III Quart. range	Statistical[a] significance
Rat kidney					
15	4	6	7.85	6.14-10.66	$p < 0.002$
30	4	6	11.84	10.07-14.59	$p < 0.002$
60	4	6	15.71	7.44-19.42	$p < 0.004$
Cumulative controls		6	3.61	2.11-3.92	-
Mice bone marrow					
30	24	6	5.50	4.20-6.49	$p = 0.002$
Controls		8	0.90	0.39-1.16	
Human cell line HuF_{22}					
0.3[b]	2	6	9.48	8.07-10.07	$p < 0.002$
Controls		5	3.55	1.75-3.61	-

Treatment was performed with Auramine O as received from Merck.
[a]Probability (two-tailed) that treated samples ≠ from their own control set, according to the nonparametric Mann-Withney test (Siegel, 1956); N.S. = $p > 0.1$.
[b]Final concentration in mmoles.

RESULTS

DNA Fragmentation

LD_{50} of Auramine O, after i.p. injection of a single dose, was equal to 135 mg/kg, 95% confidence limits: 107-171 mg/kg.

Figure 1 shows dose and time dependence of DNA damage induced in liver after a single i.p. injection. The doses given were: 15, 30, 60, and 90 mg/kg. From Fig. 1a it appears that there is a clear dose dependence of DNA damage on commercial product treatment up to 60 mg/kg. Damage is maximal at 60 mg/kg and decreases slightly at 90 mg/kg, probably because there is some saturation of the metabolic system. The relationship between amount of DNA damage and time, for a dosage of 30 mg/kg, is shown in Fig. 1b; DNA fragmentation remains high for the first 4 h, but is reduced to control levels within 8-24 h after treatment.

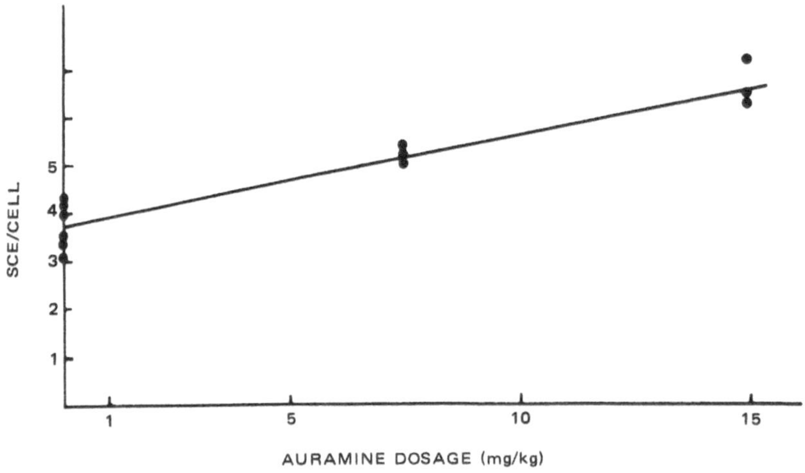

Fig. 2. Dependence of SCE number on Auramine O dosage in bone marrow cells of male Swiss mice. Animals were killed 24 h after treatment. Regression line: 3.75 + 0.19 (dosage in mg/kg): correlation coefficient $r < 0.95$ p, that $r = 0$, <0.001. Calculated according to Snedecor and Cochran (1977).

In Table 1 we report median K values, I-III quartile ranges, and statistical significance for alkaline DNA fragmentation induced by the commercial product in kidney of male rats and bone marrow of male mice, and in the human cell line HuF_{22}.

In order to investigate if the commercial product was active after treatment <u>in vitro</u> without a specific liver activating metabolic system, the human cell line HuF_{22} was also examined. At a concentration of Auramine 3×10^{-4} M, which, as a first approximation, is of the same order as the mg/kg dosage given <u>in vivo</u>, the amount of damage was statistically significant and clearly positive and practically superimposable with the amount of damage induced by the treatment <u>in vivo</u> (see Fig. 1 and Table 1).

The purified Auramine was assayed for liver DNA damage at two different dosages; 30 mg/kg and 60 mg/kg, and the animals were sacrificed 4 h after treatment. In both cases a negative result was obtained.

The major contaminant, Michler's ketone, was also assayed for liver DNA damage, at two different dosages (7.5 mg/kg and 15 mg/kg), and the animals were sacrificed 4 h after treatment. In both cases a positive result was obtained ($K = 1.30 \times 10^{-2}$ for controls, $K = 2.47 \times 10^{-2}$ for 7.5 mg/kg, $K = 4.32 \times 10^{-2}$ for 15 mg/kg).

Table 2. Induction of SCEs in Bone Marrow Cells

Compound	Dosage mg/kg	No. of exp.	SCE average No.	Statistical[a] significance
Controls		8	3.5	
Auramine O	7.5	3	5.2	$p < 0.006$
	15	3	6.6	$p < 0.006$
Purified Auramine O	15	5	3.6	N.S.
Michler's ketone	7.5	3	5.2	$p < 0.006$
	15	3	5.3	$p < 0.006$
	30	1	9.8[b]	

[a]Probability (two-tailed) that treated samples ≠ from their own control set, according to the nonparametric Mann-Withney test (Siegel, 1956); N.S. = $p > 0.1$.
[b]Mitoses could be found in a single animal over five tested.

Induction of SCEs

a) Commercial Auramine O: the results obtained in bone marrow cells after treatment of male Swiss mice are shown in Table 2. The animals were treated at two different dosage levels (7.5 and 15 mg/kg). There is a clear and statistically significant increase of the number of SCEs with respect to controls (1.7 and 3.1 SCEs over control, respectively, for the two different dosages). The increase appeared dose dependent (see Fig. 2). At higher dosages the depression of bone marrow cell replication by Auramine O was already very great, making it extremely difficult to find metaphases.

b) Purified Auramine O: Table 2 shows no increase of SCE induction after a single i.p. injection of 15 mg/kg.

c) Michler's ketone: the Michler's ketone was assayed for SCE induction in bone marrow cells at 7.5, 15, and 30 mg/kg. There was a clear increase in the number of SCEs. At the highest dosage the number of SCEs was almost three times that in controls, but it was extremely difficult to find metaphases. The results are shown in Table 2.

DISCUSSION

Data by many authors (Bonser et al., 1956; Williams and Bonser, 1962) indicate that Auramine O, of unknown purity, is carcinogenic in experimental animals. Given orally, it has produced liver tumors in mice and rats.

An epidemiological study (Case and Pearson, 1954) showed a relatively high incidence of bladder tumors in workers engaged in the manufacture of Auramine O, with a latent period ranging from 9 to 28 years.

The mutagenicity of Auramine O was determined in the standard S. typhimurium microsome test (McCann et al., 1975; Rosenkranz et al., 1976) Rosenkranz and Poirier, 1979; Simmon, 1979a) with and without the liver microsomal activating system; the data were essentially negative (up to a concentration of 1000 μg per plate of Auramine). Growth inhibition was studied in normal (pol A^+) and DNA-polymerase 1-deficient (pol A^-) E. coli strains with and without metabolic activation (Rosenkranz et al., 1976; Rosenkranz and Poirier, 1979). In this study Auramine O was also tested with the intraperitoneal host mediated assay for recombinogenic activity of S. cerevisiae D_3 and showed genetic activity in this strain (Simmon, 1979b; Simmon et al., 1979). In the sporulation system of B. subtilis 168 (McGregor and Sacks, 1976) Auramine O, tested both with and without the microsomal metabolizing system, was negative (the absolute number of mutants was not increased over controls). Auramine O, caused recessive lethal mutation in Drosophila and chromosome aberrations in Vicia faba (Landa et al., 1965). In a bioassay for morphological transformation in hamster embryo cells, Auramine O showed transforming activity (Pienta et al., 1978) after metabolic activation.

Auramine O was also positive in inducing liver preneoplastic nodules after treatment in vivo in the rat, associating the treatment with partial hepatectomy, dietary 2 acetylaminofluorene, and a single necrogenic dose of CCl_4 (Tsuda et al., 1980).

The Michler's ketone was found positive as a hepatocarcinogen in rats and mice (Carcinogenesis Testing Program: NCI bioassay; 1979). It was found negative in the Ames test both with and without metabolic activation (Scribner et al., 1980). It was capable of forming adducts with rat liver DNA (Scribner et al., 1980).

Our results show that commercial Auramine O is positive in inducing DNA fragmentation and SCE increase. A metabolic activation specific for the liver is perhaps not required because damage was found after direct incubation of HuF_{22} cells. However, Auramine O is probably not the compound responsible for DNA fragmentation and SCE induction. In fact, clearly negative results were obtained with the purified compound. One of the major contaminants was Michler's ketone. The Michler's ketone was clearly positive both for DNA fragmentation and SCE induction. We are well aware that other contaminants could be responsible, at least in part, for the observed biological effects.

It is suggested that Auramine O is perhaps not the compound responsible for the carcinogenicity of the commercial preparation. It is worthwhile to note that commercial Auramine O and the Michler's ketone are both hepatocarcinogens.

ACKNOWLEDGMENT

This research was supported by Grants from Consiglio Nazionale delle ricerche No. 80.01650.96 and 80.0168.96, Special Research Project "Control of Neoplastic Growth."

REFERENCES

The Aldrich Library of Infrared Spectra, 2nd Edition, 2:963 A (1975).
The Aldrich Library of NMR Spectra, 7:103 C (1974).
Allen, Y. W., Shuler, C. F., Mendes, L. W., and Lott, S. A., Cytogenet. Cell Genet., 18:231-237 (1977).
Bonser, G. M., Clayson, D. B., and Yull, Y. W., Brit. J. Cancer, 10: 653-667 (1956).
Carcinogenesis Testing Program, National Cancer Institute, National Cancer Institute Carcinogenesis Technical Report Series, No. 181, National Institute of Health Publication No. 79-1737 (1979).
Case, R. A. M., and Pearson, Y. T., Brit. J. Industr. Med., 11:213 (1954).
CRC Handbook of Chemistry and Physics, 60th edition, C 201 (1979).
Holmes, W. C., and Darling, J. F., J. Am. Chem. Soc., 46:2344-2346 (1924).
IARC Monographs on the Evaluation of the Carcinogenic Risk of Chemicals to Humans, 1:69-73 (1972).
Kissane, Y. M., and Robbins, E., J. Biol. Chem., 233:184-188 (1958).
Kohn, K. W., Erickson, L. C., Ewing, R. A. G., and Friedman, C. A., Biochemistry, 15:4629-4637 (1976).
Landa, Z., Klonda, P., and Pleskotowa, D., Induction of Mutation Process, Publishing House of the Czechoslovak Academy of Sciences, Prague (1965), p. 116-122.
McCann, Y., Choi, E., Yamasaki, E., and Ames, B. N., Proc. Natl. Acad. Sci. USA, 72:5135-5139 (1975).
MacGregor, Y. T., and Sacks, L. E., Mutat. Res., 38:271-286 (1976).
Parodi, S., Taningher, M., Santi, L., Cavanna, M., Sciabà, L., Maura, A., and Brambilla, G., Mutat. Res., 54:39-46 (1978).
Pienta, R. J., Poiley, J. A., and Lebherz, W. B., II, Prev. Detect. Cancer, Proc. Int. Symp. 3rd; Vol. 1, Issue No. 2, 1993-2011 (1978).
Report of an IARC Working Group, IARC monographs, Vols. 1-20, Cancer Res., 40:1-12 (1980).
Rosenkranz, H. S., Gutter, B., and Speck, W. T., Mutat. Res., 41: 61-70 (1976).
Rosenkranz, H. S., and Poirier, L. A., J. Natl. Cancer Inst., 62: 873-891 (1979).

Scribner, J. D., Koponen, G., Fisk, S. R., and Woodworth, B., Cancer Letters, 9:117-121 (1980).
Siegel, S., Nonparametric statistics for the behavioral sciences. McGraw-Hill Book Company, Inc., New York (1956), p. 116-127.
Simmon, W. F., J. Natl. Cancer Inst., 62:893-899 (1979a).
Simmon, W. F., J. Natl. Cancer Inst., 62:901-909 (1979b).
Simmon, W. F., Rosenkranz, H. S., Zeiger, E., and Poirer, L. A., J. Natl. Cancer Inst., 62:911-918 (1979).
Snedecor, G. V., and Cochran, V. G., Iowa State University Press, Ames (1977), p. 135-179,
Tsuda, H., Lee, G., and Farber, E., Cancer Res., 40:1157-1164 (1980).
Weil, G. S., Biometrics, 8:249-263 (1952).
Williams, M. H. C., and Bonser, G. M., Brit. J. Cancer, 16:87-91 (1962).

AN ATTEMPT TO DETERMINE THE ORIGIN OF DNA SINGLE-STRAND BREAKS OBSERVED AFTER TREATMENT OF MAMMALIAN CELLS WITH ALKYLATING AGENTS

A. Abbondandolo,[1] E. Dogliotti,[2]
P. H. M. Lohman,[3] and F. Berends[3]

[1]Istituto di Mutagenesi e Differenziamento CNR
Pisa, Italy

[2]Istituto Superiore di Sanità
Rome, Italy

[3]Medical Biological Laboratory TNO
Rijswijk, The Netherlands

Upon exposure of DNA to alkylating agents a number of different lesions are produced, either directly or as a consequence of secondary modifications of the original alkylation. We have investigated the formation of one of these second lesions, single-strand DNA breaks (ssb), after treatment of cultured Chinese hamster ovary cells with four different ethylating agents: N-ethyl-N'-nitro-N-nitrosoguanidine (ENNG), N-ethyl-N-nitrosourea (ENU), ethylmethanesulfonate (EMS), and diethyl sulfate (DES).

Sedimentation analysis in alkaline sucrose gradients was used for detecting ssb. By this method, the following lesions should in principle be detected: a) transient nicks in the sugar-phosphate backbone that appear during the course of excision repair events, as a result of endonucleolytic action [1]; b) alkali-labile alkylphosphotriesters [2]; c) alkali-labile apurinic/apyrimidinic sites that result from loss of alkylated bases through enzymic or chemical hydrolysis of the glycosidic bond [1, 3].

In an attempt to estimate the contribution of alkali-labile sites to the total amount of ssb measured, the kinetics of induction of ssb as a function of lysis time was determined for two of the ethylating agents under study. Cells treated with two concentrations of ENNG or DES were layered on top of sucrose gradients with lysis buffer (1 M NaOH, 10 mM EDTA; 20°C) and the number of ssb was mea-

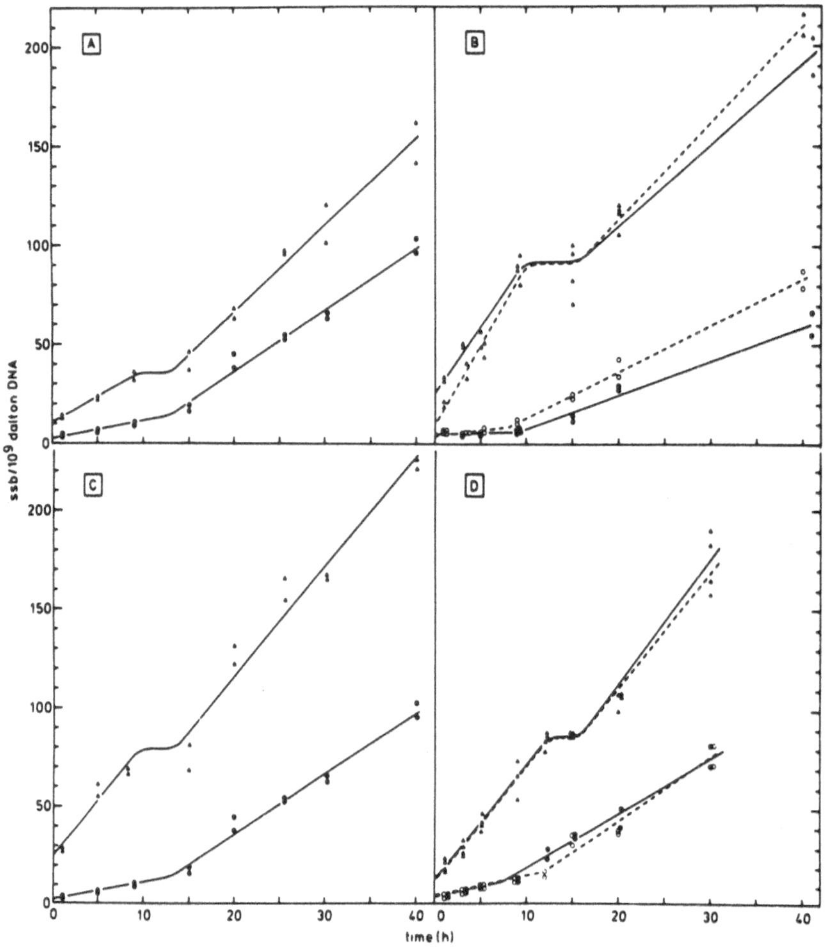

Fig. 1. The induction of single-strand breaks (ssb) in DNA of CHO cells by ENNG and DES as a function of lysis time. A) 25 μM ENNG; B) 75 μM ENNG; C) 3 mM DES; D) 2 mM DES. Black triangles; cells treated for 1 h with the agent; black circles; untreated cells; open triangles; treatment followed by a 24 h repair period; open circles; control cells after 24 h additional incubation. Dashed lines refer to open symbols. Sloping straight lines were obtained by regression analysis of the points between 0-10 h and 12-40 h of alkaline incubation, respectively.

sured after different time intervals. As shown in Fig. 1, for treated cells the number of ssb increased linearly for about 10 h; then it levelled off, but a few hours later formation of ssb started again and continued for the remaining incubation time.

Breaks at apurinic sites are known to be introduced at a high rate in alkaline conditions, such as were used in our assay, so that the process of conversion of apurinic sites into ssb should be completed before the first measurement (after 1 h lysis). Therefore, the zero intercept of curves in Fig. 1 should give the sum of ssb generated at apurinic sites by both enzymic and alkaline hydrolysis. Alkylphosphotriesters are known to be stable _in vivo_ [2, 4]. Chain breaks at phosphotriesters should then not be present at the end of treatment and should not contribute to the ssb measured at the intercept. However, they might well account for the increase in ssb observed in alkali after zero time, as will be discussed later.

By extrapolating the curves in Fig. 1 to zero time and subtracting the control values, 8.1 and 20.6 ssb/10^9 dalton of DNA were calculted for the treatment with 25 and 75 μM ENNG, respectively. For 2 and 3 mM DES the values were 10.0 and 22.1 ssb/10^9 dalton. As proposed above, these figures should be an estimate of ssb arising from apurinic sites by both intracellular action of endonucleases and alkaline hydrolysis. The relative contribution of these two causes of DNA breakage to the measured ssb will depend on the time-sequence of repair events during treatment. An important factor will be the interval between the induction of the lesion and the moment of ssb measurement. This interval may vary between 0 and 60 min, the duration of treatment. When the induction of lesions occurred at a constant rate over this period, the effect of the variation in time available for repair would be the same for all agents. If, however, the agents are degraded during the treatment period, as is to be expected, the extent to which repair processes may influence the original lesions will vary with the rate of degradation. In order to estimate the degradation of the ethylating agent during the treatments, they were incubated under the same conditions as were used in the standard assay; at intervals samples were removed and tested for their capacity to induce ssb. The degradation of the compounds was thus expressed by the exponential decrease observed in the production of ssb. From the results of this experiment, the following half-life values were derived: 180 min for EMS, 53 min for ENNG, 9.7 min for DES, and 9.5 min for ENU.

With the rapidly degraded compounds, the ssb estimated at the end of exposure originate from base alkylations which were predominantly produced early during mutagenic treatment. With the more stable compounds, on the other hand, a substantial number of alkylated bases is still being produced when the treatment is interrupted. With the latter compounds, then, a larger fraction of the induced alkylations (those produced late during treatment time) will have had no chance to be converted by enzyme action into ssb or apurinic sites before the moment of lysis. Consequently, it is to be expected that an increase in the time available for repair after the end of treatment should result in a decrease of ssb, which will be more pronounced for long-living than for short-living compounds.

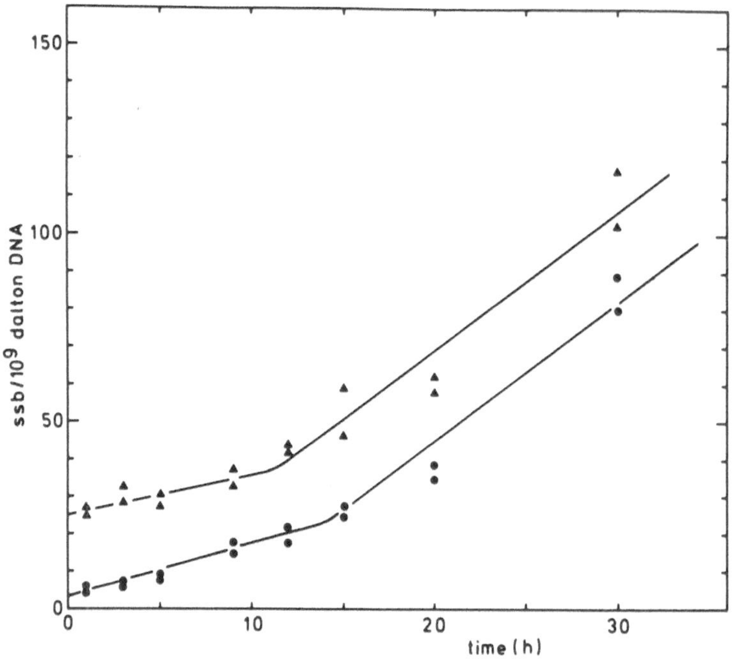

Fig. 2. The induction of single-strand breaks (ssb) in DNA of CHO cells by γ-rays as a function of lysis time. Black triangles; 7 krad ^{60}C-γ-rays, black circles, unirradiated cells. Sloping straight lines were obtained by regression analysis of the points between 0-9 h and 12-30 h of alkaline incubation, respectively.

Ssb were therefore measured after a 24 h post-treatment incubation in medium at 37°C. As shown in Fig. 1 (dashed lines), after exposure to 75 μM ENNG this incubation substantially reduced the number of ssb found at the beginning of the alkaline incubation; the extrapolated value for zero lysis time decreased from 20.6 to 5.3 ssb/10^9 dalton DNA. After 2 mM DES, however, no difference was found between ssb measured without or with the post-treatment incubation. These results are compatible with the idea that repair of the lesions induced by DES already occurred during the treatment period, which appears possible since most of the alkylation took place in the beginning of the exposition.

It follows from these considerations that about 75% of ssb measured at zero time of lysis after ENNG treatment represents transient lesions, presumably repair intermediates. No such lesions were observed after DES treatment. Therefore, it makes no sense to compare the effect of these two agents after a fixed treatment time unless conditions have been realized to maintain a constant concentration of agent. A more meaningful comparison would involve measurement of ssb after allowing optimal time for repair, with both compounds. Under these conditions, only alkaline hydrolysis of nonrepairable apurinic sites will be estimated.

The shape of the curves in Fig. 1 describing the kinetics of induction of ssb during alkaline incubation of DNA is rather puzzling. The production of ssb during alkaline incubation of alkylated DNA has been studied by Shooter [5], who obtained results basically similar to those presented here. The main difference between Shooter's and our results is the short plateau that in our curves separates the two phases of curves obtained with treated cells. To investigate whether the shape of our curves was due to the particular experimental procedures used, a similar experiment was performed with γ-rays as a DNA damaging agent. As shown in Fig. 2, there was no indication of a plateau. This indicates that the complex shape of the curves in Fig. 1 is not due to technical artefacts, and must be caused by the presence of alkylated sites in treated DNA.

Shooter [5] attributes the initial rapid increase in ssb to the hydrolysis of phosphotriesters, and the difference between treated and control DNA in the second phase to sensitization of DNA by alkylation. Accordingly, the first phase of curves in Fig. 1 should be due to the hydrolysis of phosphotriesters, and attainment of the plateau then indicates the completion of this process. When the increase in ssb is corrected for control values, the following approximate figures are obtained for breaks presumably resulting from phosphotriester hydrolysis: 17 and 66 ssb/10^9 dalton DNA after 25 and 75 μM ENNG; 43 and 45 ssb/10^9 dalton after 2 and 3 mM DES.

The following conclusions may be drawn from the results of our study:

1. Ssb determined, by alkaline sucrose gradient centrifugation, at an arbitrary moment after the start of chemical treatment is a poor measure for the total number of alkyl-adducts that are repaired via an intermediate ssb or alkali-labile site.

2. However, such measurements can be useful for a comparative study of akylating agents, provided the collected data pertain to comparable conditions of treatment, including time available for repair.

3. In this context the degradation of the agent should be taken into account. In general, exposures should be kept as short as possible. But variations in the drop of concentration during treatment can be minimized by renewing the exposition medium at intervals prescribed by the half-life of the agent.

4. Differences in possibilities for repair can also be minimized by measuring ssb after completion of repair. The obvious alternative, namely, to exclude repair, e.g., by low temperature or the presence of inhibitors, does not appear very suitable.

5. The ssb determination applied after different periods of repair and different times of exposure of DNA to alkali can give useful information about various lesions introduced by alkylating agents, but should preferably be combined with other methods which can contribute to the characterization of lesions (chromatographic or immunological identification of number and type of alkyl-adducts).

ACKNOWLEDGMENTS

This investigation was carried out at the Medical Biological Laboratory TNO, Rijswijk, The Netherlands. It was supported by EEC Contracts 192-77-1 ENV N, 266-77-1 ENV I, and 177-77-1 ENV I. The participation of one of the authors (E. Dogliotti) was made possible through a grant from the Scientific and Technical Training Program of the Commission of the European Communities.

REFERENCES

1. T. Lindahl, in: "Progress in Nucleic Acid Research and Moleculare Biology, Vol. 22," W. E. Cohn, ed., Academic Press, p. 135 (1979).
2. P. Bannon and W. Verly, Eur. J. Biochem., 31:103 (1972).
3. K. V. Shooter and R. K. Merrifield, Chem. Biol. Interactions, 13:223 (1976).
4. W. Warren, A. R. Crathorn, and K. V. Shooter, Biochim. Biophys. Acta, 563:82 (1979).
5. K. V. Shooter, Chem. Biol. Interactions, 13:151 (1976).

LOCALIZATION OF GENES INVOLVED IN DNA REPAIR ON HUMAN CHROMOSOMES BY USING CELL FUSION

M. Stefanini*, W. Keijzer, A. J. J. Reuser,
A. Geurts Van Kessel, T. Verkerk, A. Westerveld,
J. F. Jongkind, and D. Bootsma

Department of Cell Biology and Genetics
Erasmus University
Rotterdam, The Netherlands

The use of somatic cell hybrids in human gene mapping is based on the fact that human chromosomes are preferentially lost in proliferating hybrids formed between human cells and tissue culture adapted rodent cells. When it is possible to discriminate between homologous human and rodent gene products, correlation of the expression of the human phenotype in the hybrids with their human chromosome pattern allows the assignment of genes to a specific chromosome. In the case of DNA repair, the gene products are unknown and the analysis has to rely on less specific characteristics and differences between the human and rodent repair systems, like the level of repair DNA synthesis. We report differences in repair systems between normal human and Chinese hamster cells and analysis of the repair capacity of proliferating human-Chinese hamster cells.

The UV-induced repair activity was analyzed in Chinese hamster Wg3-h, E36, and CHO cells. We found that the level of repair DNA synthesis (Unscheduled DNA synthesis UDS) measured by autoradiography in these three Chinese hamster cell lines was about 50% of that observed in normal human fibroblasts (Fig. 1).

We have used this difference in our studies of DNA repair in proliferating hybrid cells: these hybrids can be used to localize

---

*M.Stefanini was supported by the EMBO fellowship ALTF/68/1979.
Present address: Istituto di Genetica Biochimica ed Evoluzionistica, C.N.R., Via S. Epifanio, 14-27100 Pavia, Italy.

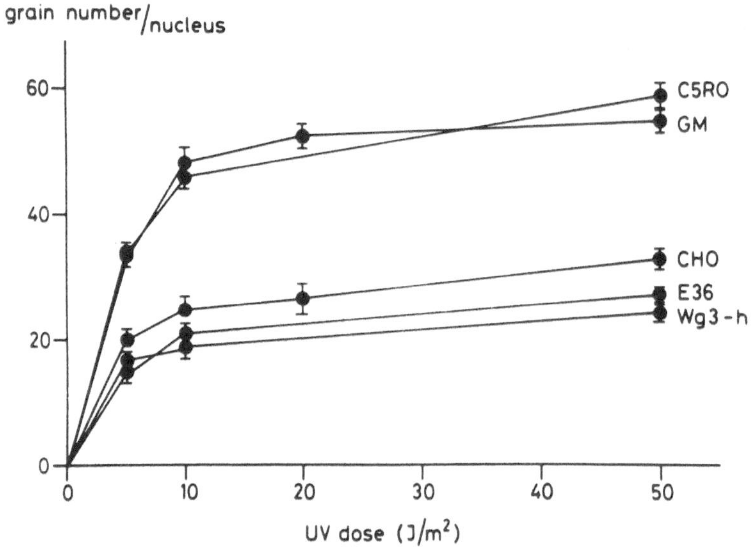

Fig. 1. Repair synthesis as a function of UV dose in two normal human fibroblast strains (C5RO, GM) and in three Chinese hamster cell lines (CHO, E36, Wg3-h). Repair synthesis is expressed as mean number of autoradiographic grains over nuclei in G_1 and G_2 phase. The arrows indicate the standard error of the mean. The cells were incubated in the presence of ^{3}H-thymidine 1 h and 2 h after UV-irradiation. Autoradiographic preparations were made as described in reference 9.

human repair genes if it is possible to differentiate between human and rodent components in the repair capacity of the hybrid cells.

The level of repair as a function of UV dose in normal human fibroblasts, Chinese hamster cells and two human-Chinese hamster hybrids is shown in Fig. 2. These hybrids have intermediate levels of repair. UDS was measured in a total of 8 proliferating hybrids between E36 and normal human cells and variable repair levels were found between those of the Chinese hamster and human cells.

Different UDS values were measured in hybrids with different human chromosome content but, taking into account the heterogeneity observed within the same hybrid population, the differences are too small to be correlated directly with the presence or the absence of a specific human chromosome. Furthermore, the repair activity in the hybrids turned out to depend also on the Chinese hamster DNA content: in fact we observed that the UDS level in Chinese hamster tetraploid cells was about twice as high as in diploid cells obtained from an asynchronous population by flow sorting.

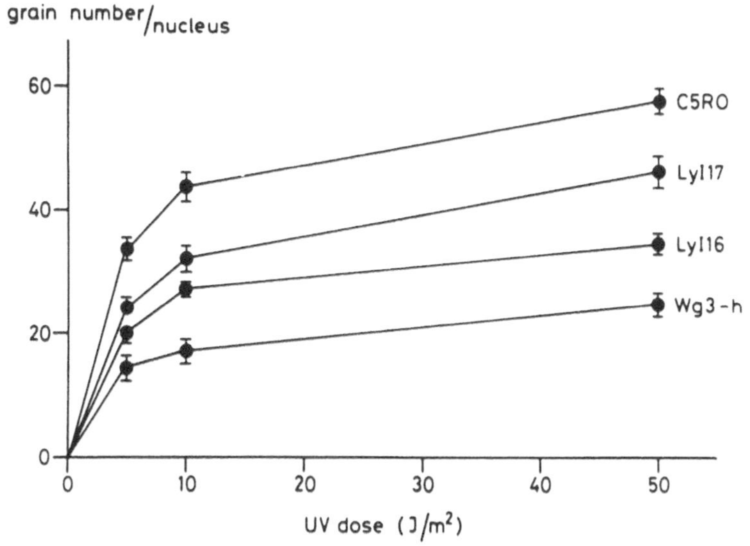

Fig. 2. Repair synthesis as a function of UV dose in normal human fibroblasts (C5RO), in Chinese hamster cells (Wg3-h) and in two hybrids between human and Wg3-h (LyI16, LyI17). For UDS analysis see legend of Fig. 1.

From these findings we concluded that on the basis of different levels of UDS, proliferating human-Chinese hamster hybrid cells cannot be used for the assignment of DNA repair genes on human chromosomes.

Isolation and Characterization of Chinese Hamster Repair Mutants

A more specific approach for the localization of DNA repair genes in the human genome makes use of rodent cells which are repair deficient as a result of mutation. The UDS analysis in hybrids between normal human and repair deficient Chinese hamster cells may allow the mapping of human gene(s) which complement the repair defect in the Chinese hamster mutants. Furthermore, complementation analysis between the rodent mutants and cells from xeroderma pigmentosum (XP) patients, the human repair mutants (for a review see [1-2]), can be carried out. In the case of absence of complementation between a Chinese hamster mutant and one XP complementation group, these mutants can probably be used for mapping the XP mutation by somatic cell fusion.

Several laboratories have reported the *in vitro* isolation of radiation or carcinogen sensitive mammalian cells (most recent references: [3-5]). We worked out a new procedure to obtain UV sensitive mutants of CHO cells. This procedure employs conventional mutagenesis followed by enrichment for UV sensitive mutants and then identification and isolation of the repair deficient clones using replica plating (Stefanini et al., in preparation). The enrichment relies upon the incorporation of bromodeoxyuridine by repair proficient cells after UV-irradiation, rendering these cells sensitive to photolysis by black light. The photolysis is potentiated by use of the bisbendimidazole dye Hoechst 33258. The surviving colonies in each culture dish were replicated using a filter paper. The colonies in the master plate were screened for their ability to perform unscheduled DNA synthesis after UV irradiation. Once identified on the master, the corresponding repair deficient clones were isolated from the replica. CHO mutants were isolated which have a strongly reduced UDS activity in combination with increased UV sensitivity.

To characterize these mutants, the possibility of a genetic defect similar to that present in XP was investigated. Hybridization experiments were performed using XP cells belonging to different complementation groups and the level of UDS in heterokaryons after fusion was measured. The results obtained so far suggest complementation between the CHO mutants and XP complementation groups A and C.

Complementation and Mapping of Genes Involved in Deficient DNA Repair in XP Cells

In 1974 Giannelli and Pawsey [6] presented evidence for the existence of rapid and slow complementing varieties in XP after fusion of XP fibroblasts with normal human fibroblasts. This difference in complementation pattern was also observed in crosses between different XP strains [7]; the kinetics with which the defect is complemented by fusion turned out to be a specific feature of the complementation group to which the XP strain is assigned [8].

Later experiments performed by Matsukuma et al. [9] indicated that complementation of the A group defect in XP occurred extremely fast: normal UDS levels were observed in the XP nuclei within 2 h after fusion of UV irradiated XP cells with unirradiated normal human cells.

We investigated the kinetics of complementation after fusion of UV exposed XP complementation group A (XPA) cells with Chinese hamster Wg3-h cells. The heterokaryons were identified by labelling the parental cells with latex beads of two different sizes. The UDS analysis performed on the heterokaryons (identified as binuclear cells containing beads of both size) showed absence of a complementing effect of the hamster genome within the first five hours after fusion. However, this analysis was complicated by a very low frequency of heterokaryon formation and by the presence of nuclei in

S-phase in many of these binuclear cells. In order to simplify this type of analysis we investigated the possibility of using so-called cybrids (cells fused with cytoplasts of other cells) instead of heterokaryons. Experiments carried out by W. Keijzer et al. (manuscript in preparation) had already shown that the fast complementation pattern, being characteristic for XPA cells, could also be obtained after fusion of irradiated XPA cells with cytoplasts derived from normal human cells. In these experiments the cytoplasts were isolated by labeling the cells with fluorescent beads, followed by treatment with cytochalasin B, nuclear staining with Hoechst and sorting in a FACS II cell sorter. About 100% pure cytoplast preparations were obtained that were used for fusion with UV irradiated XP cells.

Similar experiments were performed by isolating cytoplasts of Chinese hamster cells. These were fused with UV exposed XPA cells and UDS was studied starting immediately after fusion up to 8 h. The results confirmed unequivocally our heterokaryon data: the Chinese hamster cytoplast was unable to complement the XPA defect. The fast complementation pattern shown after fusion with cytoplasts of normal human cells was not observed with the Chinese hamster cytoplasts.

Since this difference in complementation kinetics between normal human and Chinese hamster cells in fusion with XPA cells seems to be specific for the A group mutation and can be demonstrated clearly, it was used as a parameter in cybrids after fusion of XP cells with cytoplasts of Chinese-hamster human hybrid cells.

The Chinese hamster genome in the hybrid cells acts as incubator for selected groups of human chromosomes to be tested for complementation with the XP mutation. The advantage of this "backcross" system is that complementation, when it occurs, is the result of interaction between human gene products and therefore specific for the repair mutation in the XP parental cell.

The presence or absence of fast complementation in the cybrids is correlated with the presence or absence of a particular human chromosome in the hybrids.

Cytoplasts from hybrid cells containing different sets of human chromosomes were fused with UV-irradiated XPA cells and the analysis of the kinetics of repair was performed in cybrids. Preliminary results indicate that this approach can be used for mapping on a human chromosome the gene involved in the fast complementation kinetics of the XPA defect.

REFERENCES

1. Bootsma, D., in: "DNA REpair Mechanisms, P. C. Hanawalt, E. C. Friedberg, and C. F. Fox, eds., p. 589-601 (1978).
2. Kraemer, K. H., in: "Clinical Dermatology," D. J. Demis, R. L. Dobson, and J. Mc Guire, eds., New York, 4:1-33 (1980).
3. Bush, D. B., Cleaver, J. E., and Glaser, D. A., Somat. Cell Genet., 6:407-418 (1980).
4. Thompson, L. H., Rubin, J. S., Cleaver, J. E., Whitmore, G. F., and Brookman, W., Somat. Cell Genet., 6:391-405 (1980).
5. Chang, C. C., Boesi, J. A., Warren, S. T., Sabourin, C. L. K., Liu, P. K., Glatzer, L., and Trosko, J. E., Somat. Cell Genet., 7:235-253 (1981).
6. Giannelli, F., and Pawsey, S. A., J. Cell Sci., 15:163-176 (1974).
7. Giannelli, F., and Pawsey, S. A., J. Cell Sci., 20:207-213 (1976).
8. Pawsey, S. A., Magnus, I. A., Ramsay, C. A., Benson, P. F., and Giannelli, F., Quart. J. Med., 48:179-210 (1979).
9. Matsukuma, S., Zelle B., Keijzer, W., Berends, F., and Bootsma, D., Exp. Cell Res., 134:103-112 (1981).

IN VITRO STUDIES ON CHEMICAL CARCINOGENESIS IN BALB/c 3T3 CELLS

Enrico Cortesi

Laboratory of Experimental Pathology
Division of Cancer Cause and Prevention
National Cancer Institute
Frederick, Maryland 21701

INTRODUCTION

During the last decade many in vitro systems have been developed as short-term tests for chemical, viral and physical carcinogenesis. A complete battery of such tests should include bacterial and mammalian mutagenesis, chromosome tests, DNA repair and cell transformation. These tests have been developed on the assumption that the oncogenic event is based on a genotoxic mechanism, the endpoint of which is detectable in a qualitative or quantitative way in each system.

Most of the transformation systems applied to carcinogen screening use fibroblast cultures (primary or secondary) and measure a morphological alteration of the cells, which in most tests (SHE, 10T-1/2, BALB/c 3T3, BHK 21) is well correlated with their malignancy.

In our laboratory we are studying, in various biological target systems, the combined effects of concurrent exposure to low doses of different carcinogens, which could result in a synergistic, inhibitory or additive response. The Salmonella/Ames test (1) and the BALB/c 3T3 morphological transformation assay were selected as the initial models for these studies (2).

The BALB/c 3T3 is a mouse embryo fibroblast cell line originated after a rigid passage schedule, with characteristics that make it a useful system to study neoplastic transformation in vitro (3). This cell line exhibits a high sensitivity to density dependent inhibition of cell division, but when untreated in relatively early passages it shows no anchorage independent growth, nor tumorigenicity when injected into a suitable host.

The BALB/c 3T3 cells, when treated with a carcinogenic agent, need at least one cell division to fix the initial genotoxic damage as a heritable property; the phenotypic expression of this damage takes about four additional weeks and includes a proliferative phase followed by a resting phase during which transformed foci develop. Morphologically transformed cells, piled-up in a criss-cross fashion, form foci overlying the monolayer of contact-inhibited normal cells. These foci can be easily scored in a qualitative and quantitative manner (7). The transformed cells grow in soft agar and, when injected in a syngeneic host, are tumorigenic in 90% of cases (4-7). Several sub-clones of the BALB/c 3T3 cell line are currently used in different laboratories (7-10).

EXPERIMENTS STUDIES

Clone A 31-1-1, selected by Dr. T. Kakunaga (8) was chosen because preliminary studies on this clone showed a low spontaneous transformation frequency and a high transformation rate after exposure to a range of chemical carcinogens. We evaluated different batches of cells from this clone and different batches of fetal and newborn calf serum for cytotoxicity and transformation.

For the purposes of our study we required an in vitro transformation system with such characteristics as the possibility of quantifying the activity of the test compound in a dose-response manner, good sensitivity to treatment at low doses, consistency of the reproducibility of results and a wide range of sensitivity to different chemical classes.

For these reasons preliminary dose-response studies were conducted with carcinogens requiring different metabolic pathways: the polynuclear aryl hydrocarbons, 3-methylcholanthrene and benzo(a)pyrene (MCA and B[a]P), which require preferentially the P_1-450 form of the cytochrome system and epoxide hydrase; an aromatic amine, benzidine (BZ), which recent studies (11) suggest to be metabolized through a radical pathway involving prostaglandine hydroperoxidase independently of mixed function oxidase activities; a natural product, aflatoxin B_1 (AFB_1), which require the P-450 form of the cytochrome system; and a direct acting alkylating agent N-methyl-N'-nitro-N-nitrosoguanidine (MNNG).

Some dose-response studies (BZ, MNNG, AFB) were repeated at different time intervals in order to establish the effectiveness and reproducibility of this cell transformation system and to determine the optimal conditions for its use in our laboratory.

Experimental protocols generally followed the procedures established by Kakunaga (7) and were previously described (12). Stock and experimental cultures were maintained in MEM supplemented with 10% fetal calf serum, and used at passages 7 to 13. Carcinogens were dissolved in dimethylsulfoxide (DMSO) at a final concentration of 0.2% DMSO in the culture medium. Cytotoxicity and transformation assays were performed concomitantly; relative cloning efficiency (C.E.) was determined after 8 days and transformation frequency (T.F.) per cell at risk after 4-5 weeks (12).

We obtained clear positive dose-response related transforming activity for all five substances, and additional experiments performed with MNNG and BZ showed quantitative reproducibility within a narrow range. A comparison of the dose-related effects on a molar basis showed a range of responses within three orders of magnitude: B[a]P resulted in the highest level of effect, BZ in the lowest, while AFB_1, MCA, and MNNG fell into an intermediate range.

DISCUSSION

The most important requirement for a cell transformation system is the stability and uniformity of the cell population and the reproducibility of results. We found that such reproducibility is quantitatively consistent within the same laboratory and protocol conditions, and qualitatively also among different laboratories.

AFB_1 and BZ gave a clear dose-dependent transformation effect (12), previously unreported in the BALB/c 3T3 system. In a recent test, in cells of the related A31-1 clone, AFB_1 did not induce type III transformation foci up to 1 mM concentration after a 24 h treatment, unless a microsomal (S9) preparation was added for metabolic activation (Schechtman et al., personal communication). These investigators however confirmed our quantitative results by the treatment of A31-1-1 cells with AFB_1 up to 72 h.

The results we obtained with B[a]P and MCA confirm qualitatively those reported by Kakunaga for clone A31-714 (7) and by Sivak for clone A31-1-13(9); MNNG induced a well reproducible dose-response relationship. Similar quantitative results were obtained with the same carcinogens by Schechtman et al. (personal communication) in clone A31-1 and more recently in the same clone A31-1-1.

The BALB/c 3T3 clone A31-1-1 cell line, as used in our laboratory, provided the metabolic activation pathways required to induce transformation, since no separate metabolic activation system was added in these experiments. Our results suggest that the present clone could be used, in comparison with the other BALB/c 3T3 clones, for studies on the combined effects of different classes of carcinogens and their requirements for metabolic activation (12).

Some problems are not yet resolved concerning the quantitative assessment of transformation. The transformation frequency, detertermined as a function of the number of viable cells after treatment, is calculated on the basis of the viability index which could vary depending on the chemical carcinogen and the method used for determining cell survival (cloning efficiency, trypsinization and cell count). The transformation frequency could also be dependent on the initial target cell density, so that some protocols indicate that the number of target cells should be adjusted on the basis of the expected cytotoxicity.

The transformation frequency for both treated and control groups could vary with the use of different batches of serum, with cell passage, and with different laboratory practices.

Our experiments, showing a clear dose related response of this system to different classes of carcinogens. indicates that the BALB/c 3T3 clone A31-1-1 cell transformation system is reliable for testing a wide range of chemicals, provided that experimental variables are closely controlled. The major problem of <u>in vitro</u> transformation systems is often the fact that specific quantitative results are not reproducible among different laboratories. Therefore, caution should be used in the interpretation of activity comparisons based on tests done by different laboratories or in somewhat different conditions of use.

REFERENCES

1. B. N. Ames, J. McCann, and E. Yamasaki, Methods for detecting carcinogens and mutagens with the Salmonella/mammalian-microsome mutagenicity test, Mut. Res., 31:347 (1975).
2. U. Saffiotti, P. J. Donovan, J. M. Rice, and E. Cortesi, Mutual synergism in Salmonella mutagenesis by aflatoxin B_1, benzidine, benzo[a]pyrene and safrole, Teratogenesis, Carcinogenesis, and Mutagenesis (in press).
3. S. A. Aaronson and G. J. Todaro, Development of 3T3-like lines from BALB/c mouse embryo cultures: transformation susceptibility to SV 40, Science, 162:1024 (1968).
4. J. A. Di Paolo, K. Takano, and N. C. Popescu, Quantitation of chemically induced neoplastic transformation of BALB/3T3 cloned cell lines, Cancer Res., 32:2686 (1970).
5. T. Kakunaga and J. Kamohora, Process of neoplastic transformation of cultured mammalian cell by chemical carcinogens, J. Cancer Assoc. Proc. Symp. 29th, p. 42 (1970).
6. T. Kakunaga and K. Miyashita, The involvement of DNA lesions and repair system in the cell transformation by chemical carcinogens, Symp. Cell Biol., Vol. 23:95 (1972).
7. T. Kakunaga, A quantitative system for assay of maligant transformation by chemical carcinogens using a clone derived from BALB/3T3, Int. J. Cancer, 12:463 (1973).
8. T. Kakunaga and J. D. Crow, Cell variants showing differential susceptibility to ultraviolet light-induced transformation, Science, 209:505 (1980).

9. A. Sivak et al., BALB/c-3T3 cells as target cells for chemically induced neoplastic transformation, Adv. Environ. Toxicol. (in press).
10. L. M. Schechtman and R. E. Kouri, Control of benzo(a)pyrene induced mammalian cell cytotoxicity, mutagenesis, and transformation by exogenous enzyme fractions, Progress in Genetic Toxicology:307 (1977).
11. T. V. Zenser, M. B. Mattammal, H. J. Armbrecht, and B. B. David, Benzidine binding to nucleic acids mediated by the peroxidative activity of prostaglandin endoperoxidase synthetase, Cancer Res., 40:2839 (1980).
12. E. Cortesi, U. Saffiotti, P. J. Donovan, J. M. Rice, and T. Kakunaga, Dose-response studies on neoplastic transformation of BALB/c 3T3 clone A31-1-1 cells by aflatoxin B_1, benzidine, benzo(a)pyrene, 3-methylcholantrene and N-methyl-N'-nitro-N-nitrosoguanidine, Teratogenesis, Carcinogenesis, and Mutagenesis (in press).

THE CHEMICAL HAZARD OF ANTI-IMPLANTATION ASSESSED AND ANALYZED BOTH *IN VITRO* AND *IN VIVO*

D. Michael Pugh and Hector S. Sumano

Department of Medicine and Pharmacology
Faculty of Veterinary Medicine
University College Dublin
Ballsbridge, Dublin 4

INTRODUCTION

I was tempted to offer this paper for several reasons. The term hazard describes the nature of something undesirable which may happen to an individual or population while the term risk describes the probability that the hazard will happen. Plainly identification of the hazard has to precede the assessment of risk. My paper describes a novel *in vitro* technique for the demonstration of and quantitation of the hazard of oestrogenicity using the maturation and implantation of the developing mouse embyro.

We have so far been much concerned with the hazard of neoplasia and with identifying the characteristics of neoplastic transformation. Perhaps it is superfluous for me to remind you all of the very many parallels between a foetus implanting in and growing in utero and a tumor. Both are immunologically privileged and both grow at the expense of these hosts. To take a more specific parallel, some embryologists use the term transformation to describe the spectrum of changes which the embryo undergoes while it is preparing to implant in the uterine wall. Many of the changes described in Dr. Borek's paper as characteristic of transformed cells are also characteristic of activated pre-implantation embryos.

I would like to present some results in which good agreement is shown between *in vitro* and *in vivo* experiments aimed at identifying the causative basis of one particular hazard to pregnancy in the mouse. Such agreement validates *in vitro* experimentation and should always be established so as to substantiate conclusions drawn from studies on isolated cells.

We are interested in the process of implantation of the developing embryo and especially in the control of those changes at the trophoblastic surface of the blastocyst which adapt it for the apposition and adhesion phases of implantation. In the mouse mated at 0 h, it is known that the embryo enters the uterus as an immature blastocyst 75-80 h later. After a 20 h free-living phase the now fully-expanded, activated blastocyst adheres to the endometrium and implantation begins. The late pre-implantation blastocyst sticks to glassware and its surface coat is able to bind colloidal iron. This change in trophoblastic cell surface coat properties, referred to as the surface coat change (SCC), is a prerequisite to implantation.

Oestradiol is a drug relevant to this topic because it triggers activation and implantation of the preimplantation blastocyst [1]. Again Dr. Borek referred to ability of oestrogens to increase transformations.

The second drug to interest us is tamoxifen because it prevents implantation in mice [2]. It was especially exciting when in confirming its anti-implantation effect in mice, we showed that the blastocysts from tamoxifen treated mice were not activated and had not undergone the SCC [3]. Tamoxifen is I know of interest to at least 2 groups of participants at this meeting in relation to its use in the treatment of breast cancer in man.

It was at this point that we were struck by a paradox. Oestrogens caused blastocyst activation while we had shown that tamoxifen, claimed also as an oestrogen in the mouse [2], prevented blastocyst activation. We were of course, tempted to explore this problem.

EXPERIMENTAL FINDINGS

To eliminate the interpretational problems created by the need to administer drugs to embryos via the mother we simply flushed 80 h blastocysts and grew them in culture in a fully chemically defined medium both with and without a collagen layer. As already reported elsewhere we showed that only when oestradiol was added, did the surface coat change take place [4]. Furthermore, this action of oestradiol was blocked in a concentration dependent manner by tamoxifen [5]. It was possible to claim then, that to mouse eggs *in vitro*, tamoxifen acted as an antioestrogen, i.e., it blocked the ability of oestradiol to initiate blastocyst activation and implantation.

We decided to reappraise the claimed ability of Tamoxifen (1 mg/kg oral, 50 h post coitum) to accelerate tubal transport in mice [2]. This we achieved by killing mice both untreated and tamoxifen treated, at 2 hourly intervals between 66 and 76 h post coitum and flushing separately their uteri and oviducts. The numbers, locations and morphological normality of the embryos were assessed and

Table 1. The Effect of a Single Oral Dose of Tamoxifen (1 mg/kg at 50 h p.c.) on the Numbers and Locations of Embryos in the Reproductive Tracts of Mice Killed between 16 and 26 h Later

Mouse	Dose of tamoxifen	Flushed at hours post coitum	No. of eggs in uterus	No. of eggs in oviduct	No. of eggs morpho. normal
1	0.00	66	0	10	10
2	0.00	68	0	12	10
3	0.00	70	1	11	11
4	0.00	72	3	8	9
5	0.00	74	6	5	8
6	0.00	76	8	2	9
1	1.00	66	4	3	3
2	1.00	68	4	2	2
3	1.00	70	6	2	3
4	1.00	72	5	1	3
5	1.00	74	5	0	1
6	1.00	76	7	1	2

are recorded in Table 1. The data show that tamoxifen caused embryos to be present in the uterus earlier than was the case in the control group and therefore substantiated the claim that tamoxifen could cause accelerated tubal transport in the mouse.

Because the drug also had caused a reduction in the number of embryos recoverable from treated mice we decided to run a second experiment in which the effect of the dosage of tamoxifen on the number of eggs recovered was to be assessed. In addition the eggs, collected this time at 100 h post coitum were to be examined for the presence or absence of the SCC. The data from this experiment are presented in Table 2. It is apparent that higher doses of tamoxifen cause a marked loss of embryos as well as suppressing absolutely the SCC in the survivors. As the dose is reduced, embryo numbers collected rise to more or less normal levels and an increasing proportion have undergone the SCCH. This experiment shows that the ability of tamoxifen to suppress blastocyst activation persists at a dose level which no longer causes reduction in embryo collections, i.e., at a dose level which is without major effect on the rate of tubal transport.

It was at this point valid to undertake the decisive experiment in which threshold doses of both tamoxifen and oestradiol would be

Table 2. The Effect of a Range of Single Oral Doses of Tamoxifen at 50 h p.c. on the Recovery and Trophoblastic Surface Coat Changes of Morphologically Normal Mouse Embryos

No. of animals	Tamoxifen mg/kg 50 h p.c. per os.	No. of blastocysts recovered	No. of blastocysts with TSCC	% of prevention of blasts, TSCC
4	3	1	0	100
4	2	3	0	100
4	1	11	0	100
4	0.9	12	0	100
5	0.8	21	0	100
4	0.7	19	0	100
4	0.6	21	0	100
4	0.5	20	0	100
5	0.4	36	0	100
5	0.3	34	2	94.11
5	0.2	39	3	92.30
4	0.1	39	6	84.61
5	0.05	34	8	76.47
5	0.04	31	22	29.04
4	0.03	40	38	5.00
5	0.025	40	39	2.5
4	0.01	38	38	0
5	0	48	48	0

given to the same animal and the character of their interaction on the embryo assessed [6].

Tamoxifen was given by mouth at 50 h p.c. at 0.4 mg/kg, the dose rate shown in the previous experiment to be just sufficient to abolish blastocyst activation, and, in a parallel experiment, to abolish implantation. The data from this latter experiment is summarized in Table 3.

Oestradiol was administered subcutaneously at 84 h p.c. at a dose rate previously shown to be sufficient to induce an implantation score of about 25% in post-coitally ovariectomized, progesterone maintained mice [7].

One group of mice received tamoxifen alone and a second group received tamoxifen and oestradiol. All mice were killed and inspected for implantation sites on day 6 of pregnancy. Table 4 displays the implantation scores recorded. Tamoxifen alone had caused

Table 3. The Relationship between the Dose of Tamoxifen (single, oral dose at 50 h p.c.) and the Inhibition of Implantation of the Embryo in Mice 7 Days Pregnant. @ Control, 0.1 ml of Solvent Vehicle Only (0.5% Tween 80 per os.)

No. of animals	Dose of tamoxifen mg/kg	Implantations $\bar{x}$ ± S.D.	Inhibition
3 @	0.0	10 ± 0.65	0
3	0.7	0	100
3	0.6	0	100
3	0.5	0	100
3	0.4	0	100
3	0.3	0.33 ± .57	96.67
3	0.2	1.00 ± 1.00	90.00
3	0.1	2.00 ± 1	80.00
3	0.050	3.00 ± 1	70.00
3	0.040	3.66 ± 1.15	63.34
3	0.030	5.66 ± 0.57	43.34
3	0.025	9.00 ± 1	10.00
3	0.010	9.66 ± 0.57	3.34

Table 4. The Reversal of the Anti-Implantation Effect of Tamoxifen in Mice by Oestradiol

Tamoxifen 50 h p.c. µg/kg	Oestradiol 84 h p.c. µg/kg	Implantations per mouse	$\bar{x}$ Implantations per mouse
400	0	0	
400	0	0	
400	0	0	0
400	0	0	
400	0	0	
400	0.333	7	
400	0.333	8	
400	0.333	7	7.6 ± 0.54
400	0.333	8	
400	0.333	8	

its customary total prevention of implantation. In those mice which received tamoxifen followed by oestradiol, the mean implantation score of 7.6 is compatible with the number of normal blastocysts which the chosen dose of tamoxifen would have allowed to enter the uterus.

These experiments have shown that although tamoxifen can bring about an antifertility effect by causing an oestrogen-like acceleration of tubal transport of embryos, it can also cause a suppression of blastocyst activation which both in vitro and in vivo can be overcome by oestradiol.

It is therefore possible to claim that tamoxifen can bring about both oestrogenic and antioestrogenic responses in the reproductive tract of the mouse, both of which can be expressed as a failure of implantation. This mixed effect is compatible with the behavior of a drug which is a persistent, weak agonist.

Why, in conclusion, have I presented these results of a study at first sight unrelated to the meeting's main theme of carcinogenicity risk assessment. One reason is that the findings have exemplified the value of an in vitro study not only in mimicking conveniently the in vivo situation but also in analyzing and adding to the conclusions of earlier in vivo studies on the mode of action of tamoxifen. Secondly, the mouse embryo in vitro system is at present under evaluation at ISPRA for its utility as a system in which to look for evidence of general toxicity of chemical substances. Thirdly, it seems to me that the late-preimplantation surface coat change of the embryo in vitro should be evaluated as a model in which to screen for carcinogenicity. We have already shown that certain cytostatic agents will prevent the SCC and implantation in vitro [7] and it is now our intention to look at the effects of known carcinogens in the system.

REFERENCES

1. P. V. Holmes and A. D. Dickson, Estrogen-induced surface and enzyme changes in the implantating mouse blastocyst, J. Embryol. Exp. Morphol., 29:639-645 (1973).
2. M. J. K. Harper and A. L. Walpole, A new derivative of triphenylethylene: effect on implantation and mode of action in rats, J. Reprod. Fertil., 13:101-119 (1967).
3. P. W. Bloxham, D. M. Pugh, and S. C. Sharma, An effect of tamoxifen (I.C.I. 46, 474) on the surface of the late preimplantation mouse blastocyst, J. Reprod. Fertil., 45:181-183 (1975).
4. P. W. Bloxham and D. M. Pugh, Tamoxifen inhibition of an in vitro oestradiol-induced surface coat change on mouse blastocysts, Br. J. Pharmacol., 60:517-520 (1977).

5. D. M. Pugh and H. S. Sumano, The effects of oestradiol-17B and tamoxifen on the development of mouse embryos cultured over collagen, Br. J. Pharmacol., 67:458P (1979).
6. D. M. Pugh and H. S. Sumano, The anti-implantation action of tamoxifen in mice, Paper presented to the European Society for Toxicology, Dublin, August 1981.
7. H. S. Sumano, The late pre-implantation surface coat change of the mouse embryo, Ph.D. Thesis, Trinity College, Dublin (1979).

CELLULAR SPECIFICITY IN DNA DAMAGE, REPAIR, AND REPLICATION DURING CHRONIC CARCINOGEN EXPOSURE

James G. Lewis,[1] Mary A. Bedell, Kathyrn C. Billings, and James A. Swenberg

Departments of Pathology, Duke University Medical Center,[1] Durham, NC 27710 and the Chemical Industry Institute of Toxicology, RTP, NC 27709

In order to make rational use of human cells and tissues in the evaluation of risk from chemical or physical agents, it is crucial that a better understanding of the molecular events leading to malignant transformation be reached. It is of little use simply to replace studies on animal cells with human cells unless it is known which molecular processes and changes are relevant and should be quantified. In this paper, we present data in support of the hypothesis that the replication of DNA which contains promutagenic DNA damage is necessary for the initiation of carcinogenesis. If this hypothesis is true, and the relevant types of DNA damage can be identified and monitored in human cells, the possibility of quantitatively assessing risk using human cells will be greatly enhanced.

The concept that the replication of damaged DNA is an important event in tumor development is widely held although the role of specific forms of DNA damage in tumor induction remains uncertain. Several potent carcinogens such as the nitrosamines, nitrosamides, and hydrazine derivatives are thought to effect neoplastic change through the alkylation of DNA (1). A significant amount of evidence has been gathered that suggests that methylation or ethylation of the oxygen atom at the 6 position of guanine is involved in both mutagenesis and carcinogenesis (1,2,3). Alkylation of the nitrogen atom at the 7 position of guanine is the most abundant adduct formed by most alkylating agents but alkylation at this position has little correlation with carcinogenesis. Agents such as methyl methanesulfonate (MMS) which induce high levels of 7-methylguanine (7MG) but low levels of 06 methylguanine (06MG), are weak carcinogens, whereas agents such as methylnitrosourea (MNU) which form much higher amounts of 06MG in relation to 7MG are potent carcinogens (1).

In vitro DNA replication studies have shown that 06MG will readily mispair with thymidine, thereby inducing mutations in the daughter strand (4,5). It has also been demonstrated that 06 alkylguanine is actively repaired by both bacterial and eukaryotic cells and that this capacity varies in different tissues (6,7,8). In addition, this repair capacity can be induced by exposure to alkylating agents (9). The exact nature of the mechanism of this repair is uncertain but recent studies have suggested that the methyl group is selectively removed leaving the unmodified guanine in the DNA (7,8,10).

Several in vivo studies have demonstrated correlations between the ability of various alkylating carcinogens to cause 06 alkylation and accumulation in the DNA of a particular organ with the induction of tumors in that organ (11,12). Other investigators have not found accumulation of 06AG in the DNA of the target organ (13). Studies on cell replication utilizing [^{3}H] - thymidine incorporation have shown cell specific effects of alkylating carcinogens but no in vivo studies have quantified both promutagenic damage and cell replication in the actual target cells within the target organ. This is particularly important in studying liver carcinogensis. While hepatocytes make up over 90% of the liver mass, they only account for 60-70% of the cell numbers (14). The remaining 30-40% of the cells are the nonparenchymal cells (NPC) which are composed mostly of sinusoidal endothelial cells and Kupffer cells (14). It is impossible to discern cell specific promutagenic DNA damage in determinations made on whole organ DNA preparations.

In order to study this problem, we have taken advantage of the cellular specificity of 1,2-dimethylhydrazine (SDMH). Unlike some hepatocarcinogens such as diethylnitrosamine (DEN), which induce hepatocellular carcinomas when given to rats at low doses in the drinking water, SDMH induces malignant hemangioendotheliomas, tumors arising from liver sinusoidal cells (15,16). Both DEN and SDMH alkylate hepatic DNA at the 06 position, and the 06AG induced is rapidly repaired (6,17). However, little information is available on the cellular location of the 06AG or the rate of de novo DNA synthesis of the cells containing 06AG. We have previously shown that after 2 doses of ^{14}C-SDMH, 06MG accumulates in the target cell population and not in hepatocytes (18). By chronically exposing rats to SDMH (30 ppm in the drinking water) and separating the liver cells into hepatocytes and nonparenchymal cells (NPC), we now demonstrate that SDMH induces a specific, striking increase in de novo DNA synthesis in the NPC and that 06MG accumulates in the target cell population (NPC), but is rapidly removed by hepatocytes.

MATERIALS AND METHODS

Animals. All animals were male CDF® (F-344)/CrlBR rats that weighed between 150-250 g at the beginning of the experiments.

Materials. Bromodeoxyuridine (BrdU), SDMH-dihydrochloride, and

Type 1 collagenase were obtained from Sigma Chemical Co., St. Louis, MO and [^{3}H]-Thymidine (specific activity 21 Ci/mM) was obtained from New England Nuclear, Boston, MA.

<u>Carcinogen Exposures</u>. Rats were weighed and housed 3 per cage and water consumption measured for 7 days. Then SDMH - 2 HCl was added to deionized drinking water. The dose of SDMH (free base) was approximately 3 mg/kg/day based on average weight and water consumption for cell replication studies, and 2.5 mg/kg/day for alkylation studies.

<u>Cell Separation</u>. Liver cells were separated into hepatocytes and NPC by elutrition centrifugation as previously described (18). Briefly, the livers were perfused *in situ* with collagenase and the resultant mixed liver cell suspension (MLCS) washed 3 times in Hanks balanced salt solution without Ca^{++} and Mg^{++}. The MLCS was then introduced into the Beckman J-6 elutriator rotor at 4°C with a flow rate of 18 ml/min and a rotor speed of 1500 rpm. At these settings, the NPC wash through and the hepatocytes are retained in the separation chamber. After 200 ml of effluent containing the NPC was collected, the hepatocytes were flushed from the rotor at a flow rate of 100 ml/min. Cells were frozen for later analysis.

EXPERIMENTAL DESIGN

<u>DNA alkylation and repair studies</u>. Groups of 3 animals each were exposed to SDMH for 1,2,3,4,6,8,12,16 and 28 days. The livers were perfused, the cells separated, the DNA purified by hydroxyapatite chromatography (19) and hydrolyzed in 0.1 N HCl at 80°C for 30 minutes. The normal and methylated purines were separated by HPLC and quantified by U.V. absorbance (adenine, guanine, and 7MG) and fluorescence (O6MG) (20). Briefly, adenine, guanine, and 7MG were quantified by chromatographing a small portion of the hydrolysates using 2 Partisil 10-SCX columns in series. The purines were eluted isocratically with 75 mM $NH_4H_2PO_4$ (pH 2.0) and were quantified using U.V. absorbance at a sensitivity of 0.01 A.U.F.S. The remainder of the hydrolysates were chromatographed using a single Parisil 10-SCX column with 50 mM $NH_4H_2PO_4$ + 12% MeOH (pH 2.0) as the eluent in order to quantify O6MG. O6MG peaks were detected with a Perkin-Elmer 650-10 fluorescence spectrophotometer using an excitation wavelength of 295 nM and an emission wavelength of 370 nM. All U.V. and fluorescence peaks were integrated using a chromatograph control module (CCM, Laboratory Data Control). The limits of detection were 70 pmoles of 7MG and 0.5 pmoles of O6MG.

<u>Cell replication experiments</u>. Groups of 3 animals were exposed to SDMH for 1.5,4,8,16, and 28 days. De novo DNA synthesis was separated from unscheduled DNA synthesis as previously described (21). Briefly, on the morning of sacrifice a 300 mg pellet of BrdU was inserted subcutaneously. After 1 hour, 5 hourly injections of [^{3}H] - thymidine were given i.p. to a final dose of .5 uCi/g of body weight. One hour after the last injection, the livers were perfused, the cells separated, and the DNA purified

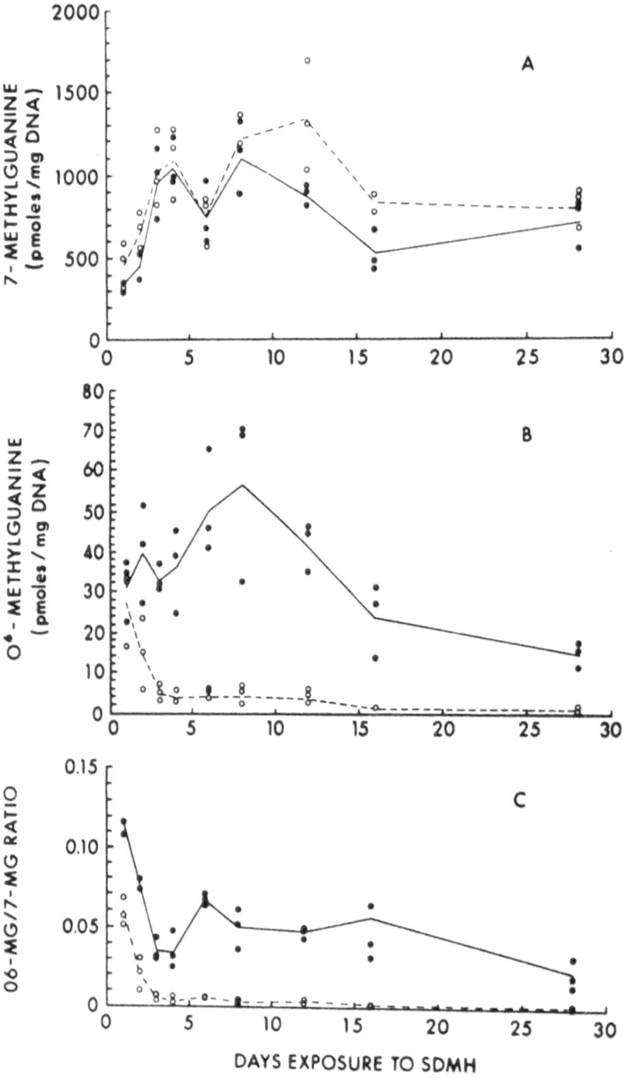

Figure 1

Normalized concentrations of 7MG (panel A), 06MG (panel B) and the ratios of 06/N7-methylguanine (panel C) in nonparenchymal cells (●——●) and hepatocytes (0---0) during chronic exposure to SDMH. Data points from individual animals are plotted and the curves represent the means of three animals. Significant differences ($p < 0.05$) exist between cell types at days 12 and 16 for 7MG, at all time points except day 1 for 06MG, and at all time points for the 06/N7 ratios. (Reprinted with permission of Cancer Research).

as described above. The DNA was then centrifuged in CsCl gradients (density 1.72 g/ml) in a Tv 850 vertical rotor (DuPont Instruments) at 40,000 rpm (129,000 rcf) for at least 40 hours. The gradients were fractionated from the top and the radioactivity in the normal density DNA defined as unscheduled DNA synthesis and that in the more dense DNA (BrdU labelled) defined as de novo DNA synthesis.

Integration of the initiation index curves was performed with a Zeiss Vidioplan.

RESULTS

7MG accumulated in hepatocytes and NPC reaching a maximum of 1100 pmoles/mg DNA in NPC by 8 days and a maximum of 1300 pmoles/mg DNA in hepatocytes by 12 days (Figure 1, Panel A). After reaching the respective peak values, 7MG slowly declined in both cell populations reaching nearly identical values by 28 days (750 pmoles/mg DNA).

In contrast to 7MG, 06MG selectively accumulated in NPC and rapidly disappeared from the DNA and hepatocytes (Figure 1, Panel B). Following one day of exposure, the amount of 06MG was similiar in both cell populations (28 pmoles/mg DNA), but by 3 days 06 methylation in hepatocytes had decreased to 4 pmoles/mg DNA, and by 16 days dropped to one pmole/mg DNA. NPC accumulated 06MG over the first 8 days of exposure reaching a maximum concentration of 60 pmoles/mg DNA at 8 days. This represented a 13 fold increase in concentration of 06MG in NPC over hepatocytes at that time point. After 8 days, the concentration of 06MG slowly declined in NPC and by 28 days 15 pmoles/mg DNA remained.

The specificity of the removal of 06MG by hepatocytes is reflected in the extremely low 06MG/7MG ratios in hepatocyte DNA compared to NPC (Figure 1, Panel C). After 3 days of exposure, the 06MG/7MG ratio in hepatocytes never exceeded .006, while the ratios in NPC ranged from .014-.07. This represents a 2.3-11.6 fold increase in the 06MG/7MG ratio in NPC over hepatocytes from 3-28 days of exposure.

Figure 2 shows representative U.V. and radioactive profiles of gradients containing DNA from NPC and hepatocytes from a control animal and one exposed to SDMH for 8 days. All of the radioactivity in DNA of control animals sedimented to a more dense position in the gradient. Radioactivity in the NPC of control animals was 2 fold higher than that in control hepatocytes. Following 8 days administration of SDMH there was a modest increase in the radioactivity in the more dense DNA of hepatocytes and a small but measurable peak of radioactivity appeared in the normal density DNA. In contrast, the NPC exhibited a striking increase in radioactivity in the density labeled DNA and no peak was observed in the normal density DNA.

DPM/mg of total DNA in the replicated DNA (Brdu labeled) from NPC and hepatocytes after exposure to SDMH for various times is presented in Figure 3. Control animals are represented by 0 days exposure. De novo DNA synthesis in NPCs exposed to SDMH was markedly increased over both control NPC and the corresponding treated hepatocytes at all time points. De novo synthesis in NPC was 11 fold higher than hepatocytes after 8 days of treatment and reached a maximum level at 16 days which persisted through 28 days. There was a small but significant increase in de novo DNA synthesis in treated hepatocytes over controls at 1.5 days of exposure. This returned to control levels by 8 days but by 16 days the rate of de novo DNA synthesis in treated hepatocytes again increased relative to control hepatocytes.

Significant increases in radioactivity in the normal density DNA of treated cells over that of control was only observed

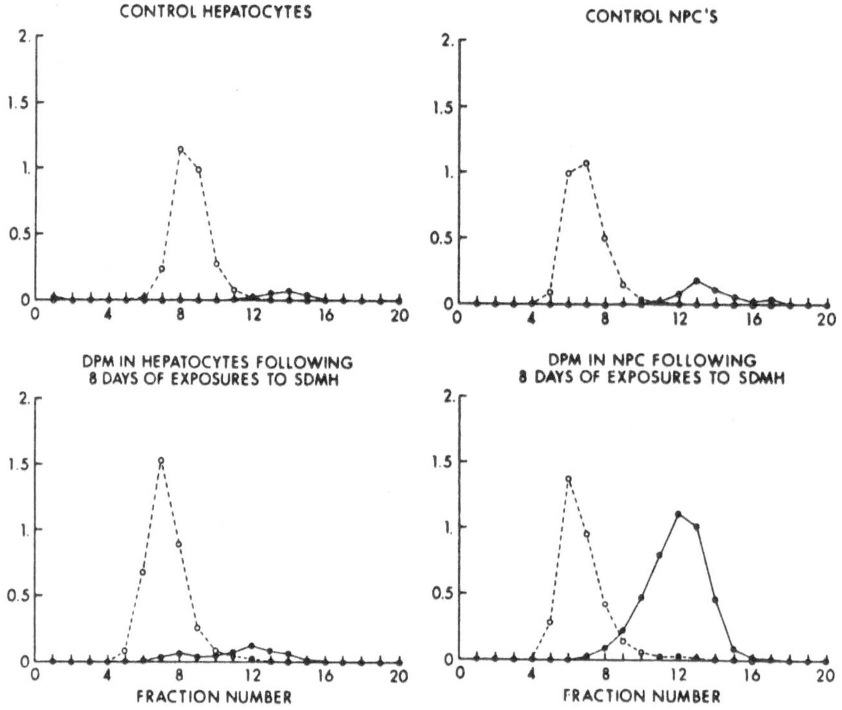

Figure 2

Representative U.V. (0---0) and radioactive (●—●) profiles of CsCl gradients harvested from the top containing DNA from hepatocytes and NPC. Presented are profiles of a control animal and one exposed to SDMH (3 mg/kg/day) in the drinking water for 8 days. On the morning of sacrifice, liver cell DNA was labeled with BrdU and [^{3}H]-thymidine <u>in vivo</u> as described in materials and methods. Hepatocytes and NPC were separated by centrifugal elutriation, and the replicated (BrdU labeled) DNA was separated in CsCl gradients. Data are normalized to 1 mg of DNA for comparison. (Reprinted with permission of Cancer Research).

in hepatocytes after 1.5,4,8, and 16 days of exposure to SDMH (Table 1). This was interpreted as unscheduled DNA synthesis and was increased over both control hepatocytes and the corresponding NPC. There were no significant differences between treated and control NPC at any time point. Unscheduled synthesis in exposed hepatocytes returned to control levels by 28 days.

DISCUSSION

The hypothesis addressed in this paper states that a critical form of DNA damage present in DNA during replication is involved in the initiation of carcinogenesis. Furthermore, if 06MG is a critical lesion in DNA it should be present in the actual target cells of the carcinogen and these cells should repli-

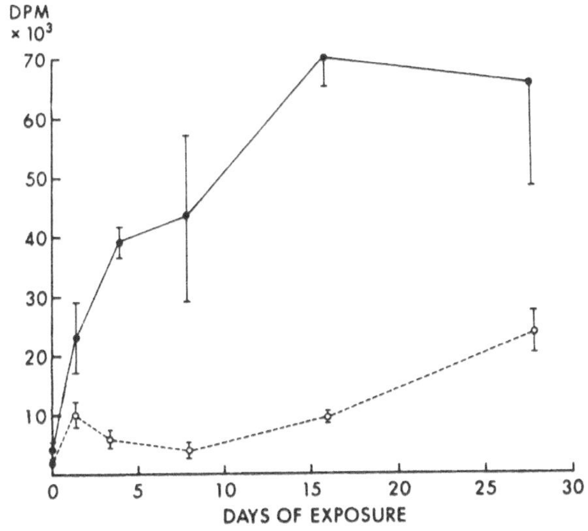

Figure 3

DPM/mg DNA in the replicated, (BrdU labeled) DNA of hepatocytes (0---0) and NPC (●——●) from animals exposed to SDMH in the drinking water (3 mg/kg/day) for various times. On the morning of the sacrifice, liver cell DNA was labeled with BrdU and [^{3}H]-thymidine _in vivo_ as described in materials and methods. Hepatocytes and NPC were separated by centrifugal elutriation and the replicated (BrdU labeled) DNA separated in CsCl gradients as described in materials and methods. Activity is expressed as DPM/mg total DNA in the more dense DNA. 0 time represents control values. Mean ± S.E.M. for 3 animals at each time point. (Reprinted with permission of _Cancer_ Research).

Table 1. The effect of SDMH administration on unscheduled DNA synthesis in hepatocytes and NPC

Carcinogen	Days of Exposure	DPM/mg DNA NPC	DPM/mg DNA Hepatocyte
Control	0	95 ± 26[a]	71 ± 31
SDMH	1.5	87 ± 68	2027 ± 147[b,c]
(3 mg/kg/day	4	0	718 ± 218[b,c]
in the drinking	8	47 ± 22	1277 ± 256[b,c]
water)	16	0	1307 ± 215[b,c]
	28	267 ± 90	191 ± 64

[a]Mean ± S.E.M.
[b]Significantly different than control ($p < 0.05$)
[c]Significantly different than corresponding treated cell type ($p < 0.05$) (Reprinted with permission of Cancer Research).

cate. Abanobi *et al.* have demonstrated that hepatic DNA actually containing 06MG is replicated following partial hepatectomy and it is in a stable, S_1 nuclease resistant conformation (22). We now show that following chronic administration of SDMH in a manner which induces malignant hemangioendotheliomas of the liver, 06MG accumulates in the NPC. Furthermore, SDMH specifically induced large increases in de novo DNA synthesis in NPC during the time of maximal 06 methylation. In contrast, hepatocytes rapidly removed 06MG and only modest increases in cell replication occurred in response to SDMH. It is unclear from this data whether the increases in cell replication seen in hepatocytes are in response to the SDMH or the loss at the vascular lining cells.

Only the hepatocytes exhibited unscheduled DNA synthesis after exposure to SDMH. It is important to note that unscheduled DNA synthesis returned to control levels after 28 days of exposure. This is a time when the hepatocytes have a very low level of 06MG, and are therefore repairing it as fast as it is formed. This suggests that unscheduled DNA synthesis may not be directly involved in repair of 06MG. These data are consistent with repair of 06MG by a specific demethylase since [^{3}H] - thymidine would not be incorporated (10).

Assuming that 06MG is the major promutagenic lesion in DNA, it becomes possible to analyze these data quantitatively to assess the likelihood of initiation. Figure 4 compares the "initiation index" of NPC to hepatocytes. The initiation index is defined as the DPM/mg DNA in the more dense DNA multiplied by the number of pmoles of 06MG/mg DNA. The initiation index, therefore, is a value which considers both the presence of promutagenic DNA damage and cell replication. Integration of these curves and comparison of the areas gives the relative probability of initiation occuring in the two cell populations. The area under the initiation index curve is 33 times greater for NPC than for hepatocytes. This represents a 33 fold higher probability of initiation occurring in NPC as opposed to hepatocytes after the 28 days of carcinogen exposure. This is consistent with and offers a possible explanation for the marked cellular specificity of SDMH when administered at low doses, chronically in the drinking water.

The techniques and experimental approach used in these experiments are directly applicable to the study of human cells in both in vivo and in vitro systems. The preparation of purified or enriched populations of cells can be applied to human tissue samples obtained at surgery or autopsy. Michalopoulos obtained

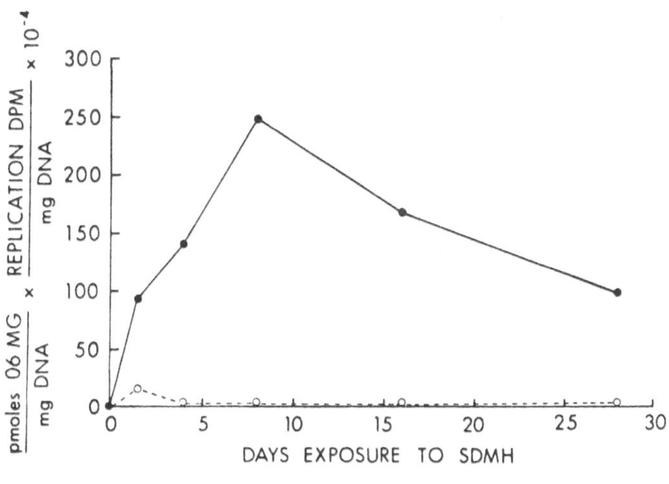

Figure 4

Initiation index of NPC (●——●) and hepatocytes (0---0) following exposure to SDMH for various times. The initiation index equals the DPM/mg DNA in the BrdU labeled DNA multiplied by the pmoles of 06MG (ordinate) present at each time of exposure (abscissa). (Reprinted with permission of Cancer Research).

viable cultures of human hepatocytes from surgical biopsies which retained the ability to metabolize several carcinogens and undergo unscheduled DNA synthesis (23). Autrup et al have cultured human alveolar macrophages from lungs obtained at autopsy. These cells were able to metabolize benzo[a]pyrene and when co-cultured with human bronchi, led to increased covalent binding of metabolites to DNA in the bronchial epithelium (24). The ability to separate and culture pure populations of human and animal cells make direct comparisons of data possible. This may provide an approach for a more thorough evaluation of the relevance of data obtained in animal studies to human exposure.

Techniques such as fluorometric or immunological detection of modified DNA (20,25) negate the need for radioactively labeled carcinogens. This offers the opportunity to directly quantify DNA lesions in cells obtained from human subjects exposed to the compound under study. By sensitive quantification of promutagenic DNA damage and repair in specific human cell types, a more quantitative approach can be taken in risk assessment.

REFERENCES

1. Pegg, A.E. Adv. Cancer Res. 25, 195-267, 1977.

2. Margison, G.P. and O'Conner, P.J. In "Chemical Carcinogens and DNA, Vol. 1" (Grover, P.L., ed.), pp. 111-159. CRC Press Inc., Boca Raton, 1979.

3. Loveless, A. Nature 223, 206-207, 1969.

4. Lawley, P.D. and Martin, C.N. Biochem. J. 145, 85-91, 1975.

5. Gerchman, L.L. and Ludlum, D.B. Biochem. Biophys. Acta, 308, 310-316, 1973.

6. Pegg, A.E. and Nicoll, J.W. In "Screening Tests in Chemical Carcinogens" (Montesano, R., ed.), pp. 571-592. IARC Scientific Publication, No. 12, Lyon, France 1976.

7. Karran, P. and Lindahl, T. Nature 280, 76-78, 1979.

8. Robins, R. and Cairns, J. Nature 280, 74-76, 1979.

9. Montesano, R., Bresil, H., Planche-Martel, G., Margison, G.P., and Pegg, A.E. Cancer Res. 40, 452-458, 1980.

10. Pegg, A.E. Biochem. Biophys. Res. Commun. 84, 166-173, 1978.

11. Margison, G.P. and Kleihues, P. Biochem. J. 148, 521-525, 1975.

12. Cooper, H.K., Hauenstein, E., Kolar, G.F., and Kleihues, P. Acta Neuropath. (Berl) 43, 105-109, 1978.

13. Margison, G.P., Margison, J.M., and Montesano, R. Biochem. J. 165, 463-468, 1977.

14. Wisse, E. and Knook, D.L. In "Progress in Liver Disease" Vol. 16 (Popper, Id. and Schaffuer F., eds.) pp 153-171, Grune and Stratton, NY 1979.

15. Druckrey, H. In "Topics in Chemical Carcinogenesis" (Nakahara, W., Takayama, S., Sugimura, T., and Odashina, S., eds.), pp. 73-151 University Park Press, Tokyo, 1972.

16. Weisburger, J.H., Madison, R.M., Warel, J.M., Vigueva, C., and Weisburger, E.K. J. Natl. Cancer Inst. 54, 1185-1188, 1975.

17. Rogers, K.J. and Pegg, A.E. Cancer Res. 37, 4082-4087, 1977.

18. Lewis, J.G. and Swenberg, J.A. Nature 288, 185-187, 1980.

19. Beland, F.A., Dooley, K.L., and Casciano, D.A. J. Chromat. 174, 177-186, 1979.

20. Bedell, M.A., Lewis, J.G., Billings, K.C., and Swenberg, J.A. Cancer Res. In Press.

21. Lewis, J.G. and Swenberg, J.A. Cancer Res. 82, 87-92, 1982.

22. Abanobi, S.E., Columbano, A., Mulivor, R.A., Rajalakshmi, S., and Sarma, D.S. Biochem. 19, 1382-1387, 1980.

23. Michalopoulos, G. Personnal Communication.

24. Autrup, H., Harris, C.C., Stoner, G.D., Selkirk, J.K., Schafer, P.W., and Trump, B.F. Lab. Invest. 38, 217-224, 1978.

25. Muller, R. and Rajewsky, M.F. Cancer Res. 40, 887-896, 1980.

THE PROBLEM OF SPECIFICITY IN THE ASSESSMENT OF RISK FROM CHEMICALS AND RADIATION-BREAST CANCER MODELS

Michael N. Gould

University of Wisconsin
Department of Human Oncology, WCCC
Madison, WI 53792

INTRODUCTION

In estimating the risk to man from radiation or chemicals one has to be concerned with specificity. These specificities include: species specificity - can we extrapolate our finding from rodents to man? organ specificity - if it can be shown that a chemical will not cause liver cancer, can we be sure that it will not cause breast cancer? individual specificity - will all women respond to breast carcinogens in a similar manner? If not, how can we identify susceptible women? I feel that many of these questions can be approached by studying primary cells *in vitro* from specific organs of both rodents and man. In the following discussion, I will give examples from our work to demonstrate how these questions can be examined. I will emphasize the problem of etiology of breast cancer.

ORGAN SPECIFICITY

Chemicals

We know from studies with rodents that certain chemicals will cause cancer in some organs and not others. For example, Aflatoxin B_1 (Afl), a very potent hepatocarcinogen, does not cause mammary carcinomas when tested in rats. On the other hand, the mammary gland is much more susceptible than the liver to neoplastic transformation by hydrocarbons such as 7,12 dimethylbenzanthracene (DMBA) or benzo (a)pyrene (BP). Within the rodent mammary gland, DMBA is a much more potent carcinogen than BP. These observations are made *in vivo*. What can be gained by employing *in vitro* systems? First, it is easier to examine responsible mechanisms for this phenomenon in the simpler and more manipulatable *in vitro* system. Second, if the *in vivo* rodent phenomena can be reproduced using rodent cells *in vitro*, we may be able to study human cells *in vitro* to answer questions about potential carcinogens where *in vivo* experiments obviously cannot be approached.

In order to explore the problem of mammary specific responses to chemicals, we have started by determining whether metabolic activation of procarcinogens is organ specific. We employ a mammary cell mediated mutagenesis system for this. In this system, mammary cells are co-cultured with a Chinese hamster cell line (V79) which has lost the ability to activate carcinogens. If the mammary cell can activate the carcinogen, it passes the active product to the V-79 cells, the V-79 cells then can be assayed for specific locus mutations such as resistance to 6-thioguanine or ouabain (1). In order to examine the ability of Sprague-Dawley rat mammary cells to activate carcinogens, we have separated the mammary cells into a stromal and epithelial fraction and find that both mammary cell populations can activate the strong mammary carcinogen DMBA while neither can activate the hepatocarcinogen Afl. However, the weak mammary carcinogen BP is activated by the stromal cells and not by the epithelial cells which give rise to mammary tumors (Table I). Thus we see both a inter- and intra-organ specificity in the activation of chemical carcinogens in the rat mammary gland (1,2).

Radiation

Unlike the hydrocarbon carcinogens, ionizing radiation is directly acting. We know both from experimental studies with rodents and from the human data obtained from the Japanese bomb survivors that radiation is an organ specific carcinogen. In man, we know that bone marrow, thyroid, and breast are highly susceptible to radiation carcinogenesis while other organs such as skin, liver, and brain are resistant (3). We have asked the question of whether there is a organ specific response for radiation induced cytotoxicity in the rat. We have found an organ specific response for both high and low LET radiation. For photon irradiation (x-rays and γ-rays) we found that bone marrow (4) was more sensitive than mammary gland (5,6). Thyroid (7) was more resistant than mammary gland while liver (8) was more resistant than thyroid. For high LET radiation (14.3 MeV neutrons) again mammary (9) was more resistant than bone marrow (10) and liver (11) was more resistant than mammary (Table II). We thus see organ specific responses for a directly acting carcinogen.

SPECIES SPECIFICITY

The mammary cell mediated assay as described above can also be used to compare the ability of rat and human mammary cells to activate carcinogens. We can prepare human mammary cells by obtaining mammary tissue from pre-menopausal women. We have successfully cultured mammary cells obtained from both fresh autopsy material and

TABLE I

Inter- and Intra-Organ Specificity of Carcinogen Activation

Carcinogen	In Vivo Mammary Carcinogenicity	Induced Mutants Per 10^6 Surviving Cells (1 μg/ml Carcinogen)	
		Stromal	Epithelial
DMBA	+++++	499 ± 44	486 ± 23
BP	+	131 ± 9.5	7 ± 10
Afl	-	2 ± 4	2 ± 5

TABLE II

Sensitivity to Radiation Induced Cytotoxicity

Organ	D_o* X-Ray (rad)	D_o Neutron (14-15 MeV) (rad)
Bone Marrow (Mouse)	82	68
Mammary (Rat)	127	97
Thyroid (Rat)	200	N.A.
Liver (Rat)	249	135**

*D_o is inversely proportional to radiosensitivity
**Preliminary estimate

from residual surgical material. The minced tissue is treated with a mixture of collagenase, hyaluronidase, and DNAse. After enzyme treatment, the cells can be separated into stromal or epithelial enriched cells by a combination of techniques. These include selective adhesion to plastic, selective centrifugation (velocity), and selective filtration.

In preliminary experiments, we have demonstrated that both human mammary stromal and epithelial enriched populations can activate DMBA to an active mutagen as assayed in a mediated V-79 mutagenesis assay. Resistance to 6-thioguanine was the locus tested.

INDIVIDUAL SPECIFICITY

One important aim of our work with mammary cells is to screen individual women for their susceptability to breast cancer. An important approach will be to examine breast epithelial cells from individual women for a variety of end points that relate to the carcinogenic process, e.g. ability to activate carcinogens, specific locus mutations, sister chromated exchange, unscheduled DNA synthesis, etc. A simple method of obtaining mammary cells from individual women would be to culture cells from milk samples.

In order to model individual specificity we are currently screening relevant cellular endpoints in rat models. We are using two models, the outbred rat model developed by Huggins and associates (12) which uses Sprague-Dawley rats which are susceptible to DMBA mammary carcinogenesis and Long Evans rats which are resistant. We are also developing models with inbred rats employing Fischer F344 rats which are resistant to DMBA mammary carcinogenesis and Wistar-Furth rats which are sensitive to this agent.

We have asked the question of whether the reason that Long Evans rats are more resistant to DMBA carcinogenesis than are Sprague-Dawley rats is because they have a diminished ability to activate carcinogens. We found that both the stromal and parenchymal cells of each strain had very similar abilities to activate both DMBA and BP. We are currently using these rodent models to further examine other steps in the process of neoplastic transformations in the hope of identifying the process(s) responsible for this differential sensitivity.

SUMMARY

Employing some of our work on the etiology of breast cancer, I have tried to point out the importance of specificity in the processes of neoplastic transformation. I feel that it will be crucial to account for both species, organ, and individual specificity when screening for environmental pollutants for the purpose of risk assessment.

ACKNOWLEDGEMENT

This work is supported in part by PHS Grants CA 28954, CA 30295, and CA 19278 awarded by the National Cancer Institute.

REFERENCES

1. Gould, M.N., Mammary Gland Cell Mediated Mutagenesis of Mammalian Cells by Organ Specific Carcinogens, Cancer Res. 40:1836-1841 (1980).
2. Gould, M.N., Chemical Carcinogen Activation in the Rat Mammary Gland: Intra-Organ Cell Specificity, Manuscript submitted (1981).
3. United Nations Scientific Committee on the Effects of Atomic Radiation, Sources, and Effects of Ionizing Radiation. United Nations, NY 1977.

4. Thomas, F. and Gould, M.N., Evidence for the Repair of Potentially Lethal Damage in Irradiated Bone Marrow, Manuscript submitted (1981).
5. Gould, M.N. and Clifton, K.H., The Survival of Mammary Cells Following Irradiation In Vivo: A Directly Generated Single-Dose Survival Curve, Radiat. Res. 72:343-352 (1977).
6. Gould, M.N. and Clifton, K.H., The Survival of Rat Mammary Gland Cells Following Irradiation In Vivo Under Different Endocrinological Conditions, J. Radiat. Oncol. Biol. Phy. 4:629-673 (1978).
7. Mulcahy, R.T., Gould, M.N. and Clifton, K.H., Survival of Thyroid Cells: In Vivo Irradiation and In Situ Repair, Radiat. Res. 84:523-528 (1980).
8. Jirtle, R.L., Michalopoulous, G., McClain, J.R. and Crowley, J., The Survival of Parenchymal Hepatocytes Exposed to Ionizing Radiation, Cancer Res., in press (1981).
9. Mahler, P.A., Gould, M.N., Pearson, D.W., DeLuca, P.M. and Clifton, K.H., Rat Mammary Survival Following Irradiation with 14.3 MeV Neutrons, Radiat. Res., in press (1981).
10. Duncan, W., Green, D., Howard, A. and Massey, J.B., The RBE of 14 MeV Neutrons: Observations on Colony Forming Units in Mouse Bone Marrow, Int. J. Radiat. Biol. 15:397-403 (1969).
11. Jirtle, R.L., DeLuca, P.M. and Gould, M.N., Manuscript in Preparation (1981).
12. Huggins, C.B., Experimental Leukemia and Mammary Cancer, The University of Chicago Press, 1979.

AUTHOR INDEX

SUBJECT INDEX